Breast Cancer—
Therapeutic Challenges,
Research Strategies
and Novel Diagnostics

Breast Cancer—Therapeutic Challenges, Research Strategies and Novel Diagnostics

Editor

Naiba Nabieva

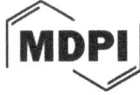

Basel • Beijing • Wuhan • Barcelona • Belgrade • Novi Sad • Cluj • Manchester

Editor
Naiba Nabieva
Department of Gynecology
and Obstetrics
Friedrich-Alexander
University Erlangen-Nürnberg
Erlangen
Germany

Editorial Office
MDPI
St. Alban-Anlage 66
4052 Basel, Switzerland

This is a reprint of articles from the Special Issue published online in the open access journal *Cancers* (ISSN 2072-6694) (available at: www.mdpi.com/journal/cancers/special_issues/Breast_Cancer_Therapeutic_Challenges_Research_Strategies_and_Novel_Diagnostics).

For citation purposes, cite each article independently as indicated on the article page online and as indicated below:

Lastname, A.A.; Lastname, B.B. Article Title. *Journal Name* **Year**, *Volume Number*, Page Range.

ISBN 978-3-0365-9443-9 (Hbk)
ISBN 978-3-0365-9442-2 (PDF)
doi.org/10.3390/books978-3-0365-9442-2

© 2023 by the authors. Articles in this book are Open Access and distributed under the Creative Commons Attribution (CC BY) license. The book as a whole is distributed by MDPI under the terms and conditions of the Creative Commons Attribution-NonCommercial-NoDerivs (CC BY-NC-ND) license.

Contents

About the Editor vii

Preface ix

Naiba Nabieva
Editorial for the Special Issue "Breast Cancer—Therapeutic Challenges, Research Strategies and Novel Diagnostics"
Reprinted from: *Cancers* 2023, 15, 4611, doi:10.3390/cancers15184611 1

Naiba Nabieva and Peter A. Fasching
CDK4/6 Inhibitors—Overcoming Endocrine Resistance Is the Standard in Patients with Hormone Receptor-Positive Breast Cancer
Reprinted from: *Cancers* 2023, 15, 1763, doi:10.3390/cancers15061763 4

Andreina Giustiniani, Laura Danesin, Rachele Pezzetta, Fabio Masina, Giulia Oliva and Giorgio Arcara et al.
Use of Telemedicine to Improve Cognitive Functions and Psychological Well-Being in Patients with Breast Cancer: A Systematic Review of the Current Literature
Reprinted from: *Cancers* 2023, 15, 1353, doi:10.3390/cancers15041353 22

Maggie Banys-Paluchowski, Thorsten Kühn, Yazan Masannat, Isabel Rubio, Jana de Boniface and Nina Ditsch et al.
Localization Techniques for Non-Palpable Breast Lesions: Current Status, Knowledge Gaps, and Rationale for the MELODY Study (EUBREAST-4/iBRA-NET, NCT 05559411)
Reprinted from: *Cancers* 2023, 15, 1173, doi:10.3390/cancers15041173 42

Louiza S. Velentzis, Victoria Freeman, Denise Campbell, Suzanne Hughes, Qingwei Luo and Julia Steinberg et al.
Breast Cancer Risk Assessment Tools for Stratifying Women into Risk Groups: A Systematic Review
Reprinted from: *Cancers* 2023, 15, 1124, doi:10.3390/cancers15041124 66

Vivek P. Chavda, Lakshmi Vineela Nalla, Pankti Balar, Rajashri Bezbaruah, Vasso Apostolopoulos and Rajeev K. Singla et al.
Advanced Phytochemical-Based Nanocarrier Systems for the Treatment of Breast Cancer
Reprinted from: *Cancers* 2023, 15, 1023, doi:10.3390/cancers15041023 94

Gabriella Bentley, Osnat Zamir, Rawan Dahabre, Shlomit Perry, Evangelos C. Karademas and Paula Poikonen-Saksela et al.
Protective Factors against Fear of Cancer Recurrence in Breast Cancer Patients: A Latent Growth Model
Reprinted from: *Cancers* 2023, 15, 4590, doi:10.3390/cancers15184590 121

Xiangling Li, Shilong Jiang, Ting Jiang, Xinyuan Sun, Yidi Guan and Songqing Fan et al.
LEM Domain Containing 1 Acts as a Novel Oncogene and Therapeutic Target for Triple-Negative Breast Cancer
Reprinted from: *Cancers* 2023, 15, 2924, doi:10.3390/cancers15112924 135

Luca Nicosia, Anna Carla Bozzini, Filippo Pesapane, Anna Rotili, Irene Marinucci and Giulia Signorelli et al.
Breast Digital Tomosynthesis versus Contrast-Enhanced Mammography: Comparison of Diagnostic Application and Radiation Dose in a Screening Setting
Reprinted from: *Cancers* 2023, 15, 2413, doi:10.3390/cancers15092413 152

Izzet Dogan, Sercan Aksoy, Burcu Cakar, Gul Basaran, Ozlem Ercelep and Nil Molinas Mandel et al.
Demographic and Clinical Features of Patients with Metastatic Breast Cancer: A Retrospective Multicenter Registry Study of the Turkish Oncology Group
Reprinted from: *Cancers* **2023**, *15*, 1667, doi:10.3390/cancers15061667 . . . . **164**

Josip Vrdoljak, Zvonimir Boban, Domjan Barić, Darko Šegvić, Marko Kumrić and Manuela Avirović et al.
Applying Explainable Machine Learning Models for Detection of Breast Cancer Lymph Node Metastasis in Patients Eligible for Neoadjuvant Treatment
Reprinted from: *Cancers* **2023**, *15*, 634, doi:10.3390/cancers15030634 . . . . **183**

Reshma Mahtani, Alexander Niyazov, Bhakti Arondekar, Katie Lewis, Alex Rider and Lucy Massey et al.
BRCA1/2 Mutation Testing in Patients with HER2-Negative Advanced Breast Cancer: Real-World Data from the United States, Europe, and Israel
Reprinted from: *Cancers* **2022**, *14*, 5399, doi:10.3390/cancers14215399 . . . . **200**

Dominik Dannehl, Tobias Engler, Lea L. Volmer, Annette Staebler, Anna K. Fischer and Martin Weiss et al.
Recurrence Score® Result Impacts Treatment Decisions in Hormone Receptor-Positive, HER2-Negative Patients with Early Breast Cancer in a Real-World Setting—Results of the IRMA Trial
Reprinted from: *Cancers* **2022**, *14*, 5365, doi:10.3390/cancers14215365 . . . . **214**

Chengcheng Gong, Cheng Liu, Zhonghua Tao, Jian Zhang, Leiping Wang and Jun Cao et al.
Temporal Heterogeneity of HER2 Expression and Spatial Heterogeneity of ^{18}F-FDG Uptake Predicts Treatment Outcome of Pyrotinib in Patients with HER2-Positive Metastatic Breast Cancer
Reprinted from: *Cancers* **2022**, *14*, 3973, doi:10.3390/cancers14163973 . . . . **225**

Yizhao Xie, Xinyue Du, Yannan Zhao, Chengcheng Gong, Shihui Hu and Shuhui You et al.
Chemotherapy Shows a Better Efficacy Than Endocrine Therapy in Metastatic Breast Cancer Patients with a Heterogeneous Estrogen Receptor Expression Assessed by ^{18}F-FES PET
Reprinted from: *Cancers* **2022**, *14*, 3531, doi:10.3390/cancers14143531 . . . . **244**

Wuzhen Chen, Baizhou Li, Fang Jia, Jiaxin Li, Huanhuan Huang and Chao Ni et al.
High PANX1 Expression Leads to Neutrophil Recruitment and the Formation of a High Adenosine Immunosuppressive Tumor Microenvironment in Basal-like Breast Cancer
Reprinted from: *Cancers* **2022**, *14*, 3369, doi:10.3390/cancers14143369 . . . . **253**

About the Editor

Naiba Nabieva

Naiba Nabieva is an office-based gynecologist and assistant professor at the Department of Gynecology and Obstetrics of the Friedrich-Alexander University in Erlangen, Germany. She graduated from the Faculty of Medicine of the same university, where she later received her PhD degree. Dr. Nabieva trained in gynecology and obstetrics at the university clinic in Erlangen, Germany, and has more than twelve years of experience in clinical cancer research. She is interested in gynecological cancers in general and breast cancer in particular. On this topic, Dr. Nabieva has published over 30 peer-reviewed original articles and reviews in renowned international journals. Her research is focused on the endocrine treatment of breast cancer patients and the associated adherence to therapy. Currently, Dr. Nabieva also works as a researcher in the pharmaceutical industry.

Preface

Thanks to the breast cancer research of recent decades, effective methods and strategies have been established, allowing the mortality rates of breast cancer patients to decrease more and more.

Compared with other subtypes, triple-negative breast cancer remains one of the most aggressive cancers. However, modern therapeutics, such as immune checkpoint inhibitors and antibody–drug conjugates, are currently changing the treatment landscape for this disease. In HER2-positive breast cancer patients, who had once been patients with an extremely poor prognosis, targeted therapies have reduced mortality rates immensely. Research has gone so far that, even decades after the discovery of the HER2 receptor, its differentiation to zero, low, or positive has now gained importance for specific novel treatments. Additionally, when it comes to hormone-receptor-positive breast cancer, it is the class of CDK4/6 inhibitors that, after almost half a century of single-endocrine treatment, has changed usual treatment patterns and was the first to be successfully combined even in the early therapy stage.

Despite all these advancements, we still face many challenges in breast cancer research.

On a molecular basis, the role of intrinsic subtypes, certain biomarkers, or mutations is still not clear for treatment and surveillance. Novel drugs, including those mentioned above, are often associated with a different spectrum of adverse events than that seen for conventional therapies, accordingly having an impact on patients' compliance behaviors. In breast cancer surgery, in some cases, the question remains whether to escalate or deescalate. Additionally, with regard to diagnostics, in a digitalized world, home-based tools and therapy monitoring options are of high importance, especially under the tough conditions and supply problems seen during the COVID-19 pandemic.

This Special Issue gathers original research articles and reviews demonstrating therapeutic challenges, current research strategies, and novel diagnostics in breast cancer.

Naiba Nabieva
Editor

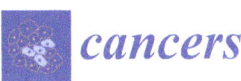

Editorial

Editorial for the Special Issue "Breast Cancer—Therapeutic Challenges, Research Strategies and Novel Diagnostics"

Naiba Nabieva [1,2]

1 Department of Gynecology and Obstetrics, Friedrich-Alexander-Universität Erlangen-Nürnberg, 91054 Erlangen, Germany; naiba.nabieva@fau.de
2 GynPraxis, 91054 Erlangen, Germany

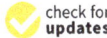

Citation: Nabieva, N. Editorial for the Special Issue "Breast Cancer—Therapeutic Challenges, Research Strategies and Novel Diagnostics". *Cancers* 2023, *15*, 4611. https://doi.org/10.3390/cancers15184611

Received: 28 August 2023
Accepted: 30 August 2023
Published: 18 September 2023

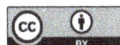

Copyright: © 2023 by the author. Licensee MDPI, Basel, Switzerland. This article is an open access article distributed under the terms and conditions of the Creative Commons Attribution (CC BY) license (https:// creativecommons.org/licenses/by/ 4.0/).

Worldwide, breast cancer affects over 2 million women a year, with a rising burden [1]. Thanks to the breast cancer research of recent decades, effective methods have been established, allowing the mortality rates of patients with this disease to decrease more and more. The aim of this Special Issue was to gather original articles and reviews demonstrating therapeutic challenges, research strategies and novel diagnostics in breast cancer.

In a retrospective multicenter registry, the Turkish Oncology Group evaluated time-related differences in treatment patterns and outcome in a real-world patient population with metastatic breast cancer (mBC) over a ten-year timeframe. Due to the incorporation of novel agents, the HER2+ subgroup showed a significant survival benefit, while triple-negative mBC (TNBC) patients still have the worst prognosis [2].

Gong et al. analyzed the impact of temporal and spatial tumor heterogeneity assessed using the discordance between primary and metastatic immunohistochemistry results and the 18F-FDG uptake on PET/CT, respectively, on the treatment outcome of patients with HER2+ mBC treated with pyrotinib. The results showed that temporal and spatial HER2 heterogeneity were predictive of poorer outcomes of pyrotinib treatment [3]. Xie et al. found that the novel 18F-FES PET/CT method could also identify mBC patients with heterogeneity in estrogen receptor expression. In these patients, chemotherapy showed a better efficacy compared with endocrine treatment [4]. However, the best method to evaluate tumor heterogeneity in clinical practice still needs to be identified.

Since TNBC shows the worst prognosis and limited treatment options, exploring novel molecular targets is urgently needed. Li et al. demonstrated that the novel oncogene LEM Domain Containing 1 (LEMD1) is highly expressed in TNBC and could act as a therapeutic target as its knockdown renders TNBC cells more sensitive to paclitaxel [5]. Also, Pannexin 1 (PANX1) has been found to be a poor prognostic factor in breast cancer; however, its role remains unknown. Chen et al. could show that PANX1 had high expression in basal-like breast cancer, and this in turn is associated with high tumor-associated neutrophil infiltration and adenosine production to induce local immunosuppression in tumor microenvironment [6].

Furthermore, it is interesting to learn more about the worldwide situation on *BRCA1/2* germline mutation testing. According to Mahtani et al., real-world data from the United States, Europe and Israel reveal that 73%, 42% and 99% of HER2− advanced breast cancer (aBC) patients were tested for *BRCA1/2*, respectively. In the US and Europe, patients who were not tested versus those who were tested were older, more likely to have HR+/HER2− aBC than TNBC and less likely to have a known family history of *BRCA1/2*-related cancer. Efforts should be made to improve *BRCA1/2* testing rates in affected countries [7].

In early breast cancer (eBC), advancements in diagnostic and localization methods are of special interest. Early detection of breast cancer in asymptomatic women through screening is an important strategy in reducing its burden. The systematic review by Velentzis et al. assessed, using a variety of methods, how accurately breast cancer risk assessment tools can group women eligible for screening within a population, into risk groups, so that each group could potentially be offered a screening protocol with more benefits and less harm compared to current age-based screening [8]. Nicosia et al. compared the diagnostic performance of Contrast-Enhanced Mammography (CEM) versus Digital Mammography (DM), and of CEM versus DM + Digital Breast Tomosynthesis (DBT), performed in the same group of patients over the same period of time in a screening setting. CEM offered a lower average glandular dose than DM protocols with added tomosynthesis. Its diagnostic performance was no less than that of DM + DBT letting the use of CEM appear promising in screening settings in dense breasts and high-risk patients [9]. Furthermore, artificial intelligence will play an important role in the detection of lesions. Vrdoljak et al. trained and evaluated several machine-learning models with the aim of predicting breast cancer lymph node metastases in patients eligible for neoadjuvant treatment. According to the authors, the models achieved a good performance in assessing the lymph node status so that such an approach could lead to more accurate disease stage prediction and consecutively better treatment selection, especially for NST patients where radiological and clinical findings are often the only method of lymph node assessment [10]. Regarding localization methods, the review of Banys-Paluchowski et al. provides an overview of current localization techniques for non-palpable breast lesions, associated knowledge gaps and potential methods to close these [11].

When it comes to HR+ breast cancer, CDK4/6 inhibitors are the first substances in almost two decades to substantially change the standard of care not only for aBC patients, but also for those with an early disease stage. In their review, Nabieva et al. discuss the recent history, current role, future directions and opportunities of this substance class [12]. However, despite advancements in endocrine treatment, especially in HR+ eBC patients often the question arises of whether treatment escalation in terms of a chemotherapy is necessary. Dannehl et al. assessed whether the multigene-expression assay Oncotype DX® that has been validated in two large clinical phase III trials, effectively reduces treatment escalation in a real-world setting. The authors could demonstrate that, using Oncotype DX®, absolute adjuvant chemotherapy recommendation can be reduced by nearly 15% [13].

And while chemically produced drugs are the standard of care, Chavda et al. emphasize in their review the anticancer activity of phytochemical-instigated and phytochemical-loaded nanocarriers against breast cancer both in vitro and in vivo. The authors discuss the selective targeted delivery of phytofabricated nanocarriers to cancer cells and consider research gaps, recent developments and the drugability of phytoceuticals [14].

Having spoken intensively about the therapy of breast cancer patients, it has to be mentioned that a well-treated patient is not automatically a healthy one. A lot depends also on cognitive and psychological well-being. Having undergone the pandemic and living in a world becoming more and more digitalized, telemedicine approaches are gaining more interest. Giustiniani et al. conducted a systematic review to clarify the effectiveness of telerehabilitation for treating the cognitive and psychological difficulties of breast cancer patients [15].

In conclusion, the collection of articles in the Special Issue "Breast Cancer—Therapeutic Challenges, Research Strategies and Novel Diagnostics" has made substantial contributions to our comprehension of breast cancer. The authors shed light on known as well as emerging diagnostic and therapeutic approaches, and various other aspects associated with this global disease burden. I hope that healthcare professionals and researchers working in this field will find it helpful.

Conflicts of Interest: Naiba Nabieva is an employee of Novartis Pharma GmbH, Nuremberg, Germany.

References

1. Heer, E.; Harper, A.; Escandor, N.; Sung, H.; McCormack, V.; Fidler-Benaoudia, M.M. Global burden and trends in premenopausal and postmenopausal breast cancer: A population-based study. *Lancet Glob. Health* **2020**, *8*, e1027–e1037. [CrossRef] [PubMed]
2. Dogan, I.; Aksoy, S.; Cakar, B.; Basaran, G.; Ercelep, O.; Molinas Mandel, N.; Korkmaz, T.; Gokmen, E.; Sener, C.; Aydiner, A.; et al. Demographic and Clinical Features of Patients with Metastatic Breast Cancer: A Retrospective Multicenter Registry Study of the Turkish Oncology Group. *Cancers* **2023**, *15*, 1667. [CrossRef] [PubMed]

3. Gong, C.; Liu, C.; Tao, Z.; Zhang, J.; Wang, L.; Cao, J.; Zhao, Y.; Xie, Y.; Hu, X.; Yang, Z.; et al. Temporal Heterogeneity of HER2 Expression and Spatial Heterogeneity of 18F-FDG Uptake Predicts Treatment Outcome of Pyrotinib in Patients with HER2−Positive Metastatic Breast Cancer. *Cancers* **2022**, *14*, 3973. [CrossRef] [PubMed]
4. Xie, Y.; Du, X.; Zhao, Y.; Gong, C.; Hu, S.; You, S.; Song, S.; Hu, X.; Yang, Z.; Wang, B. Chemotherapy Shows a Better Efficacy Than Endocrine Therapy in Metastatic Breast Cancer Patients with a Heterogeneous Estrogen Receptor Expression Assessed by 18F-FES PET. *Cancers* **2022**, *14*, 3531. [CrossRef] [PubMed]
5. Li, X.; Jiang, S.; Jiang, T.; Sun, X.; Guan, Y.; Fan, S.; Cheng, Y. LEM Domain Containing 1 Acts as a Novel Oncogene and Therapeutic Target for Triple-Negative Breast Cancer. *Cancers* **2023**, *15*, 2924. [CrossRef] [PubMed]
6. Chen, W.; Li, B.; Jia, F.; Li, J.; Huang, H.; Ni, C.; Xia, W. High PANX1 Expression Leads to Neutrophil Recruitment and the Formation of a High Adenosine Immunosuppressive Tumor Microenvironment in Basal-like Breast Cancer. *Cancers* **2022**, *14*, 3369. [CrossRef] [PubMed]
7. Mahtani, R.; Niyazov, A.; Arondekar, B.; Lewis, K.; Rider, A.; Massey, L.; Lux, M.P. BRCA1/2 Mutation Testing in Patients with HER2−Negative Advanced Breast Cancer: Real-World Data from the United States, Europe, and Israel. *Cancers* **2022**, *14*, 5399. [CrossRef] [PubMed]
8. Velentzis, L.S.; Freeman, V.; Campbell, D.; Hughes, S.; Luo, Q.; Steinberg, J.; Egger, S.; Mann, G.B.; Nickson, C. Breast Cancer Risk Assessment Tools for Stratifying Women into Risk Groups: A Systematic Review. *Cancers* **2023**, *15*, 1124. [CrossRef] [PubMed]
9. Nicosia, L.; Bozzini, A.C.; Pesapane, F.; Rotili, A.; Marinucci, I.; Signorelli, G.; Frassoni, S.; Bagnardi, V.; Origgi, D.; De Marco, P.; et al. Breast Digital Tomosynthesis versus Contrast-Enhanced Mammography: Comparison of Diagnostic Application and Radiation Dose in a Screening Setting. *Cancers* **2023**, *15*, 2413. [CrossRef] [PubMed]
10. Vrdoljak, J.; Boban, Z.; Barić, D.; Šegvić, D.; Kumrić, M.; Avirović, M.; Perić Balja, M.; Periša, M.M.; Tomasović, Č.; Tomić, S.; et al. Applying Explainable Machine Learning Models for Detection of Breast Cancer Lymph Node Metastasis in Patients Eligible for Neoadjuvant Treatment. *Cancers* **2023**, *15*, 634. [CrossRef] [PubMed]
11. Banys-Paluchowski, M.; Kühn, T.; Masannat, Y.; Rubio, I.; de Boniface, J.; Ditsch, N.; Karadeniz Cakmak, G.; Karakatsanis, A.; Dave, R.; Hahn, M.; et al. Localization Techniques for Non-Palpable Breast Lesions: Current Status, Knowledge Gaps, and Rationale for the MELODY Study (EUBREAST-4/iBRA-NET, NCT 05559411). *Cancers* **2023**, *15*, 1173. [CrossRef] [PubMed]
12. Nabieva, N.; Fasching, P.A. CDK4/6 Inhibitors—Overcoming Endocrine Resistance Is the Standard in Patients with Hormone Receptor-Positive Breast Cancer. *Cancers* **2023**, *15*, 1763. [CrossRef] [PubMed]
13. Dannehl, D.; Engler, T.; Volmer, L.L.; Staebler, A.; Fischer, A.K.; Weiss, M.; Hahn, M.; Walter, C.B.; Grischke, E.-M.; Fend, F.; et al. Recurrence Score® Result Impacts Treatment Decisions in Hormone Receptor-Positive, HER2−Negative Patients with Early Breast Cancer in a Real-World Setting—Results of the IRMA Trial. *Cancers* **2022**, *14*, 5365. [PubMed]
14. Chavda, V.P.; Nalla, L.V.; Balar, P.; Bezbaruah, R.; Apostolopoulos, V.; Singla, R.K.; Khadela, A.; Vora, L.; Uversky, V.N. Advanced Phytochemical-Based Nanocarrier Systems for the Treatment of Breast Cancer. *Cancers* **2023**, *15*, 1023. [CrossRef] [PubMed]
15. Giustiniani, A.; Danesin, L.; Pezzetta, R.; Masina, F.; Oliva, G.; Arcara, G.; Burgio, F.; Conte, P. Use of Telemedicine to Improve Cognitive Functions and Psychological Well-Being in Patients with Breast Cancer: A Systematic Review of the Current Literature. *Cancers* **2023**, *15*, 1353. [CrossRef] [PubMed]

Disclaimer/Publisher's Note: The statements, opinions and data contained in all publications are solely those of the individual author(s) and contributor(s) and not of MDPI and/or the editor(s). MDPI and/or the editor(s) disclaim responsibility for any injury to people or property resulting from any ideas, methods, instructions or products referred to in the content.

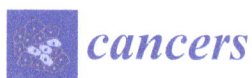

Review

CDK4/6 Inhibitors—Overcoming Endocrine Resistance Is the Standard in Patients with Hormone Receptor-Positive Breast Cancer

Naiba Nabieva [1,2] and Peter A. Fasching [1,*]

1 Department of Gynecology and Obstetrics, Erlangen University Hospital,
Comprehensive Cancer Center Erlangen-EMN, Friedrich-Alexander Universität Erlangen-Nürnberg, 91054 Erlangen, Germany
2 GynPraxis Dr. Ernst and Colleagues, 91054 Erlangen, Germany
* Correspondence: peter.fasching@uk-erlangen.de; Tel.: +49-9131-85-36167; Fax: +49-9131-85-33988

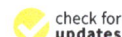

Citation: Nabieva, N.; Fasching, P.A. CDK4/6 Inhibitors—Overcoming Endocrine Resistance Is the Standard in Patients with Hormone Receptor-Positive Breast Cancer. *Cancers* 2023, *15*, 1763. https://doi.org/10.3390/cancers15061763

Academic Editor: Andrea Manni

Received: 28 February 2023
Revised: 11 March 2023
Accepted: 13 March 2023
Published: 14 March 2023

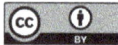

Copyright: © 2023 by the authors. Licensee MDPI, Basel, Switzerland. This article is an open access article distributed under the terms and conditions of the Creative Commons Attribution (CC BY) license (https://creativecommons.org/licenses/by/4.0/).

Simple Summary: Abemaciclib, dalpiciclib, palbociclib and ribociclib have all demonstrated significant improvements in progression-free survival in advanced disease. However, to date, abemaciclib and ribociclib are the only CDK4/6 inhibitors shown to improve the overall survival in patients with metastatic breast cancer. Moreover, abemaciclib is the first CDK4/6 inhibitor to also reduce the risk of recurrence in those with early-stage disease. Thus, achieving significant improvements in survival rates in the advanced and early breast cancer treatment setting, CDK4/6 inhibitors are the first substances in almost two decades to substantially change the standard of care for advanced breast cancer patients. This review is designed to discuss the recent history, current role, future directions and opportunities of this substance class.

Abstract: Purpose of review: Tamoxifen and aromatase inhibitors can be considered as some of the first targeted therapies. For the past 30 years, they were the endocrine treatment standard in the advanced and early breast cancer setting. CDK4/6 inhibitors, however, are the first substances in almost two decades to broadly improve the therapeutic landscape of hormone receptor-positive breast cancer patients for the upcoming years. This review is designed to discuss the recent history, current role, future directions and opportunities of this substance class. Recent findings: The CDK4/6 inhibitors abemaciclib, dalpiciclib, palbociclib and ribociclib have all demonstrated a statistically significant improvement in progression-free survival in advanced disease. However, to date, abemaciclib and ribociclib are the only CDK4/6 inhibitors to have shown an improvement in overall survival in patients with metastatic breast cancer. Moreover, abemaciclib is the first CDK4/6 inhibitor to also reduce the risk of recurrence in those with early-stage disease. Further CDK inhibitors, treatment combinations with other drugs and different therapy sequences are in development. Summary: Achieving significant improvements in survival rates in the advanced and early breast cancer treatment setting, CDK4/6 inhibitors have set a new standard of care for patients with advanced breast cancer. It remains important to better understand resistance mechanisms to be able to develop novel substances and treatment sequences.

Keywords: breast cancer; endocrine treatment; CDK4/6 inhibitor; abemaciclib; dalpiciclib; palbociclib; ribociclib

1. Introduction

The development of endocrine treatment (ET) for breast cancer (BC) patients started at the end of the 19th century when Sir George Thomas Beatson found out that a bilateral oophorectomy results in an improvement in advanced breast cancer (aBC) lesions [1]. However, the discovery and investigation of drugs targeting the hormone receptor took almost 80 years. Thus, in the 1970s, with tamoxifen as a selective estrogen receptor modulator

(SERM), the first target therapy was approved for the treatment of hormone receptor-positive BC patients [2]. Two decades later, in the 1990s, a group of further substances—the aromatase inhibitors (AIs) anastrozole, exemestane and letrozole—received approval status as, compared to tamoxifen, they improved the outcome of postmenopausal women with aBC [3,4]. These were followed soon by the approval of fulvestrant in 2002, a selective estrogen receptor degrader (SERD) that led to a longer duration of response than anastrozole in postmenopausal patients [5]. Due to positive study results, all of the abovementioned therapeutics but fulvestrant reached the treatment setting of non-advanced BC [6,7]. Therefore, being successful in the therapy of advanced as well as early breast cancer (eBC) patients, tamoxifen and AIs have set the ET standard for the past 30 years and were later only complemented by potential additional ovarian function suppression (OFS) with a gonadotropin-releasing hormone agonist to further reduce hormone blood levels in premenopausal women [8].

The introduction of everolimus represents a milestone in the treatment of hormone receptor-positive, HER2-negative BC patients. For the first time, endocrine resistance could be overcome for patients with advanced disease [9]. Furthermore, Alpelisib was the second therapy to show that endocrine resistance could be overcome in patients with *PIK3CA*-mutated hormone receptor-positive, HER2-negative aBC [10]. However, everolimus did not achieve an improvement in outcomes in the early therapy setting [11]. Figure 1 shows the diverse pathways within the cell cycle that are potential contributors to ET resistance.

Inhibitors of the cyclin-dependent kinase 4/6 (CDK4/6i) are the first substances in almost two decades to be effective in both advanced and early BC patients. Having improved survival outcomes in stage IV disease first and being later additionally successful in the therapy of stage II and III BC, CDK4/6i in combination with ET substantially improved the therapeutic landscape of hormone receptor-positive disease and became the new standard of care [12,13].

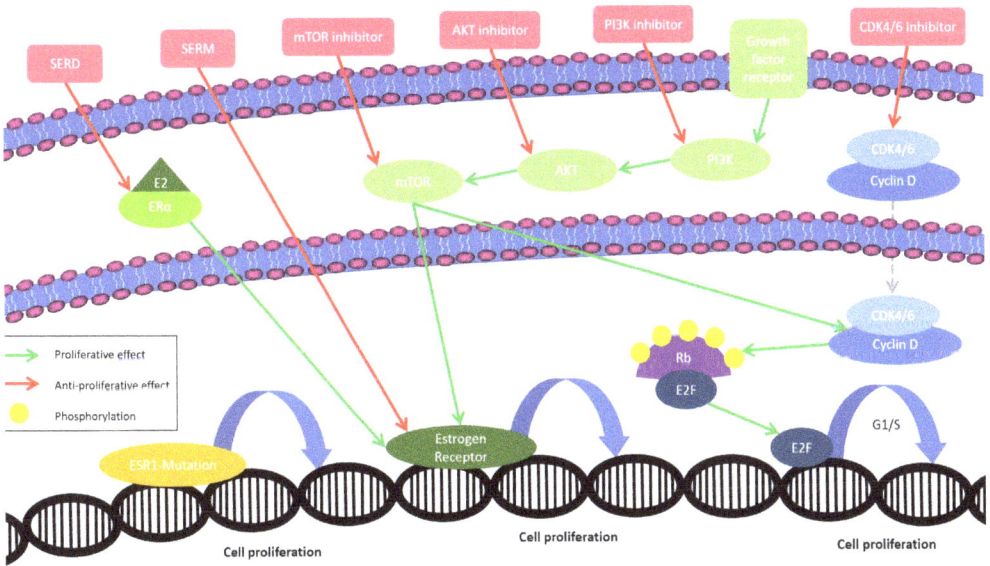

Figure 1. Pathways potentially contributing to endocrine treatment resistance (simplified representation) [14,15]. AKT: AKT murine thymoma viral oncogene; CDK4/6: cyclin-dependent kinase 4/6;

E2: estradiol; E2F: transcription factor; ERalpha: estrogen receptor alpha; ESR1: estrogen receptor 1 gene; mTOR: mammalian target of rapamycin; PI3K: phosphatidylinositol 3-kinase; Rb: retinoblastoma protein; SERD: selective estrogen receptor degrader; SERM: selective estrogen receptor modulator. In HR-positive BC cells, different mechanisms may lead to hyperactivation of the cyclin D-CDK4/6-retinoblastoma pathway. The activation of the PI3K-AKT-mTOR pathway can increase cyclin D levels or enhance its activity through post-translational mechanisms. Moreover, in contrast to triple-negative BC cells, where Rb is mostly absent or dysfunctional, in HR-positive BC cells, it is usually retained. Genomic factors, which encode for the endogenous inhibition of the CDK4/6 or are involved in the transcription of the estrogen receptor, explain why CDK4/6 plays a significant role in HR-positive BC in special. Regarding resistance mechanisms, mutations (e.g., *FAT1*) and a loss of functional Rb in particular are discussed to be associated with de novo and acquired CDK4/6i resistance [16].

2. The Early Development of CDK4/6 Inhibitors in Patients with Hormone Receptor-Positive, HER2-Negative Advanced Breast Cancer

2.1. Impact on Progression-Free Survival

The first CDK4/6i to be tested in human breast cancer cell lines was palbociclib (Ibrance®, PD-0332991, Pfizer, New York, NY, USA). It showed an effect, especially in hormone receptor-positive and HER2-amplified cell lines, which was the reason for its further development [17]. In two randomized phase III trials, it later demonstrated a statistically significant prolongation of progression-free survival (PFS), changing the standard-of-care treatment of women with hormone receptor-positive, HER2-negative aBC [18,19]. Soon after, two other substances inhibiting the CDK4/6 could show similar results. In several trials, abemaciclib (Verzenio®, LY2835219, Lilly, Indianapolis, IN, USA) and ribociclib (Kisqali®, LEE011, Novartis, Basel, Switzerland) also significantly improved the PFS of women suffering from aBC [20–24]. Later, dalpiciclib (Ai Rui Kang, SHR6390, Jiangsu Hengrui, Lianyungang, Jiangsu Province, China)—a fourth drug from this family—could also show a benefit with regard to PFS [25,26]. In some of those trials, especially in the first line, patients using CDK4/6i were free from disease progression for up to 30 months (Table 1).

Table 1. Efficacy of CDK4/6 inhibitors in hormone receptor-positive, HER2-negative aBC phase III trials (in alphabetical and numerical order; adapted and updated from [27]).

	Study Name	ET Partner	Sample Size	Randomization	Median PFS in Months (PFS = Primary Endpoint)					Median OS in Months (OS = Secondary Endpoint)				
					with CDK4/6 Inhibitor	without CDK4/6 Inhibitor	HR	95% CI	Statistically Significant as per Protocol	with CDK4/6 Inhibitor	without CDK4/6 Inhibitor	HR	95% CI	Statistically Significant as per Protocol
ET +/− Abemaciclib	MONARCH-2 [24,28]	Fulvestrant	669	2:1	16.4	9.3	0.55	0.45–0.68	yes	45.8	37.3	0.78	0.64–0.96	yes
	MONARCH-3 [23,29]	AI	493	2:1	28.2	14.8	0.54	0.42–0.70	yes	67.1	54.5	0.75	0.58–0.97	Final analys is not reported yet [1]
ET +/− Dalpiciclib	DAWNA-1 [26]	Fulvestrant	361	2:1	13.6 [2]	7.7 [2]	0.45 [2]	0.32–0.64 [2]	yes [2]	Final analys is not reported yet				
	DAWNA-2 [25]	AI	456	2:1	30.6	18.2	0.51	0.38–0.69	yes	Final analys is not reported yet				
ET +/− Palbociclib	PALOMA-2 [18,30]	AI	666	2:1	24.8	14.5	0.58	0.46–0.72	yes	53.9	51.2	0.96	0.78–1.18	no
	PALOMA-3 [19,31]	Fulvestrant	521	2:1	9.5	4.6	0.46	0.36–0.59	yes	34.9	28.0	0.81	0.64–1.03	no
ET +/− Ribociclib	MONALEESA-2 [22,32]	AI	668	1:1	25.3	16.0	0.57	0.46–0.70	yes	63.9	51.4	0.76	0.63–0.93	yes
	MONALEESA-3 [21,33]	Fulvestrant	726	2:1	20.5	12.8	0.59	0.48–0.73	yes	53.7	41.5	0.73	0.59–0.90	yes
	MONALEESA-7 [20,34]	OFS plus tamoxifen or AI	672	1:1	23.8	13.0	0.55	0.44–0.69	yes	58.7	48.0	0.76	0.61–0.96	yes

aBC: advanced breast cancer; AI: aromatase inhibitor; CI: confidence interval; ET: endocrine treatment; HR: hazard ratio; OFS: ovarian function suppression; OS: overall survival; PFS: progression-free survival; Tam: Tamoxifen. [1] An interim analysis has been reported [29]. [2] As assessed by an independent review committee.

2.2. Improvement in Overall Survival

Despite a partly diverse side effect profile between the substances, the positive PFS results throughout all trials implied a CDK4/6i class effect. This was questioned when overall survival (OS) outcomes in the advanced setting and outcome differences in the early treatment setting were reported. To date, OS results have been published for palbociclib, abemaciclib, and ribociclib [30–35], while those for dalpiciclib are yet to come. With a hazard ratio (HR) of 0.81 and a 95% confidence interval (CI) of 0.64–1.03 in the PALOMA-3 [31], and a HR of 0.96 and a 95% CI of 0.78–1.18 in the PALOMA-2 trial [30], palbociclib failed to show any OS benefit in both studies. While abemaciclib has already proven its efficacy regarding the OS in the MONARCH-2 study (HR 0.78; 95% CI 0.64–0.96) when being combined with fulvestrant in women who had not received chemotherapy and had a maximum of one prior ET for aBC [28], results from the MONARCH-3 trial in first-line patients are pending. For ribociclib, a consistent, statistically significant OS benefit could be shown in all three MonaLEEsa studies that is independent from the menopausal status or the ET partner (AI or fulvestrant) [32–34]. In the MonaLEEsa-2 trial, for instance, postmenopausal aBC patients treated with ribociclib and letrozole as first-line therapy achieved, with a median OS of 63.9 months, an OS prolongation of more than 12 months compared to the 51.4 months under endocrine monotherapy (HR 0.76; 95% CI 0.63–0.93) [32] (Table 1). It is of interest why these CDK4/6 inhibitors, despite being from the same drug family, lead to significantly different OS results. Potential reasons that are discussed are differences in the study designs and patient populations, but also in the substances' pharmacology, affinity or in the binding to a specific side (more CDK4 than CDK6 and vice versa, for instance) [36].

2.3. CDK4/6i vs. Chemotherapy

The introduction of CDK4/6i led to a shift in the 1st and 2nd treatment lines of the therapeutic landscape. While, according to a German breast cancer registry, in 2015, almost 40% of the first-line patients received chemotherapy, this rate was significantly reduced by 2018 to 25% when all three inhibitors were available [37]. Three years later, in 2021, already, almost 75% of the first-line population was treated with a CDK4/6i and only 15% with chemotherapy [38]. This rapid implementation of CDK4/6i in the treatment of aBC caused further investigations regarding its comparability to chemotherapy. With regards to the PFS, it could be shown that no chemotherapy regimen with or without targeted therapy is significantly better than CDK4/6i in the 1st and 2nd treatment lines [39]. The above-mentioned German breast cancer registry could even demonstrate, in a recent analysis, that compared to patients treated with CDK4/6i or an ET monotherapy, those under chemotherapy in the first line had the most unfavorable prognosis regarding both the PFS and the OS. One possible reason for this outcome might also be that patients who are selected to receive chemotherapy as first-line treatment are those with a worse prognosis [38]. The PEARL trial was primarily designed to show the superiority of a palbociclib-based regimen compared to capecitabine. However, statistical significance could not be demonstrated, neither regarding the PFS nor the OS [40,41]. The RIGHT Choice study specifically analyzed the situation of pre- and perimenopausal women with aggressive disease, defined mostly by visceral metastases or rapid disease progression. In this patient population, it compared, as the first prospective trial, a ribociclib-based regimen to combinational chemotherapy in the first-line treatment setting. Ribociclib + ET could show a statistically significant PFS benefit of almost one year over chemotherapy (24.0 vs. 12.3 months; HR 0.54; 95% CI 0.36–0.79) [42]. On the basis of a better toxicity profile and quality of life (QoL) and at least similar or even better efficacy compared to chemotherapy, ET-based regimens in combination with CDK4/6i became the preferred treatment choice, even in patients with aggressive disease [12].

2.4. Resistance Mechanisms and Mutations

The question remains as to which resistance mechanisms lead to disease progression under CDK4/6i (Figure 1), how to treat these patients afterwards and whether a therapy with another CDK4/6i beyond progression makes sense. Novel treatment combinations will be discussed in Section 5. One study, however, that addressed the question on treatment beyond progression is MAINTAIN, a randomized, phase II trial of fulvestrant or exemestane, with or without ribociclib, after progression on CDK4/6i-based therapy in patients with aBC. Thus, 84% of the study population received palbociclib (n = 100), 11% ribociclib (n = 13) and 2% abemaciclib (n = 2) prior to the study treatment. Patients randomized to ribociclib plus fulvestrant or exemestane had, compared to those under ET without a CDK4/6i, a statistically significant PFS improvement (median PFS 5.33 months vs. 2.76 months; HR 0.59; 95% CI 0.38–0.91). At one year, 25% of the women on ribociclib + ET were still free from disease progression vs. only 7% of those on placebo + ET. Data on OS are pending [43]. This approach shows that even after disease progression on the first CDK4/6i, there is still some significant efficacy under a subsequent one. However, it is unclear whether this effect is restricted to the specific sequence of ribociclib being the second CDK4/6i. The phase III postMONARCH study (NCT05169567) is currently enrolling patients who progressed on a CDK4/6i, either in the adjuvant setting or as initial therapy for advanced disease, to be randomly assigned to fulvestrant plus abemaciclib or placebo [44]. The phase II PALMIRA study (NCT03809988) investigates the option of a palbociclib rechallenge in patients pre-treated with palbociclib [44].

Another trial found out that the ET partner for CDK4/6i also plays a significant role regarding the patients' outcome. Women with aBC who were under an AI and palbociclib were screened in the PADA-1 study for a bESR1 mutation and then randomized 1:1 to either a continuation of the previous treatment with palbociclib plus the AI or to palbociclib plus fulvestrant instead of the AI. Median PFS from random assignment was 11.9 months in the palbociclib and fulvestrant group vs. 5.7 months in the palbociclib and AI group (HR 0.61; 95% CI 0.43–0.86). This way, PADA-1 was the first randomized prospective trial to show, in bESR1-mutated patients, that the type of ET a CDK4/6i is combined with has a relevant impact on the patients' prognosis [45].

These examples demonstrate that further investigations are needed to better understand resistance mechanisms associated with the progression on ET in combination with CDK4/6i. Phase IV trials, such as CAPTOR (NCT05452213) with ribociclib or Minerva (NCT05362760) with abemaciclib, for instance, are designed to analyze biomarkers influencing the efficacy and resistance in aBC patients treated with each CDK4/6i [44].

3. Advancements in the Endocrine Treatment of Hormone Receptor-Positive, HER2-Negative Early-Stage Breast Cancer Patients

As mentioned above, ET consisting of Tamoxifen and AIs (+/− OFS) has been the standard of care in eBC patients for the past few decades. Mostly, a drug that is successful in the therapy of advanced disease is investigated in the early stage, too. Thus, due to the positive results in aBC, several studies analyzed the efficacy of CDK4/6i in eBC (Table 2).

Table 2. Efficacy of CDK4/6 inhibitors in hormone receptor-positive, HER2-negative eBC phase III trials at the latest analysis (in alphabetical order).

	Study Name	ET Partner	Sample Size	Rando-mization	Duration of CDK4/6 Inhibitor Therapy	DFS Rate					Statistically Significant as per Protocol
						Latest Analysis	with CDK4/6 Inhibitor	without CDK4/6 Inhibitor	HR	95% CI	
ET +/− Abemaciclib	monarchE [46]	AI or Tam +/− OFS	5637	1:1	2 years	year 4	85.8%	79.4%	0.66	0.58–0.76	yes
ET +/− Dalpiciclib	SHR6390-III-303 [44]	-[1]	4350	1:1	-[1]			not reported yet			
ET +/− Palbociclib	PALLAS [47]	AI or Tam +/− OFS	5796	1:1	2 years	year 4	84.2%	84.5%	0.96	0.81–1.14	no
	Penelope-B [48]	AI or Tam +/− OFS	1250	1:1	1 year	year 3	81.2%	77.7%	0.93	0.74–1.17	no
ET +/− Ribociclib	NATALEE	AI +/− OFS	5101	1:1	3 years			not reported yet			

AI: aromatase inhibitor; CI: confidence interval; DFS: disease-free survival; eBC: early breast cancer; ET: endocrine treatment; HR: hazard ratio; OFS: ovarian function suppression; Tam: Tamoxifen. [1] Data unknown at time of manuscript writing.

3.1. Palbociclib Failing to Improve Invasive-Disease-Free Survival

As palbociclib was the first inhibitor from this family to be developed for the indication of metastatic BC, it was also the first one to be investigated in the early treatment setting. The multi-center phase III PALLAS trial enrolled 5796 patients with stage II and III disease to be randomly assigned to ET plus two years of additional palbociclib or ET alone. In the second planned interim analysis, no difference could be seen between the two treatment arms with regards to the 3-year invasive-disease-free survival (iDFS), so that the regimen was not recommended for this indication [49]. The results were confirmed by the final analysis at year four [47]. Another phase III study, Penelope-B, was investigated in parallel to the PALLAS palbociclib in patients with residual disease after neoadjuvant chemotherapy (NACT) and a high risk of recurrence defined by the CPS-EG score (clinical pathological staging-estrogen receptor grading score). In total, 1250 patients were randomized to ET plus either 13 cycles of palbociclib or placebo. However, similar to the PALLAS outcome, Penelope-B could not show any improvement in the iDFS in patients under additional palbociclib [48], making this CDK4/6i mainly a player in stage IV disease. Further studies with smaller sample sizes, such as the Appalaches (NCT03609047) comparing ET plus palbociclib to chemotherapy in elderly patients, the POLAR study (NCT03820830) investigating the efficacy of the same treatment combination in patients with isolated locoregional BC recurrence or the TRAK-ER (NCT04985266) treating ctDNA positive patients with palbociclib plus fulvestrant vs. standard ET, are ongoing [44].

3.2. Abemaciclib as the First New Drug in Two Decades to Complement Curative ET in Node-Positive Patients

Assuming, based on the exceptional OS improvement with ribociclib and abemaciclib in advanced disease, that the ET of the woman with eBC is also on the brink of a new era, this theory was first proven using abemaciclib. The monarchE, a multi-center randomized phase III trial, demonstrated, at an interim analysis in 5637 node-positive patients, a significant benefit of the addition of two years of abemaciclib to ET compared to ET alone. Further, 2-year iDFS rates were 92.2% vs. 88.7%, respectively (HR 0.75; 95% CI, 0.60–0.93) [50], resulting in an absolute delta of 3.5% between the study arms. As in other trials, such as Penelope-B, for instance, survival curves seemed to separate during the first few years but united at a later stage; further results from monarchE were awaited to see a clearer difference. At the 4-year analysis, the CDK4/6i again showed a better iDFS rate compared to the control arm (85.8% vs. 79.4%, respectively; HR 0.66; 95% CI 0.58–0.76) and the benefit even deepened over time, so that the absolute improvement grew to 6.4% [46]. Abemaciclib was approved by the FDA in 2021 in combination with ET for the therapy of node-positive patients with eBC and a high risk of recurrence [51]. A recent prespecified exploratory analysis from monarchE, looking mainly at patients who received NACT, could even extend the positive data situation for abemaciclib. Out of a total of 2056 node-positive patients pre-treated with NACT, the 2-year iDFS rate in the CDK4/6i arm was 6.6% better than in the control arm without the CDK4/6i (87.2% vs. 80.6%, respectively; HR 0.61; 95% CI 0.47–0.80), resulting in a 39% relative reduction in the risk of developing an iDFS event [52]. Thus, abemaciclib is not only the first CDK4/6i but, in general, the first drug in more than 20 years since the approval of AIs to be effective in hormone receptor-positive, HER2-negative eBC. While final OS results from the monarchE are pending, other trials that aim to analyze the role of abemaciclib in specific patient cohorts are ongoing. The ADAPTlate (NCT04565054), for instance, was designed to show whether abemaciclib added to an ongoing ET one to six years after BC diagnosis, i.e., "late", is still effective. The POETIC-A (NCT04584853), however, is targeting postmenopausal women whose Ki-67 is persistently high after neoadjuvant ET, indicating endocrine resistance. In both trials, patients were randomized 1:1 to adjuvant ET alone or in combination with two years of abemaciclib [44].

3.3. Ribociclib with the Potential of Covering the Unmet Need in Stage II Disease

The third CDK4/6i ribociclib is also being investigated in the curative adjuvant setting within the multi-center phase III NATALEE (NCT03701334) trial. In total, 5101 patients with stage II and III disease were enrolled in the study to be randomly assigned to three years of ribociclib + ET vs. ET monotherapy [44]. In contrast to the above-mentioned trials with other CDK4/6i, ribociclib is not only used in a smaller dose in eBC than in aBC (400 mg vs. 600 mg, respectively) but is also a CDK4/6i that is combinable only with AI +/− OFS due to a prolongation of the QT interval when combined with tamoxifen [20]. However, a recent meta-analysis of 7030 premenopausal women from four randomized trials found out that, compared to tamoxifen + OFS, premenopausal women with a higher risk of recurrence have a better outcome under AI + OFS. The rate of BC recurrence was lower for women under an AI (rate ratio = RR 0.79; 95% CI 0.69–0.90) [53], so that the treatment combination from the NATALEE trial in stage II and III patients with an increased risk of recurrence seems feasible and logical. The main difference between the NATALEE and the monarchE trials is that, while the monarchE investigated only patients with axillary lymph node metastases, in case of positive study results from NATALEE, ribociclib could be used not only in node-positive but also in node-negative patients (partly with additional risk criteria), covering the currently unmet need in this population, too. Study results are expected to be presented in the near future. Meanwhile, the ADAPTcycle (NCT04055493) compares ET plus 600 mg of ribociclib to chemotherapy in women with an intermediate risk of recurrence according to the Oncotype DX recurrence score. It is one of few trials in the curative treatment setting comparing an ET-based regimen directly to chemotherapy [44].

3.4. CDK4/6i as Neoadjuvant Therapy

Some trials have investigated the role of CDK4/6i also in neoadjuvant therapy. In the single-arm NeoPalAna trial, patients with stage II and III BC received palbociclib plus anastrozole after four weeks of anastrozole monotherapy and underwent serial biopsies prior to breast surgery. The complete cell cycle arrest (CCCA) rate at C1D15 of palbociclib was significantly higher than under anastrozole alone at C1D1 (87% vs. 26%, respectively, $p < 0.001$) [54]. In the randomized phase II NeoPal study, 106 patients with stage II and III disease were enrolled, but this time, they were randomized to be treated with neoadjuvant palbociclib plus ET vs. chemotherapy. Both arms led to poor pathological complete response (pCR) rates (3.8% under ET + palbociclib and 5.9% under chemotherapy) and the study did not meet its primary endpoint [55]. Recently published survival outcomes did not differ between both arms, suggesting that a neoadjuvant letrozole-palbociclib strategy may allow chemotherapy to be spared in some patients [56]. Similar trials were performed with abemaciclib and ribociclib. In neoMonarch, patients treated with neoadjuvant abemaciclib achieved significant CCCA rates compared to those treated with anastrozole alone [57]. The phase II CORALLEEN trial compared six cycles of neoadjuvant letrozole and ribociclib to four cycles of chemotherapy and could show, with the help of PAM50 before–after analyses, that some patients with high-risk BC treated with ribociclib could achieve molecular downstaging at the time of surgery [58]. These results show that there is some potential for CDK4/6i also in the neoadjuvant treatment as it seems to have a certain impact on cell proliferation in eBC.

4. Impact on Patients' Adherence and Quality of Life

No treatment is useful if patients' adherence and QoL suffer significantly. It is well-known, especially in the adjuvant ET setting, that adherence rates under AIs, for instance, decrease over the course of treatment, mainly due to adverse events (AEs) or certain characteristics [59,60]. However, despite having a life-threatening disease, even women with aBC terminate ET prematurely because of AEs [61]. As non-compliance and non-persistence are associated with a worse prognosis in BC patients [62] and any disease progression is, in turn, associated with a reduction in QoL [63], adherence and QoL under the combination of ET and CDK4/6i, that bring their own side effect profile with them, are of special interest.

The randomized trials in aBC have shown, across all CDK4/6i, that the QoL is either not significantly affected by the CDK4/6i or is even improved [64–70]. Analyses from the MonaLEEsa-2, -3 and -7 studies have, moreover, demonstrated that required dose modifications of ribociclib have no negative influence on survival outcomes [71,72]. Thus, doubts regarding patients' outcome should not hinder physicians in reducing the medication in case of AEs, as the latter might result in patients' non-persistence, leading to a worse prognosis.

Studies in eBC have further described patients' adherence under CDK4/6i. In the PALLAS trial, 42.2% stopped palbociclib before two years of treatment were completed, out of which the majority, namely 27.2%, discontinued due to AEs. However, ET non-persistence rates did not differ between the two treatment arms [73]. Penelope-B confirmed discontinuation rates within one year of treatment with palbociclib. Overall, 17.5% terminated study treatment (3.0% because of AEs) and only 5.1% ET [48]. In the monarchE study, 25.8% of patients discontinued abemaciclib for reasons other than recurrence, including 18.5% due to AEs. Most of those who terminated CDK4/6i treatment continued receiving ET, while 6.5% discontinued both the CDK4/6i and the ET partner because of AEs. In the control arm, only 1.1% was non-persistent with ET [74], indicating that the combinational treatment seems to be associated with a higher risk of discontinuing the complete therapy. The dose-escalation study TRADE (NCT number not known at time of manuscript writing) will investigate the question of whether a titration of abemaciclib results in better adherence rates and less premature treatment discontinuations. Data from the NATALEE trial will reveal more about persistence rates and QoL outcomes under ribociclib in eBC setting.

When a decision is to be made between the substances, the treating physician must not only consider the survival and QoL data of each CDK4/6i but also the patients' perspective of associated AEs. A survey among 209 oncologists and 304 patients was performed to see which AEs are key drivers for their therapy preferences. Among other risks, such as the risk of dose reduction due to AEs, risk of abdominal pain and the need for electrocardiogram monitoring, both groups rated risks of diarrhea (25% each) and grade 3/4 neutropenia (20% and 24%, respectively) as the most important attributes for treatment choice [75]. Figure 2 provides an overview of the most relevant AEs under the treatment with a CDK4/6i according to the phase III trials.

Despite ET adherence rates in need of improvement, in general, the treatment remains one of the best tolerable cancer therapies available. Still, the addition of a further substance such as the CDK4/6i to ET complicates patients' adherence. Those at risk of early treatment discontinuation, e.g., because of deteriorating AEs, should, therefore, be more in focus to ensure timely side effect management, potential dose modification and patients' compliance. Adherence programs in terms of digital health solutions might be one possible option to enable fast communication between the patient and the treating physician.

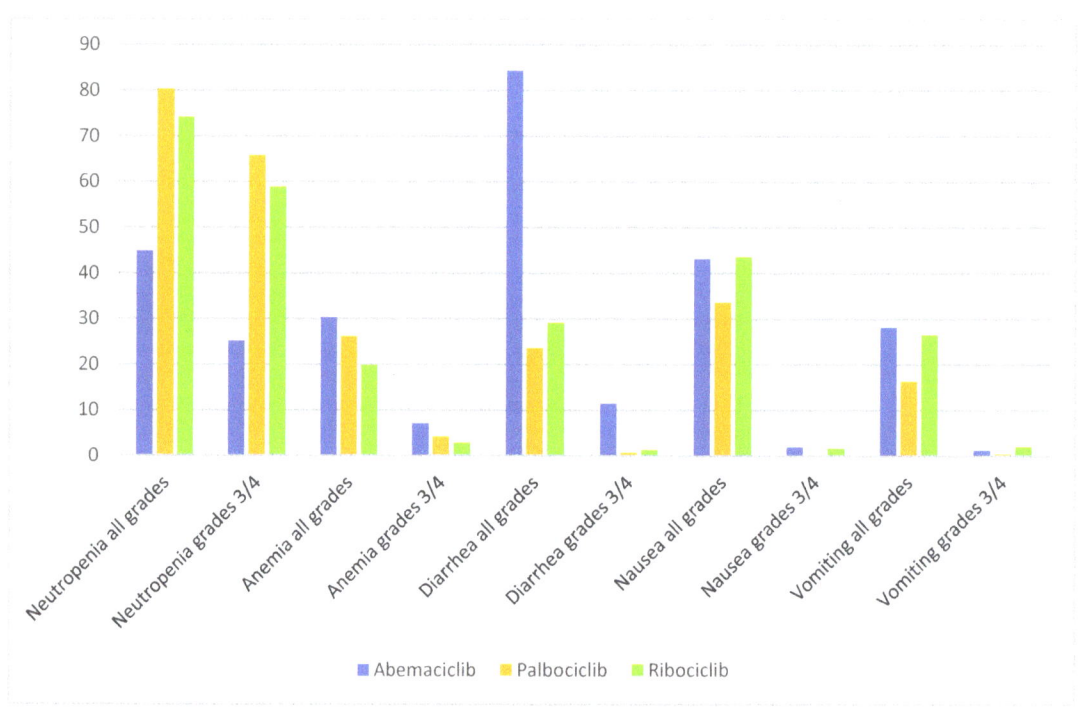

Figure 2. Relevant adverse events from phase III trials MONARCH-2 and -3 [23,24], PALOMA-2 and -3 [18,19] and MONALEESA-2, -3 and -7 [20–22] on average in percent.

5. Modern Therapy Approaches and New Opportunities

5.1. The Role of HER2

HER2 positivity seems to be associated with higher levels of CDK4/6 activity, enabling response to CDK4/6i in this BC subtype [76]. In the primary preclinical cell culture experiments, a reasonable response to palbociclib was seen in both HER2-positive and hormone receptor-positive BC cell lines [17]. Several trials have, therefore, analyzed the role of CDK4/6i in HER2-positive BC. Early-phase studies with trastuzumab in combination with palbociclib or ribociclib, respectively, demonstrated, in general, a working treatment concept with good tolerability [77,78]. The MonarcHER, a phase II trial with a total of 237 patients, compared, in a three-arm design, a treatment with abemaciclib, trastuzumab and fulvestrant to abemaciclib with trastuzumab to standard-of-care chemotherapy with trastuzumab. The combination of abemaciclib, trastuzumab and fulvestrant significantly improved PFS compared to chemotherapy with trastuzumab (8.3 months and 5.7 months, respectively; HR 0.67; 95% CI 0.45–1.00), while there was no difference between abemaciclib with trastuzumab and chemotherapy with trastuzumab (HR 0.94; 95% CI 0.64–1.38) [79], also meaning that the ET backbone plays a significant role for the efficacy of a CDK4/6i.

Patients with HER2-positive aBC previously treated with trastuzumab and a taxane received, in further trials, T-DM1 combined with a CDK4/6i. Again, a good safety profile was seen, demonstrating that with an antibody–drug conjugate, even more aggressive treatment partners can be added to a CDK4/6i without safety concerns [80,81]. However, due to a fast-changing treatment landscape and extraordinary results from novel anti-HER2 therapies, such as trastuzumab-deruxtecan and tucatinib [82], late-phase trials with CDK4/6i for HER2-positive aBC are not being performed for every CDK4/6i. Currently, palbociclib and ribociclib are being investigated in triple-positive aBC within the phase III trials PATINA (NCT02947685), PATRICIA II (NCT02448420) and DETECT V/CHEVENDO

(NCT02344472), respectively [44]. While results from the first two studies are expected to be presented in future, an interim analysis from the DETECT V study (triple-positive aBC patients randomized to trastuzumab + pertuzumab in combination with ribociclib + ET versus trastuzumab + pertuzumab in combination with chemotherapy followed by ribociclib + ET as maintenance treatment) was presented recently and showed no difference between a chemotherapy-containing and a chemotherapy-free regimen, neither regarding the PFS nor the OS. However, the tolerability was significantly better in the chemotherapy-free arm, so this phase III study is the first to demonstrate that CDK4/i—ribociclib in this case—in combination with antibodies is not inferior compared to chemotherapy and may, therefore, be an effective and safe treatment option for triple-positive BC patients [83].

Furthermore, since the introduction of multigene assays, it has been known that there is not only the BC subtype defined by immunohistochemistry (IHC) but also the one seen as the intrinsic subtype. Hence, intrinsic subtypes may differ from their immunohistochemical classification, which may also be associated with a switch in their risk categorization [84]. Luminal intrinsic subtypes have, in general, a better prognosis than HER2-enriched (HER2e) or basal-like ones, and it could be shown that, despite an immunohistochemically HER2-negative status, patients with intrinsic HER2e disease benefit from anti-HER2 treatments [85]. Therefore, it was again of special interest whether this also applies to a therapy with CDK4/6i, as these seem to have a certain efficacy in immunohistochemically HER2-positive BC, as mentioned above. To date, some studies have demonstrated efficacy of ribociclib in HER2e aBC patients, and not only across the MonaLEEsa study program [86] but also in a retrospective real-world analysis in comparison with palbo- and abemaciclib [87]. To further investigate the role of CDK4/6i in HER2e aBC, the ongoing randomized HARMONIA trial (NCT05207709) was set up and will analyze the efficacy of ribociclib versus palbociclib in this specific patient population [44]. Data from this study could help in defining the role of intrinsic subtypes for the treatment decision.

5.2. Novel Combination Partners

CDK4/6i have also been combined with novel substances from other drug families. Knowing that hormone receptor-positive, HER2-negative BC is generally a tumor with less immunoactivity, it is of interest whether the addition of checkpoint inhibitors, which usually trigger immune response, is feasible and effective in BC patients under CDK4/6i treatment. The phase II PACE trial randomized patients who progressed on CDK4/6i to fulvestrant +/− palbociclib +/− avelumab, an anti-PD-L1 antibody. While the 12-month PFS rates were 17.5% and 13.1% in the fulvestrant and fulvestrant + palbociclib arms, respectively, in the arm with the additional PD-L1 inhibitor avelumab, the rate was 35.6%. This resulted in an OS of 27.5 and 24.6 months in the fulvestrant and fulvestrant + palbociclib arms, and a total of 42.5 months in the fulvestrant + palbociclib + avelumab arm. Rates of immune related toxicities under avelumab were low [88]. Other studies with abemaciclib and pembrolizumab, palbociclib and nivolumab, or ribociclib and spartalizumab demonstrated high grade 3 AE rates, especially for enhanced transaminases and inflammatory lung disease/pneumonitis, indicating that such combinations cannot be developed further. Thus, the PACE trial showed, for the first time in a CDK4/6i pre-treated population, a feasible therapy combination with a checkpoint inhibitor beyond progression on CDK4/6i.

Further combination partners are the novel group of oral SERDs as well as new SERMs. Several ongoing phase III studies, such as the SERENA-4 and -6 with camizestrant (NCT04711252 and NCT04964934), the persevERA with giredestrant (NCT04546009) and the EMBER-3 with imlunestrant (NCT04975308), evaluate the benefit of the according oral SERD in combination with CDK4/6i [44]. The ELAINE 2, a phase II study with the novel SERM lasofoxifene, could show, in combination with abemaciclib in patients, whose metastatic disease had progressed on hormonal therapy +/− CDK4/6i, a good safety profile and a certain efficacy, with a median PFS of 13.9 months [89]. The outcomes of late-phase trials will show whether these novel substances are effective combination partners for CDK4/6i.

5.3. Further CDK Inhibitors

There are also novel inhibitors of the CDK currently under development. Among others, with dalpiciclib, birociclib and lerociclib, there is a range of new CDK4/6i being evaluated in patients with hormone receptor-positive, HER2-negative aBC within phase III studies in China [44]. Trilaciclib, also a CDK4/6i, is even being investigated in patients with triple-negative BC, with promising results [90]. Dinaciclib, in contrast, inhibits the CDK1/2/5/9 and is also of interest for BC treatment [91].

All these advancements show that CDK's role for the cell cycle is various and complex bearing high potential for further development.

6. Conclusions

The substance class of CDK4/6i has substantially improved the treatment landscape of hormone receptor-positive, HER2-negative BC patients. Achieving significant improvements in the survival rates in aBC patients and being the first substances in more than 20 years to improve DFS rates in eBC, CDK4/6i have set the new standard of care for patients suffering from this disease. The drugs have not only convinced researchers with better survival outcomes but also with manageable side effect profiles, as well as satisfying QoL data. Thanks to worldwide digitalization, nowadays, there is also more hope for better ET adherence rates using digital health solutions. For what happens after a CDK4/6i has been used, it remains important to better understand the mechanisms resulting in higher survival rates, but most of all, those that end in disease progression, to be able to develop novel substances on this basis. Further CDK inhibitors, treatment combinations with other drugs and different therapy sequences are under development, possibly leading to even more personalized BC treatment.

Author Contributions: Conceptualization, N.N.; methodology, N.N.; investigation, N.N.; writing—original draft preparation, N.N.; writing—review and editing, N.N. and P.A.F.; visualization, N.N.; supervision, N.N. and P.A.F.; project administration, N.N. and P.A.F. All authors have read and agreed to the published version of the manuscript.

Funding: This research received no external funding.

Institutional Review Board Statement: Not applicable.

Informed Consent Statement: Not applicable.

Data Availability Statement: Not applicable.

Conflicts of Interest: N.N. is currently an employee of Novartis and has received travel support from Novartis and TEVA in the past. P.A.F. reports personal fees from Novartis, grants from Biontech, grants and personal fees from Pfizer, personal fees from Daiichi-Sankyo, personal fees from Astra Zeneca, personal fees from Eisai, personal fees from Merck Sharp & Dohme, grants from Cepheid, personal fees from Lilly, personal fees from Pierre Fabre, personal fees from SeaGen, personal fees from Roche, personal fees from Agendia, personal fees from Sanofi Aventis and personal fees from Gilead.

References

1. Beatson, G. On the Treatment of Inoperable Cases of Carcinoma of the Mamma: Suggestions for a New Method of Treatment, with Illustrative Cases. *Lancet* **1896**, *148*, 162–165. [CrossRef]
2. Cole, M.P.; Jones, C.T.; Todd, I.D. A new anti-oestrogenic agent in late breast cancer. An early clinical appraisal of ICI46474. *Br. J. Cancer* **1971**, *25*, 270–275. [CrossRef]
3. Nabholtz, J.M.; Buzdar, A.; Pollak, M.; Harwin, W.; Burton, G.; Mangalik, A.; Steinberg, M.; Webster, A.; von Euler, M. Anastrozole is superior to tamoxifen as first-line therapy for advanced breast cancer in postmenopausal women: Results of a North American multicenter randomized trial. Arimidex Study Group. *J. Clin. Oncol.* **2000**, *18*, 3758–3767. [CrossRef]

4. Mouridsen, H.; Gershanovich, M.; Sun, Y.; Perez-Carrion, R.; Boni, C.; Monnier, A.; Apffelstaedt, J.; Smith, R.; Sleeboom, H.P.; Janicke, F.; et al. Superior efficacy of letrozole versus tamoxifen as first-line therapy for postmenopausal women with advanced breast cancer: Results of a phase III study of the International Letrozole Breast Cancer Group. *J. Clin. Oncol.* **2001**, *19*, 2596–2606. [CrossRef]
5. Osborne, C.K.; Pippen, J.; Jones, S.E.; Parker, L.M.; Ellis, M.; Come, S.; Gertler, S.Z.; May, J.T.; Burton, G.; Dimery, I.; et al. Double-blind, randomized trial comparing the efficacy and tolerability of fulvestrant versus anastrozole in postmenopausal women with advanced breast cancer progressing on prior endocrine therapy: Results of a North American trial. *J. Clin. Oncol.* **2002**, *20*, 3386–3395. [CrossRef]
6. Early Breast Cancer Trialists' Collaborative, G.; Dowsett, M.; Forbes, J.F.; Bradley, R.; Ingle, J.; Aihara, T.; Bliss, J.; Boccardo, F.; Coates, A.; Coombes, R.C.; et al. Aromatase inhibitors versus tamoxifen in early breast cancer: Patient-level meta-analysis of the randomised trials. *Lancet* **2015**, *386*, 1341–1352.
7. Early Breast Cancer Trialists' Collaborative, G. Effects of chemotherapy and hormonal therapy for early breast cancer on recurrence and 15-year survival: An overview of the randomised trials. *Lancet* **2005**, *365*, 1687–1717.
8. Pagani, O.; Francis, P.A.; Fleming, G.F.; Walley, B.A.; Viale, G.; Colleoni, M.; Lang, I.; Gomez, H.L.; Tondini, C.; Pinotti, G.; et al. Absolute Improvements in Freedom From Distant Recurrence to Tailor Adjuvant Endocrine Therapies for Premenopausal Women: Results from TEXT and SOFT. *J. Clin. Oncol.* **2020**, *38*, 1293–1303. [CrossRef]
9. Baselga, J.; Campone, M.; Piccart, M.; Burris, H.A., 3rd; Rugo, H.S.; Sahmoud, T.; Noguchi, S.; Gnant, M.; Pritchard, K.I.; Lebrun, F.; et al. Everolimus in postmenopausal hormone-receptor-positive advanced breast cancer. *N. Engl. J. Med.* **2012**, *366*, 520–529. [CrossRef]
10. Andre, F.; Ciruelos, E.; Rubovszky, G.; Campone, M.; Loibl, S.; Rugo, H.S.; Iwata, H.; Conte, P.; Mayer, I.A.; Kaufman, B.; et al. Alpelisib for PIK3CA-Mutated, Hormone Receptor-Positive Advanced Breast Cancer. *N. Engl. J. Med.* **2019**, *380*, 1929–1940. [CrossRef]
11. Bachelot, T.; Cottu, P.; Chabaud, S.; Dalenc, F.; Allouache, D.; Delaloge, S.; Jacquin, J.P.; Grenier, J.; Venat Bouvet, L.; Jegannathen, A.; et al. Everolimus Added to Adjuvant Endocrine Therapy in Patients with High-Risk Hormone Receptor-Positive, Human Epidermal Growth Factor Receptor 2-Negative Primary Breast Cancer. *J. Clin. Oncol.* **2022**, *40*, 3699–3708. [CrossRef]
12. Gennari, A.; Andre, F.; Barrios, C.H.; Cortes, J.; de Azambuja, E.; DeMichele, A.; Dent, R.; Fenlon, D.; Gligorov, J.; Hurvitz, S.A.; et al. ESMO Clinical Practice Guideline for the diagnosis, staging and treatment of patients with metastatic breast cancer. *Ann. Oncol.* **2021**, *32*, 1475–1495. [CrossRef]
13. Ditsch, N.; Wocke, A.; Untch, M.; Jackisch, C.; Albert, U.S.; Banys-Paluchowski, M.; Bauerfeind, I.; Blohmer, J.U.; Budach, W.; Dall, P.; et al. AGO Recommendations for the Diagnosis and Treatment of Patients with Early Breast Cancer: Update 2022. *Breast Care* **2022**, *17*, 403–420. [CrossRef]
14. Brufsky, A.M.; Dickler, M.N. Estrogen Receptor-Positive Breast Cancer: Exploiting Signaling Pathways Implicated in Endocrine Resistance. *Oncologist* **2018**, *23*, 528–539. [CrossRef]
15. Mills, J.N.; Rutkovsky, A.C.; Giordano, A. Mechanisms of resistance in estrogen receptor positive breast cancer: Overcoming resistance to tamoxifen/aromatase inhibitors. *Curr. Opin. Pharmacol.* **2018**, *41*, 59–65. [CrossRef]
16. Watt, A.C.; Goel, S. Cellular mechanisms underlying response and resistance to CDK4/6 inhibitors in the treatment of hormone receptor-positive breast cancer. *Breast Cancer Res.* **2022**, *24*, 17. [CrossRef]
17. Finn, R.S.; Dering, J.; Conklin, D.; Kalous, O.; Cohen, D.J.; Desai, A.J.; Ginther, C.; Atefi, M.; Chen, I.; Fowst, C.; et al. PD 0332991, a selective cyclin D kinase 4/6 inhibitor, preferentially inhibits proliferation of luminal estrogen receptor-positive human breast cancer cell lines in vitro. *Breast Cancer Res.* **2009**, *11*, R77. [CrossRef]
18. Finn, R.S.; Martin, M.; Rugo, H.S.; Jones, S.; Im, S.A.; Gelmon, K.; Harbeck, N.; Lipatov, O.N.; Walshe, J.M.; Moulder, S.; et al. Palbociclib and Letrozole in Advanced Breast Cancer. *N. Engl. J. Med.* **2016**, *375*, 1925–1936. [CrossRef]
19. Cristofanilli, M.; Turner, N.C.; Bondarenko, I.; Ro, J.; Im, S.A.; Masuda, N.; Colleoni, M.; DeMichele, A.; Loi, S.; Verma, S.; et al. Fulvestrant plus palbociclib versus fulvestrant plus placebo for treatment of hormone-receptor-positive, HER2-negative metastatic breast cancer that progressed on previous endocrine therapy (PALOMA-3): Final analysis of the multicentre, double-blind, phase 3 randomised controlled trial. *Lancet Oncol.* **2016**, *17*, 425–439.
20. Tripathy, D.; Im, S.A.; Colleoni, M.; Franke, F.; Bardia, A.; Harbeck, N.; Hurvitz, S.A.; Chow, L.; Sohn, J.; Lee, K.S.; et al. Ribociclib plus endocrine therapy for premenopausal women with hormone-receptor-positive, advanced breast cancer (MONALEESA-7): A randomised phase 3 trial. *Lancet Oncol.* **2018**, *19*, 904–915. [CrossRef]
21. Slamon, D.J.; Neven, P.; Chia, S.; Fasching, P.A.; De Laurentiis, M.; Im, S.A.; Petrakova, K.; Bianchi, G.V.; Esteva, F.J.; Martin, M.; et al. Phase III Randomized Study of Ribociclib and Fulvestrant in Hormone Receptor-Positive, Human Epidermal Growth Factor Receptor 2-Negative Advanced Breast Cancer: MONALEESA-3. *J. Clin. Oncol.* **2018**, *36*, 2465–2472. [CrossRef]
22. Hortobagyi, G.N.; Stemmer, S.M.; Burris, H.A.; Yap, Y.S.; Sonke, G.S.; Paluch-Shimon, S.; Campone, M.; Petrakova, K.; Blackwell, K.L.; Winer, E.P.; et al. Updated results from MONALEESA-2, a phase III trial of first-line ribociclib plus letrozole versus placebo plus letrozole in hormone receptor-positive, HER2-negative advanced breast cancer. *Ann. Oncol.* **2018**, *29*, 1541–1547. [CrossRef]
23. Johnston, S.; Martin, M.; Di Leo, A.; Im, S.A.; Awada, A.; Forrester, T.; Frenzel, M.; Hardebeck, M.C.; Cox, J.; Barriga, S.; et al. MONARCH 3 final PFS: A randomized study of abemaciclib as initial therapy for advanced breast cancer. *NPJ Breast Cancer* **2019**, *5*, 5. [CrossRef]

24. Sledge, G.W., Jr.; Toi, M.; Neven, P.; Sohn, J.; Inoue, K.; Pivot, X.; Burdaeva, O.; Okera, M.; Masuda, N.; Kaufman, P.A.; et al. MONARCH 2: Abemaciclib in Combination With Fulvestrant in Women With HR+/HER2− Advanced Breast Cancer Who Had Progressed While Receiving Endocrine Therapy. *J. Clin. Oncol.* **2017**, *35*, 2875–2884. [CrossRef]
25. Xu, B.; Zhang, Q.Y.; Zhang, P.; Tong, Z.; Sun, T.; Li, W.; Ouyang, Q.; Hu, X.; Cheng, Y.; Yan, M.; et al. LBA16 Dalpiciclib plus letrozole or anastrozole as first-line treatment for HR+/HER2- advanced breast cancer (DAWNA-2): A phase III trial. *Ann. Oncol.* **2022**, *33*, S1384–S1385. [CrossRef]
26. Xu, B.; Zhang, Q.; Zhang, P.; Hu, X.; Li, W.; Tong, Z.; Sun, T.; Teng, Y.; Wu, X.; Ouyang, Q.; et al. Dalpiciclib or placebo plus fulvestrant in hormone receptor-positive and HER2-negative advanced breast cancer: A randomized, phase 3 trial. *Nat. Med.* **2021**, *27*, 1904–1909. [CrossRef]
27. Nabieva, N.; Fasching, P.A. Endocrine Treatment for Breast Cancer Patients Revisited—History, Standard of Care, and Possibilities of Improvement. *Cancers* **2021**, *13*, 5643. [CrossRef]
28. Sledge, G.; Toi, M.; Neven, P.; Sohn, J.; Inoue, K.; Pivot, X.; Okera, M.; Masuda, N.; Kaufman, P.A.; Koh, H.; et al. Final Overall Survival Analysis of MONARCH-2: A Phase 3 trial of Abemaciclib Plus Fulvestrant in Patients with Hormone Receptor-positive, Human Epidermal Growth Factor Receptor 2-Negative Advanced Breast Cancer. In Proceedings of the 2022 San Antonio Breast Cancer Symposium, San Antonio, TX, USA, 6–10 December 2022.
29. Goetz, M.P.; Toi, M.; Huober, J.; Sohn, J.; Tredan, O.; Park, I.H.; Campone, M.; Chen, S.C.; Manso Sanchez, L.M.; Paluch-Shimon, S.; et al. LBA15 MONARCH 3: Interim overall survival (OS) results of abemaciclib plus a nonsteroidal aromatase inhibitor (NSAI) in patients (pts) with HR+, HER2- advanced breast cancer (ABC). *Ann. Oncol.* **2022**, *33*, S1384. [CrossRef]
30. Finn, R.S.; Rugo, H.S.; Dieras, V.C.; Harbeck, N.; Im, S.-A.; Gelmon, K.A.; Walshe, J.M.; Martin, M.; Gregor, M.C.M.; Bananis, E.; et al. Overall survival (OS) with first-line palbociclib plus letrozole (PAL + LET) versus placebo plus letrozole (PBO + LET) in women with estrogen receptor–positive/human epidermal growth factor receptor 2–negative advanced breast cancer (ER+/HER2− ABC): Analyses from PALOMA-2. *J. Clin. Oncol.* **2022**, *40*, LBA1003.
31. Turner, N.C.; Slamon, D.J.; Ro, J.; Bondarenko, I.; Im, S.A.; Masuda, N.; Colleoni, M.; DeMichele, A.; Loi, S.; Verma, S.; et al. Overall Survival with Palbociclib and Fulvestrant in Advanced Breast Cancer. *N. Engl. J. Med.* **2018**, *379*, 1926–1936. [CrossRef]
32. Hortobagyi, G.N.; Stemmer, S.M.; Burris, H.A.; Yap, Y.S.; Sonke, G.S.; Hart, L.; Campone, M.; Petrakova, K.; Winer, E.P.; Janni, W.; et al. Overall Survival with Ribociclib plus Letrozole in Advanced Breast Cancer. *N. Engl. J. Med.* **2022**, *386*, 942–950. [CrossRef]
33. Slamon, D.J.; Neven, P.; Chia, S.; Jerusalem, G.; De Laurentiis, M.; Im, S.; Petrakova, K.; Valeria Bianchi, G.; Martin, M.; Nusch, A.; et al. Ribociclib plus fulvestrant for postmenopausal women with hormone receptor-positive, human epidermal growth factor receptor 2-negative advanced breast cancer in the phase III randomized MONALEESA-3 trial: Updated overall survival. *Ann. Oncol.* **2021**, *32*, 1015–1024. [CrossRef]
34. Tripathy, D.; Im, S.-A.; Colleoni, M.; Franke, F.; Bardia, A.; Harbeck, N.; Hurvitz, S.; Chow, L.; Sohn, J.; Lee, K.S.; et al. Abstract PD2-04: Updated overall survival (OS) results from the phase III MONALEESA-7 trial of pre- or perimenopausal patients with hormone receptor positive/human epidermal growth factor receptor 2 negative (HR+/HER2−) advanced breast cancer (ABC) treated with endocrine therapy (ET) ± ribociclib. *Cancer Res.* **2021**, *81*, PD2-04.
35. Sledge, G.W., Jr.; Toi, M.; Neven, P.; Sohn, J.; Inoue, K.; Pivot, X.; Burdaeva, O.; Okera, M.; Masuda, N.; Kaufman, P.A.; et al. The Effect of Abemaciclib Plus Fulvestrant on Overall Survival in Hormone Receptor-Positive, ERBB2-Negative Breast Cancer That Progressed on Endocrine Therapy-MONARCH 2: A Randomized Clinical Trial. *JAMA Oncol.* **2020**, *6*, 116–124. [CrossRef] [PubMed]
36. George, M.A.; Qureshi, S.; Omene, C.; Toppmeyer, D.L.; Ganesan, S. Clinical and Pharmacologic Differences of CDK4/6 Inhibitors in Breast Cancer. *Front. Oncol.* **2021**, *11*, 693104. [CrossRef] [PubMed]
37. Schneeweiss, A.; Ettl, J.; Luftner, D.; Beckmann, M.W.; Belleville, E.; Fasching, P.A.; Fehm, T.N.; Geberth, M.; Haberle, L.; Hadji, P.; et al. Initial experience with CDK4/6 inhibitor-based therapies compared to antihormone monotherapies in routine clinical use in patients with hormone receptor positive, HER2 negative breast cancer—Data from the PRAEGNANT research network for the first 2 years of drug availability in Germany. *Breast* **2020**, *54*, 88–95.
38. Engler, T.; Fasching, P.A.; Luftner, D.; Hartkopf, A.D.; Muller, V.; Kolberg, H.C.; Hadji, P.; Tesch, H.; Haberle, L.; Ettl, J.; et al. Implementation of CDK4/6 Inhibitors and its Influence on the Treatment Landscape of Advanced Breast Cancer Patients—Data from the Real-World Registry PRAEGNANT. *Geburtshilfe Frauenheilkd.* **2022**, *82*, 1055–1067. [CrossRef]
39. Giuliano, M.; Schettini, F.; Rognoni, C.; Milani, M.; Jerusalem, G.; Bachelot, T.; De Laurentiis, M.; Thomas, G.; De Placido, P.; Arpino, G.; et al. Endocrine treatment versus chemotherapy in postmenopausal women with hormone receptor-positive, HER2-negative, metastatic breast cancer: A systematic review and network meta-analysis. *Lancet Oncol.* **2019**, *20*, 1360–1369. [CrossRef]
40. Martin, M.; Zielinski, C.; Ruiz-Borrego, M.; Carrasco, E.; Turner, N.; Ciruelos, E.M.; Munoz, M.; Bermejo, B.; Margeli, M.; Anton, A.; et al. Palbociclib in combination with endocrine therapy versus capecitabine in hormonal receptor-positive, human epidermal growth factor 2-negative, aromatase inhibitor-resistant metastatic breast cancer: A phase III randomised controlled trial-PEARL. *Ann. Oncol.* **2021**, *32*, 488–499. [CrossRef]
41. Martin, M.; Zielinski, C.; Ruiz-Borrego, M.; Carrasco, E.; Ciruelos, E.M.; Munoz, M.; Bermejo, B.; Margeli, M.; Csoszi, T.; Anton, A.; et al. Overall survival with palbociclib plus endocrine therapy versus capecitabine in postmenopausal patients with hormone receptor-positive, HER2-negative metastatic breast cancer in the PEARL study. *Eur. J. Cancer* **2022**, *168*, 12–24. [CrossRef]

42. Lu, Y.-S.; Bin Mohd Mahidin, E.I.; Azim, H.; Eralp, Y.; Yap, Y.-S.; Im, S.-A.; Rihani, J.; Bowles, J.; Alfaro, T.D.; Wu, J.; et al. Primary Results From the Randomized Phase II RIGHT Choice Trial of Premenopausal Patients with Aggressive HR+/HER2− Advanced Breast Cancer Treated with Ribociclib + Endocrine Therapy vs Physician's Choice Combination Chemotherapy. In Proceedings of the 2022 San Antonio Breast Cancer Symposium, San Antonio, TX, USA, 6–10 December 2022.
43. Kalinsky, K.; Accordino, M.K.; Chiuzan, C.; Mundi, P.S.; Trivedi, M.S.; Novik, Y.; Tiersten, A.; Raptis, G.; Baer, L.N.; Oh, S.Y.; et al. A randomized, phase II trial of fulvestrant or exemestane with or without ribociclib after progression on anti-estrogen therapy plus cyclin-dependent kinase 4/6 inhibition (CDK 4/6i) in patients (pts) with unresectable or hormone receptor–positive (HR+), HER2-negative metastatic breast cancer (MBC): MAINTAIN trial. *J. Clin. Oncol.* **2022**, *40*, LBA1004.
44. Clinicaltrials.gov. Available online: https://clinicaltrials.gov/ (accessed on 15 December 2022).
45. Bidard, F.C.; Hardy-Bessard, A.C.; Dalenc, F.; Bachelot, T.; Pierga, J.Y.; de la Motte Rouge, T.; Sabatier, R.; Dubot, C.; Frenel, J.S.; Ferrero, J.M.; et al. Switch to fulvestrant and palbociclib versus no switch in advanced breast cancer with rising ESR1 mutation during aromatase inhibitor and palbociclib therapy (PADA-1): A randomised, open-label, multicentre, phase 3 trial. *Lancet Oncol.* **2022**, *23*, 1367–1377. [CrossRef] [PubMed]
46. Johnston, S.; Toi, M.; O'Shaughnessy, J.; Rastogi, P.; Campone, M.; Neven, P.; Huang, C.-S.; Huober, J.; Jaliffe, G.G.; Cicin, I.; et al. Abemaciclib plus endocrine therapy for HR+, HER2−, node-positive, high-risk early breast cancer: Results from a pre-planned monarchE overall survival interim analysis, including 4-year efficacy outcomes. In Proceedings of the 2022 San Antonio Breast Cancer Symposium, San Antonio, TX, USA, 6–10 December 2022.
47. Gnant, M.; Dueck, A.C.; Frantal, S.; Martin, M.; Burstein, H.J.; Greil, R.; Fox, P.; Wolff, A.C.; Chan, A.; Winer, E.P.; et al. Adjuvant Palbociclib for Early Breast Cancer: The PALLAS Trial Results (ABCSG-42/AFT-05/BIG-14-03). *J. Clin. Oncol.* **2022**, *40*, 282–293. [CrossRef]
48. Loibl, S.; Marme, F.; Martin, M.; Untch, M.; Bonnefoi, H.; Kim, S.B.; Bear, H.; McCarthy, N.; Mele Olive, M.; Gelmon, K.; et al. Palbociclib for Residual High-Risk Invasive HR-Positive and HER2-Negative Early Breast Cancer-The Penelope-B Trial. *J. Clin. Oncol.* **2021**, *39*, 1518–1530. [CrossRef] [PubMed]
49. Mayer, E.L.; Dueck, A.C.; Martin, M.; Rubovszky, G.; Burstein, H.J.; Bellet-Ezquerra, M.; Miller, K.D.; Zdenkowski, N.; Winer, E.P.; Pfeiler, G.; et al. Palbociclib with adjuvant endocrine therapy in early breast cancer (PALLAS): Interim analysis of a multicentre, open-label, randomised, phase 3 study. *Lancet Oncol.* **2021**, *22*, 212–222. [CrossRef]
50. Johnston, S.R.D.; Harbeck, N.; Hegg, R.; Toi, M.; Martin, M.; Shao, Z.M.; Zhang, Q.Y.; Martinez Rodriguez, J.L.; Campone, M.; Hamilton, E.; et al. Abemaciclib Combined With Endocrine Therapy for the Adjuvant Treatment of HR+, HER2−, Node-Positive, High-Risk, Early Breast Cancer (monarchE). *J. Clin. Oncol.* **2020**, *38*, 3987–3998. [CrossRef] [PubMed]
51. Royce, M.; Osgood, C.; Mulkey, F.; Bloomquist, E.; Pierce, W.F.; Roy, A.; Kalavar, S.; Ghosh, S.; Philip, R.; Rizvi, F.; et al. FDA Approval Summary: Abemaciclib with Endocrine Therapy for High-Risk Early Breast Cancer. *J. Clin. Oncol.* **2022**, *40*, 1155–1162. [CrossRef]
52. Martin, M.; Hegg, R.; Kim, S.B.; Schenker, M.; Grecea, D.; Garcia-Saenz, J.A.; Papazisis, K.; Ouyang, Q.; Lacko, A.; Oksuzoglu, B.; et al. Treatment with Adjuvant Abemaciclib Plus Endocrine Therapy in Patients with High-risk Early Breast Cancer Who Received Neoadjuvant Chemotherapy: A Prespecified Analysis of the monarchE Randomized Clinical Trial. *JAMA Oncol.* **2022**, *8*, 1190–1194. [CrossRef]
53. Early Breast Cancer Trialists' Collaborative, G. Aromatase inhibitors versus tamoxifen in premenopausal women with oestrogen receptor-positive early-stage breast cancer treated with ovarian suppression: A patient-level meta-analysis of 7030 women from four randomised trials. *Lancet Oncol.* **2022**, *23*, 382–392.
54. Ma, C.X.; Gao, F.; Luo, J.; Northfelt, D.W.; Goetz, M.; Forero, A.; Hoog, J.; Naughton, M.; Ademuyiwa, F.; Suresh, R.; et al. NeoPalAna: Neoadjuvant Palbociclib, a Cyclin-Dependent Kinase 4/6 Inhibitor, and Anastrozole for Clinical Stage 2 or 3 Estrogen Receptor-Positive Breast Cancer. *Clin. Cancer Res.* **2017**, *23*, 4055–4065. [CrossRef]
55. Cottu, P.; D'Hondt, V.; Dureau, S.; Lerebours, F.; Desmoulins, I.; Heudel, P.E.; Duhoux, F.P.; Levy, C.; Mouret-Reynier, M.A.; Dalenc, F.; et al. Letrozole and palbociclib versus chemotherapy as neoadjuvant therapy of high-risk luminal breast cancer. *Ann. Oncol.* **2018**, *29*, 2334–2340. [CrossRef]
56. Delaloge, S.; Dureau, S.; D'Hondt, V.; Desmoulins, I.; Heudel, P.E.; Duhoux, F.P.; Levy, C.; Lerebours, F.; Mouret-Reynier, M.A.; Dalenc, F.; et al. Survival outcomes after neoadjuvant letrozole and palbociclib versus third generation chemotherapy for patients with high-risk oestrogen receptor-positive HER2-negative breast cancer. *Eur. J. Cancer* **2022**, *166*, 300–308. [CrossRef]
57. Hurvitz, S.A.; Martin, M.; Press, M.F.; Chan, D.; Fernandez-Abad, M.; Petru, E.; Rostorfer, R.; Guarneri, V.; Huang, C.S.; Barriga, S.; et al. Potent Cell-Cycle Inhibition and Upregulation of Immune Response with Abemaciclib and Anastrozole in neoMONARCH, Phase II Neoadjuvant Study in HR(+)/HER2(−) Breast Cancer. *Clin. Cancer Res.* **2020**, *26*, 566–580. [CrossRef] [PubMed]
58. Prat, A.; Saura, C.; Pascual, T.; Hernando, C.; Munoz, M.; Pare, L.; Gonzalez Farre, B.; Fernandez, P.L.; Galvan, P.; Chic, N.; et al. Ribociclib plus letrozole versus chemotherapy for postmenopausal women with hormone receptor-positive, HER2-negative, luminal B breast cancer (CORALLEEN): An open-label, multicentre, randomised, phase 2 trial. *Lancet Oncol.* **2020**, *21*, 33–43. [CrossRef] [PubMed]
59. Nabieva, N.; Kellner, S.; Fehm, T.; Haberle, L.; de Waal, J.; Rezai, M.; Baier, B.; Baake, G.; Kolberg, H.C.; Guggenberger, M.; et al. Influence of patient and tumor characteristics on early therapy persistence with letrozole in postmenopausal women with early breast cancer: Results of the prospective Evaluate-TM study with 3941 patients. *Ann. Oncol.* **2018**, *29*, 186–192. [CrossRef]

60. Nabieva, N.; Fehm, T.; Haberle, L.; de Waal, J.; Rezai, M.; Baier, B.; Baake, G.; Kolberg, H.C.; Guggenberger, M.; Warm, M.; et al. Influence of side-effects on early therapy persistence with letrozole in post-menopausal patients with early breast cancer: Results of the prospective EvAluate-TM study. *Eur. J. Cancer* **2018**, *96*, 82–90. [CrossRef] [PubMed]
61. Wallwiener, M.; Nabieva, N.; Feisst, M.; Fehm, T.; de Waal, J.; Rezai, M.; Baier, B.; Baake, G.; Kolberg, H.C.; Guggenberger, M.; et al. Influence of patient and tumor characteristics on therapy persistence with letrozole in postmenopausal women with advanced breast cancer: Results of the prospective observational EvAluate-TM study. *BMC Cancer* **2019**, *19*, 611. [CrossRef] [PubMed]
62. Chirgwin, J.H.; Giobbie-Hurder, A.; Coates, A.S.; Price, K.N.; Ejlertsen, B.; Debled, M.; Gelber, R.D.; Goldhirsch, A.; Smith, I.; Rabaglio, M.; et al. Treatment Adherence and Its Impact on Disease-Free Survival in the Breast International Group 1-98 Trial of Tamoxifen and Letrozole, Alone and in Sequence. *J. Clin. Oncol.* **2016**, *34*, 2452–2459. [CrossRef]
63. Muller, V.; Nabieva, N.; Haberle, L.; Taran, F.A.; Hartkopf, A.D.; Volz, B.; Overkamp, F.; Brandl, A.L.; Kolberg, H.C.; Hadji, P.; et al. Impact of disease progression on health-related quality of life in patients with metastatic breast cancer in the PRAEGNANT breast cancer registry. *Breast* **2018**, *37*, 154–160. [CrossRef]
64. Kaufman, P.A.; Toi, M.; Neven, P.; Sohn, J.; Grischke, E.M.; Andre, V.; Stoffregen, C.; Shekarriz, S.; Price, G.L.; Carter, G.C.; et al. Health-Related Quality of Life in MONARCH 2: Abemaciclib plus Fulvestrant in Hormone Receptor-Positive, HER2-Negative Advanced Breast Cancer after Endocrine Therapy. *Oncologist* **2020**, *25*, e243–e251. [CrossRef]
65. Goetz, M.P.; Martin, M.; Tokunaga, E.; Park, I.H.; Huober, J.; Toi, M.; Stoffregen, C.; Shekarriz, S.; Andre, V.; Gainford, M.C.; et al. Health-Related Quality of Life in MONARCH 3: Abemaciclib plus an Aromatase Inhibitor as Initial Therapy in HR+, HER2− Advanced Breast Cancer. *Oncologist* **2020**, *25*, e1346–e1354. [CrossRef]
66. Harbeck, N.; Franke, F.; Villanueva-Vazquez, R.; Lu, Y.S.; Tripathy, D.; Chow, L.; Babu, G.K.; Im, Y.H.; Chandiwana, D.; Gaur, A.; et al. Health-related quality of life in premenopausal women with hormone-receptor-positive, HER2-negative advanced breast cancer treated with ribociclib plus endocrine therapy: Results from a phase III randomized clinical trial (MONALEESA-7). *Ther. Adv. Med. Oncol.* **2020**, *12*. [CrossRef] [PubMed]
67. Fasching, P.A.; Beck, J.T.; Chan, A.; De Laurentiis, M.; Esteva, F.J.; Jerusalem, G.; Neven, P.; Pivot, X.; Bianchi, G.V.; Martin, M.; et al. Ribociclib plus fulvestrant for advanced breast cancer: Health-related quality-of-life analyses from the MONALEESA-3 study. *Breast* **2020**, *54*, 148–154. [CrossRef]
68. Verma, S.; O'Shaughnessy, J.; Burris, H.A.; Campone, M.; Alba, E.; Chandiwana, D.; Dalal, A.A.; Sutradhar, S.; Monaco, M.; Janni, W. Health-related quality of life of postmenopausal women with hormone receptor-positive, human epidermal growth factor receptor 2-negative advanced breast cancer treated with ribociclib + letrozole: Results from MONALEESA-2. *Breast Cancer Res. Treat.* **2018**, *170*, 535–545. [CrossRef]
69. Rugo, H.S.; Dieras, V.; Gelmon, K.A.; Finn, R.S.; Slamon, D.J.; Martin, M.; Neven, P.; Shparyk, Y.; Mori, A.; Lu, D.R.; et al. Impact of palbociclib plus letrozole on patient-reported health-related quality of life: Results from the PALOMA-2 trial. *Ann. Oncol.* **2018**, *29*, 888–894. [CrossRef]
70. Harbeck, N.; Iyer, S.; Turner, N.; Cristofanilli, M.; Ro, J.; Andre, F.; Loi, S.; Verma, S.; Iwata, H.; Bhattacharyya, H.; et al. Quality of life with palbociclib plus fulvestrant in previously treated hormone receptor-positive, HER2-negative metastatic breast cancer: Patient-reported outcomes from the PALOMA-3 trial. *Ann. Oncol.* **2016**, *27*, 1047–1054. [CrossRef]
71. Hart, L.L.; Bardia, A.; Beck, J.T.; Chan, A.; Neven, P.; Hamilton, E.P.; Sohn, J.; Sonke, G.S.; Bachelot, T.; Spring, L.; et al. Impact of ribociclib (RIB) dose modifications (mod) on overall survival (OS) in patients (pts) with HR+/HER2- advanced breast cancer (ABC) in MONALEESA(ML)-2. *J. Clin. Oncol.* **2022**, *40*, 1017. [CrossRef]
72. Burris, H.A.; Chan, A.; Bardia, A.; Thaddeus Beck, J.; Sohn, J.; Neven, P.; Tripathy, D.; Im, S.A.; Chia, S.; Esteva, F.J.; et al. Safety and impact of dose reductions on efficacy in the randomised MONALEESA-2, -3 and -7 trials in hormone receptor-positive, HER2-negative advanced breast cancer. *Br. J. Cancer* **2021**, *125*, 679–686. [CrossRef] [PubMed]
73. Mayer, E.L.; Fesl, C.; Hlauschek, D.; Garcia-Estevez, L.; Burstein, H.J.; Zdenkowski, N.; Wette, V.; Miller, K.D.; Balic, M.; Mayer, I.A.; et al. Treatment Exposure and Discontinuation in the PALbociclib CoLlaborative Adjuvant Study of Palbociclib With Adjuvant Endocrine Therapy for Hormone Receptor-Positive/Human Epidermal Growth Factor Receptor 2-Negative Early Breast Cancer (PALLAS/AFT-05/ABCSG-42/BIG-14-03). *J. Clin. Oncol.* **2022**, *40*, 449–458.
74. Rugo, H.S.; O'Shaughnessy, J.; Boyle, F.; Toi, M.; Broom, R.; Blancas, I.; Gumus, M.; Yamashita, T.; Im, Y.H.; Rastogi, P.; et al. Adjuvant abemaciclib combined with endocrine therapy for high-risk early breast cancer: Safety and patient-reported outcomes from the monarchE study. *Ann. Oncol.* **2022**, *33*, 616–627. [CrossRef]
75. Maculaitis, M.C.; Liu, X.; Will, O.; Hanson, M.; McRoy, L.; Berk, A.; Crastnopol, M. Oncologist and Patient Preferences for Attributes of CDK4/6 Inhibitor Regimens for the Treatment of Advanced/Metastatic HR Positive/HER2 Negative Breast Cancer: Discrete Choice Experiment and Best-Worst Scaling. *Patient Prefer Adherence* **2020**, *14*, 2201–2214. [CrossRef]
76. Sinclair, W.D.; Cui, X. The Effects of HER2 on CDK4/6 Activity in Breast Cancer. *Clin. Breast Cancer* **2022**, *22*, e278–e285. [CrossRef] [PubMed]
77. Ciruelos, E.; Villagrasa, P.; Pascual, T.; Oliveira, M.; Pernas, S.; Pare, L.; Escriva-de-Romani, S.; Manso, L.; Adamo, B.; Martinez, E.; et al. Palbociclib and Trastuzumab in HER2-Positive Advanced Breast Cancer: Results from the Phase II SOLTI-1303 PATRICIA Trial. *Clin. Cancer Res.* **2020**, *26*, 5820–5829. [CrossRef] [PubMed]
78. Goel, S.; Pernas, S.; Tan-Wasielewski, Z.; Barry, W.T.; Bardia, A.; Rees, R.; Andrews, C.; Tahara, R.K.; Trippa, L.; Mayer, E.L.; et al. Ribociclib Plus Trastuzumab in Advanced HER2-Positive Breast Cancer: Results of a Phase 1b/2 Trial. *Clin. Breast Cancer* **2019**, *19*, 399–404. [CrossRef]

79. Tolaney, S.M.; Wardley, A.M.; Zambelli, S.; Hilton, J.F.; Troso-Sandoval, T.A.; Ricci, F.; Im, S.A.; Kim, S.B.; Johnston, S.R.; Chan, A.; et al. Abemaciclib plus trastuzumab with or without fulvestrant versus trastuzumab plus standard-of-care chemotherapy in women with hormone receptor-positive, HER2-positive advanced breast cancer (monarcHER): A randomised, open-label, phase 2 trial. *Lancet Oncol.* **2020**, *21*, 763–775. [CrossRef] [PubMed]
80. Spring, L.M.; Clark, S.L.; Li, T.; Goel, S.; Tayob, N.; Viscosi, E.; Abraham, E.; Juric, D.; Isakoff, S.J.; Mayer, E.; et al. Phase 1b clinical trial of ado-trastuzumab emtansine and ribociclib for HER2-positive metastatic breast cancer. *NPJ Breast Cancer* **2021**, *7*, 103. [CrossRef] [PubMed]
81. Haley, B.; Batra, K.; Sahoo, S.; Froehlich, T.; Klemow, D.; Unni, N.; Ahn, C.; Rodriguez, M.; Hullings, M.; Frankel, A.E. A Phase I/Ib Trial of PD 0332991 (Palbociclib) and T-DM1 in HER2-Positive Advanced Breast Cancer after Trastuzumab and Taxane Therapy. *Clin. Breast Cancer* **2021**, *21*, 417–424. [CrossRef]
82. Thill, M.; Luftner, D.; Kolberg-Liedtke, C.; Albert, U.S.; Banys-Paluchowski, M.; Bauerfeind, I.; Blohmer, J.U.; Budach, W.; Dall, P.; Fallenberg, E.M.; et al. AGO Recommendations for the Diagnosis and Treatment of Patients with Locally Advanced and Metastatic Breast Cancer: Update 2022. *Breast Care* **2022**, *17*, 421–429. [CrossRef]
83. Janni, W.; Fehm, T.; Müller, V.; Schochter, F.; De Gregorio, A.; Decker, T.; Hartkopf, A.; Just, M.; Sagasser, J.; Schmidt, M.; et al. Omission of chemotherapy in the treatment of HER2-positive and hormone-receptor positive metastatic breast cancer—Interim results from the randomized phase 3 DETECT V trial. In Proceedings of the 2022 San Antonio Breast Cancer Symposium, San Antonio, TX, USA, 6–10 December 2022.
84. Canino, F.; Piacentini, F.; Omarini, C.; Toss, A.; Barbolini, M.; Vici, P.; Dominici, M.; Moscetti, L. Role of Intrinsic Subtype Analysis with PAM50 in Hormone Receptors Positive HER2 Negative Metastatic Breast Cancer: A Systematic Review. *Int. J. Mol. Sci.* **2022**, *23*, 7079. [CrossRef]
85. Prat, A.; Cheang, M.C.; Galvan, P.; Nuciforo, P.; Pare, L.; Adamo, B.; Munoz, M.; Viladot, M.; Press, M.F.; Gagnon, R.; et al. Prognostic Value of Intrinsic Subtypes in Hormone Receptor-Positive Metastatic Breast Cancer Treated With Letrozole With or Without Lapatinib. *JAMA Oncol.* **2016**, *2*, 1287–1294. [CrossRef]
86. Jacobson, A. Ribociclib Improves Overall Survival in HR+/HER2− Metastatic Breast Cancer Across Common Genomic and Clinical Subtypes. *Oncologist* **2022**, *27*, S11–S12. [CrossRef] [PubMed]
87. Martínez-Sáez, O.; Tolosa, P.; Sánchez De Torre, A.; Pascual, T.; Brasó-Maristany, F.; Rodriguez Hernandez, A.; Parrilla, L.; Roncero, A.M.; Ruano, Y.; Chic, N.; et al. 23P CDK4/6 inhibition and endocrine therapy (ET) in the HER2-enriched subtype (HER2-E) in hormone receptor-positive/HER2-negative (HR+/HER2−) advanced breast cancer (ABC): A retrospective analysis of real-world data. *Ann. Oncol.* **2021**, *32*, S30. [CrossRef]
88. Mayer, E.; Ren, Y.; Wagle, N.; Mahtani, R.; Ma, C.; DeMichele, A.; Cristofanilli, M.; Meisel, J.; Miller, K.D.; Jolly, T.; et al. PACE: Palbociclib After CDK and Endocrine Therapy A Randomized Phase II Study of Fulvestrant +/− Palbociclib after Progression on CDK4/6 inhibitor for HR+/HER2− Metastatic Breast Cancer. In Proceedings of the 2022 San Antonio Breast Cancer Symposium, San Antonio, TX, USA, 6–10 December 2022.
89. Damodaran, S.; Plourde, P.V.; Moore, H.C.F.; Anderson, I.C.; Portman, D.J. Open-label, phase 2, multicenter study of lasofoxifene (LAS) combined with abemaciclib (Abema) for treating pre- and postmenopausal women with locally advanced or metastatic ER+/HER2− breast cancer and an ESR1 mutation after progression on prior therapies. *J. Clin. Oncol.* **2022**, *40*, 1022. [CrossRef]
90. Tan, A.R.; Wright, G.S.; Thummala, A.R.; Danso, M.A.; Popovic, L.; Pluard, T.J.; Han, H.S.; Vojnovic, Z.; Vasev, N.; Ma, L.; et al. Trilaciclib Prior to Chemotherapy in Patients with Metastatic Triple-Negative Breast Cancer: Final Efficacy and Subgroup Analysis from a Randomized Phase II Study. *Clin. Cancer Res.* **2022**, *28*, 629–636. [CrossRef] [PubMed]
91. Tsao, A.N.; Chuang, Y.S.; Lin, Y.C.; Su, Y.; Chao, T.C. Dinaciclib inhibits the stemness of two subtypes of human breast cancer cells by targeting the FoxM1 and Hedgehog signaling pathway. *Oncol. Rep.* **2022**, *47*, 105. [CrossRef]

Disclaimer/Publisher's Note: The statements, opinions and data contained in all publications are solely those of the individual author(s) and contributor(s) and not of MDPI and/or the editor(s). MDPI and/or the editor(s) disclaim responsibility for any injury to people or property resulting from any ideas, methods, instructions or products referred to in the content.

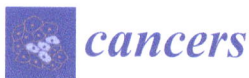

Review

Use of Telemedicine to Improve Cognitive Functions and Psychological Well-Being in Patients with Breast Cancer: A Systematic Review of the Current Literature

Andreina Giustiniani *, Laura Danesin , Rachele Pezzetta, Fabio Masina , Giulia Oliva , Giorgio Arcara, Francesca Burgio and Pierfranco Conte *

IRCCS San Camillo Hospital, 30126 Venice, Italy
* Correspondence: andreina.giustiniani@hsancamillo.it (A.G.); pierfranco.conte@hsancamillo.it (P.C.)

Simple Summary: Breast cancer is one of the most frequently diagnosed cancers among women. This diagnosis is accompanied by many psychological implications as well as cognitive consequences due to both the cancer itself and cancer treatments. Recently, telemedicine approaches have been used to provide support to these patients. We conducted a systematic review to clarify the effectiveness of telerehabilitation for treating the cognitive and psychological difficulties of breast cancer patients. The literature suggests that telerehabilitation may represent a promising approach for breast cancer patients, but more studies are needed that address the role of telerehabilitation, especially for cognitive symptoms.

Abstract: The diagnosis and side effects of breast cancer (BC) treatments greatly affect the everyday lives of women suffering from this disease, with relevant psychological and cognitive consequences. Several studies have reported the psychological effects of receiving a diagnosis of BC. Moreover, women undergoing anticancer therapies may exhibit cognitive impairment as a side effect of the treatments. The access to cognitive rehabilitation and psychological treatment for these patients is often limited by resources; women of childbearing age often encounter difficulties in completing rehabilitation programs requiring access to care institutions. Telemedicine, which provides health services using information and communication technologies, is a useful tool to overcome these limitations. In particular, telemedicine may represent an optimal way to guarantee cognitive rehabilitation, psychological support, and recovery to BC patients. Previous studies have reviewed the use of telemedicine to improve psychological well-being in BC patients, and a few have investigated the effect of telerehabilitation on cognitive deficits. This study systematically reviewed the evidence on the cognitive and psychological effects of telemedicine in BC patients. Current evidence suggests that telemedicine may represent a promising tool for the management of some psychological problems experienced by breast cancer patients, but more controlled studies are needed to clarify its effectiveness, especially for cognitive deficits. The results are also discussed in light of the intervening and modulating factors that may mediate both side effect occurrence and the success of the interventions.

Keywords: oncology; telemedicine; telerehabilitation; psychological well-being; cognitive impairment; rehabilitation; cancer side effects

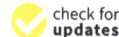

Citation: Giustiniani, A.; Danesin, L.; Pezzetta, R.; Masina, F.; Oliva, G.; Arcara, G.; Burgio, F.; Conte, P. Use of Telemedicine to Improve Cognitive Functions and Psychological Well-Being in Patients with Breast Cancer: A Systematic Review of the Current Literature. *Cancers* 2023, 15, 1353. https://doi.org/10.3390/cancers15041353

Academic Editors: Stefan Ambs and Naiba Nabieva

Received: 18 January 2023
Revised: 13 February 2023
Accepted: 17 February 2023
Published: 20 February 2023

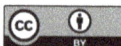

Copyright: © 2023 by the authors. Licensee MDPI, Basel, Switzerland. This article is an open access article distributed under the terms and conditions of the Creative Commons Attribution (CC BY) license (https://creativecommons.org/licenses/by/4.0/).

1. Introduction

Breast cancer is the most frequently diagnosed cancer among women and, in spite of an increasing curability, still ranks as the primary cause of cancer-related death [1,2]. The number of women diagnosed with breast cancer is dramatically increasing, and survivors must face many challenges while they continue with their lives during and after cancer treatment. In particular, several studies have reported the occurrence of cognitive and psychological difficulties in breast cancer patients [3,4]. Indeed, a new generation of hormone therapies, targeted therapies, and immunotherapy have resulted in improved survival rates, but an increasing number of studies are reporting the impact of pharmacological therapies and of cancer itself on cognitive functions [5]. Cognitive difficulties have become a growing area of clinical concern, and they occur in about 25% of patients with cancer before pharmacological treatment, in about 75% of patients during treatment, and in about 35% of patients post-treatment [6]. There is considerable variability regarding the severity and the duration of cognitive impairment, with the most impaired cognitive domains usually being memory [7], processing speed [8], attention, and executive functions [9]. The variability may depend on factors such as the type of pharmacological therapy, the woman's age and body mass index, and other disease-related biological factors such as inflammatory cytokine dysregulation, oxidative stress, DNA damage, or genetic polymorphisms and microvascular injury [10–12].

Psychological problems are common in breast cancer, and they have been shown to affect cognitive functioning [13]. Psychological difficulties are related to the fact that a breast cancer diagnosis is a stressful experience, causing significant psychosocial concerns such as marital problems or occupational difficulties [14], which vary along the disease trajectory. As is easily conceivable, patients may first develop depression and anxiety due to uncertainty as well as anger, sadness, and fear of death [15–18]. When the diagnosis comes during a phase of life in which women are developing their careers and having children, the psychological scenario is even worse [19]. In this context, in addition to anxiety and depression, women experience the emergence of negative feelings such as stress in significant relationships, sexual problems, separation anxiety, and fear of losing love, interest, support, and approval [20]. Furthermore, difficulties in managing health care while carrying on daily activities have important consequences for the quality of life, sleep quality, cognitive functioning, and even disease progression. Furthermore, the combination of cognitive and psychological problems may in turn influence women's functioning at work, thus resulting in a vicious cycle that enhances negative emotions and cognitive impairment. Of note, while psychological dysfunctions are prominent in patients during breast cancer therapy and tend to decrease in survivors, cognitive impairment remains after treatment cessation [21]. In this situation, psychological support is pivotal immediately after the diagnosis and during treatment, and, in parallel, the rehabilitation of cognitive impairment becomes particularly relevant in both patients and survivors.

Long-term care and health management in breast cancer are easier when the patient is an active manager of their own health. A promising resource for promoting this attitude is telemedicine, a method of providing health care services using information communication technologies (ICTs). These technologies offer the opportunity to overcome the patient's mobility problems and reduce costs for the national health system. To date, telemedicine has been widely used with promising results in terms of cost-effectiveness, in mental health, and in cognitive impairment [22–25]. Among the telemedicine approaches, telerehabilitation provides the delivery of rehabilitation programs through ICT. Telerehabilitation programs are used for home rehabilitation to improve motor, cognitive, or psychological dysfunctions with several advantages. Indeed, these programs also provide the opportunity to access rehabilitation for patients who cannot reach care centers, allow for the continuity of care over time and space, reduce care costs, and improve comfort for the patients, thus reducing the drop-out rates.

Telemedicine and telerehabilitation offer several advantages when used with breast cancer patients in which they have positive effects on both cancer-related and treatment-related psychological conditions [20]. Previous studies have reported improvements after telemedicine interventions in the quality of life (QoL), anxiety and depression, psychological distress, social functioning, and fatigue in patients with many different diseases including breast cancer, respiratory diseases, and diabetes [20,26]. However, very few studies have investigated the effects of telerehabilitation on cognition [21–23]. Overall, in spite of some inconsistencies [27], improvements in verbal fluency, processing speed, cognitive flexibility, memory, and working memory as well as in subjective cognitive functioning have been reported [28,29].

A previous review focused on the effect of telemedicine on mental problems experienced by breast cancer patients. The present study aims at expanding the current literature by reviewing studies on the effects of telemedicine on the psychological and cognitive difficulties experienced by breast cancer patients, and also by considering the role that specific mediating factors may play in the success rate of these techniques, highlighting future directions and needs. Because of the close relationship between the cognitive and psychological domains in breast cancer patients, it is important to clarify whether telemedicine and telerehabilitation can represent an effective approach to a comprehensive management of both psychological wellness and cognitive difficulties. In the present study, we therefore reviewed the research focused on the effect of telemedicine on psychological and/or cognitive functioning, providing an overview of factors that can play a role in the success rate of these interventions.

2. Materials and Methods

This study was conducted by following the Preferred Reporting Items for Systematic Reviews and Meta-Analyses (PRISMA) [30]. We systematically searched the following databases: Scopus, PubMed, and Embase from January 2000 to September 2022. We used the following keywords: "telemedicine", "e-health", "telerehabilitation", "breast cancer", "cognit*", "psycholog*". The six terms were combined using appropriate Boolean operators for search.

- To be eligible, studies had to meet the following criteria:
- Being concluded or planned randomized controlled trials (RCTs);
- Assessing the impact of telemedicine in patients treated for early breast cancer or breast cancer survivors after the completion of treatment;
- Reporting a cognitive test or psychological scales as primary or secondary outcomes;
- Using telemedicine for evaluation or rehabilitation;
- Being written in English;
- Being published in an English language journal after 2000.

Candidate studies were excluded when they were published in non-scientific journals, were not conducted on humans, used rehabilitation protocols other than telehealth, telemedicine, web-based therapy, online therapy, and did not use cognitive or psychological tests as the primary or secondary outcome. Duplicate studies were excluded using the Mendeley reference tool. Other reviews were inspected to extract possible eligible papers.

Six authors (AG, LD, FB, RP, FM, GO) independently screened the titles and abstracts of articles collected from the database search. Only articles meeting the inclusion criteria were selected. Any disagreement in study selection was discussed and resolved among all the authors.

The remaining articles were read by five authors (AG, LD, RP, FM, GO) who extracted relevant information following a modified version of the PICO guidelines: participants, methodology, comparisons, outcomes. Additional data on the sample's demographic were extracted.

3. Results

Our search initially identified 260 records. After the removal of duplicates, 209 articles remained. During the abstract screening process, 186 studies were excluded and 23 studies were selected for the full text reading. During the full text reading, 16 records were determined to meet the inclusion criteria. Among these, four records were RCT study protocols (Figure 1).

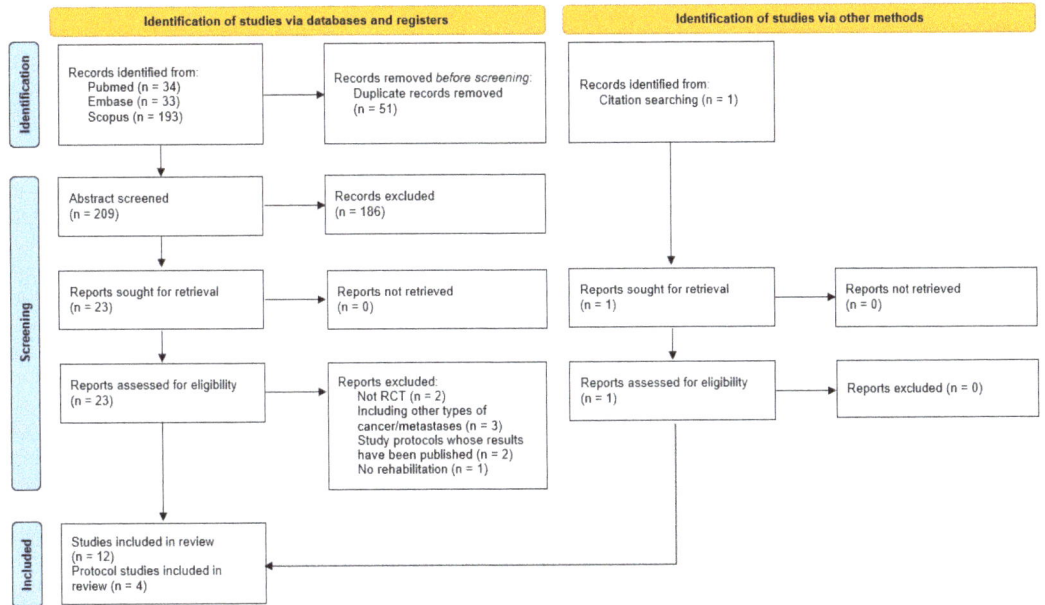

Figure 1. Search strategy used for the selection of studies included in the review.

3.1. Included Studies and Protocols-Sample Characteristics

From the reviewed studies, a total of 1754 participants constituted the sample. The women's ages varied from 30 to 70 years, with only one study recruiting participants older than 70 years [31]. A total of 2898 participants were included in the study protocols (Table 1).

3.1.1. Patients' Cancer Stages in the Included Studies

Among the included records, one completed study recruited women with stage I–III primary breast cancer starting adjuvant therapy [31], and 11 studies recruited women during or after the completion of adjuvant endocrine therapy [27,29,32–40]. Moreover, four study protocols that planned to enroll patients who would start [41–43] or would complete [44] adjuvant or neoadjuvant therapies were included. Only one study and one study protocol reported some information on the molecular subtypes of breast cancer: the study from Zachariae [37] included 80% of patients with luminal tumors, and the protocol from Carlson [41] will include all subtypes except for HER2+ disease.

3.1.2. Characteristics of the Telemedicine Programs and of the Control Conditions Applied in the Included Studies

Overall, the type of telerehabilitation employed in the included studies ranged from programs on physical fitness to psycho-education, cognitive behavioral therapy (CBT), mindfulness, and cognitive training. Similarly, the duration of these programs was heterogeneous, with most of the studies applying a 6–12 weeks of training.

Two studies used the E-CUIDATE program to improve QoL, pain, muscle strength, and fatigue [35,36]. This system consists of an interface in which patients perform tailored exercises consisting of a warm-up routine, resistance and aerobic exercise training, and a cool-down phase. The training consisted of three sessions per week. Each session lasted about 90 min and the entire training lasted 8 weeks.

Table 1. Characteristic of the (**A**) included studies and (**B**) included study protocols [21,23,25–29,31–38].

(A)

Author and Year	Sample Size	Age	Cancer Stage	Treatment	Type of Telemedicine Applied	Control	Duration	Outcome Variables	Results
Admiraal et al., 2017 [27]	139	C: 53.2 ± 8.5; T: 53.1 ± 9.8	I–III	Completed curative-intent primary treatment (surgery + chemotherapy) within the past six months	ENCOURAGE program: Psycho-education, problem-solving strategies for coping	Standard care	12 weeks	EORTC, QoL_Questionnaire, optimism and control over the future scale, Dutch Distress Thermometer, 47-item problem list	Increased optimism and control over the future
Bandani-Susan et al., 2021 [31]	38	46.34 ± 9.96 (C: 45.89 ± 7.64; T: 46.79 ± 12.28)	NA	Ongoing chemotherapy, radiotherapy, hormone therapy and/or brachytherapy	Educational messages, cognitive behavioral therapy for improving body image, and cognitive restructuring	Waitlist	49 days	CFS; Body Image Concern Inventory	Significant difference in quality of life (body image and cancer-related fatigue)
Damholdt et al., 2016 [21]	157	C: 54.56 ± 8.74; T: 54.98 ± 8.51	0–III	Ongoing chemotherapy, radiotherapy, or hormonal therapy	HappyNeuron Pro: Web-based program for cognitive training focused on six cognitive domains (attention, processing speed, learning, memory, working memory, problem-solving)	Waitlist	6 weeks	PASAT, RAVLT, Digit Span Forwards, Digit Span Backwards, Digit Ordering, Letter Fluency Test, 20 Questions Test, Cognitive Estimation Task, BDI, Whitely-7, SCL-ANX4 from Symptoms Checklist-92, self-reported benefit from the training	Improvements in verbal learning and working memory
Freeman et al., 2014 [23]	102	C: 55.28 ± 7.90; LD: 55.44 ± 8.08; T: 55.57 ± 9.88	0–IV	Completed main treatment from at least 6 weeks	Videoconference groups, education on the mind-body connection and on mental imagery	Live delivered (LD) psycho-educational groups; waitlist	5 weeks	Medical Outcomes Study survey (SF-36); FACT-B; FACIT-Fatigue Scale; FACT-Cog; Functional Assessment of Chronic Illness Therapy; Brief Symptom Inventory-GSI; Pittsburgh Sleep Quality Index	Improvement in fatigue, cognitive dysfunction, sleep disturbance, and health-related and breast cancer-related QoL for LD and TD groups compared to waitlist

Table 1. Cont.

(A)

Author and Year	Sample Size	Age	Cancer Stage	Treatment	Type of Telemedicine Applied	Control	Duration	Outcome Variables	Results
Galiano-Castillo et al., 2016 [29]	81	C: 49.2 ± 7.9; T: 47.4 ± 9.6	I-III	Completed adjuvant therapy except hormone treatment	e-CUIDATE: Online system for the remote administration of physical exercises focused on resistance, aerobic, mobility, and stretching	Written recommendation on stress management, physical fitness	8 weeks	EORTC QLQ-C30; Brief Pain Inventory short form; Piper Fatigue Scale-revised	Improvements in global health status, pain severity, interference, and total fatigue
Galiano-Castillo et al., 2017 [28]	81	48.30 ± 8.80	I-III	Completed adjuvant therapy except hormone treatment	e-CUIDATE: Online system for the remote administration of physical	Written recommendation on stress management, physical fitness	8 weeks	6 Min Walk Test; Auditory Consonant Trigrams; TMT	Improvements in functional capacity and cognitive functioning maintained at 6 months
Krzyzanowska et al., 2021 [25]	561	55.7 *	I-IV	Starting adjuvant or neoadjuvant chemotherapy	Symptom Self-Management Booklet-patient edition + follow-up calls to address the presence of chemotherapy side effects	Standard care	Duration of chemotherapy cycle	NCI PRO-CTCAE; Stanford self-management self-efficacy scale; European quality-of-life; Patient Health Questionnaire 9; VAS; Generalized anxiety disorder; FACT-B	No differences in self-efficacy, anxiety, or depression
Lozano-Lozano et al., 2020 [34]	80	C: 49.76 ± 8.42; T: 53.40 ± 8.66	I-III	Completed adjuvant therapy except hormonal therapy	BENECA mHEALTH + rehabilitation: Supervised used of the BENECA app occupational therapy focused on reduction of fatigue and improvement of processing speed, working memory, and attention	BENECA mHEALTH: App for recommendation on physical activity and nutrition	8 weeks	EORTC- QoL Questionnaire; Breast Cancer-Specific Quality of Life Questionnaire;	Improvement in QoL, maintained after 6 months

Table 1. Cont.

(A)

Author and Year	Sample Size	Age	Cancer Stage	Treatment	Type of Telemedicine Applied	Control	Duration	Outcome Variables	Results
Lozano-Lozano et al., 2022 [26]	80	C: 49.76 ± 8.42; T: 53.40 ± 8.66	I-III	Completed chemotherapy, could continue therapy with hormone	BENECA mHEALTH + rehabilitation: Supervised used of the BENECA app for recommendation on physical activity and nutrition; occupational therapy focused on reduction of fatigue and improvement of processing speed, working memory and attention	BENECA mHEALTH: App for recommendation on physical activity and nutrition	8 weeks	TMT; WAIS; Hospital Anxiety and Depression Scale; Brief pain inventory; Piper Fatigue Scale-revised; 6 Min Walk Test	Greater improvements in selective attention, working memory, and processing speed, anxiety, and functional capacity at 8 weeks and 6 months. Fatigue perception and pain were also improved
Oswald et al., 2022 [33]	30	58.44 ± 9.22 (C: 56.90 ± 8.91; T: 59.98 ± 9.58)	NA	Completed primary cancer treatment	CBT-I: Group sessions of cognitive behavioral therapy focused on sleep education, sleep restriction, stimulus control, sleep hygiene, and sleep medications, cognitive restructuring, and relapse prevention	Waitlist	6 weeks	Treatment Perceptions Questionnaire; 7-item Insomnia Severity Index; Pittsburgh Sleep Quality Index	Improvements in insomnia symptoms, sleep disturbance, and sleep efficiency compared to the control group

Table 1. Cont.

(A)

Author and Year	Sample Size	Age	Cancer Stage	Treatment	Type of Telemedicine Applied	Control	Duration	Outcome Variables	Results
van den Berg et al., 2015 [32]	150	C: 50.18 ± 9.15; T: 51.44 ± 8.30	NA	Completed primary cancer treatment (surgery plus adjuvant chemotherapy and/or radiotherapy)	BREATH: Cognitive behavioral therapy online self-help program for the four phases of adjustment to breast cancer (looking back, emotional processing, strengthening, and looking ahead)	Standard care	16 weeks	Symptom Checklist-90; Cancer Empowerment Questionnaire; Hospital Anxiety and Depression Scale; EORTC Quality of Life Questionnaire Core 30; Distress Thermometer; Illness Cognitions Questionnaire; Remoralization Scale; Mastery Scale; Positive Adjustment Questionnaire; Self-Efficacy Scale; Cancer Worry Scale; Cancer Acceptance Scale; Checklist Individual Strength-Fatigue; Openness to discuss hereditary cancer in the family; Big Five Inventory	Reduced distress. Not persistent at follow-up
	255	53.1 ± 8.8 (C: 52.9 ± 8.9; T: 53.2 ± 8.8)	I-II	Ongoing chemotherapy, radiotherapy, or endocrine therapy	SHUTi: Automated interactive cognitive behavioral therapy for insomnia focused on sleep restriction and stimulus control, cognitive restructuring, sleep hygiene, and relapse prevention	Waitlist	6 weeks	Sleep diary; Insomnia Severity Index; Pittsburgh Sleep Quality Index; Functional Assessment of Chronic Illness Therapy for Fatigue	iCBT-I groups showed improvements in sleep-related outcomes which were maintained at 15 weeks follow-up

Table 1. *Cont.*

(B)

Author and Year	Sample Size	Age	Cancer Stage	Treatment	Type of Telemedicine Applied	Control	Duration	Outcome Variables
Carlson et al., 2019 [35]	178	>18	I–III	Scheduled for chemotherapy	Mindfulness-based cancer recovery, online group	Standard care, waitlist	12 weeks	Brief Screen for Cognitive Impairment; Functional Assessment of Chronic Illness Therapy—Fatigue; Pittsburgh Sleep Quality Index; Brief Pain Inventory; Osoba Nausea and Vomiting Module; FACT—General; Calgary Symptoms of Stress Inventory; Profile of Mood States—Short Form; FACT—Cog; Sustained Attention to Response Task; blood counts
González-Santos et al., 2022 [36]	98	>18	I–III	Scheduled for chemotherapy	e-OTCAT program: Cognitive training using paper-pencil exercises and the NeuroNation mobile app	Standard care, provision of educational handbook on cancer treatment side effects	12 weeks	FACT-Cog; TMT; WAIS; Hospital Anxiety and Depression Scale; Piper Fatigue Scale-Revised; Pittsburgh Sleep Quality Index; EORTC-Quality of Life Questionnaire Core; Canadian Occupational Performance Measure
Krusche et al., 2019 [38]	2500	>18	NA	Finished primary cancer treatment within prior ten years	Renewed: Software addressing four main areas (physical activity, stress reduction, diet improvement, weight loss)	Standard care, provision of educational resources	NA	QoL; fear of relapses; anxiety and depression; website satisfaction and usage
Lidington et al., 2020 [37]	122	>18	Early stage	Non-specified anticancer treatment	OWise: Online tool offering tailored medical information, medical terms glossary, useful links to local resources, tracking tool for symptoms, and a consultation recording device	Standard care, provision of educational resources	NA	Hospital Anxiety and Depression Scale; EORTC QLQ C-30; EuroQol 5-Dimension 5-Level questionnaire (EQ-5D-5L)

Notes for (A): Quality of Life (QoL); Cancer Fatigue Scale (CSF); Beck Depression Inventory (BDI); Global Severity Index (GSI); Rey Auditory Verbal Learning Test (RAVLT); National Cancer Institute Patient Reported Outcomes version of the Common Terminology Criteria for Adverse Events (NCI PRO-CTCAE); Trail making test (TMT); Visual Analogue Scale (VAS); Functional Assessment of Cancer Therapy for Patients with Breast Cancer (FACT-B); European Organization for Research and Treatment of Cancer (EORTC); Wechsler Adult Intelligence Scale (WAIS); * Median. Notes for (B): Functional Assessment of Cancer Therapy for Patients with Breast Cancer (FACT-cog).

Four studies applied CBT to improve sleep disturbances [37,40] and psychological well-being [38,39]. Oswald performed CBT through weekly 90-min educational group sessions for 6 weeks over a videoconference. The group received information about sleep education, hygiene, and medications as well as on cognitive restructuring [40]. Zachariae used the CBT program for an individual delivery of six psycho-educational themes: introduction and treatment rationale, sleep restriction, stimulus control, cognitive reconstruction, sleep hygiene, and relapse prevention [37]. Each theme was studied by participants in a 45–60 min session. Van den Berg used a system named BREATH to improve psychological well-being. The therapy included information, assignments (48 tasks), assessment of the difficulties, and educational video. BREATH is a pure self-help program without therapist contact [39]. The training lasted 16 weeks. Bandani-Susan performed a group online intervention with the aim of helping patients to manage cancer-related fatigue and body image and to encourage positive feelings [38]. The program consisted of 7 weeks of educational approaches, supervised physical activity, religious messages, cognitive therapy to improve body image and cognitive restructuring, and meditation.

Three studies provided psychoeducational material via telemedicine [29,31,34]. Specifically, in the Krzyzanowska study, patients were given a booklet for the management of common side effects of chemotherapy (e.g., nausea, vomiting, pain, fatigue) and received two structured follow-up calls during the cycle of chemotherapy to assess the frequency and severity of such symptoms [31]. In the study by Freeman and colleagues, the patients received four group sessions comprising didactic education on mind–body connection, mental imagery, and physiological processes followed by a discussion of the presented material [29]. Admiraal and colleagues asked participants to perform the ENCOURAGE program for 12 weeks, receiving psychoeducational material, coping strategies, and hyperlinks to address emotional and physical problems related to cancer [34].

One study applied a cognitive training program (i.e., HappyNeuron Pro) to improve cognitive functioning [27]. The program consisted of several tasks centered on attention, processing speed, learning, memory, working memory, and problem solving. Tasks were structured as a computerized game with different levels of difficulty. Each participant trained 30 min/day, 5 days/week, for 6 weeks. The program was performed online and accompanied by telephone and email-based support.

Lozano-Lozano combined in-person occupational sessions with the BENECA app, which provided nutritional recommendations to improve mood, cognitive functions, and physical functions in breast cancer survivors [32]. The BENECA app is a validated mobile health application that monitors the energy balance of individuals in terms of physical activity and diet and provides recommendations for improvement. The original BENECA program was extended by including exercises based on occupational therapy and on cognitive training. In another study by the same author, the same program was used to improve the quality of life.

With respect to the inclusion of a control group, four studies compared the telerehabilitation program with a waitlist group [27,37,38,40]. Three studies used patients undergoing standard care as a control group [31,34,39]. Three studies provided written recommendations to the control group on health and nutrition [39] and stress management [35,36]. One study also compared the efficacy of telerehabilitation with the delivery of the same program in person [29]. Finally, two studies used telerehabilitation as the control for an integrated approach combining telemedicine and face-to-face rehabilitation [32,33].

Concerning the study protocols, two studies will provide psychological and medical education on cancer [43,44]. One study protocol will use a mindfulness-based program to address psychological recovery in cancer patients [41]. Finally, Gonzales-Santos [42] will use a cognitive training program (E-OTCAT) focusing on attention, memory, and processing speed.

3.2. Effects on Cognition

Seven of the included studies investigated the effect of telerehabilitation programs on cognition after cancer treatment [27,29,33,35,36,41,42]. Five studies were original articles [27,29,33,35,36], and two were study protocols describing ongoing RCT [41,42].

Among the original articles, two studies exclusively considered objective neuropsychological assessment [33,35], two focused on subjective cognitive functioning [29,36], and the remaining one investigated both self-reported and objectively assessed cognitive functioning [27]. The two protocol papers will investigate self-reported and objectively assessed cognitive functioning [41,42]. All of the included studies focused on the cognitive domains most frequently reported to be impaired after cancer treatments such as executive functioning, working memory, attention, and information processing. One research study also examined verbal memory and learning as secondary outcomes [27].

Freeman and colleagues investigated the impact of an imagery-based group intervention delivered through telemedicine on self-reported cognitive functioning, which was assessed with the cognitive subscale of the Functional Assessment of Cancer Therapy (FACT-Cog version 2) at baseline, 1-, and 3-months follow-up. Results revealed an improvement in subjective cognitive functioning after both telerehabilitation and live-delivered interventions compared to the waiting list control group. The improvement detected in cognition was considered clinically significant and was maintained at the 3-month follow-up [29].

Similarly, Galiano-Castillo and colleagues investigated the effect of an 8-week Internet-based, tailored physical exercise program (E-CUIDATE) on the quality of life, pain, muscle strength, and fatigue in patients who had completed adjuvant therapy compared to a control group receiving basic recommendations on physical exercise [28]. The European Organization for Research and Treatment of Cancer Quality-of-Life Questionnaire Core 30 was administered, which assesses various aspects of the quality of life and includes two items about self-reported cognitive functioning. The authors found an improvement in self-reported cognitive functioning for the telerehabilitation group compared to the control group, which was maintained at a 6-month follow-up.

In a secondary analysis of data from this previous study, Galiano-Castillo found mixed results. The authors examined the efficacy of the E-CUIDATE in improving the functional and cognitive abilities in breast cancer survivors. In this case, cognitive functioning was assessed by the objective measures of short-term memory, attention, information processing, and mental flexibility. A lasting improvement was found for the group receiving telerehabilitation only in information processing and not in other cognitive domains [35].

In a recent study, Lozano-Lozano and colleagues examined the efficacy of the BENECA app combined with in-person occupational sessions on cognition, mood, and physical function. The authors found that selective attention (assessed with the Trail Making Test [45]) was significantly higher after the combined intervention compared to the control group that received the BENECA app alone, with a moderate-to-large effect size for TMT-A, working memory, and processing speed (assessed through the WAIS-IV), at 2 and 6 months after the intervention [33].

Damholdt found the opposite result. Indeed, the author reported no changes in working memory and attention in a group of breast cancer patients receiving a web-based telerehabilitation program with telephone support compared to a waiting list control group. The primary outcome of cognitive functioning was assessed with the Paced Auditory Sequence Test (PASAT [46]), a working memory and attentional span test. Of note, in this study, the authors compared the differences between self-reported and objectively measured cognitive functions. Other neuropsychological measures were verbal learning, working memory, and executive functioning indices. No statistical changes were found in the former nor in the latter. However, a small improvement was found in verbal learning and in the working memory tests post-intervention and at the 5-month follow-up [27].

Effects on Cognition: Study Protocols

Two of the included studies were RCT study protocols [41,42] aiming at investigating the efficacy of two different telemedicine approaches in preventing and mitigating the cognitive and psychological (i.e., anxiety and depression) and other common consequences of breast cancer and chemotherapy such as fatigue, pain, sleep disturbances, nausea/vomiting, and quality of life. Regarding cognition, both studies will investigate self-reported and objective cognitive functioning (see Table 1).

The more recent study designed an RCT protocol aiming to investigate the efficacy of videoconference-based cognitive adaptive training (eOCTAT) in preventing cancer-related cognitive impairment in patients with breast cancer undergoing chemotherapy [42]. Participants will be randomized to either the experimental group that will receive the e-OTCAT program for 12 consecutive weeks from the beginning of chemotherapy or the control group, which will receive an educational handbook and the usual care. Assessment will focus on cognitive functioning and psychological distress, fatigue, sleep disturbance, quality of life, and occupational performance will be investigated. Subjective cognitive complaints will be measured with the Cog-FACT [47]. Assessments will be conducted before chemotherapy (baseline) and at 6 and 12 months after the baseline.

Similarly, Carlson and colleagues designed an RCT aiming to determine the efficacy of an online mindfulness group for breast cancer patients during chemotherapy in 12 real-time interactive weekly sessions [41]. In this case, the online intervention will be aimed at primarily managing fatigue and other common post-chemotherapy symptoms (i.e., sleep disturbance, pain, nausea/vomiting, mood, stress, quality of life), whereas cognition will be explored as a secondary outcome. Patients will be randomized to the experimental group or a waiting list control group, with assessments at four time points: baseline (pre-chemotherapy), post-rehabilitation, post-chemotherapy, and 12 months post-baseline. Self-reported cognitive functioning will be assessed with the Cog-FACT [47], while objective cognitive functioning will be assessed through the Sustained Attention to Response Task, a computer-based go/no-go task designed to measure working memory, sustained attention, and impulse/inhibitory control. If effective, both of these ongoing RCTs will provide support and more evidence about the implementation of telemedicine approaches in oncological care.

3.3. Psychological Effects
3.3.1. Quality of Life

Three of the included studies investigated the clinical implications and benefits of telemedicine for the general QoL of breast cancer patients (see Table 1).

Among these, Admiraal and colleagues reported no differences between psycho-educational approaches and standard care in problem-solving strategies and other psychological outcomes measured at the baseline, 6, and 12 weeks (see Table 1) [34]. An unplanned subgroup analysis showed that in clinically distressed patients (n = 57), participation in the web-based program resulted in more optimism and control over the future at 12 weeks than the control group patients, suggesting that the lack of effects between groups might be due to some patients being unable to further increase their optimism.

Lozano-Lozano and colleagues [32] compared the effect of the mobile BENECA app combined with a supervised rehabilitation program versus the BENECA app alone. In this study, patients were assessed with questionnaires at the baseline, 2-months post-intervention, and 6-month follow-up. Both rehabilitation programs improved the QoL, with global QoL significantly better with the BENECA app plus rehabilitation than with the BENECA program alone, with a moderate-to-large effect size. The clinically significant effect on QoL was maintained during the follow-up.

Galiano-Castillo and colleagues compared a telerehabilitation group (8-week Internet-based intervention) with a control group at the baseline, after 8 weeks and at a 6-month follow-up. Results showed that the telerehabilitation group improved regarding the QoL, which was maintained during the follow-up check [36].

As shown by Freeman and colleagues, an aspect that seems crucial in the effectiveness of treatment is the web-mediated interaction with a therapist who actively interacts with the patient [29]. The aim of this study was to compare the effects of an imagery-based behavioral intervention delivered live or via telemedicine compared to a waitlist control on the QoL of breast cancer survivors. Their system consisted of videoconferencing software that enabled the therapist to view and interact with the patient. Their results revealed the beneficial effects of the intervention for improving QoL in cancer survivors. Remarkably, it seems that involvement in the telemedicine-delivered intervention did not result in different outcomes compared to the intervention delivered with a therapist physically present.

3.3.2. Sleep

Several authors developed web-based interventions for sleep disturbances on the basis of CBT with the aim of enabling patients to cope with problems related to the diagnosis or the administration of cancer treatments. Following the application of web-based CBT programs to treat sleep disturbance, Zachariae and colleagues [37], and later Oswald and colleagues, proposed two RCTs to assess the efficiency of this type of rehabilitation in breast cancer survivors [40] (see Table 1).

In the former, women with breast cancer who experienced clinically significant sleep disturbance were randomly allocated to a CBT program or to a waitlist control group. Insomnia severity, sleep quality, and fatigue measures were collected at the baseline, post-intervention (9 weeks), and follow-up (15 weeks). Breast cancer survivors following the CBT program showed reduced insomnia severity and improved the overall sleep quality. Indeed, significant effects were found for all sleep-related outcomes from pre- to post-intervention. Furthermore, improvements were maintained for outcomes measured at follow-up. Similarly, in the study of Oswald and colleagues, the breast cancer survivors were randomized to a CBT group to treat insomnia or to a waitlist control for 6 weeks. Results showed that post-intervention, there were medium-to-large group differences for secondary outcomes of interest such as insomnia symptoms, sleep disturbance, and sleep efficiency, with CBT showing a preliminary efficiency compared to the control group. In addition, group differences after intervention indicated that participants who reported clinically significant symptomatology all favored the eHealth CBT condition, with small/medium to medium/large effect sizes. Limitations of this study included the use of a waitlist control group instead of a robust attention-control comparison.

3.3.3. Fatigue

Besides investigating insomnia and general sleep quality, Zachariae and colleagues also assessed the levels of fatigue of groups of women with breast cancer experiencing clinically significant sleep disturbance, finding benefits in terms of reduced fatigue in those who followed CBT, compared to the waitlist [37].

In a recent study conducted by Bandani-Susan and colleagues, the efficacy of a mobile health educational intervention in improving cancer fatigue and body image was investigated [38]. Results showed that the mobile intervention improved the levels of fatigue and body image among breast cancer survivors. Limitations concerning the small sample size were highlighted (see Table 1).

Furthermore, Galiano-Castillo and colleagues demonstrated that the telerehabilitation intervention improved aspects of the QoL compared to the control group, and that it improved the general levels of fatigue perception. Of note, these improvements were maintained at the follow-up [36].

3.3.4. Anxiety, Depression, and Distress

A few studies have investigated the effects of using mobile interventions on improving mood, depression or anxiety feelings, and distress in patients with breast cancer.

Similar to previous interventions, van den Berg and colleagues developed a web-based self-management intervention based on the principles of CBT to reduce distress and improve empowerment [39]. Patients could choose to access a wide range of materials (assignments, self-assessments, and videos) that were released on a website. Since the intervention was a self-management program, it did not require real interaction or contact with a therapist. The findings indicated that the intervention contributed to reducing the level of distress in patients without affecting empowerment.

Finally, studies investigating the effects on anxiety and depression did not report any significant improvement after treatment delivered through telemedicine [31].

3.3.5. Pain

We only found one study investigating the effect of telerehabilitation on pain perception. In this study, it was shown that the telerehabilitation group improved regarding aspects of pain severity and pain interference; the results for the pain interference effects, but not pain severity, were maintained during the follow-up [36].

3.3.6. Psychological Effects: Study Protocols

Four of the included studies were RCT study protocols, therefore the results are not available yet.

In two of these studies, the interventions were developed to promote, through interactive programs of telerehabilitation, a healthy lifestyle, together with other typical outcomes such as QoL, fatigue, anxiety, and depression [42,44].

Carlson and colleagues plan to apply a mindfulness-based intervention. This program will be administered during chemotherapy in 12 real-time interactive weekly sessions with the principal aim of managing fatigue, and in addition to this primary outcome, insomnia, pain, nausea/vomiting, mood, distress, and QoL. Crucial in this intervention are the recommendations for patients to practice mindfulness exercises for 30–45 min per session [41].

Lidington and colleagues will explore the effectiveness of a mobile application for self-monitoring symptoms and managing care in patients with breast cancer (see Table 1) The authors will investigate whether using the application may affect QoL, health status, and distress [43].

González-Santos and colleagues are conducting an RCT aimed at investigating the effects of a videoconference cognitive-adaptive training (e-OTCAT) for 12 weeks from the beginning of chemotherapy. Outcomes will be the cognitive function, psychological distress, fatigue, sleep disturbance, QoL, and occupational performance, measured at the baseline, after 12 weeks, and 6 months of post-randomization. The authors are interested in understanding whether the telemedicine approach can prevent cognitive impairments and other effects of cancer and its treatment [42].

4. Discussion

The aim of the present paper was to systematically review the literature on the current telemedicine interventions applied to improve psychological and/or cognitive functions in breast cancer patients both during and after pharmacological therapies. Only RCT studies were considered to define the state-of-the-art, and the study protocols were included to shed light on possible future paths and fields of investigation in both clinical and scientific practices. In particular, we were interested in understanding whether telemedicine can represent a valuable option for the rehabilitation of breast cancer patients as it allows for the combination of both psychological support and cognitive rehabilitation, which are two crucial needs of breast cancer patients and survivors.

Contrary to our expectations, only a few studies have investigated both the cognitive and psychological effects of telerehabilitation. Among these, only one used a telerehabilitation program with the specific aim of improving both psychological and cognitive functions [32]. The other studies were aimed at improving either the cognitive or the psychological effects. Overall, these three studies highlight that combining telerehabilitation with the presence of a therapist led to the best results, whereas not explicitly providing participants with the opportunity to contact the therapist in case of need led to the worst results, namely, inconsistent improvement in working memory tests with no changes in all the other trained domains [27]. However, in this latter study, an important issue that may have limited the significance of the results was that the neuropsychological assessment was conducted via telephone.

Of note, in all of the included studies but one [27], cognitive performance was measured as a primary or secondary outcome after treatments that were only partially focused on cognitive tasks and mostly based on occupational therapy, psycho-educational approaches, physical activity, and body exercises.

Overall, some considerations arose from these studies. First, in each study, cognitive domains were assessed with many different neuropsychological tests, which may have distinct levels of sensitivity to cognitive impairments, thus leading to heterogeneous and variable findings. Similarly, the methodology used for the neuropsychological assessment varied among studies, with some studies reporting a face-to-face assessment and other studies reporting telephonically conducted neuropsychological interviews. To complicate the matter further, information was generally lacking about whether rehabilitation programs were individualized based on the patients' specific deficits. This aspect is crucial for cognitive rehabilitation to have meaningful clinical results and should be addressed when considering experimental findings. Another concern was that cognitive deficits were reported as either objectively measured or self-assessed by the patients. There can be a great discrepancy between deficits measured by a professional and deficits reported by the patient, with the latter being even more susceptible to intervening psychological factors. More studies should compare the effects of telerehabilitation in terms of the perceived and objectively measured cognitive impairment to clarify this issue. Furthermore, there was wide variability with respect to the employed telerehabilitation programs, with the one used by Lozano and colleagues being the most effective, which induced a stable improvement in all the studied domains [32]. On the other hand, in this study, we could not exclude that the strong presence of face-to-face support for the patients during the training might have played a role in modulating the observed results.

Finally, an important consideration is that to date, only a few studies using telemedicine have focused the intervention on both cognitive and psychological factors, thus suggesting that the interaction between these aspects has not been fully addressed. Indeed, in many of the included studies, the observed results on the psychological and cognitive factors were maintained separately. In contrast, even with a lack of effect, the role of one or the other should be considered and discussed as these two aspects often influence each other [48,49].

In the present study, we found that the domain that benefitted the most from telemedicine is probably the QoL. Indeed, an improvement in QoL was reported in almost all of the reviewed studies. Of note, the improvement substantially remained at follow-up, that is, it remained, despite cancer progression and treatment side effects. For instance, a long-lasting (i.e., 6 months) improvement in QoL was observed with long (i.e., 8 weeks) treatment durations [32,35]. Unfortunately, other psychological aspects were not investigated in these two studies.

Overall, the research findings prove that telemedicine practices have an impact on the QoL of breast cancer patients. Among the psycho-education approaches, BENECA [32] and imagery-based behavioral interventions [29] were the most effective. The lack of effect reported by only one of the studies reviewed here [34] might have depended on the general ineffectiveness of problem-solving oriented programs, even when targeted at the patients' needs. However, other factors may have played a role such as the cancer stages and the different symptoms experienced by patients due to different pharmacological treatments.

Sleep problems are often a major complaint of breast cancer patients, and they are usually treated on the basis of CBT. We found only two studies that applied web-based CBT, reporting that it may be an efficacious treatment option for breast cancer survivors with robust and clinically relevant effects. Similarly, telemedicine has been proven to be effective in reducing fatigue when related to sleep difficulties [37,40]. However, more studies are needed to replicate these promising and encouraging results.

Conversely, less encouraging were the results with respect to anxiety and depression. Indeed, where a general reduction in distress levels was reported by previous studies [39], no effects were reported on the anxiety and depression levels [31]. These findings are in contrast to a previous review reporting that technology-based interventions were effective for depressive symptoms and anxiety experienced by women with breast cancer [26]. The discrepancy between this previous study and our findings is probably due to the fact that in the former, RCTs were included as well as studies focusing on specific ethnic populations. On the other hand, our results were limited by the low number of included studies. Therefore, more controlled studies are needed to clarify this issue.

Pain is another common side effect of both surgery and hormonal therapies in breast cancer patients. In particular, after breast cancer surgery, the pain levels experienced by patients are high, so they often use opioids for pain reduction. Similarly, patients receiving aromatase inhibitors generally report arthralgia and myalgia [36]. The studies included in the present review suggested that telemedicine-based interventions, by teaching patients strategies to manage pain, could be useful to reduce pain perception and opioid use. Therefore, these interventions should be integrated in standard programs to enhance recovery and complement medical treatments. However, these results were limited, being based on only two studies. More studies are needed to investigate the effect of telemedicine on pain, taking into account other factors that are reported to influence pain perception such as menopause [36].

However, another consideration concerns the lack of a gold standard with respect to the use of telemedicine in breast cancer patients. Indeed, clarification is needed as to which program would be most effective based on the patients' specific needs.

These programs should be targeted specifically at psychological and/or cognitive functioning and should follow a precise cognitive and psychological assessment. Overall, based on the current literature, reliable cognitive telerehabilitation should include cognitive tasks as well as psycho-educational intervention to train cognitive functioning and provide patients with information related to the treatment side effects. This training should not last less than 3 weeks, and ideally, it should be performed until the end of the breast cancer therapy and include a follow-up evaluation. Similarly, the current literature suggests that to maximize the benefits of psychological interventions, programs should be based on CBT and include both individual and group sessions in which patients ideally are provided with information about their status as well as cognitive restructuring. In this case, the remote on-demand presence of a therapist will be pivotal. Regarding cognitive training, psychological support should be provided from the diagnosis to the end of chemotherapy.

There are many other difficulties that patients experience after a breast cancer diagnosis such as sexual problems [50], which can benefit from a telemedicine approach. Studies are needed investigating this field.

5. Considerations on Mediating Factors and Unmet Needs

Understanding the factors that may contribute to the development of cognitive and psychological problems in patients treated for breast cancer was behind the purpose of the present review. However, factors involved in the emergence of such deficits may also contribute to their maintenance and can affect the success rate of both psychological and cognitive telemedicine-based interventions. These factors may be related to (1) cancer subtypes (luminal, HER2+, triple negative) and treatments (chemotherapy, hormonal therapies, biological therapies); (2) patient lifestyles; (3) biological factors (i.e., inflammation, oxidative stress, DNA damage and repair, genetic susceptibility, decreased telomere length and cell senescence [51]); (4) psychological factors and distress levels; (5) genetic variations; and (6) demographic factors. First, stronger cognitive dysfunctions have been reported for breast cancer patients exposed to both chemotherapy and hormone therapy than for patients exposed to chemotherapy only [52]. This observation holds true, especially for postmenopausal women [53]. The pivotal role played by estrogens in cognitive performance and psychological aspects might explain the potential negative effect of hormone therapies on both the cognition and psychological well-being of breast cancer patients. Similarly, the estrogen depletion induced by hormonal therapies might account for the possible reduced effects of concurrent cognitive rehabilitation and psychological treatments.

Several biological factors may play a role in both the occurrence of cognitive symptoms and in the effect of cognitive rehabilitation. Systemic inflammation can cross the blood–brain barrier and have a deleterious effect on the central nervous system [54], thus inducing cognitive impairment [55]. Anticancer treatment-induced cytokine storms may hamper or annul the beneficial effects of treatment.

Furthermore, elevated levels of C-reactive protein reflecting chronic inflammation may also play a role in cognitive problems [56], and the levels of this protein, together with other biological factors, may impact the efficacy of telerehabilitation and psychological telemedicine.

Genetic factors have been suggested to play a role in cognitive dysfunctions. For instance, variants of genes encoding apolipoprotein E (ApoE) and catechol-O-methyltransferase (COMT) have both been associated with age-related cognitive decline in the general population [57].

Finally, demographic factors may contribute to cognitive impairment and psychological symptoms. In particular, age (with older patients who are likely more vulnerable to pre- and post-treatment cancer-related side effects), race, and education have been shown to be associated with the presence of impairment in breast cancer patients [58]. Similarly, these factors may affect the success of the rehabilitation.

Psychological and emotional stress can alter the sympathetic nervous system and, in turn, the immune system [59]. In other words, psychological distress consequent to cancer treatment and side effects may trigger biologic alterations in the brain. These modifications may create long-term homeostatic changes that are responsible for the neuroplastic alterations leading to cognitive dysfunctions. Neuroplasticity is a crucial process underlying the effects of cognitive rehabilitation [60]. Altered or absent neuroplastic processes prevent training-related cognitive changes and may be responsible for the lack of improvement observed after cognitive rehabilitation in some of the studies reviewed here. Similarly, after breast cancer diagnosis, patients may experience post-traumatic growth [61], an experience that should be monitored during psychological treatment because of the confounding impact it can have on the effects of psychological telemedicine interventions. Finally, we must acknowledge that nowadays, breast cancer diagnosis includes several pathological conditions with very different natural histories, treatments, and prognoses. Each of these factors may affect the patients' psychological conditions, needs, and responses to interventions, and should therefore be addressed in future studies.

6. Conclusions and Future Perspectives

In general, the current literature highlights the need for more controlled studies that are designed based on the general guidelines on breast cancer [62]. These guidelines should be updated in order to consider both the cognitive and psychological difficulties exhibited by breast cancer patients. With respect to cognitive evaluation and rehabilitation, a standard neuropsychological assessment including ad hoc testing as well as a standard procedure for test administration is currently lacking. Additionally, a distinction should be made between the self-assessment and objectively measured deficits as these are both important but not directly comparable. Similarly, with respect to psychological concerns, novel telemedicine-based approaches are needed that focus on specific interventions related to the wide range of difficulties experienced by breast cancer patients, namely, depression and anxiety, and the patients' demographics should be the focus of new RCT studies. Along these lines, further studies should target both cognitive and psychological factors with specific telemedicine-based protocols that also consider the molecular classification and new standard of therapy. Moreover, it must be highlighted that while most studies have shown that psycho-educational approaches improve cognitive functions, future studies should apply dedicated cognitive telerehabilitation programs.

In conclusion, evidence is promising with respect to the use of telemedicine in breast cancer patients; however, current evidence also poses the need for more controlled studies to clarify the effectiveness of telemedicine, especially for cognitive deficits, but also for psychological problems (e.g., anxiety and depression).

Author Contributions: Conceptualization, A.G., R.P., F.M., G.A., F.B. and P.C.; Methodology, A.G., R.P., F.M., G.A., F.B. and P.C. Data curation, A.G., L.D., G.O., F.M. and R.P., Writing—original draft preparation, A.G., L.D., R.P., F.M. and G.O.; Writing—review and editing, A.G., G.A., F.B. and P.C.; Supervision, P.C. All authors have read and agreed to the published version of the manuscript.

Funding: This research was funded by the Italian Ministry of Health, Ricerca corrente 2022.

Conflicts of Interest: The authors declare no conflict of interest.

References

1. Azamjah, N.; Soltan, Y.-Z.; Zayeri, F. Global Trend of Breast Cancer Mortality Rate: A 25-Year Study. *Asian Pac. J. Cancer Prev.* **2019**, *20*, 2015–2020. [CrossRef] [PubMed]
2. Miller, K.D.; Nogueira, L.; Mariotto, A.B.; Rowland, J.H.; Yabroff, K.R.; Alfano, C.M.; Jemal, A.; Kramer, J.L.; Siegel, R.L. Cancer treatment and survivorship statistics, 2019, CA. Cancer treatment and survivorship statistics, 2019. *CA Cancer J. Clin.* **2019**, *69*, 363–385. [CrossRef] [PubMed]
3. Oh, P.J.; Cho, J.R. Changes in Fatigue, Psychological Distress, and Quality of Life after Chemotherapy in Women with Breast Cancer: A Prospective Study. *Cancer Nurs.* **2018**, *43*, E54–E60. [CrossRef] [PubMed]
4. Wefel, J.S.; Vardy, J.; Ahles, T.; Schagen, S.B. International Cognition and Cancer Task Force recommendations to harmonise studies of cognitive function in patients with cancercancer. *Lancet Oncol.* **2011**, *12*, 703–708. [CrossRef]
5. Zwart, W.; Terra, H.; Linn, S.C.; Schagen, S.B. Cognitive effects of endocrine therapy for breast cancer: Keep calm and carry on? *Nat. Rev. Clin. Oncol.* **2015**, *12*, 597–606. [CrossRef]
6. Buchanan, N.D.; Dasari, S.; Rodriguez, J.L.; Smith, J.L.; Hodgson, M.E.; Weinberg, C.R.; Sandler, D.P. Post-treatment Neurocognition and Psychosocial Care among Breast Cancer Survivors. *Am. J. Prev. Med.* **2015**, *49*, S498–S508. [CrossRef]
7. Berndt, U.; Leplow, B.; Schoenfeld, R.; Lantzsch, T.; Grosse, R.; Thomssen, C. Memory and Spatial Cognition in Breast Cancer Patients Undergoing Adjuvant Endocrine Therapyy. *Breast Care* **2016**, *11*, 240–246. [CrossRef]
8. Collins, B.; Mackenzie, J.; Stewart, A.; Bielajew, C.; Verma, S. Cognitive effects of hormonal therapy in early stage breast cancer patients: A prospective study. *Psychooncology* **2008**, *18*, 811–821. [CrossRef]
9. Chen, X.; Li, J.; Zhang, J.; He, X.; Zhu, C.; Zhang, L.; Hu, X.; Wang, K. Impairment of the executive attention network in premenopausal women with hormone receptor-positive breast cancer treated with tamoxifen. *Psychoneuroendocrinology* **2017**, *75*, 116–123. [CrossRef]
10. Asegaonkar, S.B.; Asegaonkar, B.N.; Takalkar, U.V.; Advani, S.; Thorat, A.P. C-Reactive Protein and Breast Cancer: New Insights from Old Molecule. *Int. J. Breast Cancer* **2015**, *2015*, 145647. [CrossRef]
11. Cheung, Y.T.; Lim, S.R.; Ho, H.K.; Chan, A. Cytokines as mediators of chemotherapy-associated cognitive changes: Current evidence, limitations and directions for future research. *PLoS ONE* **2013**, *8*, e81234. [CrossRef]
12. Gaman, A.M.; Uzoni, A.; Popa, A.-W.; Andrei, A.; Petcu, E.B. The role of oxidative stress in etiopathogenesis of chemotherapy induced cognitive impairment (CICI)-"Chemobrain" *Aging Dis.* **2016**, *7*, 307–317. [CrossRef] [PubMed]
13. Pullens, J.J.M.; De Vries, J.; Roukema, J.A. Subjective cognitive dysfunction in breast cancer patients: A systematic reviewreview. *Psychooncology* **2010**, *19*, 1127–1138. [CrossRef] [PubMed]
14. Leedham, B.; Ganz, P.A. Psychosocial concerns and quality of life in breast cancer survivors. *Cancer Investig.* **1999**, *17*, 342–348. [CrossRef] [PubMed]
15. van Helmondt, S.J.; van der Lee, M.L.; van Woezik, R.A.M.; Lodder, P.; de Vries, J. No effect of CBT-based online self-help training to reduce fear of cancer recurrence: First results of the CAREST multicenter randomized controlled trial. *Psychooncology* **2019**, *29*, 86–97. [CrossRef] [PubMed]
16. Lueboonthavatchai, P. Prevalence and psychosocial factors of anxiety and depression in breast cancer patients. *J. Med Assoc. Thail.* **2007**, *90*, 2164–2174.
17. Tsaras, K.; Papathanasiou, I.V.; Mitsi, D.; Veneti, A.; Kelesi, M.; Zyga, S.; Fradelos, E.C. Assessment of depression and anxiety in breast cancer patients: Prevalence and associated Factors. *Asian Pac. J. Cancer Prev.* **2018**, *19*, 1661–1669. [CrossRef]
18. Izci, F.; Ilgun, A.S.; Findikli, E.; Ozmen, V. Psychiatric Symptoms and Psychosocial Problems in Patients with Breast Cancer. *J. Breast Health* **2016**, *12*, 94–101. [CrossRef]
19. Triberti, S.; Savioni, L.; Sebri, V.; Pravettoni, G. eHealth for improving quality of life in breast cancer patients: A systematic review. *Cancer Treat. Rev.* **2019**, *74*, 1–14. [CrossRef]

20. Perez-Tejada, J.; Labaka, A.; Pascual-Sagastizabal, E.; Garmendia, L.; Iruretagoyena, A.; Arregi, A. Predictors of psychological distress in breast cancer survivors: A biopsychosocial approach. *Eur. J. Cancer Care* **2019**, *28*, e13166. [CrossRef]
21. Whittaker, A.L.; George, R.P.; O'Malley, L. Prevalence of cognitive impairment following chemotherapy treatment for breast cancer: A systematic review and meta-analysis. *Sci. Rep.* **2022**, *12*, 1–22. [CrossRef]
22. Oksman, E.; Linna, M.; Hörhammer, I.; Lammintakanen, J.; Talja, M. Cost-effectiveness analysis for a tele-based health coaching program for chronic disease in primary care. *BMC Heal. Serv. Res.* **2017**, *17*, 1–7. [CrossRef] [PubMed]
23. Ambrosino, N.; Fracchia, C. The role of tele-medicine in patients with respiratory diseases. *Expert Rev. Respir. Med.* **2017**, *11*, 893–900. [CrossRef]
24. Maresca, G.; Maggio, M.G.; De Luca, R.; Manuli, A.; Tonin, P.; Pignolo, L.; Calabrò, R.S. Tele-Neuro-Rehabilitation in Italy: State of the Art and Future Perspectives. *Front. Neurol.* **2020**, *11*. [CrossRef] [PubMed]
25. von Storch, K.; Graaf, E.; Wunderlich, M.; Rietz, C.; Polidori, M.C.; Woopen, C. Telemedicine-Assisted Self-Management Program for Type 2 Diabetes Patients. *Diabetes Technol. Ther.* **2019**, *21*, 514–521. [CrossRef] [PubMed]
26. Koç, Z.; Kaplan, E.; Tanrıverdi, D. The effectiveness of telehealth programs on the mental health of women with breast cancer: A systematic review. *J. Telemed. Telecare* **2022**. [CrossRef] [PubMed]
27. Damholdt, M.; Mehlsen, M.; O'Toole, M.; Andreasen, R.; Pedersen, A.; Zachariae, R. Web-based cognitive training for breast cancer survivors with cognitive complaints—A randomized controlled trial. *Psychooncology* **2016**, *25*, 1293–1300. [CrossRef]
28. Galiano-Castillo, N.; Ariza-García, A.; Cantarero-Villanueva, I.; Fernández-Lao, C.; Díaz-Rodríguez, L.; Legerén-Alvarez, M.; Sánchez-Salado, C.; Del-Moral-Avila, R.; Arroyo-Morales, M. Telehealth system (e-CUIDATE) to improve quality of life in breast cancer survivors: Rationale and study protocol for a randomized clinical trial. *Trials* **2013**, *14*, 187. [CrossRef]
29. Freeman, L.W.; White, R.; Ratcliff, C.G.; Sutton, S.; Stewart, M.; Palmer, J.L.; Link, J.; Cohen, L. A randomized trial comparing live and telemedicine deliveries of an imagery-based behavioral intervention for breast cancer survivors: Reducing symptoms and barriers tocare. *Psychooncology* **2014**, *24*, 910–918. [CrossRef]
30. Page, M.J.; E McKenzie, J.; Bossuyt, P.M.; Boutron, I.; Hoffmann, T.C.; Mulrow, C.D.; Shamseer, L.; Tetzlaff, J.M.; Moher, D. Updating guidance for reporting systematic reviews: Development of the PRISMA 2020 statement. *J. Clin. Epidemiol.* **2021**, *134*, 103–112. [CrossRef]
31. Krzyzanowska, M.K.; A Julian, J.; Gu, C.-S.; Powis, M.; Li, Q.; Enright, K.; Howell, D.; Earle, C.C.; Gandhi, S.; Rask, S.; et al. Remote, proactive, telephone based management of toxicity in outpatients during adjuvant or neoadjuvant chemotherapy for early stage breast cancer: Pragmatic, cluster randomised trial. *BMJ* **2021**, *375*, e066588. [CrossRef] [PubMed]
32. Lozano-Lozano, M.; Martín-Martín, L.; Galiano-Castillo, N.; Fernández-Lao, C.; Cantarero-Villanueva, I.; López-Barajas, I.B.; Arroyo-Morales, M. Mobile health and supervised rehabilitation versus mobile health alone in breast cancer survivors: Randomized controlled trial. *Ann. Phys. Rehabil. Med.* **2019**, *63*, 316–324. [CrossRef] [PubMed]
33. Lozano-Lozano, M.; Galiano-Castillo, N.; Gonzalez-Santos, A.; Ortiz-Comino, L.; Sampedro-Pilegaard, M.; Martín-Martín, L.; Arroyo-Morales, M. Effect of mHealth plus occupational therapy on cognitive function, mood and physical function in people after cancer: Secondary analysis of a randomized controlled trial. *Ann. Phys. Rehabil. Med.* **2023**, *66*, 101681. [CrossRef] [PubMed]
34. Admiraal, J.M.; van der Velden, A.W.; Geerling, J.I.; Burgerhof, J.G.; Bouma, G.; Walenkamp, A.M.; de Vries, E.; Schröder, C.P.; Reyners, A.K. Web-Based Tailored Psychoeducation for Breast Cancer Patients at the Onset of the Survivorship Phase: A Multicenter Randomized Controlled Trial. *J. Pain Symptom Manag.* **2017**, *54*, 466–475. [CrossRef] [PubMed]
35. Galiano-Castillo, N.; Arroyo-Morales, M.; Lozano-Lozano, M.; Fernández-Lao, C.; Martín-Martín, L.; Del-Moral-Ávila, R.; Cantarero-Villanueva, I. Effect of an Internet-based telehealth system on functional capacity and cognition in breast cancer survivors: A secondary analysis of a randomized controlled trial. *Support. Care Cancer* **2017**, *25*, 3551–3559. [CrossRef]
36. Galiano-Castillo, N.; Cantarero-Villanueva, I.; Fernández-Lao, C.; Ariza-García, A.; Díaz-Rodríguez, L.; Del-Moral-Ávila, R.; Arroyo-Morales, M. Telehealth system: A randomized controlled trial evaluating the impact of an internet-based exercise intervention on quality of life, pain, muscle strength, and fatigue in breast cancer survivors. *Cancer* **2016**, *122*, 3166–3174. [CrossRef] [PubMed]
37. Zachariae, R.; Amidi, A.; Damholdt, M.F.; Clausen, C.D.R.; Dahlgaard, J.; Lord, H.; Thorndike, F.P.; Ritterband, L.M. Internet-Delivered Cognitive-Behavioral Therapy for Insomnia in Breast Cancer Survivors: A Randomized Controlled Trial. *Gynecol. Oncol.* **2018**, *110*, 880–887. [CrossRef]
38. Bandani-Susan, B.; Montazeri, A.; Haghighizadeh, M.H.; Araban, M. The effect of mobile health educational intervention on body image and fatigue in breast cancer survivors: A randomized controlled trial. *Ir. J. Med Sci.* **2021**, *191*, 1599–1605. [CrossRef]
39. Berg, S.W.V.D.; Gielissen, M.F.; Custers, J.A.; Van Der Graaf, W.T.; Ottevanger, P.B.; Prins, J.B. BREATH: Web-Based Self-Management for Psychological Adjustment after Primary Breast Cancer—Results of a Multicenter Randomized Controlled Trial. *J. Clin. Oncol.* **2015**, *33*, 2763–2771. [CrossRef]
40. Oswald, L.B.; Morales-Cruz, J.; Eisel, S.L.; Del Rio, J.; Hoogland, A.I.; Ortiz-Rosado, V.; Soto-Lopez, G.; Rodriguez-Rivera, E.; Savard, J.; Castro, E.; et al. Pilot randomized controlled trial of eHealth cognitive-behavioral therapy for insomnia among Spanish-speaking breast cancer survivors. *J. Behav. Med.* **2022**, *45*, 503–508. [CrossRef]
41. Carlson, L.E.; Subnis, U.B.; Piedalue, K.L.; Vallerand, J.; Speca, M.; Lupichuk, S.; Tang, P.; Faris, P.; Wolever, R.Q. The ONE-MIND Study: Rationale and protocol for assessing the effects of ONlinE MINDfulness-based cancer recovery for the prevention of fatigue and other common side effects during chemotherapy. *Eur. J. Cancer Care* **2019**, *28*, e13074. [CrossRef] [PubMed]

42. González, Á.S.; Lopez-Garzon, M.; Sánchez-Salado, C.; Postigo-Martin, P.; Lozano-Lozano, M.; Galiano-Castillo, N.; Fernández-Lao, C.; Castro-Martín, E.; Gallart-Aragón, T.; Legerén-Álvarez, M.; et al. A Telehealth-Based Cognitive-Adaptive Training (e-OTCAT) to Prevent Cancer and Chemotherapy-Related Cognitive Impairment in Women with Breast Cancer: Protocol for a Randomized Controlled Trial. *Int. J. Environ. Res. Public Health* **2022**, *19*, 7147. [CrossRef] [PubMed]
43. Lidington, E.; E McGrath, S.; Noble, J.; Stanway, S.; Lucas, A.; Mohammed, K.; van der Graaf, W.; Husson, O. Evaluating a digital tool for supporting breast cancer patients: A randomized controlled trial protocol (ADAPT). *Trials* **2020**, *21*, 1–10. [CrossRef] [PubMed]
44. Krusche, A.; Bradbury, K.; Corbett, T.; Barnett, J.; Stuart, B.; Yao, G.L.; Bacon, R.; Böhning, D.; Cheetham-Blake, T.; Eccles, D.; et al. Renewed: Protocol for a randomised controlled trial of a digital intervention to support quality of life in cancer survivors. *BMJ Open* **2019**, *9*, e024862. [CrossRef]
45. Tombaugh, T.N. Trail Making Test A and B: Normative data stratified by age and education. *Arch. Clin. Neuropsychol.* **2004**, *19*, 203–214. [CrossRef] [PubMed]
46. Crawford, J.R.; Obonsawin, M.C.; Allan, K.M. PASAT and Components of WAIS-R Performance: Convergent and Discriminant Validity. *Neuropsychol. Rehabil.* **1998**, *8*, 255–272. [CrossRef]
47. Jacobs, S.R.; Jacobsen, P.B.; Booth-Jones, M.; Wagner, L.I.; Anasetti, C. Evaluation of the Functional Assessment of Cancer Therapy Cognitive Scale with Hematopoetic Stem Cell Transplant Patients. *J. Pain Symptom Manag.* **2007**, *33*, 13–23. [CrossRef]
48. Scott, J.; Teasdale, J.D.; Paykel, E.S.; Johnson, A.L.; Abbott, R.; Hayhurst, H.; Moore, R.; Garland, A. Effects of Cognitive Therapy on Psychological Symptoms and Social Functioning in Residual Depression. *Focus* **2005**, *3*, 122–130. [CrossRef]
49. Bourne, L.E., Jr.; Yaroush, R.A. Stress and cognition: A cognitive psychological perspective. *NASA Tech. Reports Serv.* **2003**.
50. Fobair, P.; Stewart, S.L.; Chang, S.; D'Onofrio, C.; Banks, P.J.; Bloom, J.R. Body image and sexual problems in young women with breast cancer. *Psychooncology* **2005**, *15*, 579–594. [CrossRef]
51. Carroll, J.E.; Van Dyk, K.; Bower, J.E.; Scuric, Z.; Ms, L.P.; Schiestl, R.; Irwin, M.; Ganz, P.A. Cognitive performance in survivors of breast cancer and markers of biological aging. *Cancer* **2018**, *125*, 298–306. [CrossRef] [PubMed]
52. Wagner, A.D. Sex differences in cancer chemotherapy effects, and why we need to reconsider BSA-based dosing of chemotherapy. *ESMO Open* **2020**, *5*, e000770. [CrossRef] [PubMed]
53. Ganz, P.A.; Van Dyk, K. Cognitive Impairment in Patients with Breast Cancer: Understanding the Impact of Chemotherapy and Endocrine Therapy. *J. Clin. Oncol.* **2020**, *38*, 1871–1874. [CrossRef]
54. Cheung, Y.T.; Ng, T.; Shwe, M.; Ho, H.K.; Foo, K.M.; Cham, M.T.; Lee, J.A.; Fan, G.; Tan, Y.P.; Yong, W.S.; et al. Association of proinflammatory cytokines and chemotherapy-associated cognitive impairment in breast cancer patients: A multi-centered, prospective, cohort study. *Ann. Oncol.* **2015**, *26*, 1446–1451. [CrossRef] [PubMed]
55. Meyers, C.A.; Albitar, M.; Estey, E. Cognitive impairment, fatigue, and cytokine levels in patients with acute myelogenous leukemia or myelodysplastic syndrome. *Cancer* **2005**, *104*, 788–793. [CrossRef]
56. Carroll, J.E.; Nakamura, Z.M.; Small, B.J.; Zhou, X.; Cohen, H.J.; Ahles, T.A.; Ahn, J.; Bethea, T.N.; Extermann, M.; Graham, D.; et al. Elevated C-Reactive Protein and Subsequent Patient-Reported Cognitive Problems in Older Breast Cancer Survivors: The Thinking and Living with Cancer Study. *J. Clin. Oncol.* **2023**, *41*, 295–306. [CrossRef]
57. Asher, A.; Myers, J.S. The effect of cancer treatment on cognitive function. *Clin. Adv. Hematol. Oncol.* **2015**.
58. Mandelblatt, J.S.; Stern, R.A.; Luta, G.; McGuckin, M.; Clapp, J.D.; Hurria, A.; Jacobsen, P.B.; Faul, L.A.; Isaacs, C.; Denduluri, N.; et al. Cognitive Impairment in Older Patients with Breast Cancer before Systemic Therapy: Is There an Interaction between Cancer and Comorbidity? *J. Clin. Oncol.* **2014**, *32*, 1909–1918. [CrossRef]
59. Irwin, M.R.; Cole, S.W. Reciprocal regulation of the neural and innate immune systems. *Nat. Rev. Immunol.* **2011**, *11*, 625–632. [CrossRef]
60. Mishra, J.; Gazzaley, A. Harnessing the neuroplastic potential of the human brain & the future of cognitive rehabilitation. *Front. Hum. Neurosci.* **2014**, *8*, 218. [CrossRef]
61. Koutrouli, N.; Anagnostopoulos, F.; Potamianos, G. Posttraumatic Stress Disorder and Posttraumatic Growth in Breast Cancer Patients: A Systematic Review. *Women Health* **2012**, *52*, 503–516. [CrossRef] [PubMed]
62. Runowicz, C.D.; Leach, C.R.; Henry, N.L.; Henry, K.S.; Mackey, H.T.; Cowens-Alvarado, R.L.; Cannady, R.S.; Pratt-Chapman, M.; Edge, S.B.; Jacobs, L.A.; et al. American Cancer Society/American Society of Clinical Oncology Breast Cancer Survivorship Care Guideline. *CA A Cancer J. Clin.* **2015**, *66*, 43–73. [CrossRef] [PubMed]

Disclaimer/Publisher's Note: The statements, opinions and data contained in all publications are solely those of the individual author(s) and contributor(s) and not of MDPI and/or the editor(s). MDPI and/or the editor(s) disclaim responsibility for any injury to people or property resulting from any ideas, methods, instructions or products referred to in the content.

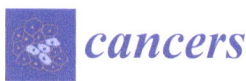

Review

Localization Techniques for Non-Palpable Breast Lesions: Current Status, Knowledge Gaps, and Rationale for the MELODY Study (EUBREAST-4/iBRA-NET, NCT 05559411)

Maggie Banys-Paluchowski [1,*], Thorsten Kühn [2], Yazan Masannat [3], Isabel Rubio [4], Jana de Boniface [5,6], Nina Ditsch [7], Güldeniz Karadeniz Cakmak [8], Andreas Karakatsanis [9,10], Rajiv Dave [11], Markus Hahn [12], Shelley Potter [13], Ashutosh Kothari [14], Oreste Davide Gentilini [15], Bahadir M. Gulluoglu [16], Michael Patrick Lux [17], Marjolein Smidt [18], Walter Paul Weber [19], Bilge Aktas Sezen [20], Natalia Krawczyk [21], Steffi Hartmann [22], Rosa Di Micco [15], Sarah Nietz [23], Francois Malherbe [24], Neslihan Cabioglu [25], Nuh Zafer Canturk [26], Maria Luisa Gasparri [27,28,29], Dawid Murawa [30] and James Harvey [31]

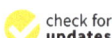

Citation: Banys-Paluchowski, M.; Kühn, T.; Masannat, Y.; Rubio, I.; de Boniface, J.; Ditsch, N.; Karadeniz Cakmak, G.; Karakatsanis, A.; Dave, R.; Hahn, M.; et al. Localization Techniques for Non-Palpable Breast Lesions: Current Status, Knowledge Gaps, and Rationale for the MELODY Study (EUBREAST-4/iBRA-NET, NCT 05559411). *Cancers* 2023, 15, 1173. https://doi.org/10.3390/cancers15041173

Academic Editors: Samuel Cos and Naiba Nabieva

Received: 28 December 2022
Revised: 7 February 2023
Accepted: 10 February 2023
Published: 12 February 2023

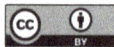

Copyright: © 2023 by the authors. Licensee MDPI, Basel, Switzerland. This article is an open access article distributed under the terms and conditions of the Creative Commons Attribution (CC BY) license (https://creativecommons.org/licenses/by/4.0/).

1. Department of Gynecology and Obstetrics, University Hospital Schleswig-Holstein, Campus Lübeck, 23538 Lübeck, Germany
2. Department of Gynecology and Obstetrics, Die Filderklinik, 70794 Filderstadt, Germany
3. Aberdeen Breast Unit, Aberdeen Royal Infirmary, Aberdeen AB25 2ZN, UK
4. Breast Surgical Oncology, Clinica Universidad de Navarra, 28027 Madrid, Spain
5. Department of Molecular Medicine and Surgery, Karolinska Institutet, 17177 Stockholm, Sweden
6. Department of Surgery, Capio St. Göran's Hospital, 11219 Stockholm, Sweden
7. Breast Cancer Center, University Hospital Augsburg, 86156 Augsburg, Germany
8. Breast and Endocrine Unit, General Surgery Department, Zonguldak BEUN The School of Medicine, Kozlu/Zonguldak 67600, Turkey
9. Department for Surgical Sciences, Faculty of Pharmacy and Medicine, Uppsala University, 75236 Uppsala, Sweden
10. Section for Breast Surgery, Department of Surgery, Uppsala University Hospital, 75236 Uppsala, Sweden
11. Nightingale & Genesis Breast Cancer Prevention Centre, Manchester University NHS Foundation Trust, Faculty of Biology, Medicine and Health, University of Manchester, Manchester M13 9PL, UK
12. Department for Women's Health, University of Tübingen, 72076 Tübingen, Germany
13. Bristol Medical School (THS), Bristol Population Health Science Institute, Bristol BS8 1QU, UK
14. Guy's & St Thomas NHS Foundation Trust, Kings College, London SE1 9RT, UK
15. Department of Breast Surgery, San Raffaele University and Research Hospital, 20132 Milan, Italy
16. Department of Surgery, Breast Surgery Unit, Marmara University School of Medicine and SENATURK Turkish Academy of Senology, Istanbul 34854, Turkey
17. Department of Gynecology and Obstetrics, St. Louise Frauen-und Kinderklinik, 33098 Paderborn, Germany
18. Department of Surgical Oncology, Maastricht University Medical Center, 6229 HX Maastricht, The Netherlands
19. Division of Breast Surgery, Department of Surgery, Basel University Hospital, 4031 Basel, Switzerland
20. European Breast Cancer Research Association of Surgical Trialists (EUBREAST), 73730 Esslingen, Germany
21. Department of Gynecology and Obstetrics, Heinrich-Heine-University Düsseldorf, 40225 Düsseldorf, Germany
22. Department of Gynecology and Obstetrics, University Hospital Rostock, 18059 Rostock, Germany
23. Department of Surgery, Faculty of Health Sciences, University of the Witwatersrand, Johannesburg 2000, South Africa
24. Breast and Endocrine Surgery Unit, Groote Schuur Hospital, University of Cape Town, Cape Town 7935, South Africa
25. Istanbul Faculty of Medicine, Department of General Surgery, Istanbul University, Istanbul 34093, Turkey
26. Department of General Surgery, Kocaeli University School of Medicine, Kocaeli 41001, Turkey
27. Department of Gynecology and Obstetrics, Ospedale Regionale di Lugano EOC, 6900 Lugano, Switzerland
28. Centro di Senologia della Svizzera Italiana (CSSI), Ente Ospedaliero Cantonale, Via Pietro Capelli 1, 6900 Lugano, Switzerland
29. Faculty of Biomedical Sciences, Università della Svizzera Italiana (USI), Via Giuseppe Buffi 13, 6900 Lugano, Switzerland
30. General Surgery and Surgical Oncology Department, Collegium Medicum, University in Zielona Gora, 65-417 Zielona Góra, Poland
31. Nightingale & Genesis Breast Cancer Prevention Centre, University Hospital of South Manchester NHS Foundation Trust, Manchester M13 9PL, UK
* Correspondence: maggie.banys-paluchowski@uksh.de

Simple Summary: Most breast cancers are small and can be treated using breast-conserving surgery. Since these tumors are non-palpable, they require a localization step that helps the surgeon to decide which tissue needs to be removed. The oldest localization technique is a guidewire placed into the tumor before surgery, usually using ultrasound or mammography. Afterwards, the surgeon removes the tissue around the wire tip. However, this technique has several disadvantages: It can cause the patient discomfort, requires a radiologist or another professional specialized in breast diagnostics to perform the procedure shortly before surgery, and 15–20% of patients need a second surgery to completely remove the tumor. Therefore, new techniques have been developed but most of them have not yet been examined in large, prospective, multicenter studies. In this review, we discuss all available techniques and present the MELODY study that will investigate their safety, with a focus on patient, surgeon, and radiologist preference.

Abstract: Background: Surgical excision of a non-palpable breast lesion requires a localization step. Among available techniques, wire-guided localization (WGL) is most commonly used. Other techniques (radioactive, magnetic, radar or radiofrequency-based, and intraoperative ultrasound) have been developed in the last two decades with the aim of improving outcomes and logistics. Methods: We performed a systematic review on localization techniques for non-palpable breast cancer. Results: For most techniques, oncological outcomes such as lesion identification and clear margin rate seem either comparable with or better than for WGL, but evidence is limited to small cohort studies for some of the devices. Intraoperative ultrasound is associated with significantly higher negative margin rates in meta-analyses of randomized clinical trials (RCTs). Radioactive techniques were studied in several RCTs and are non-inferior to WGL. Smaller studies show higher patient preference towards wire-free localization, but little is known about surgeons' and radiologists' attitudes towards these techniques. Conclusions: Large studies with an additional focus on patient, surgeon, and radiologist preference are necessary. This review aims to present the rationale for the MELODY (NCT05559411) study and to enable standardization of outcome measures for future studies.

Keywords: breast cancer; localization technique; non-palpable lesion; intraoperative ultrasound; wire-guided localization; magnetic seed; radioactive seed; radar reflector; radiofrequency identification tag

1. Introduction

Surgical excision of a non-palpable breast lesion requires some form of breast localization device. Despite multiple available solutions, a majority of units use wire-guided localization (WGL) due to the high efficacy and low cost [1,2]. Other techniques, e.g., radioactive seed localization, radio-occult lesion localization (ROLL), and intraoperative ultrasound, have become established in a smaller number of centers but have not gained widespread adoption. While WGL has clear benefits in terms of cost, efficacy, and a trained workforce, it also carries several weaknesses, including logistical difficulties due to the need of placement on the day of surgery and the potential for displacement. Despite widespread WGL use, a majority of breast surgeons have voiced a preference to switch to an alternative technique [2]. Since 2016, a new generation of localization devices has entered the market including SAVI SCOUT®, LOCalizer™, Magseed®, Pintuition®, EnVisio®, and Molli™ (Figure 1). The IDEAL framework provides a system for evaluating surgical innovations from "first in human" (stage 1), "exploration" (stage 2), and "assessment" (stage 3) to "long term study" (stage 4) [3]. Most novel techniques are moving through from a development stage into an exploratory phase, where they are becoming more standardized and replicated by others. Acknowledgement of learning curves is important [4,5].

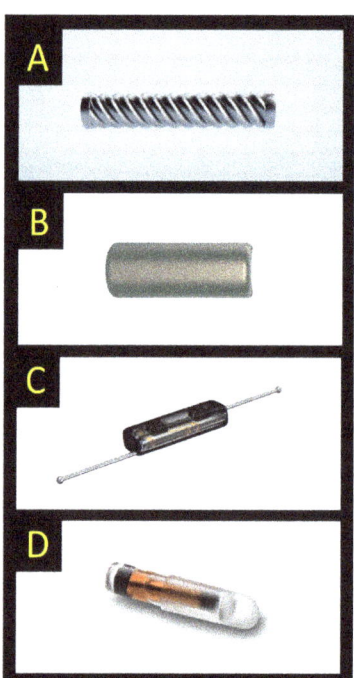

Figure 1. Examples of commercially available localization devices (the depicted size does not correctly compare the different markers shown): (**A**) Magseed (5 × 1 mm); (**B**) Sirius Pintuition (5 × 1.65 mm); (**C**) SAVI SCOUT (12 × 1.6 mm); (**D**) LOCalizer (11 × 2 mm) [reprinted with permission of manufacturers 2022: Endomag, Sirius Medical, Merit Medical, Hologic].

The European Breast Cancer Research Association of Surgical Trialists (EUBREAST) and the iBRA-NET have initiated the MELODY (Methods for Localization of Different types of breast lesions) study to assess breast localization techniques and devices from several perspectives. MELODY is a multinational prospective intergroup cohort study which enrolls breast cancer patients undergoing breast-conserving surgery using imaging-guided localization. As an IDEAL stage 2b/3 observational study, it aims to explore the safety, efficacy. and patient-/clinician-reported outcomes of different localization techniques [6]. The study is designed to ensure thorough surgical evaluation and yield high-quality evidence for both patients and clinicians, potentially allowing evidence-based adoption of these techniques by national bodies and regulatory authorities.

This narrative review aims to identify the current knowledge base of established and newer localization techniques, to help inform the MELODY (NCT05559411) study design and to enable standardisation of outcome measures for future studies.

2. Current Evidence of Different Localization Techniques

2.1. Wire-Guided Localization (WGL)

For decades, WGL was the main localization technique, and is still considered the gold standard in many countries [7,8]. Initially developed in the 1960s and popularized in the 1970s and 1980s, the technique involves a wire or a needle placed preoperatively into the lesion under sonographic or mammographic guidance, usually followed by ultrasound or radiography of the subsequently surgically removed specimen (Figure 2) [9]. Disadvantages of WGL, such as the necessity to perform the procedure on the day of surgery or—less frequently—on the day before, the possibility of wire dislocation, and patient discomfort and distress, have led to a search for alternative strategies.

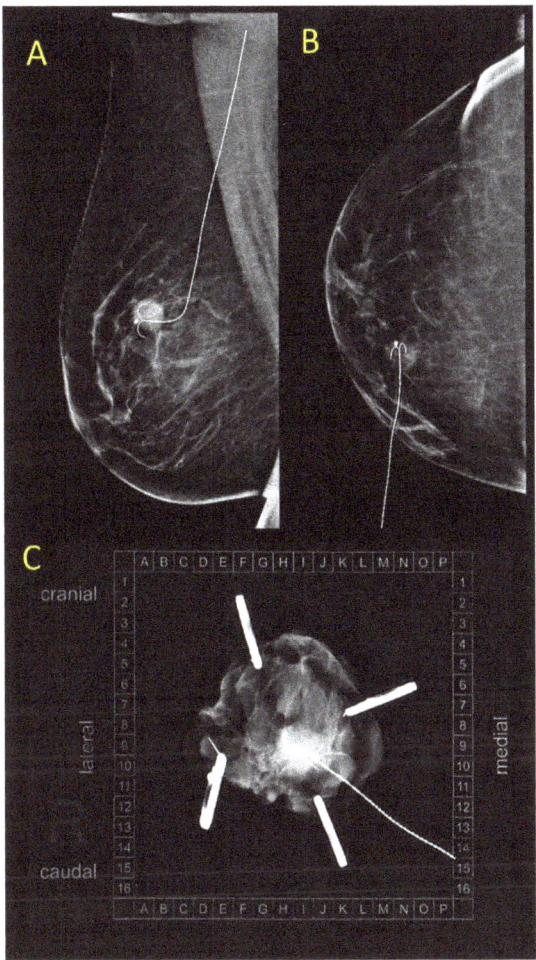

Figure 2. (**A**,**B**) Control mammography after ultrasound-guided wire placement in a patient with an invasive breast cancer, NST, max. size 11 mm. (**C**) Specimen mammography.

A recent analysis from the Netherlands including 28,370 patients showed that probe guided localization is replacing WGL, with the use of radioactive seed localization having increased from 16% to 61% between 2013 and 2018, while WGL decreased from 75% to 32% [1].

To date, all randomized controlled trials (RCTs) on newer localization techniques have compared them to the WGL (Tables 1 and 2) [8,10,11]. The positive margin rate of WGL was reported to be in the range of 15–21% [8,10,12,13]. Two network meta-analyses of RCTs showed that margin positivity and reoperation rates of all techniques were similar, except for intraoperative ultrasound that led to significantly reduced margin positivity and re-excision rates [10,11].

Table 1. Comparison of different localization methods regarding oncological outcomes.

	Successful Excision	Positive Margins [1]	Re-Operation Rate	Data Quality
Wire-guided localization (WGL)	99% [9,12]	15–21% [9,10,12,14]	14–19% [9,10]	High; Meta-analyses of RCTs available (LoE 1a)
Radioactive seed localization (RSL)	100% [9]	12–13% [9,10]	10–15% [9,10]	High; Meta-analyses of RCTs available (LoE 1a)
Radio-guided Occult Lesion Localization (ROLL)	99.5% [9]	12–17% [9,10]	9–10% [9,10]	High; Meta-analyses of RCTs available (LoE 1a)
Magseed	99.8% [12]	13.3% [12]	12% [12]	Large cohort studies [12], no RCTs (LoE 2b)
Sirius Pintuition	100% [15]	8% [15]	4% [15]	Small cohort studies, one small RCT [3] [15] (LoE 2b)
MOLLI	100% [16]	0% [16]	0% [16]	Small phase I cohort study (LoE 4)
TAKUMI	100% [17]	7.3% [17]	4.9% [17]	Small cohort study (LoE 4)
SAVI SCOUT	99.64% [4]	n.d.	12.8% [4]	Systemic review and pooled analysis [4] (LoE 2b)
LOCalizer	99.9% [18]	n.d.	13.9% [18]	Systemic review and pooled analysis [18] (LoE 2b)
EnVisio	n.d.	n.d.	n.d.	Case report [19] (LoE 5)
Intraoperative ultrasound (IOUS)	100% [8] [2]	5% [8,10,11] [2]	5–7% [8,10] [2]	High; Meta-analyses of RCTs available (LoE 1a) [2]
Carbon	79.0–99.1% [20–24]	75.0–96.4% [21,22,25]	7.1% [25]	Cohort studies, no RCTs (LoE 4)

[1] Positive margins were defined differently across studies; whenever possible, positive margin was defined as no tumor on ink. [2] Patients in RCTs on IOUS had ultrasound-visible lesions; therefore, the patient collective might be different from those in studies on other localization methods [3] The RCT studied MaMaLoc; the technology was further developed and is now available as Sirius Pintuition.

Table 2. Comparison of different localization methods used in breast cancer patients undergoing breast conserving surgery (modified after: [26]).

	Advantages	Disadvantages
Wire-guided localization (WGL)	• Well-established • Cost-effective • Marker placement under radiographic, ultrasound or MRI guidance possible → suitable for localization of lesions visible only upon mammography (e.g., microcalcifications) or MRI • Control mammogram or MRI after wire placement possible • Reposition in case of some wires possible	• Scheduling issues: the wire needs to be placed on the day of surgery or the day before • Wire dislocation possible • Patient discomfort
Radioactive seed localization (RSL)	• Well-established • Scheduling flexibility: localization can be performed several days/weeks before surgery or—in case of neoadjuvant therapy—before start of treatment • Marker placement under radiographic or ultrasound guidance possible → suitable for localization of lesions visible only upon mammography (e.g., microcalcifications) • Control mammogram after marker placement possible • Can be combined with isotope-based sentinel node biopsy	• Procedure not authorized in some countries, requires complex radiation safety procedures • Radiation exposure to patient and staff • Invasive procedure for marker placement necessary • In case of marker placement before neoadjuvant therapy signal loss possible in case of longer than planned duration of therapy • Reposition after placement not possible • Radiation safety concerns regarding MRI-guided localization (Geiger counter is MRI unsafe and cannot be used in case of seed loss in Zone IV) • Very low risk of seed rupture or transection, resulting in emergency treatment with iodine to saturate and safeguard the thyroid gland in case of ^{125}I

Table 2. Cont.

	Advantages	Disadvantages
Radio-guided Occult Lesion Localization (ROLL)	• Well-established • Marker placement under radiographic, ultrasound or MRI guidance possible → suitable for localization of lesions visible only upon mammography (e.g., microcalcifications) or MRI	• Scheduling issues: procedure needs to be performed on the day of surgery or the day before • Radiation safety procedures required • Potential radiation exposure to patient and staff • Invasive preoperative procedure necessary • Reposition after placement not possible • Control mammogram not possible unless contrast also given
Magnetic and paramagnetic localization Commercially available systems: • Magseed (Endomag) • Sirius Pintuition (formerly known as MaMaLoc; Sirius Medical) • MOLLI (MOLLI Surgical) • TAKUMI/Guiding-marker system (Hakko)	• No radioactivity involved • Marker placement under radiographic or ultrasound guidance possible → suitable for localization of lesions visible only upon mammography (e.g., microcalcifications) • Scheduling flexibility: localization can be performed several days/weeks before surgery or—in case of neoadjuvant therapy—before start of treatment • No decrease of signal over time → reliable detectability in case of longer than planned neoadjuvant therapy • Control mammogram after marker placement possible • Can be combined with magnetic tracer for sentinel node biopsy	• Concerns regarding use in patients with pacemakers and implantable defibrillators • Standard metal surgical tools may lead to interference during measurement • Large MRI artifacts • Not suitable for lesions visible only upon MRI • Higher device cost • Adequate localization may be limited in case of a large distance between marker and detection probe • Reposition after placement not possible
Radar reflector-based localization Commercially available systems: • SAVI SCOUT (Merit Medical)	• No radioactivity involved • Minimal MRI artifact • Marker placement under radiographic or ultrasound guidance possible → suitable for localization of lesions visible only upon mammography (e.g., microcalcifications) • Scheduling flexibility: localization can be performed several days/weeks before surgery or—in case of neoadjuvant therapy—before start of treatment • No decrease of signal over time → reliable detectability in case of longer than planned neoadjuvant therapy • Control mammogram after marker placement possible	• Potential signal interference with lights in the operating theatre • Small MRI artifacts • Not suitable for lesions visible only upon MRI • Higher device cost • Adequate localization may be limited in case of a large distance between marker and detection probe • Reposition after placement not possible
Radiofrequency identification tags (RFID) Commercially available systems: • LOCalizer (HOLOGIC) • EnVisio (Elucent Medical)	• No radioactivity involved • Scheduling flexibility: localization can be performed several days/weeks before surgery or—in case of neoadjuvant therapy—before start of treatment • Marker placement under radiographic or ultrasound guidance possible → suitable for localization of lesions visible only upon mammography (e.g., microcalcifications) • No decrease of signal over time → reliable detectability in case of longer than planned neoadjuvant therapy • Unique tag number → differentiation between tags possible • Control mammogram after marker placement possible	• Concerns regarding use in patients with pacemakers and implantable defibrillators • MRI artifacts • Not suitable for lesions visible only upon MRI • Higher device cost • Adequate localization may be limited in case of a large distance between marker and detection probe • Reposition after placement not possible

Table 2. *Cont.*

	Advantages	Disadvantages
Intraoperative ultrasound (IOUS)	• Direct visualization during surgery • No radioactivity involved • Patient friendly (non-invasive) • No preoperative invasive procedure necessary → scheduling flexibility • Specimen sonography is performed immediately after tissue removal → no time loss due to specimen transport • Specimen sonography performed in the operating room → exact and reliable topographic localization of close margins for immediate re-excision • Relatively low cost	• Surgeon needs to be experienced in breast ultrasound, otherwise radiologist's presence in the operating theatre necessary • Learning curve • Useful only for lesions with good sonographic visibility • Not suitable for lesions visible only upon mammography (e.g., microcalcifications) or MRI • Use in the neoadjuvant setting limited in case of complete remission due to low sonographic visibility of some tissue markers • Ultrasound machine must be available in the operating theatre during surgery • Some ultrasound machines available in operating theatres are unsuitable for breast ultrasound (frequency, transducer type) or of a much lower quality than machines in the diagnostics department • Radiogram showing lesion and marker not possible
Carbon	• No radioactivity involved • Low cost • Scheduling flexibility: localization can be performed several days/weeks before surgery or—in case of neoadjuvant therapy—before start of treatment • Marker placement under radiographic or ultrasound guidance possible • No MRI artifacts	• Marker cannot be localized without surgical exploration • Possible ink migration • Intentional or unintentional tattooing of skin • Reposition after placement not possible • Control mammogram not possible

2.2. Radioactive Localization

Radio-guided surgery is a wire-free approach to assist surgical excision of non-palpable breast lesions by using a gamma probe to detect a preinserted marker. Two forms of radioactive localization are currently in use: radioactive seed localization (RSL) is based on the detection of a small 125-iodine seed, while radioactive occult lesion localization (ROLL) relies on the identification of preinjected radiocolloid (99m Technetium) [9].

Radioactive seed localization was first described in 1999 in a pilot study that included 25 patients who underwent excisional biopsy [27]. The seed is composed of titanium containing 3.7 to 10.7 MBq ^{125}I (iodine) with a half-life of 60 days. Seeds are introduced via a needle under sonographic or mammographic guidance directed into the index lesion, and appropriate insertion is confirmed via subsequent imaging. Due to the long half-life, it is possible to insert the seed weeks or even months before the surgical intervention, making its use also an option in the neoadjuvant setting. During surgery, the seed is detected by a standard intraoperative handheld gamma probe, and the area of greatest activity projecting directly over the lesion is easily located to allow the most appropriate incision to be placed. In some countries, such as the United States, Canada, and the Netherlands, RSL is considered a standard approach [1]. Beyond localization of breast lesions, there is an increasing body of evidence for marking axillary lymph nodes with radioactive seeds [28,29].

RSL is one of the best validated wire-free localization methods. It has been investigated in several RCTs and meta-analyses [9–11]. A Cochrane review published in 2015 concluded that RSL was equally reliable compared with WGL, but the authors stressed the need for further, fully powered RCTs. Since then, more RCTs were published [30–32]. The successful excision rate, defined as removal of the index lesion with clear margins, was reported in the range of 99.4–100% [9,30,31,33,34]. In the available studies, the failure rate was comparable to that of WGL.

In the RCTs comparing RSL with WGL, the rate of positive margins was generally lower for RSL [30–35]. However, a recent network meta-analysis of RCTs evaluating optimal localization strategies for non-palpable breast cancers, including 24 studies, suggested no significant differences when comparing RSL with WGL for both margin positivity (OR: 0.677, 95% CI 0.397–1.110) and reoperation rates (OR: 0.685, 95% CI 0.341–1.260) [10]. In contrast, another meta-analysis comparing RSL with WGL, including both retrospective and prospective studies, outlined that RSL was superior to WGL by providing negative margins (RR: 0.72, 95% CI 0.56–0.92, $p = 0.01$) and lower reoperation rates (RR: 0.68, 95% CI 0.52–0.88, $p = 0.004$) [36,37].

While RSL is a popular localization method in some countries, the seeds are not approved for such use in others. Due to complex radiation safety regulations, the use of iodine seeds requires trained personnel, the implementation of standard operating procedures, and, depending on the country, a formal submission to a radiation protection agency for authorization. It may be mandatory to provide a facility diagram and description of the location(s) where the radioactive sources will be received, used, and stored. Each seed must be accounted for, and, unlike other localization devices, the loss of a seed is considered a serious breach of radiation safety. For this reason, seeds are generally implanted under ultrasound or mammographic, but not MRI, guidance. The MRI safety concern is related to the possibility of losing a seed in the MRI scan room without the option of using a hand-held Geiger counter to locate the seed [38].

Several studies analyzed the cost-effectiveness of RSL. The necessity to adhere to strict radiation safety regulations results in substantial upfront costs of RSL implementation [39]. The estimated costs per patient vary strongly between studies; while some reported slightly higher costs for RSL than for WGL (EUR 2834 vs. EUR 2,617 per patient, respectively) [39], others showed a lower average cost per patient for RSL (USD 251 compared to USD 1130 for WGL) [40]. Possibly, the cost-effectiveness of RSL depends on the health-care payment system (fee-for-service vs. bundled) [41].

Regarding MRI compatibility after placement, radioactive seeds may cause minimal and usually not clinically relevant susceptibility artifacts, similar to those observed around clips/coils [42]. Migration of implanted seeds seems rare, and was reported as 0.9 mm on average [42]. Although some early studies reported lower specimen volumes in patients receiving RSL [34], the available meta-analyses show no significant differences regarding specimen size, weight, or volume between patients undergoing RSL and WGL [10,11]. Few studies analyzed patient satisfaction with the localization procedure. In a RCT by Bloomquist et al., significantly fewer patients in the RSL arm reported moderate to severe pain during the localization procedure compared to the WGL arm, and the overall convenience of the procedure was rated as very good to excellent in 85% of RSL patients compared to 44% of WGL patients ($p < 0.0001$) [31]. No randomized data are available on surgeon or radiologist satisfaction with the technique.

The Radio-guided Occult Lesion Localization (ROLL) technique was primarily introduced by the team at the European Institute of Oncology in Milan in 1999 [13]. This procedure uses 99m Technetium-labelled colloidal human serum albumin as a radioactive tracer to label the lesion under sonographic or mammographic guidance. Similar to RSL, the tracer is localized using a handheld gamma probe and can be used for simultaneous sentinel node biopsy. The combined procedure is commonly referred to as SNOLL (Sentinel Node plus Occult Lesion Localization) [44]. The gamma radiation dose to the patient and the operators is very low and well within safe radiation regulatory limits.

Several RCTs and meta-analyses have examined the use of ROLL. A Cochrane review showed comparable rates of successful excision of the target lesion between the technique and WGL [9]. In the RCTs comparing WGL with ROLL, the rate of positive margins was reported to be higher in the WGL arm, but the differences were mostly not statistically significant [45–54]. In a recent network meta-analysis of RCTs evaluating optimal localization strategies for non-palpable breast cancers, including 24 studies, margin positivity rate was 20.1% for WGL and 17.2% for ROLL [10].

While ROLL is a popular technique in some parts of the world (Turkey, Australia, Latin America), it remains unknown in others. In clinical practice, the main disadvantage of ROLL is the necessity of the injection on the day of surgery or the day before surgery, which may be associated with difficulties in synchronizing the schedules of the nuclear medicine, radiology, and the operating room. Further, strictly seen, 99m Technetium is approved for sentinel lymph node identification, and not lesion localization, so there might be some concern regarding a potential off-label use in some countries.

The cost-effectiveness of ROLL has not been evaluated in large RCTs. In two RCTs comparing costs, ROLL (mean cost: EUR 182) was found to be slightly more expensive than WGL (mean cost: EUR 163) [10]. The technique is MRI compatible: It does not cause MRI artifacts and allows localization of lesions observed only on MRI [55]. Localization failures are rare [9]. Regarding specimen size, weight, and volumes, two recent meta-analyses reported no significant differences compared to WGL [10,11]. However, in the largest RCT, ROLL led to the excision of larger volumes [51].

Surgeon satisfaction rate was highest (98.4%) for ROLL when compared to the rate of 66% for WGL [10]. Conflicting results were reported with regard to patient pain score during the localization procedure [50,51]. No significant differences were found on patient-reported cosmetic results and pain between ROLL and WGL six months after surgery [51].

2.3. Magnetic and Paramagnetic Localization

Moving further from WGL, and in order to address the strict regulatory issues with regards to access, availability, handling, and disposal of radioactive material, several markers based on the principle of magnetic detection have been developed in recent years. The perceived advantage in such a device is that it allows for wire-free and radiation-free localization. Additionally, it yields the potential to facilitate logistics of localization, as it can be implanted many days before surgery. At present, both magnetic and paramagnetic markers are available for clinical use. Paramagnetic markers have a small susceptibility to magnetic fields and become temporarily magnetized in a presence of an externally applied magnetic field, while magnetic markers are permanent magnets. Metallic instruments may interfere with the detection of magnetic and paramagnetic markers, and both types of markers lead to significant MRI artifacts, limiting its use in the neoadjuvant setting [56].

The most well-studied marker in this category is a 5×1 mm long, steel paramagnetic marker (Magseed, Endomag, Cambridge, UK) investigated in multiple cohort studies (Figure 3) [12,57,58]. This device is licensed for both breast and axillary placement, and early studies demonstrated no migration within the breast [59]. In a recent multi-center study from the UK iBRA-NET, a total of 946 Magseed-guided excisions were compared with 1170 wire-guided excisions [12]. The authors found that the use of Magseed resulted in more successful index lesion removal (99.8% vs. 99.1%, $p = 0.048$) and fewer failed localizations (1.64% vs. 1.98%, $p = 0.032$). While it was associated with less risk of dislocation (0.4% vs. 1.4%, $p = 0.039$), the secondary outcomes (minimum margins, specimen sizes, re-excision surgery, postoperative complications) were comparable. In terms of logistics, Magseed-guided surgery had an earlier start on the day of surgery. Previous reports from the UK had shown similar results; Zacharioudakis et al. demonstrated comparable outcomes between the two techniques (n = 100 patients each arm) with regards to successful identification and removal, margin status, specimen size, and tumor-to-specimen volume ratio [58]. Micha et al. found that re-excision rates were similar in an institutional cohort study comparing Magseed (n = 100) to WGL (n = 100). The use of Magseed did not only achieve smaller specimens but also resulted in higher patient and physician satisfaction, and thus a preference for the magnetic technique [60]. Magseed localization is compromised by metal instruments and can be challenging when the seed is placed deep in the breast [61]. There is no evidence for superior cost-effectiveness or patient-reported outcomes when comparing it to other localization devices [62].

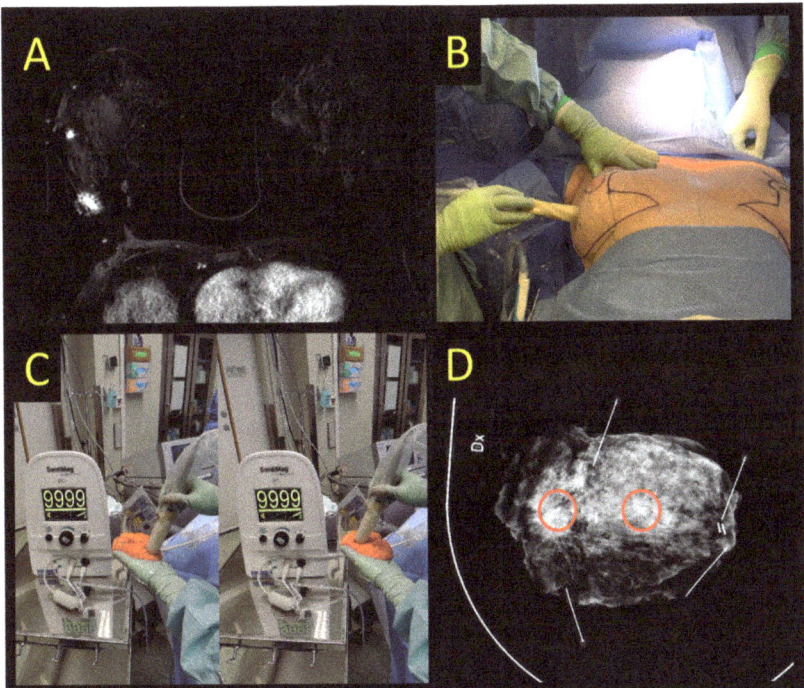

Figure 3. Magseed detection system. (**A**) Multicentric invasive lobular cancer (distance between lesions 4.7 cm). Each lesion is marked with a Magseed. Magtrace (SPIO) is injected between the lesions. (**B**) Transcutaneous detection with the probe. Mark the lack of skin discoloration after a deep Magtrace injection. (**C**) Ex vivo signal of the specimen. Both Magseeds have maximum signal. Observe the brown tissue staining at the SPIO injection site that does not affect specimen radiography. (**D**) Specimen radiography depicting the lesions with Magseeds (red circles highlight the position of Magseed markers).

2.4. Sirius Pintuition

The Magnetic Marker Localization (MaMaLoc) is a permanent magnetic marker that has been developed for breast localization. This marker has evolved with its own detection system; it is commercially available as Sirius Pintuition. The probe used for detection has an additional tool to show not only the distance to the seed, but the angle as well (Figure 4). Available data at the time of writing of this manuscript are so far limited to institutional reports presented as congress abstracts [63,64]. The originally developed device, the MaMaLoc, was compared to WGL in a small RCT (n = 70), powered to detect differences in the System Usability Scale (SUS) [15]. In this trial, all markers could be successfully retrieved. The positive margin rate was significantly lower in the magnetic marker arm (8% vs. 18% in the WGL group), but reoperation rates were similar (4% vs. 6%, respectively).

Sirius Pintuition is approved in the EU for placement for up to 180 days in any soft tissue, allowing for use in both breast and axilla. There is little evidence base to establish its migration rate, effectiveness, failure rate, cost-effectiveness, complication rates, or patient/physician satisfaction. The performance and safety of the Pintuition device is currently undergoing evaluation in a UK multi-center comparative cohort study [65].

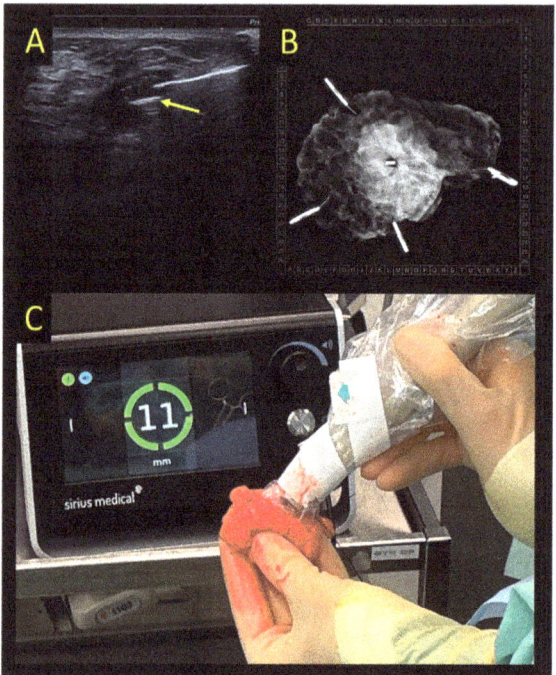

Figure 4. Sirius Pintuition system. (**A**) Ultrasound-guided placement of the marker (yellow arrow). (**B**) Intraoperative radiogram showing the marker in the center of the specimen. (**C**) Console used for detection in the OR showing 11 mm distance between probe tip and marker.

The detection probe is compatible with standard metal instruments, as long as they are not magnetized since this may lead to interference with the probe. Thus, it might be prudent to have one set of non-metallic instruments available. The main disadvantage of all magnetic markers is the creation of 5–6 cm artifacts surrounding the marker when using MRI. Therefore, if tumor response is to be assessed by MRI, magnetic markers should not be placed in the vicinity of the tumor area before neoadjuvant chemotherapy (NACT) [66].

While no such data are available regarding Sirius Pintuition localization, the abovementioned RCT on MaMaLoc vs. WGL showed comparable specimen weight and volume in both arms [15]. In this trial, patients reported more discomfort and pain during guidewire placement, but this result may be biased since patients allocated to WGL did not receive local anaesthesia whereas those allocated to the MaMaLoc did. Patients' overall satisfaction with the localization technique was rated significantly better for MaMaLoc than for WGL. Similarly, MaMaLoc localization led to higher surgeon satisfaction scores measured by a procedure-specific questionnaire, and surgeons would have preferred the MaMaLoc technique in 56% of cases. No preference was reported in 38% of cases, and WGL was preferred in only 7%.

The Magnetic Occult Lesion Localization Instrument (MOLLI) is another magnetic (not paramagnetic) marker with its own probe-based detection system. The current evidence is very limited and stems from only one feasibility study (n = 20) where all patients received a radioactive seed together with the MOLLI [16]. In this study, retrieval of the MOLLI was successful in all cases and with high physician satisfaction, but the small population studied, and study design do not allow for more robust conclusions. Finally, another magnetic marker has been developed in Japan: the Guiding-Marker System®, which is compatible with the handheld TAKUMI magnetic probe. The system has been validated in a single-arm multicenter study (n = 87), where marker retrieval was 100% and the re-excision rate was 6.1% [17].

In conclusion, magnetic guidance for tumor localization seems a promising technique, with a variety of devices that are commercially available. However, all evidence stems from non-randomized data, the only exception being a small RCT on MaMaLoc [15]. At the time of writing, a phase 3, pragmatic multicenter randomized controlled trial (MagTotal) is accruing data comparing Magseed and WGL (ISRCTN11914537). Given the differences of available devices in principle (paramagnetic vs. magnetic), probe compatibility, possibilities to utilize as a single platform for breast and axillary surgery, and the imbalance among them in terms of published data, further evaluation is needed.

2.5. Radar Reflector Localization

The SAVI SCOUT is a zero-radiation breast localization and surgical guidance system using micro-impulse radar technology for the removal of non-palpable breast lesions. It was introduced in 2015 and is approved by FDA and CE for long-term placement in breast, lymph nodes, and soft tissue. The reflector is activated by infrared light impulses generated by the console probe and uses two antennas to reflect an electromagnetic wave signal back to the handpiece. It can be placed using ultrasound or stereotactic guidance (Figure 5).

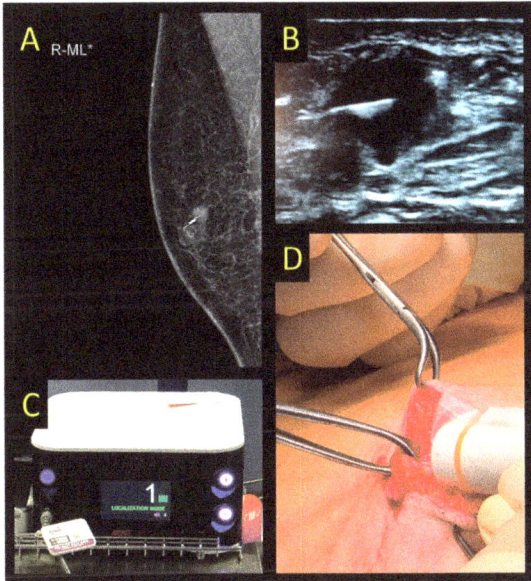

Figure 5. SAVI SCOUT system. (**A**) Control mammography after ultrasound-guided marker placement in a patient with an invasive breast cancer, NST, max. size: 12 mm. (**B**) Ultrasound of the marker and lesion. (**C**) Console used for detection in the operating room. (**D**) Intraoperative use of radar probe to guide excision.

Initial successful data from a pilot study led to a multicenter study [67]. The primary endpoints were the rates of successful reflector placement, localization, and removal in a patient cohort scheduled to have an excisional biopsy or breast-conserving surgery of a non-palpable breast lesion. SCOUT reflectors were successfully placed in 153 of 154 patients, but in one case, the reflector was placed at such a distance from the target that an additional wire had to be placed. All 154 lesions and reflectors were successfully removed during surgery [67].

A systematic review and pooled analysis of 842 cases (11 studies) revealed an overall successful deployment rate of 99.64% and a successful retrieval rate of 99.64% using the radar reflector system. A statistically significant difference in re-excision rate was found in a smaller pooled analysis conducted across four studies comparing radar reflectors and

WGL (12.9% and 21.1% respectively, $p < 0.01$) [4]. This should be interpreted with caution as each study was small, two of these studies are unpublished, and only 264 patients were included in this analysis.

The migration rate of the SCOUT reflector post-placement is low at 1.3%, and location stability was demonstrated across multiple studies up to 516 days post placement [4,67–71]. MRI artifacts may occur but are smaller than those created by magnetic or RFID markers [56,68]. There is no significant evidence evaluating the size of the surgical specimen or cost-effectiveness of the device. There is a failure rate of the device through damage of the antennae prior to surgery or by diathermy, but its magnitude and clinical impact are unclear. There is evidence demonstrating good patient, physician, and radiologist satisfaction but this is limited to a single-arm study [58].

2.6. Radiofrequency Identification Tags

Radiofrequency identification (RFID; LOCalizer, Hologic Inc., Santa Clara, CA, USA) is a relatively new but promising technology. The LOCalizer received FDA approval in April 2017 and European CE marking in October 2018, and is approved for marking of breast lesions, not axillary nodes. The RFID marker is a small radiofrequency 'tag,' identified with a small portable hand-held device which also comes with a pencil-sized single use probe (Figure 6). It displays the real-time distance to the tag in millimeters, and a unique tag identification number discerns each individual tag if more than one was inserted. [72].

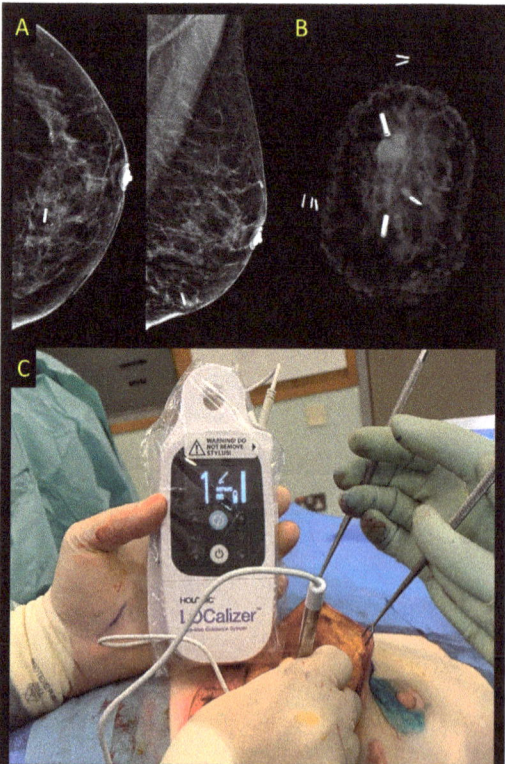

Figure 6. LOCalizer system. (**A**) Control mammography after ultrasound-guided placement of two RFID markers (one of them is near the thoracic wall and therefore not visible on the mammogram). (**B**) Specimen radiogram confirming the excision of both markers and the lesion. (**C**) Intraoperative use of the radiofrequency probe to guide excision.

The implantable seed is large compared to other markers, 11 × 2 mm, requiring a 12G needle for deployment. Since the needle is relatively blunt and does not penetrate the skin easily, a small skin incision is needed [73]. Hypothetically, the needle size may cause a wider tract that can result in seed migration. While this had not been reported in the limited literature, there are descriptions that the tag may move intraoperatively while the specimen is being retracted and mobilized [74,75]. Some also have reported loss of previously placed titanium marker clips while inserting the tags [73]. Moreover, the large needle size may pose a challenge to accurate insertion in the dense breast and in hard masses where the tag sometimes resides at the edge of the lesion [73].

An important consideration when planning for RFID are its potential interference with defibrillators and pacemakers, so RFID should be avoided in these patients [74]. Furthermore, a significant MRI artifact of about 2–2.5 cm needs to be accommodated for and is partly caused by the glass encasing [18,74]. Deep lesions in larger breasts can pose a challenge as the RFID detection range is 6 cm [72]. In available studies, patients felt that the procedure went smooth and was easier than expected, with high patient satisfaction rates [76,77], while surgeons and radiologists reported that the device was at least as fast and reliable as WGL [76] or even better [77].

The published body of evidence is limited but growing. In a recent systematic review, nine prospective and retrospective studies were included. Seven studies including 1151 patients and 1344 tags showed a pooled accurate deployment rate of 99.1%, a retrieval rate of 100%, and a re-excision rate of 13.9%. This suggests the device may not migrate although this had not been specifically investigated. Two further studies compared RFID with WGL; the pooled re-excision rate was comparable at 15.6% (20/128 vs. 44/282, respectively, $p = 0.995$) but the datasets are relatively small [18]. Furthermore there are no comparative data regarding patient, surgeon or radiologist experience, cost-effectiveness, or size of surgical specimens [78]. Most data stem from single-center, heterogeneously designed studies at risk of bias, which underlines a need for high-quality data collection to validate early, promising datasets. Although LOCalizer is only licenced for use in the breast, some have also used it to mark axillary nodes for targeted dissection [5].

2.7. Intraoperative Ultrasound

In the first publication on intraoperative ultrasound (IOUS)-guided surgery in 1988, Schwartz and colleagues found that ultrasound (US) was an accurate and effective tool for localizing breast masses, thus facilitating the surgical excision [79]. Since then, multiple manuscripts have reported on the use of IOUS to guide breast-conservative surgery in non-palpable breast cancer [80–82]. Using this technique, no preoperative localization procedure is necessary. IOUS is performed using a multifrequency probe covered in sterile sheath that ranges from 7 Mhz to 18 Mhz. Smaller probes that are easily introduced into the breast incision can be incorporated to improve visibility during surgery. The method is limited to targets visible on US (either the lesion itself or a sonographically visible marker (Figure 7)) [83]. Furthermore, an US machine needs to be available in the operating room during the procedure, and surgeon training in breast ultrasound is a requirement. A major reported benefit of IOUS is the omission of preoperative localization, which avoids the burden of an additional radiology appointment and facilitates an easy workflow towards surgery. IOUS also allows for continuous margin assessment during surgery and ex vivo margin evaluation directly after specimen removal.

The available evidence on IOUS stems from several RCTs and meta-analyses, as well as cohort studies [8,10,11]. Three RCTs compared IOUS with WGL in non-palpable breast cancer, and a further three RCTs compared IOUS with palpation-guided surgery in patients with palpable tumors [8]. The studies showed a high successful excision rate of target lesions. In addition, various meta-analyses have demonstrated that IOUS significantly increases negative margin rates when compared to WGL [8,10,11,84]. Re-excision of positive or very close margins already identified by intraoperative US reduces the need for a second surgical procedure [8,10,11]. Based on these results, the AGO Breast Committee updated its guidelines in 2022 and endorses IOUS for removal of non-palpable breast cancer with a strong level of recommendation [7,85].

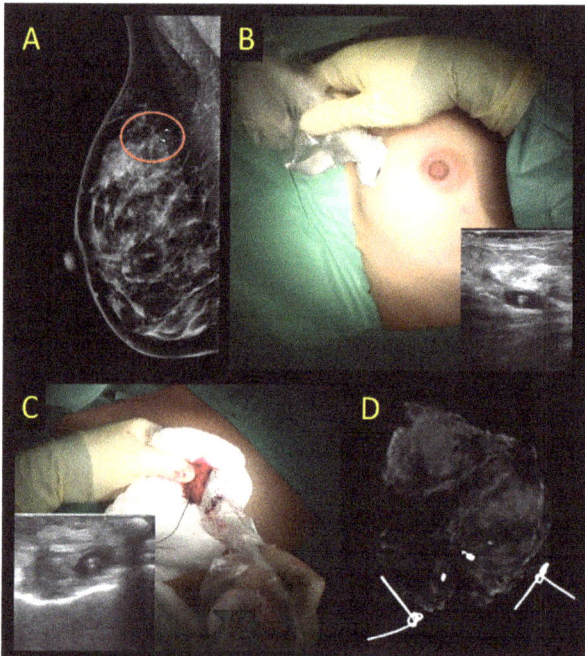

Figure 7. Ultrasound-guided excision of ductal carcinoma in situ with a preoperative placement of an US-visible marker. (**A**) Area of microcalcifications surrounding the US-visible marker seen on preoperative imaging. (**B**) Assessing marker before incision with IOUS with US-visible marker. (**C**) Specimen ultrasound after excision of the clip-marked area confirming marker removal. (**D**) Specimen radiograph to assess microcalcifications excised.

There are few cost-efficiency studies comparing IOUS and WGL, probably due to the complexity considering not only direct but also indirect costs, and their equivalence in quality-adjusted life years (QALY). Available studies show lower costs with IOUS than with WGL [86]. One study evaluated costs related to the use of US-visible clips compared with traditional clips and favored US as a means of localization when feasible. There was an estimated cost saving of USD 36,000 over the 3-year study period despite the initially higher cost of US-visible clips. US localization with US-visible markers thus appears to be cost-effective and spares patients an additional wire placement, which can evoke unnecessary stress and anxiety before surgery [87].

Another advantage of IOUS is the potential for resecting less surrounding healthy breast tissue. The randomized COBALT trial showed lower excised volumes when using IOUS when compared to palpation-guided surgery, which significantly affected cosmetic outcomes and patient satisfaction [88]. No data on surgeon satisfaction with IOUS are available. In the neoadjuvant chemotherapy (NACT) setting, where WGL traditionally has been the standard, IOUS can be used if a residual lesion or an US-visible marker is present [89,90].

Several researchers evaluated the extent of the learning curve to acquire the necessary skills for IOUS. Most surgeons reached mastering level after 7–17 cases, with an average of 11 cases [86]. Others have measured proficiency by observational studies that recorded calculated resection ratios by three surgeons performing ten cases of IOUS surgery each and found this case number to be sufficient to master the technique [91].

2.8. Carbon Suspension

The use of a sterile aqueous suspension of carbon powder for the stereotactic marking of occult breast lesions was first described in 56 patients by radiologist Gunilla Svane at Karolinska University Hospital in Sweden in 1983 [25]. The tip of the injection needle was placed in the direct vicinity of the lesion, and a technique was devised allowing the even distribution of carbon suspension over the entire length of a carbon track from lesion to skin, marking the point of entry with a small skin tattoo (Figure 8). Four lesions were missed at first operation or incompletely excised, probably owing to the fact that the concentration of the carbon solution was lower than later recommended in three cases; the fourth case was a fibroadenoma displaced by 5 mm during marking. Subsequently, the method was reported in a few publications [20,92–94]. Interruption of the carbon track between skin and lesion may occur during release of pressure after mammography if carbon is placed by stereotaxis, which makes following the carbon track more difficult than when carbon is placed by ultrasound guidance [20]. Since carbon does not yield any acoustic signal, a carbon track placed by stereotaxis entering the skin distant from the lesion location may be challenging, and US-guided placement may facilitate correct excision significantly. In contrast to ink marking, carbon does not bleed into surrounding tissue and does not migrate over time, thus making the method feasible for use before NACT. As carbon is not visible on specimen radiography, it may be combined with clip placement in neoadjuvant cases where the original lesion may undergo complete regression and thus otherwise lose visibility on imaging. The main perceived advantages of carbon localization are its low cost, easy availability, simple logistics, and durability over time, although there is poor quality data supporting its use and no comparative datasets. Currently, this remains a technique that is yet to gain widespread adoption in breast localization and offers no high-quality evidence on accuracy, margin involvement, cost-effectiveness, or patient/surgeon satisfaction.

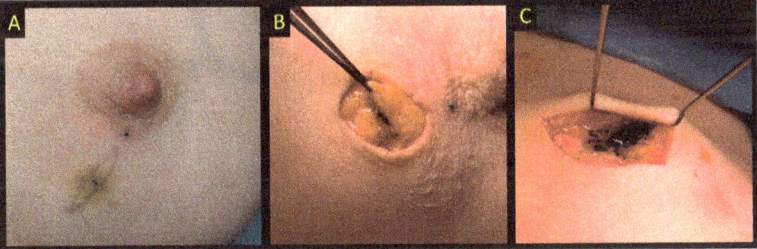

Figure 8. Carbon ink localization. (**A**) Intentional skin tattoo to mark the exact position of the lesion. (**B**,**C**) Intraoperative photos showing carbon ink in the tissue that will guide excision.

In contrast, there is a rapidly emerging use of carbon marking for axillary lymph nodes in patients receiving NACT, demonstrating 82–98% accuracy of removal of the targeted node [95–100].

3. The MELODY Study

MELODY, initiated as an intergroup study between EUBREAST and iBRA-NET, is a prospective non-interventional multicohort study aiming to evaluate different localization techniques for non-palpable breast cancer (http://melody.eubreast.com; accessed on 11 December 2022 (Figure 9)). With a target accrual of 7416 patients, the study is powered to resolve several knowledge gaps. Patients with invasive breast cancer or ductal carcinoma in situ (DCIS), confirmed by minimally invasive biopsy, and scheduled to receive breast-conserving surgery, can be enrolled. The use of NACT and preoperative endocrine therapy are allowed. Marking and localization procedures and treatment modalities are chosen at the discretion of the treating physicians and according to national and institutional guidelines. Inclusion and exclusion criteria are presented in Table 3. Patients will be followed for 30 days postoperatively for potential complications. No long-term surveillance is required.

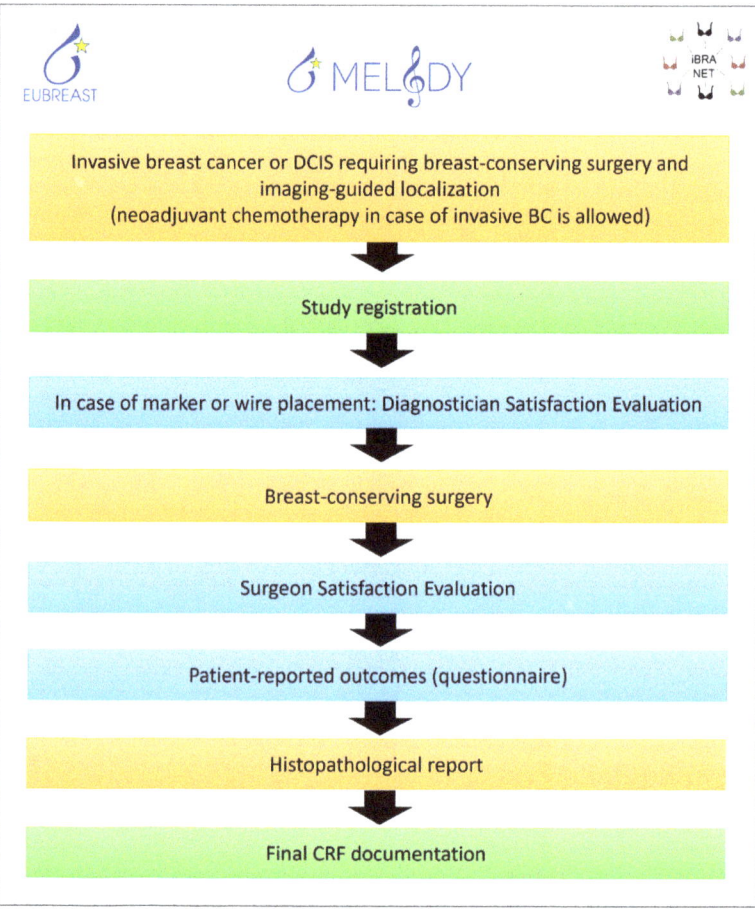

Figure 9. MELODY flow chart.

Table 3. The MELODY study: Inclusion and exclusion criteria.

Inclusion Criteria	Exclusion Criteria
<ul><li>Signed informed consent form</li><li>Malignant breast lesion requiring breast-conserving surgery and imaging-guided localization (either DCIS or invasive breast cancer; multiple or bilateral lesions and the use of neoadjuvant chemotherapy are allowed)</li><li>Planned surgical removal of the lesion using one or more of the following imaging-guided localization techniques:<ul><li>○ Wire-guided localization;</li><li>○ Intraoperative ultrasound;</li><li>○ Magnetic localization;</li><li>○ Radioactive seed localization;</li><li>○ Radio-guided Occult Lesion Localization (ROLL);</li><li>○ Radar localization;</li><li>○ Radiofrequency identification (RFID) tag localization;</li><li>○ Ink/carbon localization.</li></ul></li><li>Female/male patients ≥ 18 years old</li></ul>	<ul><li>Patients not suitable for surgical treatment</li><li>Patients requiring mastectomy as first surgery</li><li>Surgical removal without imaging-guided localization</li></ul>

MELODY is supported by the AGO-B study group, the Oncoplastic Breast Consortium (OPBC), SENATURK, AWOgyn (German Working Group for Reconstructive Surgery in Oncology-Gynecology), and German Breast Group (GBG).

Primary Study Endpoints:

1. Intended target lesion and/or marker removal, independent of margin status on final histopathology;
2. Negative resection margin rates (defined as lesion removal with no invasive or non-invasive carcinoma on ink) at first surgery.

Secondary Study Endpoints:

3. Rates of second surgery;
4. Rates of secondary mastectomy;
5. Resection ratio, defined as actual resection volume divided by the calculated optimum specimen volume;
6. Duration of surgery in BC patients, defined as time between first incision and end of skin closure (patients receiving simultaneous reconstructive, oncoplastic or contralateral surgery will be excluded from this analysis);
7. Marker dislocation rates;
8. Rates of marker placement failure, i.e., marker dislocation requiring a placement of a second marker;
9. Rates of localization failure, i.e., failed removal of marker or lesion, or necessity to switch to another intraoperative localization method;
10. Patient-reported outcomes (e.g., patient discomfort, pain level, and impairment of breathing);
11. Diagnostician/radiologist satisfaction with marking technique;
12. Surgeon satisfaction with localization technique;
13. Rates of "lost markers" (defined as markers placed prior to surgery and not retrieved at surgery);
14. Volume and weight of resected tissue;
15. Impact of experience of study sites on other outcome measures, depending on the localization technique used;
16. Impact of self-reported ethnicity on outcome measures;
17. Evaluation of surgical standards of care in different countries;
18. Evaluation of economic resources required for different localization techniques (material costs, operative time etc.);
19. Evaluation of MRI artifacts;
20. Evaluation of complication rates related to marker placement;
21. Evaluation of peri- and postoperative complication rates.

The first MELODY study site has opened in Q4 2022. Currently, 20 countries are planning to participate in the study, most of which are in the process of applying for ethical approval.

4. Conclusions

Wire-guided techniques represented the gold standard for the localization and removal of non-palpable breast lesions for more than a century. Numerous disadvantages of the procedure from a patient as well as a surgeon perspective have put this standard into question for almost two decades. The introduction of intraoperative ultrasound and probe-guided technologies provided new options that currently intensify the discussion on replacement of WGL by more sophisticated technologies. While IOUS offers favorable rates of clear margins and re-excisions compared to WGL, its use is restricted to solid masses and requires high expertise from the surgeon. Radioactive seeds are cheap and RSL has shown equivalence to WGL with regard to successful lesion localization and removal. Its use is, however, not widely available due to radiation protection regulations in many countries. Non-wire and non-radio-guided techniques using magnetic or paramagnetic markers, radar reflectors, or radiofrequency identification tags are promising in this context and provide excellent early results compared to competing technologies. The devices, however, have a high upfront cost, although the cost-effectiveness of the whole pathway is not established. Carbon localization is a cost-effective option used in some countries. Modification of treatment standards and the introduction of new and potentially more cost-intensive technologies require solid evidence with regard to clinical effectiveness as well as patient and clinician satisfaction. The MELODY study aims to close this important knowledge gap by comparing all available localization techniques in a single prospective cohort study with regard to clinically relevant endpoints.

Author Contributions: Manuscript writing: M.B.-P., T.K., Y.M., I.R., J.d.B., N.D., G.K.C., A.K. (Andreas Karakatsanis) and J.H., Manuscript editing: M.B.-P., T.K., Y.M., I.R., J.d.B., N.D., G.K.C., A.K. (Andreas Karakatsanis), R.D., M.H., S.P., A.K. (Ashutosh Kothari), O.D.G., B.M.G., M.P.L., M.S., W.P.W., B.A.S., N.K., S.H., S.N., F.M., N.C., N.Z.C., R.D.M., M.L.G., D.M. and J.H. All authors have read and agreed to the published version of the manuscript.

Funding: The MELODY study will be financially supported by: Hologic, Merit Medical, Endomag and Sirius Medical.

Conflicts of Interest: Maggie Banys-Paluchowski has received honoraria for lectures and participation in advisory boards: Roche, Novartis, Pfizer, pfm, Eli Lilly, Onkowissen, Seagen, AstraZeneca, Eisai, AstraZeneca, Amgen, Samsung, MSD, GSK, Daiichi Sankyo, Gilead, Canon, Sirius Pintuition, and Pierre Fabre; and study support from Endomag, Mammotome, MeritMedical, Gilead, ExactSciences. Ash Kothari has received a research grant from Endomag and acts as PI of the respective study. Andreas Karakatsanis has received a research grant from Endomag; acts as PI of the respective study; and recieved honoraria from Pfizer and Resitu AB. Michael P. Lux received honoraria for lectures and advisory participation from Lilly, AstraZeneca, MSD, Roche, Novartis, Pfizer, Eisai, Exact Sciences, Daiichi-Sankyo, Grünenthal, Gilead, Pierre Fabre, PharmaMar, pfm, Samantree, and Endomag; travel expenses from AstraZeneca, Roche, and Pfizer; editorial board membership for medac. Francois Malherbe received honoraria and travel support from Sysmex, the local distributor of Magseed. Dawid Murawa received honoraria for lectures from Roche, Medtronic, Stryker, Mammotome, MDT—diagnostic green, GEM-Italy, Combat-Medical. Other authors declared no conflicts of interest.

References

1. Schermers, B.; van Riet, Y.E.; Schipper, R.J.; Vrancken Peeters, M.J.; Voogd, A.C.; Nieuwenhuijzen, G.A.P.; Ten Haken, B.; Ruers, T.J.M. Nationwide registry study on trends in localization techniques and reoperation rates in non-palpable ductal carcinoma in situ and invasive breast cancer. *Br. J. Surg.* **2021**, *109*, 53–60. [CrossRef] [PubMed]
2. Somasundaram, S.K.; Potter, S.; Elgammal, S.; Maxwell, A.J.; Sami, A.S.; Down, S.K.; Dave, R.V.; Harvey, J. Impalpable breast lesion localisation, a logistical challenge: Results of the UK iBRA-NET national practice questionnaire. *Breast Cancer Res. Treat.* **2021**, *185*, 13–20. [CrossRef] [PubMed]
3. Hirst, A.; Agha, R.A.; Rosin, D.; McCulloch, P. How can we improve surgical research and innovation?: The IDEAL framework for action. *Int. J. Surg.* **2013**, *11*, 1038–1042. [CrossRef] [PubMed]
4. Kasem, I.; Mokbel, K. Savi Scout(R) Radar Localisation of Non-palpable Breast Lesions: Systematic Review and Pooled Analysis of 842 Cases. *Anticancer Res.* **2020**, *40*, 3633–3643. [CrossRef]
5. Lowes, S.; Bell, A.; Milligan, R.; Amonkar, S.; Leaver, A. Use of Hologic LOCalizer radiofrequency identification (RFID) tags to localise impalpable breast lesions and axillary nodes: Experience of the first 150 cases in a UK breast unit. *Clin. Radiol.* **2020**, *75*, 942–949. [CrossRef]
6. Ergina, P.L.; Barkun, J.S.; McCulloch, P.; Cook, J.A.; Altman, D.G.; Group, I. IDEAL framework for surgical innovation 2: Observational studies in the exploration and assessment stages. *BMJ* **2013**, *346*, f3011. [CrossRef]
7. Ditsch, N.; Woeckel, A.; Untch, M.; Jackisch, C.; Albert, U.S.; Banys-Paluchowski, M.; Bauerfeind, I.; Blohmer, J. AGO Recommendations for the Diagnosis and Treatment of Patients with Early Breast Cancer (EBC): Update 2022. *Breast Care* **2022**, *17*, 403–420. [CrossRef]
8. Banys-Paluchowski, M.; Rubio, I.T.; Karadeniz Cakmak, G.; Esgueva, A.; Krawczyk, N.; Paluchowski, P.; Gruber, I.; Marx, M.; Brucker, S.Y.; Bundgen, N.; et al. Intraoperative Ultrasound-Guided Excision of Non-Palpable and Palpable Breast Cancer: Systematic Review and Meta-Analysis. *Ultraschall Med.* **2022**, *43*, 367–379. [CrossRef]
9. Chan, B.K.; Wiseberg-Firtell, J.A.; Jois, R.H.; Jensen, K.; Audisio, R.A. Localization techniques for guided surgical excision of non-palpable breast lesions. *Cochrane Database Syst. Rev.* **2015**, *12*, CD009206. [CrossRef]

10. Davey, M.G.; O'Donnell, J.P.M.; Boland, M.R.; Ryan, E.J.; Walsh, S.R.; Kerin, M.J.; Lowery, A.J. Optimal localization strategies for non-palpable breast cancers—A network meta-analysis of randomized controlled trials. *Breast* **2022**, *62*, 103–113. [CrossRef]
11. Athanasiou, C.; Mallidis, E.; Tuffaha, H. Comparative effectiveness of different localization techniques for non-palpable breast cancer. A systematic review and network meta-analysis. *Eur. J. Surg. Oncol.* **2022**, *48*, 53–59. [CrossRef] [PubMed]
12. Dave, R.V.; Barrett, E.; Morgan, J.; Chandarana, M.; Elgammal, S.; Barnes, N.; Sami, A.; Masudi, T.; Down, S.; Holcombe, C.; et al. Wire- and magnetic-seed-guided localization of impalpable breast lesions: iBRA-NET localisation study. *Br. J. Surg.* **2022**, *109*, 274–282. [CrossRef] [PubMed]
13. Tang, S.S.; Kaptanis, S.; Haddow, J.B.; Mondani, G.; Elsberger, B.; Tasoulis, M.K.; Obondo, C.; Johns, N.; Ismail, W.; Syed, A.; et al. Current margin practice and effect on re-excision rates following the publication of the SSO-ASTRO consensus and ABS consensus guidelines: A national prospective study of 2858 women undergoing breast-conserving therapy in the UK and Ireland. *Eur. J. Cancer* **2017**, *84*, 315–324. [CrossRef] [PubMed]
14. Langhans, L.; Jensen, M.B.; Talman, M.M.; Vejborg, I.; Kroman, N.; Tvedskov, T.F. Reoperation Rates in Ductal Carcinoma In Situ vs Invasive Breast Cancer After Wire-Guided Breast-Conserving Surgery. *JAMA Surg.* **2017**, *152*, 378–384. [CrossRef]
15. Struik, G.M.; Schermers, B.; Mares, I.; Lont, H.E.; Bradshaw, J.W.; Ten Haken, B.; Ruers, T.J.M.; Mourik, J.E.M.; Birnie, E.; Klem, T. Randomized controlled trial comparing magnetic marker localization (MaMaLoc) with wire-guided localization in the treatment of early-stage breast cancer. *Breast J.* **2021**, *27*, 638–650. [CrossRef]
16. Look Hong, N.; Wright, F.C.; Semple, M.; Nicolae, A.M.; Ravi, A. Results of a phase I, non-randomized study evaluating a Magnetic Occult Lesion Localization Instrument (MOLLI) for excision of non-palpable breast lesions. *Breast Cancer Res. Treat.* **2020**, *179*, 671–676. [CrossRef]
17. Kurita, T.; Taruno, K.; Nakamura, S.; Takei, H.; Enokido, K.; Kuwayama, T.; Kanada, Y.; Akashi-Tanaka, S.; Matsuyanagi, M.; Hankyo, M.; et al. Magnetically Guided Localization Using a Guiding-Marker System((R)) and a Handheld Magnetic Probe for Nonpalpable Breast Lesions: A Multicenter Feasibility Study in Japan. *Cancers* **2021**, *13*, 2923. [CrossRef]
18. Tayeh, S.; Wazir, U.; Mokbel, K. The Evolving Role of Radiofrequency Guided Localisation in Breast Surgery: A Systematic Review. *Cancers* **2021**, *13*, 4996. [CrossRef]
19. Shaughnessy, E.; Vijapura, C.; Reyna, C.; Lewis, J.; Lewis, K.; Lee, S.J.; Sobel, L.; Wahab, R.; Rosen, L.; Brown, A. Exploiting the advantages of a wireless seed localization system that differentiates between the seeds: Breast cancer resection following neoadjuvant chemotherapy. *Cancer Rep.* **2022**, *6*, e1690. [CrossRef]
20. Arman, A.; Kilicoglu, G.; Guner, H.H.; Celik, L. Marking of nonpalpable breast lesions using a custom carbon suspension. *Acta Radiol.* **2001**, *42*, 599–601. [CrossRef]
21. Moss, H.A.; Barter, S.J.; Nayagam, M.; Lawrence, D.; Pittam, M. The use of carbon suspension as an adjunct to wire localisation of impalpable breast lesions. *Clin. Radiol.* **2002**, *57*, 937–944. [CrossRef] [PubMed]
22. Rose, A.; Collins, J.P.; Neerhut, P.; Bishop, C.V.; Mann, G.B. Carbon localisation of impalpable breast lesions. *Breast* **2003**, *12*, 264–269. [CrossRef] [PubMed]
23. Mazy, S.; Galant, C.; Berliere, M.; Mazy, G. Localization of non-palpable breast lesions with black carbon powder (experience of the Catholic University of Louvain). *J. Radiol.* **2001**, *82*, 161–164. [PubMed]
24. Riedl, C.C.; Pfarl, G.; Helbich, T.H.; Memarsadeghi, M.; Wagner, T.; Rudas, M.; Fuchsjager, M. Comparison of wire versus carbon localization of non-palpable breast lesions. *Rofo* **2002**, *174*, 1126–1131. [CrossRef]
25. Svane, G. A stereotaxic technique for preoperative marking of non-palpable breast lesions. *Acta Radiol. Diagn.* **1983**, *24*, 145–151. [CrossRef]
26. Banys-Paluchowski, M.; Gruber, I.V.; Hartkopf, A.; Paluchowski, P.; Krawczyk, N.; Marx, M.; Brucker, S.; Hahn, M. Axillary ultrasound for prediction of response to neoadjuvant therapy in the context of surgical strategies to axillary dissection in primary breast cancer: A systematic review of the current literature. *Arch. Gynecol. Obstet.* **2020**, *301*, 341–353. [CrossRef]
27. Dauway, E.L., Sanders, R.; Freidland, J. Innovative diagnostics for breast cancer: New frontiers for the new millennium using radioactive seed localization. Presented at the 85th Annual American College of Surgeons Clinical Congress, Chicago, IL, USA; 1999.
28. Simons, J.M.; van Nijnatten, T.J.; Koppert, L.B.; Van der Pol, C.C.; Van Diest, P.J.; Jager, A.; Van Klaveren, D.; Kam, B.L.R.; Lobbes, M.B.I.; De Boer, M.; et al. Radioactive Iodine Seed placement in the Axilla with Sentinel lymph node biopsy after neoadjuvant chemotherapy in breast cancer: Results of the prospective multicenter RISAS trial. In Proceedings of the San Antonio Breast Cancer Symposium 2020, Abstract GS1-10, Virtual, 8–11 December 2020.
29. Donker, M.; Straver, M.E.; Wesseling, J.; Loo, C.E.; Schot, M.; Drukker, C.A.; van Tinteren, H.; Sonke, G.S.; Rutgers, E.J.; Vrancken Peeters, M.J. Marking axillary lymph nodes with radioactive iodine seeds for axillary staging after neoadjuvant systemic treatment in breast cancer patients: The MARI procedure. *Ann. Surg.* **2015**, *261*, 378–382. [CrossRef]
30. Langhans, L.; Tvedskov, T.F.; Klausen, T.L.; Jensen, M.B.; Talman, M.L.; Vejborg, I.; Benian, C.; Roslind, A.; Hermansen, J.; Oturai, P.S.; et al. Radioactive Seed Localization or Wire-guided Localization of Nonpalpable Invasive and In Situ Breast Cancer: A Randomized, Multicenter, Open-label Trial. *Ann. Surg.* **2017**, *266*, 29–35. [CrossRef]
31. Bloomquist, E.V.; Ajkay, N.; Patil, S.; Collett, A.E.; Frazier, T.G.; Barrio, A.V. A Randomized Prospective Comparison of Patient-Assessed Satisfaction and Clinical Outcomes with Radioactive Seed Localization versus Wire Localization. *Breast J.* **2016**, *22*, 151–157. [CrossRef]

32. Taylor, D.B.; Bourke, A.G.; Westcott, E.J.; Marinovich, M.L.; Chong, C.Y.L.; Liang, R.; Hughes, R.L.; Elder, E.; Saunders, C.M. Surgical outcomes after radioactive 125I seed versus hookwire localization of non-palpable breast cancer: A multicentre randomized clinical trial. *Br. J. Surg.* **2021**, *108*, 40–48. [CrossRef]
33. Lovrics, P.J.; Goldsmith, C.H.; Hodgson, N.; McCready, D.; Gohla, G.; Boylan, C.; Cornacchi, S.; Reedijk, M. A multicentered, randomized, controlled trial comparing radioguided seed localization to standard wire localization for nonpalpable, invasive and in situ breast carcinomas. *Ann. Surg. Oncol.* **2011**, *18*, 3407–3414. [CrossRef]
34. Gray, R.J.; Salud, C.; Nguyen, K.; Dauway, E.; Friedland, J.; Berman, C.; Peltz, E.; Whitehead, G.; Cox, C.E. Randomized prospective evaluation of a novel technique for biopsy or lumpectomy of nonpalpable breast lesions: Radioactive seed versus wire localization. *Ann. Surg. Oncol.* **2001**, *8*, 711–715. [CrossRef] [PubMed]
35. Parvez, E.; Cornacchi, S.D.; Hodgson, N.; Thoma, A.; Kong, I.; Foster, G.; Cheng, J.; Goldsmith, C.H.; Dao, D.; Lovrics, P.J. A cosmesis outcome substudy in a prospective, randomized trial comparing radioguided seed localization with standard wire localization for nonpalpable, invasive, and in situ breast carcinomas. *Am. J. Surg.* **2014**, *208*, 711–718. [CrossRef] [PubMed]
36. Wang, G.L.; Tsikouras, P.; Zuo, H.Q.; Huang, M.Q.; Peng, L.; Bothou, A.; Zervoudis, S.; Tobias Teichmann, A. Radioactive seed localization and wire guided localization in breast cancer: A systematic review and meta-analysis. *J. BUON* **2019**, *24*, 48–60.
37. Pouw, B.; de Wit-van der Veen, L.J.; Stokkel, M.P.; Loo, C.E.; Vrancken Peeters, M.J.; Valdes Olmos, R.A. Heading toward radioactive seed localization in non-palpable breast cancer surgery? A meta-analysis. *J. Surg. Oncol.* **2015**, *111*, 185–191. [CrossRef] [PubMed]
38. Lee, C.; Bhatt, A.; Felmlee, J.P.; Trester, P.; Lanners, D.; Paulsen, A.; Brunette, J. How to Safely Perform Magnetic Resonance Imaging-guided Radioactive Seed Localizations in the Breast. *J. Clin. Imaging Sci.* **2020**, *10*, 19. [CrossRef] [PubMed]
39. Lindenberg, M.; van Beek, A.; Retel, V.; van Duijnhoven, F.; van Harten, W. Early budget impact analysis on magnetic seed localization for non-palpable breast cancer surgery. *PLoS ONE* **2020**, *15*, e0232690. [CrossRef]
40. Zhang, Y.; Seely, J.; Cordeiro, E.; Hefler, J.; Thavorn, K.; Mahajan, M.; Domina, S.; Aro, J.; Ibrahim, A.M.; Arnaout, A.; et al. Radioactive Seed Localization Versus Wire-Guided Localization for Nonpalpable Breast Cancer: A Cost and Operating Room Efficiency Analysis. *Ann. Surg. Oncol.* **2017**, *24*, 3567–3573. [CrossRef]
41. Loving, V.A.; Edwards, D.B.; Roche, K.T.; Steele, J.R.; Sapareto, S.A.; Byrum, S.C.; Schomer, D.F. Monte Carlo simulation to analyze the cost-benefit of radioactive seed localization versus wire localization for breast-conserving surgery in fee-for-service health care systems compared with accountable care organizations. *AJR Am. J. Roentgenol.* **2014**, *202*, 1383–1388. [CrossRef]
42. Alderliesten, T.; Loo, C.E.; Pengel, K.E.; Rutgers, E.J.T.; Gilhuijs, K.G.A.; Vrancken Peeters, M.J. Radioactive Seed Localization of Breast Lesions: An Adequate Localization Method without Seed Migration. *Breast J.* **2011**, *17*, 594–601. [CrossRef]
43. Luini, A.; Zurrida, S.; Paganelli, G.; Galimberti, V.; Sacchini, V.; Monti, S.; Veronesi, P.; Viale, G.; Veronesi, U. Comparison of radioguided excision with wire localization of occult breast lesions. *Br. J. Surg.* **1999**, *86*, 522–525. [CrossRef] [PubMed]
44. Monti, S.; Galimberti, V.; Trifiro, G.; De Cicco, C.; Peradze, N.; Brenelli, F.; Fernandez-Rodriguez, J.; Rotmensz, N.; Latronico, A.; Berrettini, A.; et al. Occult breast lesion localization plus sentinel node biopsy (SNOLL): Experience with 959 patients at the European Institute of Oncology. *Ann. Surg. Oncol.* **2007**, *14*, 2928–2931. [CrossRef]
45. Moreno, M.; Wiltgen, J.E.; Bodanese, B.; Schmitt, R.L.; Gutfilen, B.; da Fonseca, L.M. Radioguided breast surgery for occult lesion localization—Correlation between two methods. *J. Exp. Clin. Cancer Res.* **2008**, *27*, 29. [CrossRef] [PubMed]
46. Medina-Franco, H.; Abarca-Perez, L.; Ulloa-Gomez, J.L.; Romero, C. Radioguided localization of clinically occult breast lesions (ROLL): A pilot study. *Breast J.* **2007**, *13*, 401–405. [CrossRef]
47. Rampaul, R.S.; Bagnall, M.; Burrell, H.; Pinder, S.E.; Evans, A.J.; Macmillan, R.D. Randomized clinical trial comparing radioisotope occult lesion localization and wire-guided excision for biopsy of occult breast lesions. *Br. J. Surg.* **2004**, *91*, 1575–1577. [CrossRef]
48. Duarte, C.; Bastidas, F.; de los Reyes, A.; Martinez, M.C.; Hurtado, G.; Gomez, M.C.; Sanchez, R.; Manrique, J. Randomized controlled clinical trial comparing radioguided occult lesion localization with wire-guided lesion localization to evaluate their efficacy and accuracy in the localization of nonpalpable breast lesions. *Surgery* **2016**, *159*, 1140–1145. [CrossRef]
49. Ocal, K.; Dag, A.; Turkmenoglu, O.; Gunay, E.C.; Yucel, E.; Duce, M.N. Radioguided occult lesion localization versus wire-guided localization for non-palpable breast lesions: Randomized controlled trial. *Clinics* **2011**, *66*, 1003–1007. [CrossRef]
50. Kanat, N.B.; Tuncel, M.; Aksoy, T.; Firat, A.; Demirkazik, F.; Onat, D.; Caglar Tuncali, M.; Caner, B.E. Comparison of wire-guided localization and radio-guided occult lesionlocalization in preoperative localization of nonpalpable breast lesions. *Turk. J. Med. Sci.* **2016**, *46*, 1829–1837. [CrossRef]
51. Postma, E.L.; Verkooijen, H.M.; van Esser, S.; Hobbelink, M.G.; van der Schelling, G.P.; Koelemij, R.; Witkamp, A.J.; Contant, C.; van Diest, P.J.; Willems, S.M.; et al. Efficacy of 'radioguided occult lesion localisation' (ROLL) versus 'wire-guided localisation' (WGL) in breast conserving surgery for non-palpable breast cancer: A randomised controlled multicentre trial. *Breast Cancer Res. Treat.* **2012**, *136*, 469–478. [CrossRef]
52. Alikhassi, A.; Saeed, F.; Abbasi, M.; Omranipour, R.; Mahmoodzadeh, H.; Najafi, M.; Gity, M.; Kheradmand, A. Applicability of Radioguided Occult Lesion Localization for NonPalpable Benign Breast Lesions, Comparison with Wire Localization, a Clinical Trial. *Asian Pac. J. Cancer Prev.* **2016**, *17*, 3185–3190.
53. Tang, J.; Xie, X.M.; Wang, X.; Xie, Z.M.; He, J.H.; Wu, Y.P.; Fan, W.; Fu, J.H.; Yang, M.T. Radiocolloid in combination with methylene dye localization, rather than wire localization, is a preferred procedure for excisional biopsy of nonpalpable breast lesions. *Ann. Surg. Oncol.* **2011**, *18*, 109–113. [CrossRef]

54. Mariscal Martinez, A.; Sola, M.; de Tudela, A.P.; Julian, J.F.; Fraile, M.; Vizcaya, S.; Fernandez, J. Radioguided localization of nonpalpable breast cancer lesions: Randomized comparison with wire localization in patients undergoing conservative surgery and sentinel node biopsy. *AJR Am. J. Roentgenol.* **2009**, *193*, 1001–1009. [CrossRef]
55. Philadelpho Arantes Pereira, F.; Martins, G.; Gregorio Calas, M.J.; Fonseca Torres de Oliveira, M.V.; Gasparetto, E.L.; Barbosa da Fonseca, L.M. Magnetic resonance imaging-radioguided occult lesion localization (ROLL) in breast cancer using Tc-99m macro-aggregated albumin and distilled water control. *BMC Med. Imaging* **2013**, *13*, 33. [CrossRef] [PubMed]
56. Hayes, M.K. Update on Preoperative Breast Localization. *Radiol. Clin. North Am.* **2017**, *55*, 591–603. [CrossRef] [PubMed]
57. D'Angelo, A.; Trombadori, C.M.L.; Caprini, F.; Lo Cicero, S.; Longo, V.; Ferrara, F.; Palma, S.; Conti, M.; Franco, A.; Scardina, L.; et al. Efficacy and Accuracy of Using Magnetic Seed for Preoperative Non-Palpable Breast Lesions Localization: Our Experience with Magseed. *Curr. Oncol.* **2022**, *29*, 8468–8474. [CrossRef] [PubMed]
58. Zacharioudakis, K.; Down, S.; Bholah, Z.; Lee, S.; Khan, T.; Maxwell, A.J.; Howe, M.; Harvey, J. Is the future magnetic? Magseed localisation for non palpable breast cancer. A multi-centre non randomised control study. *Eur. J. Surg. Oncol.* **2019**, *45*, 2016–2021. [CrossRef]
59. Harvey, J.R.; Lim, Y.; Murphy, J.; Howe, M.; Morris, J.; Goyal, A.; Maxwell, A.J. Safety and feasibility of breast lesion localization using magnetic seeds (Magseed): A multi-centre, open-label cohort study. *Breast Cancer Res. Treat.* **2018**, *169*, 531–536. [CrossRef]
60. Micha, A.E.; Sinnett, V.; Downey, K.; Allen, S.; Bishop, B.; Hector, L.R.; Patrick, E.P.; Edmonds, R.; Barry, P.A.; Krupa, K.D.C.; et al. Patient and clinician satisfaction and clinical outcomes of Magseed compared with wire-guided localisation for impalpable breast lesions. *Breast Cancer* **2021**, *28*, 196–205. [CrossRef]
61. Morgan, J.L.; Bromley, H.L.; Dave, R.V.; Masannat, Y.; Masudi, T.; Mylvaganam, S.; Elgammal, S.; Barnes, N.; Down, S.; Holcombe, C.; et al. Results of shared learning of a new magnetic seed localisation device–A UK iBRA-NET breast cancer localisation study. *Eur. J. Surg. Oncol.* **2022**, *48*, 2408–2413. [CrossRef]
62. Powell, M.; Gate, T.; Kalake, O.; Ranjith, C.; Pennick, M.O. Magnetic Seed Localization (Magseed) for excision of impalpable breast lesions-The North Wales experience. *Breast J.* **2021**, *27*, 529–536. [CrossRef]
63. Bessems, M.; van Breest Smallenburg, V.; van Bebber, I.; van Dijk, E.; van der Giessen, A.; Schermers, B.; Malloni, M. Safety and performance of Sirius Pintuition—A novel wire-free and non-radioactive localization system for breast cancer surgery. *Eur. J. Surg. Oncol.* **2022**, *47*, E1. [CrossRef]
64. Clement, C.; Heeren, A.; den Hoed, I.; Jansen, P.; Venmans, A. First experience with Sirius Pintuition®—A novel magnetic localization system for breast cancer surgery. *Eur. J. Surg. Oncol.* **2022**, *48*, E70. [CrossRef]
65. Bromley, H.L.; Dave, R.; Holcombe, C.; Potter, S.; Maxwell, A.J.; Kirwan, C.; Mylvaganam, S.; Elgammal, S.; Morgan, J.; Down, S.; et al. A Novel Mixed-Methods Platform Study Protocol for Investigating New Surgical Devices, with Embedded Shared Learning: ibra-net Breast Lesion Localisation Study. *Int. J. Surg. Protoc.* **2021**, *25*, 26–33. [CrossRef] [PubMed]
66. Banys-Paluchowski, M.; Thill, M.; Kuhn, T.; Ditsch, N.; Heil, J.; Wockel, A.; Fallenberg, E.; Friedrich, M.; Kummel, S.; Muller, V.; et al. AGO Recommendations for the Surgical Therapy of Breast Cancer: Update 2022. *Geburtshilfe Frauenheilkd* **2022**, *82*, 1031–1043. [CrossRef] [PubMed]
67. Cox, C.E.; Russell, S.; Prowler, V.; Carter, E.; Beard, A.; Mehindru, A.; Blumencranz, P.; Allen, K.; Portillo, M.; Whitworth, P.; et al. A Prospective, Single Arm, Multi-site, Clinical Evaluation of a Nonradioactive Surgical Guidance Technology for the Location of Nonpalpable Breast Lesions during Excision. *Ann. Surg. Oncol.* **2016**, *23*, 3168–3174. [CrossRef] [PubMed]
68. Tayeh, S.; Muktar, S.; Heeney, J.; Michell, M.J.; Perry, N.; Suaris, T.; Evans, D.; Malhotra, A.; Mokbel, K. Reflector-guided Localization of Non-palpable Breast Lesions: The First Reported European Evaluation of the SAVI SCOUT(R) System. *Anticancer Res.* **2020**, *40*, 3915–3924. [CrossRef]
69. Falcon, S.; Weinfurtner, R.J.; Mooney, B.; Niell, B.L. SAVI SCOUT(R) localization of breast lesions as a practical alternative to wires: Outcomes and suggestions for trouble-shooting. *Clin. Imaging* **2018**, *52*, 280–286. [CrossRef]
70. Cox, C.E.; Garcia-Henriquez, N.; Glancy, M.J.; Whitworth, P.; Cox, J.M.; Themar-Geck, M.; Prati, R.; Jung, M.; Russell, S.; Appleton, J.; et al. Pilot Study of a New Nonradioactive Surgical Guidance Technology for Locating Nonpalpable Breast Lesions. *Ann. Surg. Oncol.* **2016**, *23*, 1824–1830. [CrossRef]
71. Hayes, M.K.; Bloomquist, E.V.; Wright, H.R. Long Term SCOUT®Placement in Breast and Axillary Node Prior to Neoadjuvant Chemotherapy. Clinical Case Review. 2018. Available online: https://www.merit.com/wp-content/uploads/2019/12/Case-Review-Long-Term-Placement-in-Breast-and-Node-Prior-to-NAC.pdf (accessed on 28 December 2022).
72. Benoy, I.H.; Elst, H.; Van der Auwera, I.; Van Laere, S.; van Dam, P.; Van Marck, E.; Scharpe, S.; Vermeulen, P.B.; Dirix, L.Y. Real-time RT-PCR correlates with immunocytochemistry for the detection of disseminated epithelial cells in bone marrow aspirates of patients with breast cancer. *Br. J. Cancer* **2004**, *91*, 1813–1820. [CrossRef]
73. Lamb, L.R.; Gilman, L.; Specht, M.; D'Alessandro, H.A.; Miles, R.C.; Lehman, C.D. Retrospective Review of Preoperative Radiofrequency Tag Localization of Breast Lesions in 848 Patients. *AJR Am. J. Roentgenol.* **2021**, *217*, 605–612. [CrossRef]
74. Dauphine, C.; Reicher, J.J.; Reicher, M.A.; Gondusky, C.; Khalkhali, I.; Kim, M. A prospective clinical study to evaluate the safety and performance of wireless localization of nonpalpable breast lesions using radiofrequency identification technology. *AJR Am. J. Roentgenol.* **2015**, *204*, W720–W723. [CrossRef] [PubMed]
75. Singh, C.; Juette, A. Radio-Frequency Identifier Devices (RFIDs): Our Experience With Wireless Localisation in Non-palpable Breast Masses at a UK Tertiary Breast Imaging Unit. *Cureus* **2022**, *14*, e22402. [CrossRef] [PubMed]

76. DiNome, M.L.; Kusske, A.M.; Attai, D.J.; Fischer, C.P.; Hoyt, A.C. Microchipping the breast: An effective new technology for localizing non-palpable breast lesions for surgery. *Breast Cancer Res. Treat.* **2019**, *175*, 165–170. [CrossRef] [PubMed]
77. Wazir, U.; Tayeh, S.; Perry, N.; Michell, M.; Malhotra, A.; Mokbel, K. Wireless Breast Localization Using Radio-frequency Identification Tags: The First Reported European Experience in Breast Cancer. *Vivo* **2020**, *34*, 233–238. [CrossRef]
78. Heindl, F.; Schulz-Wendtland, R.; Jud, S.; Erber, R.; Hack, C.C.; Preuss, C.; Behrens, A.; Poschke, P.; Emons, J. Evaluation of a Wireless Localization System for Nonpalpable Breast Lesions—Feasibility and Cost-effectiveness in Everyday Clinical Routine. *Vivo* **2022**, *36*, 2342–2349. [CrossRef]
79. Schwartz, G.F.; Goldberg, B.B.; Rifkin, M.D.; D'Orazio, S.E. Ultrasonography: An alternative to x-ray-guided needle localization of nonpalpable breast masses. *Surgery* **1988**, *104*, 870–873.
80. Rubio, I.T.; Henry-Tillman, R.; Klimberg, V.S. Surgical use of breast ultrasound. *Surg. Clin. North Am.* **2003**, *83*, 771–788. [CrossRef]
81. Karadeniz Cakmak, G.; Emre, A.U.; Tascilar, O.; Bahadir, B.; Ozkan, S. Surgeon performed continuous intraoperative ultrasound guidance decreases re-excisions and mastectomy rates in breast cancer. *Breast* **2017**, *33*, 23–28. [CrossRef]
82. Kaufman, C.S.; Jacobson, L.; Bachman, B.; Kaufman, L. Intraoperative ultrasound facilitates surgery for early breast cancer. *Ann. Surg. Oncol.* **2002**, *9*, 988–993. [CrossRef]
83. Banys-Paluchowski, M.; Paluchowski, P.; Krawczyk, N. Twinkle artifact in sonographic breast clip visualization. *Arch. Gynecol. Obstet.* **2022**. [CrossRef]
84. Pan, H.; Wu, N.; Ding, H.; Ding, Q.; Dai, J.; Ling, L.; Chen, L.; Zha, X.; Liu, X.; Zhou, W.; et al. Intraoperative ultrasound guidance is associated with clear lumpectomy margins for breast cancer: A systematic review and meta-analysis. *PLoS ONE* **2013**, *8*, e74028. [CrossRef] [PubMed]
85. Banys-Paluchowski, M.; Thill, M.; Kühn, T.; Ditsch, N.; Heil, J.; Wöckel, A.; Fallenberg, E.; Friedrich, M.; Kümmel, S.; Müller, V.; et al. *AGO Breast Committee Recommendations: Surgical Therapy Update 2022. AGO Empfehlungen zur Operativen Therapie des Mammakarzinoms: Update 2022*; GebFra: Bielefeld, Germany, 2022.
86. Esgueva, A.; Rodriguez-Revuelto, R.; Espinosa-Bravo, M.; Salazar, J.P.; Rubio, I.T. Learning curves in intraoperative ultrasound guided surgery in breast cancer based on complete breast cancer excision and no need for second surgeries. *Eur. J. Surg. Oncol.* **2019**, *45*, 578–583. [CrossRef]
87. Konen, J.; Murphy, S.; Berkman, A.; Ahern, T.P.; Sowden, M. Intraoperative Ultrasound Guidance With an Ultrasound-Visible Clip: A Practical and Cost-effective Option for Breast Cancer Localization. *J. Ultrasound Med.* **2020**, *39*, 911–917. [CrossRef]
88. Volders, J.H.; Haloua, M.H.; Krekel, N.M.; Negenborn, V.L.; Kolk, R.H.; Lopes Cardozo, A.M.; Bosch, A.M.; de Widt-Levert, L.M.; van der Veen, H.; Rijna, H.; et al. Intraoperative ultrasound guidance in breast-conserving surgery shows superiority in oncological outcome, long-term cosmetic and patient-reported outcomes: Final outcomes of a randomized controlled trial (COBALT). *Eur. J. Surg. Oncol.* **2017**, *43*, 649–657. [CrossRef] [PubMed]
89. Ramos, M.; Diaz, J.C.; Ramos, T.; Ruano, R.; Aparicio, M.; Sancho, M.; Gonzalez-Orus, J.M. Ultrasound-guided excision combined with intraoperative assessment of gross macroscopic margins decreases the rate of reoperations for non-palpable invasive breast cancer. *Breast* **2013**, *22*, 520–524. [CrossRef] [PubMed]
90. Rubio, I.T.; Esgueva-Colmenarejo, A.; Espinosa-Bravo, M.; Salazar, J.P.; Miranda, I.; Peg, V. Intraoperative Ultrasound-Guided Lumpectomy Versus Mammographic Wire Localization for Breast Cancer Patients After Neoadjuvant Treatment. *Ann. Surg. Oncol.* **2016**, *23*, 38–43. [CrossRef]
91. Krekel, N.M.; Lopes Cardozo, A.M.; Muller, S.; Bergers, E.; Meijer, S.; van den Tol, M.P. Optimising surgical accuracy in palpable breast cancer with intra-operative breast ultrasound—Feasibility and surgeons' learning curve. *Eur. J. Surg. Oncol.* **2011**, *37*, 1044–1050. [CrossRef]
92. Canavese, G.; Catturich, A.; Vecchio, C.; Tomei, D.; Estienne, M.; Moresco, L.; Imperiale, A.; Parodi, G.C.; Massa, T.; Badellino, F. Pre-operative localization of non-palpable lesions in breast cancer by charcoal suspension. *Eur. J. Surg. Oncol.* **1995**, *21*, 47–49. [CrossRef]
93. Ko, K.; Han, B.K.; Jang, K.M.; Choe, Y.H.; Shin, J.H.; Yang, J.H.; Nam, S.J. The value of ultrasound-guided tattooing localization of nonpalpable breast lesions. *Korean J. Radiol.* **2007**, *8*, 295–301. [CrossRef]
94. Mathieu, M.C.; Bonhomme-Faivre, L.; Rouzier, R.; Seiller, M.; Barreau-Pouhaer, L.; Travagli, J.P. Tattooing breast cancers treated with neoadjuvant chemotherapy. *Ann. Surg. Oncol.* **2007**, *14*, 2233–2238. [CrossRef]
95. Porpiglia, M.; Borella, F.; Chieppa, P.; Brino, C.; Ala, A.; Marra, V.; Castellano, I.; Benedetto, C. Carbon tattooing of axillary lymph nodes in breast cancer patients before neoadjuvant chemotherapy: A retrospective analysis. *Tumori* **2022**. [CrossRef] [PubMed]
96. Simons, J.M.; van Nijnatten, T.J.A.; van der Pol, C.C.; van Diest, P.J.; Jager, A.; van Klaveren, D.; Kam, B.L.R.; Lobbes, M.B.I.; de Boer, M.; Verhoef, C.; et al. Diagnostic Accuracy of Radioactive Iodine Seed Placement in the Axilla with Sentinel Lymph Node Biopsy After Neoadjuvant Chemotherapy in Node-Positive Breast Cancer. *JAMA Surg.* **2022**, *157*, 991–999. [CrossRef] [PubMed]
97. de Boniface, J.; Frisell, J.; Kuhn, T.; Wiklander-Brakenhielm, I.; Dembrower, K.; Nyman, P.; Zouzos, A.; Gerber, B.; Reimer, T.; Hartmann, S. False-negative rate in the extended prospective TATTOO trial evaluating targeted axillary dissection by carbon tattooing in clinically node-positive breast cancer patients receiving neoadjuvant systemic therapy. *Breast Cancer Res. Treat.* **2022**, *193*, 589–595. [CrossRef] [PubMed]
98. Hartmann, S.; Kuhn, T.; de Boniface, J.; Stachs, A.; Winckelmann, A.; Frisell, J.; Wiklander-Brakenhielm, I.; Stubert, J.; Gerber, B.; Reimer, T. Carbon tattooing for targeted lymph node biopsy after primary systemic therapy in breast cancer: Prospective multicentre TATTOO trial. *Br. J. Surg.* **2021**, *108*, 302–307. [CrossRef]

99. Goyal, A.; Puri, S.; Marshall, A.; Valassiadou, K.; Hoosein, M.M.; Carmichael, A.R.; Erdelyi, G.; Sharma, N.; Dunn, J.; York, J. A multicentre prospective feasibility study of carbon dye tattooing of biopsied axillary node and surgical localisation in breast cancer patients. *Breast Cancer Res. Treat.* **2021**, *185*, 433–440. [CrossRef]
100. Banys-Paluchowski, M.; Untch, M.; Krawczyk, N.; Thurmann, M.; Kuhn, T.; Sehouli, J.; Gasparri, M.L.; de Boniface, J.; Gentilini, O.D.; Stickeler, E.; et al. Current trends in diagnostic and therapeutic management of the axilla in breast cancer patients receiving neoadjuvant therapy: Results of the German-wide NOGGO MONITOR 24 survey. *Arch. Gynecol. Obstet.* **2022**. [CrossRef]

Disclaimer/Publisher's Note: The statements, opinions and data contained in all publications are solely those of the individual author(s) and contributor(s) and not of MDPI and/or the editor(s). MDPI and/or the editor(s) disclaim responsibility for any injury to people or property resulting from any ideas, methods, instructions or products referred to in the content.

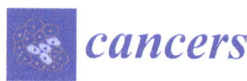

Review

Breast Cancer Risk Assessment Tools for Stratifying Women into Risk Groups: A Systematic Review

Louiza S. Velentzis [1,2,†], Victoria Freeman [1,3,†], Denise Campbell [1], Suzanne Hughes [1], Qingwei Luo [1], Julia Steinberg [1], Sam Egger [1], G. Bruce Mann [4,5] and Carolyn Nickson [1,2,*]

[1] The Daffodil Centre, The University of Sydney, A Joint Venture with Cancer Council NSW, Sydney, NSW 2011, Australia
[2] Melbourne School of Population and Global Health, University of Melbourne, Carlton, VA 3010, Australia
[3] Centre for Outcomes Research and Effectiveness, Research Department of Clinical, Educational & Health Psychology, University College London, London WC1E 7HB, UK
[4] Breast Service, The Royal Women's and Royal Melbourne Hospital, Parkville, VIC 3010, Australia
[5] Department of Surgery, University of Melbourne, Parkville, VIC 3010, Australia
* Correspondence: carolyn.nickson@nswcc.org.au
† These authors contributed equally to this work.

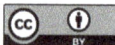

Citation: Velentzis, L.S.; Freeman, V.; Campbell, D.; Hughes, S.; Luo, Q.; Steinberg, J.; Egger, S.; Mann, G.B.; Nickson, C. Breast Cancer Risk Assessment Tools for Stratifying Women into Risk Groups: A Systematic Review. *Cancers* **2023**, *15*, 1124. https://doi.org/10.3390/cancers15041124

Academic Editor: Naiba Nabieva

Received: 1 November 2022
Revised: 31 January 2023
Accepted: 1 February 2023
Published: 9 February 2023

Copyright: © 2023 by the authors. Licensee MDPI, Basel, Switzerland. This article is an open access article distributed under the terms and conditions of the Creative Commons Attribution (CC BY) license (https://creativecommons.org/licenses/by/4.0/).

Simple Summary: Early detection of breast cancer in asymptomatic women through screening is an important strategy in reducing the burden of breast cancer. In current organized breast screening programs, age is the predominant risk factor. Breast cancer risk assessment tools are numerical models that can combine information on various risk factors to estimate the risk of being diagnosed with breast cancer within a certain time period. These tools could be used to offer risk-based screening. This systematic review assessed, using a variety of methods, how accurately breast cancer risk assessment tools can group women eligible for screening within a population, into risk groups, so that each group could potentially be offered a screening protocol with more benefits and less harms compared to current age-based screening.

Abstract: Background: The benefits and harms of breast screening may be better balanced through a risk-stratified approach. We conducted a systematic review assessing the accuracy of questionnaire-based risk assessment tools for this purpose. Methods: Population: asymptomatic women aged ≥40 years; Intervention: questionnaire-based risk assessment tool (incorporating breast density and polygenic risk where available); Comparison: different tool applied to the same population; Primary outcome: breast cancer incidence; Scope: external validation studies identified from databases including Medline and Embase (period 1 January 2008–20 July 2021). We assessed calibration (goodness-of-fit) between expected and observed cancers and compared observed cancer rates by risk group. Risk of bias was assessed with PROBAST. Results: Of 5124 records, 13 were included examining 11 tools across 15 cohorts. The Gail tool was most represented ($n = 11$), followed by Tyrer-Cuzick ($n = 5$), BRCAPRO and iCARE-Lit ($n = 3$). No tool was consistently well-calibrated across multiple studies and breast density or polygenic risk scores did not improve calibration. Most tools identified a risk group with higher rates of observed cancers, but few tools identified lower-risk groups across different settings. All tools demonstrated a high risk of bias. Conclusion: Some risk tools can identify groups of women at higher or lower breast cancer risk, but this is highly dependent on the setting and population.

Keywords: risk prediction models; breast cancer screening; risk assessment; risk-based screening

1. Introduction

Early detection of breast cancer in asymptomatic women through screening is an important strategy in reducing the burden of breast cancer. Mammographic screening programs have decreased mortality for screened women and reduced the intensity of breast cancer treatment and associated sequelae [1–4]. Nevertheless, breast screening also confers potential harms such as overdiagnosis leading to the treatment of tumours that would not have progressed to symptomatic disease within a person's lifetime, and false positive screening tests, associated with adverse psychological effects and possible reduced screening reattendance [5]. Current organised breast screening programs are directed to specific age groups, so that age is the predominant risk factor [3,6–8]. However, there are numerous other risk factors for breast cancer. More personalised, risk-based approaches to screening are expected to improve the balance of benefits and harms for identified risk groups [9,10]. This would require a rigorous and reliable method to routinely assess breast cancer risk in screening populations.

Breast cancer risk assessment tools (also known as risk prediction models) use numerical models to combine information on various risk factors (or risk predictors) to estimate the risk or probability of being diagnosed with breast cancer within a certain time period (e.g., 5 or 10 years) or from the time of assessment to older age [11]. These tools have evolved over time. Where earlier risk assessment tools considered information on reproductive factors (e.g., age at menarche/menopause, age at first live birth), family history, and breast biopsies, later tools incorporated additional lifestyle information (e.g., menopausal hormone therapy, alcohol consumption, smoking), anthropometric data (weight, height), ethnicity or/and mammographic density and various more recent tools incorporate genetic information in the form of polygenic risk scores (PRS) from analysing single-nucleotide polymorphisms associated with inherited variance in breast cancer risk [12,13]. Highly penetrant ("pathogenic") variants in BRCA1/2 or other key genes are also included in some tools, e.g., Tyrer-Cuzick and BODICEA.

While many of these tools have been developed for individual clinical applications or management of higher-risk population groups, such risk assessment tools could potentially be used to stratify screening populations into population-level risk groups, with each group offered a screening protocol to optimise the benefits and minimise the harms of screening [14]. In line with increasing interest in personalised medicine and risk-based screening over the last decade [15,16] there has been a growth in publications concerning breast cancer risk assessment tool development, validation and evaluation. The wealth of tools now available are not widely utilised for the general population mainly due to insufficient validation, lack of available resources for capturing complete risk factor information from screening participants and the need to agree on, and resource, tailored screening protocols for specific risk groups [17,18].

A critical step making the most of available tools is understanding which tools can accurately achieve population-level risk stratification, including the extent to which their accuracy can be generalised to different populations and health settings. Case-control studies frequently report improvements in the discrimination of new or revised risk assessment tools [12,19–21]; however, risk assessment tools can only be adequately assessed for the purpose of population-level implementation when they are externally validated on populations different to the study groups on which they were developed.

This systematic review aims to characterise studies which compare breast cancer risk assessment tools and assess their ability to stratify screening populations according to (i) absolute risk of breast cancer and (ii) related outcomes of breast cancer risk (expected versus observed incidence of invasive breast cancer, with or without in situ disease and incidence of breast cancer). This review was undertaken as part of the Roadmap to Optimising Screening in Australia (ROSA) project [22] funded by the Australian Government Department of Health, and includes: (i) studies that compare tools generated from, or calibrated to, a different population to the one in which the tools were applied to, i.e., the validation population of interest, and (ii) studies comparing risk assessment tools calibrated or recalibrated to the validation population of interest.

2. Methods

2.1. Study Registration

Our Patient, Intervention, Comparison, Outcomes (PICO) question is 'For asymptomatic women aged ≥40 years, how accurately do different breast cancer risk assessment tools assign women to risk groups?', where the term 'risk assessment tool' is used synonymously for risk prediction tool, prognostic model, risk prediction model, risk model, and breast cancer prediction model. The protocol for this systematic review was registered on the International Prospective Register of Systematic Reviews (PROSPERO) as part of a larger protocol exploring breast cancer risk assessment tools (CRD42020159232). We followed the requirements of the PRISMA 2020 guidelines for conducting and reporting of systematic reviews [23].

2.2. Eligibility Criteria

The current analysis was confined to articles comparing breast cancer risk assessment tools on the same study cohort; cohorts had to consist of asymptomatic women undergoing population mammographic screening. We excluded articles limited to cohorts of women undergoing diagnostic breast imaging, specific ethnic groups or women with high risk of breast cancer as these represent sub-groups of the screened population. We considered only external validation studies (so that the study cohort was different from that used to develop each tool being compared), We included randomised controlled trials, paired cohort studies or systematic reviews thereof. Due to the need for sufficient follow-up between risk assessment and cancer outcomes, we included prospective or retrospective cohort studies (based on timing of risk predictor data collection in relation to outcome occurrence). All other study designs (such as cross-sectional studies or case–control studies) were excluded.

We included risk assessment tools based on questionnaire data with or without genetic and/or breast density information, where estimated future risk was projected to a minimum of two years (in line with the most common screening interval of most population breast cancer screening programs). Tools designed to be calibrated to the target population prior to use were included if they were developed on a different population to the study cohort. Tools requiring any non-standardised input (e.g., subjective assessment by a clinician) were excluded.

We restricted our analysis to articles published from 2008, aiming to include studies likely to use more relevant imaging methods and more recent versions of risk assessment tools while not excluding relatively contemporary studies with longer periods of follow-up. Only English language peer-reviewed publications were included; conference abstracts, reviews, letters, editorials and comments were excluded.

The primary outcome was expected versus observed incidence of invasive breast cancer (with or without in situ disease). Secondary outcomes were breast cancer mortality, incidence for different types of breast cancer as defined by characteristics such as tumour subtype, grade, size, nodal involvement, and interval breast cancers (i.e., cancers diagnosed following a negative screen and before any consecutive screens). Articles that did not report expected versus observed (E/O) calibration outcomes according to risk groups determined by the risk assessment tool were excluded.

Results were excluded from the analysis if risk was projected beyond the period for which the tool was developed. Five-year risk was the primary outcome compared and reported; results for 10-year risk are included in Supplementary Materials.

We contacted corresponding authors when there was a lack of clarity around criteria for inclusion in our review, allowing two weeks for a response, after which we sent a reminder in addition to contacting other authors on the paper. If no response was received, the study was excluded. Extracted data is presented in Supplementary Dataset S1.

2.3. Information Sources and Search Strategy

An experienced systematic reviewer (VF) searched on 1 July 2021 for English-language reports published from 1 January 2008 to 29 June 2021 on the following databases: (i) Ovid Medline and Embase; (ii) The Cochrane Database of Systematic Reviews (CDSR) and (iii) PROSPERO. An updated search until 20 July 2021 was also performed for these databases. For Ovid databases, database-specific subject headings and text terms were combined for breast cancer, risk assessment and calibration terms (see Supplementary Methods). The CDSR was searched by combining "breast cancer" and "risk" text terms. Reference lists of relevant systematic reviews and full-text articles were also scanned for additional potentially relevant reports by two systematic reviewers (VF, DC). The search strategy is presented in supplementary Table S1.

2.4. Selection Process

Titles and abstracts of the articles identified via the literature searches were screened against pre-specified inclusion criteria and split equally between two reviewers (VF, DC) with 20% assessed by both reviewers. The two reviewers independently assessed full-text articles of potential or unclear relevance for inclusion using a form with pre-specified selection criteria. Reviewers were not blinded to journal titles or study authors/institutions. Disagreements were resolved by discussion or adjudication by a third reviewer (SH).

2.5. Data Collection

Two independent reviewers (VF, DC) equally split the extraction of pre-determined study characteristics and results data from each included study and then reviewed the other's extractions for accuracy. Disagreements were resolved by discussion or adjudication by a third reviewer (SH, LV or CN); experienced statisticians were consulted to advise upon or review article methodology or calculations (SE or CN).

The following information was extracted: first author, publication year, country, study design, setting, study start, participant inclusion/exclusion criteria, screening protocol, population characteristics, risk assessment tool information, follow-up duration, risk prediction interval, reported relevant outcomes, E/O estimates and 95% confidence intervals (CIs), observed rates (or if missing, the observed number of breast cancers and number of women in each risk category) and other relevant information (including methods used, factors potentially affecting risk of bias). If E/O ratios, their 95% CIs or data for observed rates were not reported, these were calculated by the systematic reviewers from available data or plots where possible (VF, DC, SE). Ninety-five percent CIs were calculated using the following formula: $E/O \times \exp\hat{}(\pm 1.96 \times \sqrt{1/O})$ [23,24]. If there was insufficient data to perform calculations, authors were contacted and if attempts to obtain data were unsuccessful, the tool or study was excluded. In addition, where a tool version remained unclear after contacting authors and major updates to risk predictors had occurred between versions, the tool was excluded. It should be noted that risk predictors may be identified as risk factors, covariates, risk indicators, prognostic factors, determinants or independent variables [24].

We also identified high, moderate and low risk groups for each tool in each cohort. These groups were dependent on the number of quantiles the cohort of interest was divided into and whether they had the equivalent number of participants in each one. In general, when the cohort was divided in equal quartiles or deciles, we assumed the high-risk group corresponded to quartile 5 or deciles 9 and 10, the low-risk group corresponded to quartile 1 or deciles 1 and 2 while moderate-risk groups correspond to the remaining quantiles (quartiles 2–4 or deciles 3–8).

2.6. Metrics for Evaluating Risk Assessment Tools and Statistical Analysis

Prior to analysis, risk assessment tool comparisons were grouped by comparator tool (which could be any version of that tool). Data was extracted into Microsoft Excel and then plotted for each tool, age range and predicted year of risk.

We generated various data presentations and metrics to help evaluate and compare studies, as follows:

A. Goodness of fit between expected (predicted) and observed outcomes:
   1. Plotted ratios of expected versus observed cancers, by population percentile. The E/O ratio (in log10 scale) with 95% confidence intervals were plotted according to risk group assignment using the mid-point percentile of each risk group in the study population. This facilitated standardisation of comparisons between tools that had a different number of risk groups and/or assigned different proportions of women to each risk group.
   2. The total number of women in each study cohort in risk groups for which the E/O 95%CIs included unity. This helped indicate the proportion of each study cohort that was well-validated by the tool, noting that this is more likely for smaller studies (and therefore wider CIs).
   3. Calibration belt goodness-of-fit tests. We assessed goodness of fit between expected (predicted) probabilities of developing breast cancer and observed data using calibration belts [25] as applied in Li et al., 2021 [26], where a p-value <0.05 indicated miscalibration by the tool [25].

B. Analysis of observed outcomes by risk group classification:
   1. Observed cancer rates (number of breast cancers divided by the number of women per 10,000 for each risk category), by mid-point percentile of each risk group in the study population. This helped to standardise comparisons.
   2. Characterisation of the functional form (curve) of observed cancer incidence rates according to increasing risk group, classified as either: 'increasing' (observed rates consistently increasing across risk categories), 'monotonic' (i.e., increasing or remaining steady across groups) or 'fluctuating' (all other options).
   3. Assessment of whether highest-risk women could be distinguished from women at more moderate-risk. We compared the observed breast cancer rate corresponding to the mid-range risk groups (usually quintiles 2–4 or deciles 3–8) with the highest risk group (quintile 5 or deciles 9–10). p-values <0.05 indicated a statistically significant difference and, therefore, good allocation of women to the highest risk group. To ensure comparability of findings, if >25% of the study cohort was allocated to the highest risk groups, p-values were reported but not taken into consideration when drawing conclusions regarding a particular tool. Consequently, mid-range risk groups would be expected to include $\geq$50% of the study cohort.
   4. Assessment of whether lowest-risk women could be distinguished from women at more moderate-risk. As for (3 above), but for the lowest risk group (quintile 1 or deciles 1–2 or the equivalent sub-groups representing $\leq$25% of cohort), compared to the remainder (quintiles 2–4 or deciles 3–8, or equivalent sub-groups representing $\leq$50% of the cohort). To ensure comparability of findings, if >25% of the study cohort was allocated in the lowest risk groups, p-values were reported but not taken into consideration when drawing conclusions regarding a particular tool.

Plots and all statistical analyses were conducted using STATA (version 17, Stata Corporation, College Station, TX, USA).

2.7. Risk of Bias Assessment

Two independent reviewers (DC, VF) assessed the risk of bias for each included study. Differences were resolved by consensus or adjudication from a third reviewer (JS). Risk of bias was assessed using the 'Prediction model Risk Of Bias ASsessment Tool' (PROBAST), specifically designed to assess the Risk of Bias for, and the applicability of, diagnostic and prognostic prediction model studies [24]. PROBAST is organised into four domains; (i) participants (assessing suitable data sources or study designs and appropriate inclusions or exclusions), (ii) predictors (assessing predictor definition and measurements, knowledge of outcome influencing predictor assessment and whether the tool is used as designed if predictors are missing at time of validation), (iii) outcome (assessing methods used to classify participants with or without outcome, pre-specified/standard definition of outcome used, predictor exclusion from outcome definition, similar definition and determination of outcome for all participants, knowledge of predictor influencing outcome assessment, time interval between predictor assessment and outcome determination), and (iv) analysis (assessing reasonable number of participants with outcome, handling of continuous and categorical predictors, enrolled participant inclusion in analysis, handling of participants with missing data, handling of data complexities, evaluation of relevant tool performance measures). Each domain contains signalling questions to facilitate a structured judgement of risk of bias; the overall rating for a domain can be classified as either "low", "high" or "unclear" risk of bias. Each study is also allocated an overall risk of bias rating: "low", if no relevant shortcomings were identified in the risk of bias assessment; "high", if at least one domain was assessed as high risk of bias and "unclear" if risk of bias was assessed as unclear for at least one domain (and no other domains assessed as high risk of bias).

For each study, a separate risk of bias assessment was conducted for each distinct risk assessment tool validated, for each individual outcome and each cohort included [24]. Outcomes with multiple time points (e.g., 5- and 10-year risk predictions) were assessed separately because ratings for signalling questions on appropriate time interval between predictor assessment and outcome determination, and reasonable number of participants with outcome, could differ. As such, it was possible for a single study to have multiple overall risk of bias assessments.

Rulings were developed where necessary to account for judgements that required topic-specific knowledge or statistical expertise. These rulings were initially trialled independently over several studies by the same two reviewers (DC, VF) with third reviewer input from a senior researcher (JS) where required. It was decided a priori that: (i) risk of bias domains that contained signalling items relating only to model development would be omitted as the primary interest of this systematic review was risk assessment tool validation and (ii) the applicability of a study would not be formally assessed by the PROBAST tool; instead, concerns would be highlighted where necessary in the discussion. We sought statistical advice to develop rulings for items in the analysis domain as suggested by PROBAST. When assessing the reasonable number of participants with outcome PROBAST recommends that validation studies should include at least 100 participants with outcomes. After consulting statistical experts (SE, DO'C), it was decided a priori that a study would qualify for a low risk of bias rating if this was the case for every risk category. Where data for observed incidence of breast cancer per risk category was provided by authors or calculated by reviewers from calibration figures, this was used to inform our ratings. Otherwise, risk of bias was appraised based on the information reported in the article and included references. For the handling of missing data, based on methodological advice (QL), it was decided a priori that a study performing multiple imputation would qualify for low risk only if <50% of values were originally missing (and thus imputed) for a predictor and the missing data were missing at random [27,28].

3. Results

3.1. Selection of Articles and Summary Characteristics

Figure 1 summarises the search process conducted. The search strategy identified a total of 5114 records of which 3405 remained after duplicates were removed. Of these, 3324 records were excluded based on title and abstract review. Full texts or records of 91 potentially relevant reports were assessed according to the eligibility criteria. This included 10 additional articles identified from citation searching of full text articles and 1 potentially eligible article from the update search conducted on the 20 July 2021. A total of 78 reports were found not to be relevant and therefore excluded. We contacted authors to confirm the eligibility of two tools for one validation cohort [29]. Common reasons for exclusion included ineligible study design, ineligible population and E/O not reported by risk category. Further details on reasons for exclusions (studies and tools) and information regarding authors contacted are details in a Supplementary List S1.

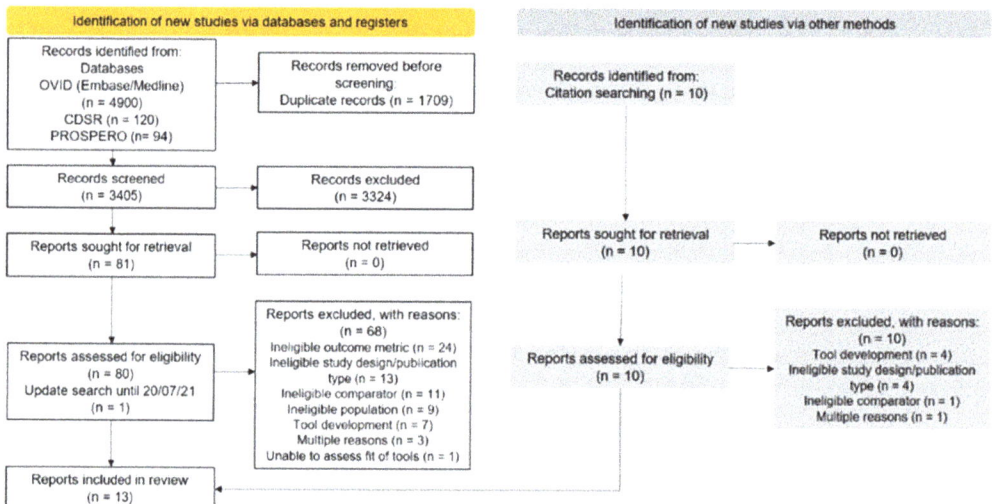

Figure 1. Flow diagram based on the PRISMA 2020 flow chart summarising the article screening process.

The remaining 13 articles included in this review examined the prediction of breast cancer across 15 cohort studies applying 11 distinct breast cancer risk assessment tools of different versions. Summary characteristics of included articles are presented in Table 1. All studies were prospective in design apart from one retrospective study [30]. Ten of the 13 articles were from North America and Europe and compared more than two risk assessment tools based on a 5-year risk prediction interval. Only two articles presented findings for 5- and 10-year tool-determined risk [31,32].

Table 1. Summary of the main characteristics of the included articles.

			Population								Outcome	
Study ID	Country	Cohort	Age Range (Median), y	N	Study Start	Screening	Tool Comparisons	FU	Calibrated to Population?	Breast Cancer	Risk Interval (y)	
Jantzen 2021 [33]	Canada	CARTaGENE	40–69 (53.1)	10,200	2009–2010	2 yearly, 50–69 y	TC v8.0b vs. BCRAT v4 [a]	5	No	Invasive	5	
Hurson 2021 [29]	UK	UK Biobank	Age subgroups <50 years: 40–49 at DNA collection; (46)	<50 years: 36,005	2006	NR	iCARE-BPC3 vs. iCARE-BPC3 + PRS	4	Yes	Invasive or DCIS	5	
			≥50 years: 50–72 at DNA collection; (61)	≥50 years: 134,920			iCARE-Lit vs. iCARE-Lit + PRS		Yes			
	USA	WGHS [b]	50–74 at DNA collection; (56)	17,001	2000	NR	iCARE-Lit vs. iCARE-Lit + PRS	21 [d]	Yes	Invasive or DCIS	5	
									Yes			
McCarthy 2020 [34]	USA	Newton-Wellesley Hospital	40–84; (53.9) [d]	35,921	2007–2009	NR	TC v7 vs. TC v8.0b BCRAT v4 [a] vs. BRCAPRO v2.1-4	6.7 [d]	No	Invasive	6	
									Yes			
Choudhury 2020 [35]	UK	Generations Study	Age subgroups <50 years: 35–49; (42)	<50 years: 28,232	2003–2012	NR	TC v8 vs. iCARE-Lit, TC v8 vs. iCARE-BPC3, BCRATv3 vs. iCARE-Lit, iCARE-BPC3 vs. iCARE-Lit aRAT [c]	5	Yes	Invasive	5	
			≥50 years: 50–74; (58)	≥50 years: 36,642					Yes			
	USA	PLCO	5(–75; (61)	48,279	1993–2001	NR	BCRAT v3 [a] vs. iCARE-Lit aRAT [c]	5	Yes	Invasive	5	

Table 1. *Cont.*

Study ID	Country	Cohort	Population Age Range (Median), y	N	Study Start	Screening	Tool Comparisons	FU	Calibrated to Population?	Breast Cancer	Outcome Risk Interval (y)
Hüsing 2020 [36]	Germany	EPIC-Germany	20–70; (40+: median 52.6)	22,098	1994–1998	NR	BCRAT v3 [a] vs. BCRmod; BCRAT v3 [a] recalibrated vs. BCRmod recalibrated	11.8	No; Yes	Invasive	5
Jee 2020 [37]	Republic of Korea	KCPS-II Biobank	Age subgroups <50 years 21–49; (38); ≥50 years 50–80; (58)	<50 years: 57,439; ≥50 years: 15,776	2004–2013	2-yearly, ≥40 years	KREA vs. KRKR (iCARE-Lit—based tools) aRAT [c]	8.6	Yes	Invasive	5
Terry 2019 [31]	USA, Canada, Australia	ProF-SC	20–70; (NR)	15,732	1992–2011	NR	BCRAT v4 [a] vs. BRCAPRO v2.1-3; TC v8.0b vs. BCRAT v4 [a]; BOADICEA v3 vs. BRCAPRO v2.1-3; BOADICEA v3 vs. BCRAT v4 [a]	11.1	No; No; No; No	Invasive	5, 10
Brentnall 2018 [38]	USA	Kaiser Permanente Washington BCSC	40–75; (50) (general population: ≥50 y; high risk: ≥40 y)	132,139	1996–2013	Annually; 50–75 y; high-risk women 40–49 y [e]	TC v7.02 vs. TC v7.02 + breast density	5.2	No	Invasive	10
Li 2018 [39]	USA	WHI	50–79; (63.2) [d]	82,319	1993–1998	NR	ER- vs. ER+ aRAT [c]	8.2 [d]	No	Invasive	5

Table 1. Cont.

Study ID	Population						Tool Comparisons	FU	Calibrated to Population?	Outcome	
	Country	Cohort	Age Range (Median), y	N	Study Start	Screening				Breast Cancer	Risk Interval (y)
Min 2014 [40]	Republic of Korea	Women's Healthcare Center of Cheil General Hospital, Seoul	<29 to ≥60; (NR)	40,229	1999–2004	NR	BCRAT v2 [a] vs. AABCS Original Korean tool vs. Updated Korean tool	NR	No Yes	Invasive	5
Powell 2014 [30]	USA	MWS	<40 to ≥80; (NR)	12,843	2003–2007	NR	BCRAT v2 or v3 [a] vs. BRCAPRO v(NR) aRAT [c]	NR	Yes	Invasive	5
Arrospide 2013 [41]	Spain	Screening in Sabadell-Cerdanyola (EDBC-SC) area in Catalonia	50–69; (57.0) [d]	13,760	1995–1998	2-yearly; 50–69 y	BCRAT v1 [a,f] vs. Chen v1	13.3	Yes	Invasive	5 [g]
Chay 2012 [32]	Singapore	SBCSP	50–64 [h]; (NR)	28,104 [i]	1994–1997 [k]	Single 2-view mammogram, 50–64 y	BCRAT v2 [a] vs. AABCS	NR	No	Invasive	5, 10

[a] Different versions of the BCRAT are labelled according to the SAS Macro version; [b] Following communication with the authors, iCare-BPC3 was excluded as part of the WGHS cohort was used for the development of this tool; [c] aRAT = Additional risk assessment tool. Additional tools were available for some studies but were excluded as they did not meet the criteria for inclusion in data synthesis, see supplementary methods for details); [d] Mean; [e] 62% of women aged <50 years at entry were low risk for breast cancer; [f] The study did not include DCIS in the outcome and women with DCIS were considered at risk of invasive breast cancer; [g] only 5-year risk data was extracted; [h] some women were older than 64 years based on screening time; [i] numbers or ages are as cited in text or tables; cannot verify accuracy due to different numbers or ages cited between the original trial and other reports; [k] organised national breast screening in Singapore was introduced in 2002. Abbreviations: AABCS = Asian American Breast Cancer Study; BCRAT = Breast cancer risk assessment tool; BCSC = Breast Cancer Surveillance Consortium; BOADICEA = Breast and Ovarian Analysis of Disease Incidence and Carrier Estimation Algorithm; DCIS = ductal carcinoma in situ; EPIC = European Investigation into Cancer and Nutrition study; ER = Estrogen receptor; i-Care-BPC3 = Individualized Coherent Absolute Risk Estimation—Breast and Prostate Cancer Cohort Consortium; iCARE-Lit = Individualized Coherent Absolute Risk Estimation—literature based tool; KCPS: Korean Cancer Prevention Study; KREA = tool using Korean incidence, mortality and risk factor distributions with European-ancestry relative risks; KRKR = tool using Korean incidence, mortality and risk factor distributions with Korean relative risks; MWS: Marin Women's Study; N = number of participants; NHS = Nurses' Health Study; NR = not reported; PLCO: Prostate, Lung, Colorectal and Ovarian Cancer Screening Trial; ProF-SC: Breast Cancer Prospective Family Study Cohort; PRS = polygenic risk score; SBCSP: Singapore Breast Cancer Screening Project; TC = Tyrer-Cuzick; v = version; WGHS: Women's Genome Health Study; WHI = Women's Health Initiative.

The tools assessed included data from questionnaires, with or without information on mammographic breast density and PRS. The number of risk predictors varied between tools, from as few as five (e.g., Chen version 1) [41] to as many as 13 (e.g., Tyrer-Cuzick version 8.0b [31] although it should be noted that some studies did not have data for all the risk predictors specified by the tool they assessed. Risk predictors considered in each tool by each study are presented in Supplementary Table S2. The Breast Cancer Risk Assessment Tool (BCRAT; also known as the Gail model), was the most frequently assessed tool in publications assessed (9 of 13 articles). This was followed by the Tyrer-Cuzick tool (also known as the IBIS risk assessment tool) in 5 articles, and BRCAPRO and iCARE-Lit in 3 articles each.

Two articles evaluated the effect of adding breast density data: McCarthy et al. [32] compared 5-year risk using Tyrer-Cuzick version 7 versus version 8.0b which had breast density incorporated within the tool and Brentnall et al. [38] assessed 10-year risk using Tyrer-Cuzick version 7.0 with and without breast density data. In two more articles, tools with integrated breast density data (Chen version 1; Tyrer-Cuzick version 8.0b) were compared to other tools; in Choudhury et al., 2020 [35] Tyrer-Cuzick version 8.0b was compared to iCARE tool variants, and in Arrospide et al. [41] Chen version 1 was compared to BCRAT version 1.

Only one study assessed the effect of PRS data on existing tools; in Hurson et al. [29] a 313-variant polygenic score was added to two iCARE risk assessment tools (iCARE-Lit and iCARE-BPC3).

Evidence was available to compare tools in terms of risk of invasive breast cancer, however, evidence was sparse for in situ breast cancer incidence, while no data was available on breast cancer incidence according to prognostic indicators (e.g., tumour subtype, grade, size, nodal). Therefore, these outcomes were not able to be assessed.

3.2. Goodness-of-Fit

Absolute risk calibration is shown for various tools and tool comparisons (along with observed rates of incident breast cancer) in Figure 2A–C and Supplementary Figure S1A–C. In terms of goodness-of-fit between estimated and observed outcomes, no risk assessment tool was identified as being consistently well-calibrated in multiple studies. As can be observed from Table 2, many tools showed good calibration in some but not all studies: namely AABCS [32,40], BCRAT version 3 [30,35,36], BCRAT version 4 [31,33,34], Tyrer-Cuzick version 8.0b [31,33–35], iCARE-Lit and iCARE-BPC3 [29,35], and BRCAPRO version 2.1 [31,34]. In contrast, some tools did not demonstrate good calibration across studies; examples include BCRAT version 2 [32,40] and Tyrer-Cuzick version 7 [31,34]. There were other tools that were applied in single cohorts within this review, and thus could only be assessed in only one population and one setting. Of these, six showed a good fit (BCRAT version 1 [41]; Chen version 1 [41]; BCRmod [36]; BCRmod recalibrated [36]; KREA for women over 50 years [37]; KRKR [37]) and five showed evidence of miscalibration (i.e., $p < 0.05$) (BOADICEA [31]; ER- [39]; ER+ [39]; KREA for women under 50 years of age [37]; original Korean tool [40]; updated Korean tool [40]).

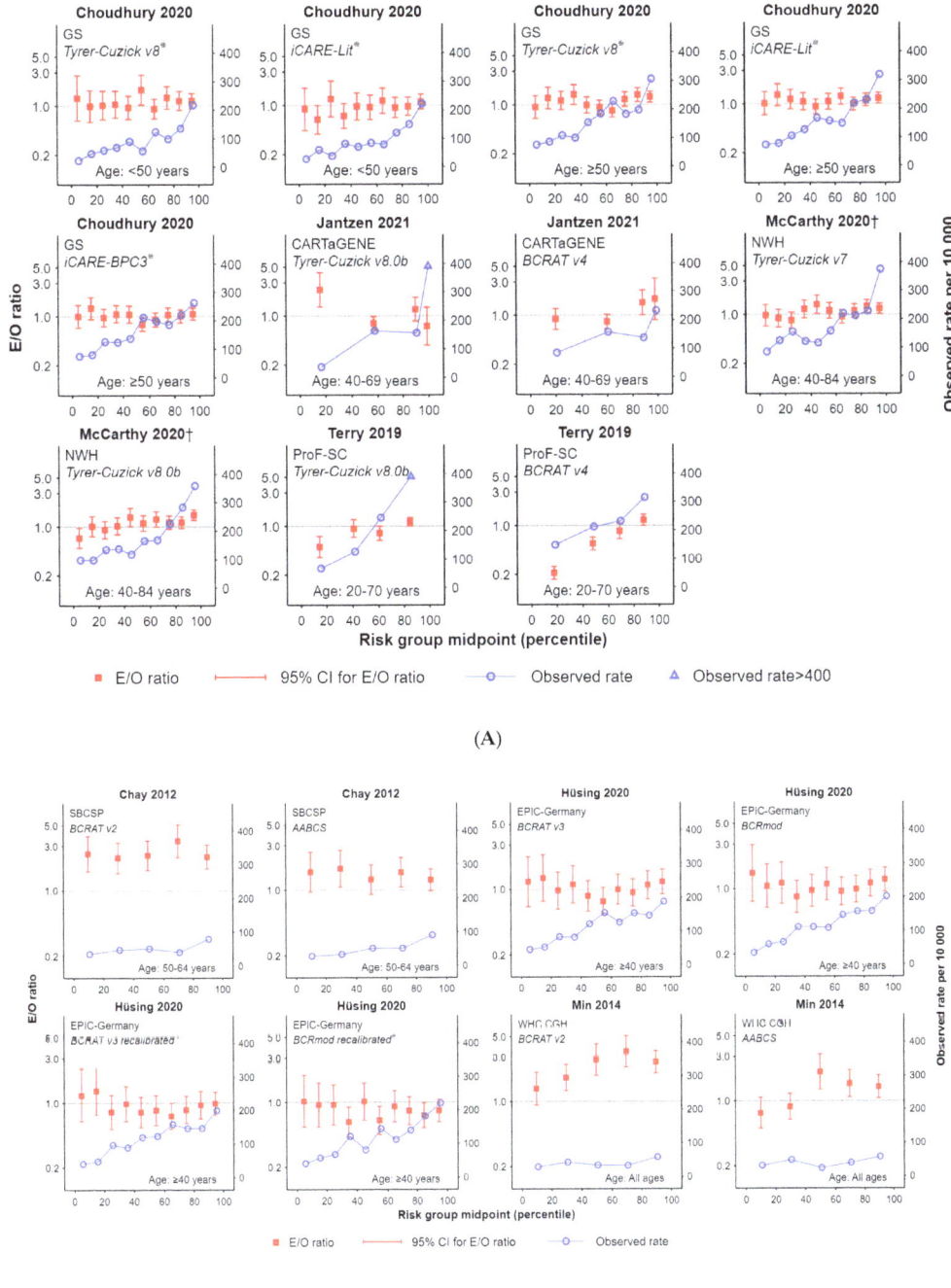

Figure 2. Cont.

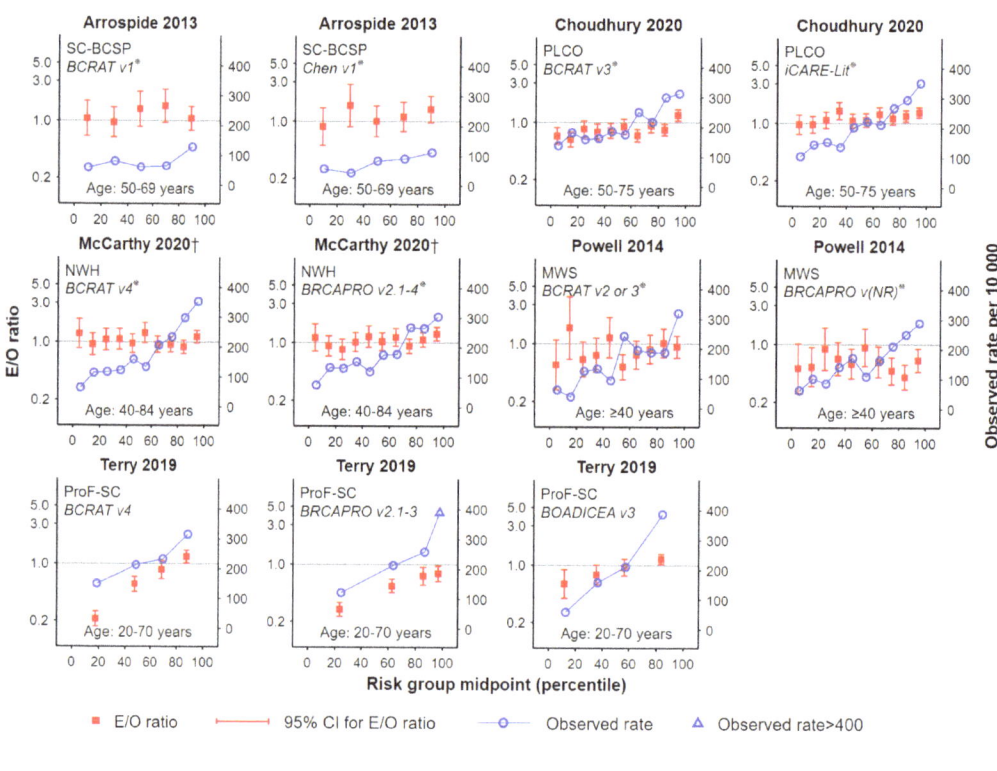

(C)

Figure 2. Absolute risk calibration and observed rate of incident breast cancer by 5-year risk. The three groups shown are: (**A**) Tyrer-Cuzick vs. BCRAT or other tool comparisons; (**B**) BCRAT vs. BCRAT modifications; (**C**) BCRAT vs. other risk assessment tools. Plots are then presented according to first author name. (The number of data points in each graph is determined by the number of risk groups that were reported in each study. To assist with comparison of studies, the x-axis shows the percentile distribution of groups being reported, with data points shown for the mid-points of each group. Red squares show the 'expected over observed' ratio for each risk group (with 95% confidence intervals shown), indicating calibration between expected and observed cancers at a risk group level. Blue circles show the corresponding observed rate of breast cancers within the study group, indicating the gradient of rates across the risk groups (expected to increase from left to right in accordance with increases in estimated breast cancer risk). Italic font indicates the risk tool being assessed, with the study cohort abbreviation also shown). * tools were calibrated to local population.

Combining breast density data with a tool score [38] or integrating breast density within a tool generating a new tool version [Tyrer-Cuzick version 7 vs. Tyrer-Cuzick version 8.0b [34]) did not improve the goodness of fit of the tool, with evidence of miscalibration in both cases.

Addition of PRS data, in the single study that evaluated a specific score [29], did not improve the goodness-of-fit of neither iCARE-Lit nor iCARE-BPC3, as assessed on different cohorts ([UK Biobank; Women's Genome Health Study (US)] (Supplementary Figure S1). For these evaluations, there was evidence of miscalibration before and after addition of PRS information ($p < 0.05$).

No change was observed in the calibration of most tools (BCRAT version 2; BCRAT version 4; BRCAPRO version 2.1; BOADICEA) for longer-term risks, with evidence of miscalibration for both 5- and 10-year risk. The only exception was the AABCS tool, for which the goodness-of-fit improved for 10-year risk [32].

Table 2. Assessment of risk assessment tools' validation using metrics for expected/observed rates and trend in observed breast cancer incidence rates.

Study (Country, Age Range)	Model	Proportion of Cohort Well-Validated [a]	Evidence of Miscalibration (p-Value)	Mis-Calibration [b]	Lower Q Compared to Middle Qs (p-Value)	Distinguishes Women in Lowest RG? [b,c]	Upper Q Compared to Middle Qs (p-Value)	Distinguishes Women in Highest RG? [b,c]	Trend in Observed Rates
Tyrer-Cuzick vs. BCRAT (5-year risk)									
Jantzen 2021, [33] (Canada, 50–69 y)	TC v8.0b	2/4 (18%)	0.045	Yes	<0.001	N/A	<0.001	N/A	Fluctuating
	BCRAT v4	3/4 (84%)	0.035	Yes	<0.001	N/A	<0.001	N/A	Fluctuating
Terry 2019 [31] (USA, Canada, Australia, 20–70 y)	TC v8.0b	2/4 (40%)	<0.001	Yes	<0.001	N/A	<0.001	N/A	Increasing
	BCRAT v4	1/4 (16%)	<0.001	Yes	0.004	N/A	0.004	N/A	Increasing
Tyrer-Cuzick vs. BCRAT (10-year risk)									
Terry 2019 [31], (USA, Canada, Australia, 20–70 y)	BCRAT v4	1/4 (26%)	<0.001	Yes	<0.001	N/A	<0.001	N/A	Increasing
	TC v8.0b	2/4 (42%)	<0.001	Yes	<0.001	N/A	<0.001	N/A	Increasing
Tyrer-Cuzick vs. its variants or other tools (5–6 year risk)									
Choudhury 2020 [35], 5 y risk (UK cohort)	TC v8 (<50 y)	9/10 (90%)	0.074	No	<0.001	Yes	<0.001	Yes	Fluctuating
	iCARE-Lit (<50 y)	10/10 (100%)	0.251	No	0.006	Yes	<0.001	Yes	Fluctuating
	TC v8 (≥50 y)	7/10 (70%)	<0.001	Yes	<0.001	Yes	<0.001	Yes	Fluctuating
	iCARE-Lit (≥50 y)	9/10 (90%)	0.010	Yes	<0.001	Yes	<0.001	Yes	Fluctuating
	iCARE-BPC3 (≥50 y)	9/10 (90%)	0.997	No	<0.001	Yes	<0.001	Yes	Fluctuating
McCarthy 2020 [34], 6 y risk (USA, 40–84 y)	TC v.7	7/10 (70%)	0.002	Yes	<0.001	Yes	<0.001	Yes	Fluctuating
	TC v8.0b	6/10 (60%)	<0.001	Yes	<0.001	Yes	<0.001	Yes	Fluctuating
Tyrer-Cuzick tool variants (10-year risk)									
Brentnall 2018 [38] 10 y risk (USA, 40–75 y)	TC v7.02	2/5 (55%)	<0.001	Yes	<0.001	N/A	<0.001	N/A	Increasing
	TC v7.02 + MD	2/5 (47%)	<0.001	Yes	<0.001	N/A	<0.001	Yes	Increasing

Table 2. Cont.

Study (Country, Age Range)	Model	Proportion of Cohort Well-Validated [a]	Evidence of Miscalibration (p-Value)	Mis-Calibration [b]	Lower Q Compared to Middle Qs (p-Value)	Distinguishes Women in Lowest RG? [b,c]	Upper Q Compared to Middle Qs (p-Value)	Distinguishes Women in Highest RG? [b,c]	Trend in Observed Rates
BCRAT vs. its modifications (5-year risk)									
Chay 2012 [32], (Singapore, 50–64 y)	BCRAT v2	0/5 (0%)	<0.001	Yes	0.269	No	0.004	Yes	Fluctuating
	AABCS	3/5 (60%)	<0.001	Yes	0.082	No	<0.001	Yes	Monotonic
	BCRAT v3	10/10 (100%)	0.918	No	<0.001	Yes	0.018	Yes	Fluctuating
	BCRmod	10/10 (100%)	0.227	No	0.002	Yes	<0.001	Yes	Fluctuating
Hüsing 2020 [36] (Germany, 20–70 y)	BCRAT v3 recalibrated	10/10 (100%)	0.324	No	<0.001	Yes	0.011	Yes	Fluctuating
	BCRmod recalibrated	7/10 (70%)	0.007	Yes	<0.001	Yes	<0.001	Yes	Fluctuating
Min 2014 [40] (Republic of Korea, >29–60 y)	BCRAT v2	1/5 (19%)	<0.001	Yes	0.333	No	0.010	Yes	Fluctuating
	AABCS	2/5 (40%)	<0.001	Yes	0.464	No	0.016	Yes	Fluctuating
BCRAT vs. its modifications (10-year risk)									
Chay 2012 [32], (Singapore, 50–64 y)	BCRAT v2	0/5 (0%)	<0.001	Yes	0.253	No	<0.001	Yes	Fluctuating
	AABCS	5/5 (100%)	0.719	No	0.007	Yes	<0.001	Yes	Increasing
BCRAT vs. other risk assessment tools (5-year risk)									
Arrospide 2013 [41] (Spain, 50–69 y)	BCRAT v1	5/5 (100%)	0.289	No	0.599	No	0.004	Yes	Fluctuating
	Chen v1	5/5 (100%)	0.124	No	0.430	No	0.060	No	Fluctuating
Choudhury 2020 [35] (USA cohort, 50–75 y)	BCRAT v3	3/10 (30%)	<0.001	Yes	0.045	Yes	<0.001	Yes	Fluctuating
	iCARE-Lit	6/10 (60%)	<0.001	Yes	<0.001	Yes	<0.001	Yes	Fluctuating
McCarthy 2020 [34] (6-year risk only)	BCRAT v4	10/10 (100%)	0.863	No	<0.001	Yes	<0.001	Yes	Fluctuating
	BRCAPRO v2.1-4	9/10 (90%)	0.061	No	<0.001	Yes	<0.001	Yes	Fluctuating
Powell 2014 [30] (USA, >40–80 y)	BCRAT v2 or 3	9/10 (90%)	0.009	Yes	<0.001	Yes	0.003	Yes	Fluctuating
	BRCAPRO v(NR)	4/10 (40%)	<0.001	Yes	0.012	Yes	<0.001	Yes	Fluctuating
Terry 2019 [31] (USA, Canada, Australia, 20–70 y)	BCRAT v4	1/4 (26%)	<0.001	Yes	0.004	N/A	<0.001	N/A	Increasing
	BRCAPRO v2.1-3	0/4 (0%)	<0.001	Yes	<0.001	N/A	<0.001	N/A	Increasing
	BOADICEA v3	2/4 (44%)	<0.001	Yes	<0.001	N/A	<0.001	N/A	Increasing

Table 2. Cont.

Study (Country, Age Range)	Model	Proportion of Cohort Well-Validated [a]	Evidence of Miscalibration (p-Value)	Mis-Calibration [b]	Lower Q Compared to Middle Qs (p-Value)	Distinguishes Women in Lowest RG? [b,c]	Upper Q Compared to Middle Qs (p-Value)	Distinguishes Women in Highest RG? [b,c]	Trend in Observed Rates
BCRAT vs. other risk assessment tools (10-year risk)									
Terry 2019 [31], (USA, Canada, Australia, 20–70 y)	BCRAT v4	1/4 (26%)	<0.001	Yes	<0.001	N/A	<0.001	N/A	Increasing
	BRCAPRO v2.1-3	1/4 (7%)	<0.001	Yes	<0.001	N/A	<0.001	N/A	Increasing
	BOADICEA v3	3/4 (66%)	<0.001	Yes	<0.001	N/A	<0.001	N/A	Increasing
Tool comparisons with and without polygenic risk scores (5-year risk)									
Hurson 2021 [29] (UK cohort)	iCARE-Lit (<50 y)	6/10 (60%)	<0.001	Yes	<0.001	Yes	<0.001	Yes	Fluctuating
	iCARE-Lit + PRS (<50 y)	8/10 (80%)	<0.001	Yes	<0.001	Yes	<0.001	Yes	Increasing
	iCARE-Lit (≥50 y)	9/10 (90%)	0.041	Yes	<0.001	Yes	<0.001	Yes	Fluctuating
	iCARE-Lit + PRS (≥50 y)	9/10 (90%)	0.004	Yes	<0.001	Yes	<0.001	Yes	Fluctuating
	iCARE-BPC3 (≥50 y)	10/10 (100%)	0.020	Yes	<0.001	Yes	<0.001	Yes	Fluctuating
	iCARE-BPC3 + PRS (≥50 y)	10/10 (100%)	0.002	Yes	<0.001	Yes	<0.001	Yes	Fluctuating

Table 2. *Cont.*

Study (Country, Age Range)	Model	Proportion of Cohort Well-Validated [a]	Evidence of Miscalibration (p-Value)	Mis-Calibration [b]	Lower Q Compared to Middle Qs (p-Value)	Distinguishes Women in Lowest RG? [b,c]	Upper Q Compared to Middle Qs (p-Value)	Distinguishes Women in Highest RG? [b,c]	Trend in Observed Rates
Other risk assessment tools (5-year risk)									
Jee 2020 [37] (Republic of Korea)	KREA (<50 y)	5/10 (50%)	0.022	Yes	<0.001	Yes	<0.001	Yes	Fluctuating
	KRKR (<50 y)	4/10 (40%)	0.383	No	<0.001	Yes	<0.001	Yes	Fluctuating
	KREA (≥50 y)	6/10 (60%)	0.341	No	0.002	Yes	0.160	No	Fluctuating
	KRKR (≥50 y)	3/10 (30%)	0.127	No	0.005	Yes	0.222	No	Fluctuating
Li 2018 [39] (USA, 50–79 y)	ER−	9/10 (90%)	0.044	Yes	0.810	No	0.380	No	Fluctuating
	ER+	9/10 (90%)	<0.001	Yes	<0.001	Yes	<0.001	Yes	Fluctuating
Min 2014 [40] (Republic of Korea, >29–60 y)	Original Korean tool	1/5 (20%)	<0.001	Yes	0.439	No	0.356	No	Fluctuating
	Updated Korean tool	2/5 (40%)	<0.001	Yes	0.640	No	0.022	Yes	Fluctuating

[a] Evaluation of well-validated risk groups is based on the corresponding 95% confidence intervals of point estimates including 1; [b] Based on *p*-value of <0.05 for statistical significance, [c] To ensure comparability of findings, if >25% of the study cohort was in the highest or/and the lowest risk groups, *p*-values were reported but were not used to determine if the tool distinguished women in highest or lowest risk groups. Abbreviations: AABCS = Asian American Breast Cancer Study; BCRAT = Breast cancer risk assessment tool; BOADICEA = Breast and Ovarian Analysis of Disease Incidence and Carrier Estimation Algorithm; ER = Estrogen receptor; i-Care-BPC3 = Individualized Coherent Absolute Risk Estimation; iCARE-Lit = Individualized Coherent Absolute Risk Estimation—literature based tool; KREA = tool using Korean incidence, mortality and risk factor distributions with European-ancestry relative risks; KRKR = tool using Korean incidence, mortality and risk factor distributions with Korean relative risks; NHS = Nurses' Health Study; PRS = polygenic risk score; Q = quartile; TC = Tyrer-Cuzick; v = version; v: version; WHI = Women's Health Initiative; y: years.

3.3. Observed Cancer Incidence by Risk Group

The majority of tools, with a few exceptions (Chen version 1 [41], ER- [39], the KREA and KRKR Korean tools [37] and the original Korean model [40]), were able to identify the broad group of women with the highest risk of breast cancer. This group always corresponded to the highest observed rates of incident breast cancer, indicating that most tools are effective in identifying women in the highest risk category in one setting (BCRAT version 1 [41]; BCRAT version 4 [34]; BCRmod and BCRmod recalibrated [36]; ER+ [39], Tyrer-Cuzick version 7 [34], updated Korean [40]) and across different settings (AABCS and BCRAT version 2 [32,40]; BCRAT v3 [35,36]; iCARE-Lit and iCARE-BPC3 [29,35]; BRCAPRO [30,34] and Tyrer-Cuzick version 8.0b [34,35]).

Some tools could consistently stratify women in the lowest categories of breast cancer risk across different settings; namely Tyrer-Cuzick version 8.0b [34,35], BCRAT version 3 [35,36], BRCAPRO [30,34], iCARE-Lit and iCARE-BPC3 [29,35]. Although additional tools could distinguish women in the lowest category of risk in a single setting (e.g., BCRAT version 4, Tyrer-Cuzick version 7, ER+, KREA, KRKR), there was not enough evidence to ascertain their performance across different settings.

The contribution of PRS to improving risk tool accuracy varied between tools and sub-groups in Hurson et al. [29]. For example, PRS improved the consistency of the graded association between risk groups and observed rates for the iCARE-Lit tool applied to a UK cohort of women aged under 50 years but did not improve the trend for women in that cohort aged 50 years or older, nor for a US cohort aged 50–74 years. Another iCARE tool variant of (iCARE-BPC3) worsened the graded association between risk groups and observe cancer rates for women aged 50 years or older in a UK cohort.

The addition of mammographic density appeared to improve some tools slightly for some risk groups. For example, the Tyrer-Cuzick tool reported in McCarthy et al. [34] improved differentiation for the higher-risk groups but worsened the graded association in lower-risk groups (Figure 2A), and Tyrer-Cuzick applied in Brentnall et al. [38] did not discernibly improve the association (Figure S1C, Supplementary Materials).

There was limited evidence to evaluate the effect of a longer risk-prediction interval on observed cancer incidence. The AABCS tool appeared to better differentiate lower and higher-risk groups at 10 years than 5 years, [32,40] and the BCRAT version 2 tool was more clearly graded with longer-term cancer incidence (Figure 2B; Supplementary Figure S1C) [32]. It was not possible to evaluate the results from the risk assessment tools reported by Terry et al. [31] due to the uneven distribution of the cohort among the five risk groups reported.

3.4. Risk of Bias Assessment

Risk of bias assessments were undertaken for each of the tools evaluated in each study. The overall risk of bias rating for all 47 risk of bias assessments undertaken was high (Table 3). The overall risk of bias for the participants domain was low for 75% of assessments. For the predictor domain, the overall rating was low for 36% of assessments, high for 36% and unclear for 28%; for the outcome domain, 66% of assessments were rated as unclear and 34% at high risk while the overall rating for the analysis domain was high risk of bias for all 47 assessments. Detailed findings listed per risk of bias domain are provided in the Supplementary Table S3.

Table 3. Summary of risk of bias of included breast cancer risk assessment tool studies for breast cancer calibration outcomes. low risk is green, high risk is red and undetermined is orange.

Study	RAT	Cohort	Year	Outcome	Participants	Predictors	Outcome	Analysis [a]	Overall RoB
Hurson 2021 [29]	iCARE BPC3	UK Biobank	5	Invasive or DCIS	LR	LR	U	HR	HR
Hurson 2021 [29]	iCARE BPC3 LR PRS	UK Biobank	5	Invasive or DCIS	LR	U	U	HR	HR
Hurson 2021 [29]	iCARE Lit	UK Biobank	5	Invasive or DCIS	LR	LR	U	HR	HR
Hurson 2021 [29]	iCARE Lit LR PRS	UK Biobank	5	Invasive or DCIS	LR	U	U	HR	HR
Hurson 2021 [29]	iCARE Lit	WGHS	5	Invasive or DCIS	LR	U	U	HR	HR
Hurson 2021 [29]	iCARE Lit LR PRS	WGHS	5	Invasive or DCIS	LR	U	U	HR	HR
Jantzen 2021 [33]	TC v8	CARTaGENE	5	Invasive	LR	LR	U	HR	HR
Jantzen 2021 [33]	BCRAT v4	CARTaGENE	5	Invasive	LR	LR	U	HR	HR
McCarthy 2020 [34]	TC v7	NWH	6	Invasive	HR	LR	U	HR	HR
McCarthy 2020 [34]	TC v8.0b	NWH	6	Invasive	HR	LR	U	HR	HR
McCarthy 2020 [34]	BCRAT v4	NWH	6	Invasive	LR	LR	U	HR	HR
McCarthy 2020 [34]	BRCAPRO v2.1HR4	NWH	6	Invasive	HR	LR	U	HR	HR
Choudhury 2020 [35]	TC v8	GS	5	Invasive	LR	U	U	HR	HR
Choudhury 2020 [35]	iCARE Lit	GS	5	Invasive	LR	U	U	HR	HR
Choudhury 2020 [35]	iCARE BPC3	GS	5	Invasive	LR	U	U	HR	HR
Choudhury 2020 [35]	BCRAT v3	PLCO	5	Invasive	LR	LR	U	HR	HR
Choudhury 2020 [35]	iCARE Lit	PLCO	5	Invasive	LR	LR	U	HR	HR
Hüsing 2020 [36]	BCRAT v3	EPICHRGermany	5	Invasive	HR	U	HR	HR	HR
Hüsing 2020 [36]	BCRmod	EPICHRGermany	5	Invasive	LR	U	HR	HR	HR
Hüsing 2020 [36]	BCRAT v3 recalibrated	EPICHRGermany	5	Invasive	HR	U	HR	HR	HR
Hüsing 2020 [36]	BCRmod recalibrated	EPICHRGermany	5	Invasive	LR	U	HR	HR	HR
Jee 2020 [37]	KREA	KCPSHRII Biobank	5	Invasive	LR	LR	U	HR	HR
Jee 2020 [37]	KRKR	KCPSHRII Biobank	5	Invasive	LR	LR	U	HR	HR
Terry 2019 [31]	BCRAT v4	ProFHRSC	5	Invasive	HR	HR	HR	HR	HR
Terry 2019 [31]	BRCAPRO v2.1HR3	ProFHRSC	5	Invasive	LR	HR	HR	HR	HR
Terry 2019 [31]	TC v8.0b	ProFHRSC	5	Invasive	LR	HR	HR	HR	HR
Terry 2019 [31]	BOADICEA v3	ProFHRSC	5	Invasive	LR	HR	HR	HR	HR
Terry 2019 [31]	BCRAT v4	ProFHRSC	10	Invasive	HR	HR	HR	HR	HR
Terry 2019 [31]	BRCAPRO v2.1HR3	ProFHRSC	10	Invasive	LR	HR	HR	HR	HR
Terry 2019 [31]	TC v8.0b	ProFHRSC	10	Invasive	LR	HR	HR	HR	HR
Terry 2019 [31]	BOADICEA v3	ProFHRSC	10	Invasive	LR	HR	HR	HR	HR
Brentnall 2018 [38]	TC v7.02	KPWHRBCSC	10	Invasive	LR	HR	U	HR	HR
Brentnall 2018 [38]	TC v7.02 LR BD	KPWHRBCSC	10	Invasive	LR	HR	U	HR	HR

Table 3. Cont.

Study	RAT	Cohort	Year	Outcome	Participants	Predictors	Outcome	Analysis [a]	Overall RoB
Li 2018 [39]	ERHR	WHI	5	Invasive	LR	U	HR	HR	HR
Li 2018 [39]	ERLR	WHI	5	Invasive	LR	U	HR	HR	HR
Min 2014 [40]	BCRAT v2	WHC CGH	5	Invasive	HR	LR	U	HR	HR
Min 2014 [40]	AABCS	WHC CGH	5	Invasive	HR	LR	U	HR	HR
Min 2014 [40]	Original Korean tool	WHC CGH	5	Invasive	HR	LR	U	HR	HR
Min 2014 [40]	Updated Korean tool	WHC CGH	5	Invasive	HR	LR	U	HR	HR
Powell 2014 [30]	BCRAT v2 or 3	MWS	5	Invasive	HR	HR	U	HR	HR
Powell 2014 [30]	BRCAPRO v(NR)	MWS	5	Invasive	LR	HR	U	HR	HR
Arrospide 2013 [41]	BCRAT v1	SCHRBCSP	5	Invasive	LR	LR	HR	HR	HR
Arrospide 2013 [41]	Chen v1	SCHRBCSP	5	Invasive	LR	HR	HR	HR	HR
Chay 2012 [32]	BCRAT v2	SBCSP	5	Invasive	LR	HR	U	HR	HR
Chay 2012 [32]	AABCS	SBCSP	5	Invasive	LR	HR	U	HR	HR
Chay 2012 [32]	BCRAT v2	SBCSP	10	Invasive	LR	HR	U	HR	HR
Chay 2012 [32]	AABCS	SBCSP	10	Invasive	LR	HR	U	HR	HR

[a] Note: Items 4.5, 4.8 and 4.9 omitted as they are signalling questions for model development and not validation; Key to domain and overall rating: High risk of bias: indicated as 'HR'; low risk of bias: indicated as 'LR'; unclear risk of bias: indicated as 'U' Abbreviations: AABCS = Asian American Breast Cancer Study; BCRAT = Breast cancer risk assessment tool; BOADICEA = Breast and Ovarian Analysis of Disease Incidence and Carrier Estimation Algorithm; DCIS = ductal carcinoma in situ; ER = Estrogen receptor; i-Care-BPC3 = Individualized Coherent Absolute Risk Estimation—Breast and Prostate Cancer Cohort Consortium; iCARE-Lit = Individualized Coherent Absolute Risk Estimation—literature based tool; KREA = tool using Korean incidence, mortality and risk factor distributions with European-ancestry relative risks; KRKR = tool using Korean incidence, mortality and risk factor distributions with Korean relative risks; N = number of participants; NHS = Nurses' Health Study; NR = not reported; ROB = risk of bias; PRS = polygenic risk score; TC = Tyrer-Cuzick; v = version; WHI = Women's Health Initiative.

Common factors that contributed to unclear or high risk of bias ratings included: handling of missing predictors at the time of validation when a tool did not allow for an unknown or missing option; specification of standard measurement of predictors at baseline; minimal reporting of predictor assessments blind to outcome; limited information provided around methods used to determine outcomes; omission of standard outcome definitions and standardised follow-up protocol and lack of clarity on the number of women who had full follow-up for the time interval between predictor assessment and outcome determination. Furthermore, the analysis domain rated poorly with all tools examining 5-year risk having <100 events across risk categories, although this was achieved for most tools assessing 10-year risk. Additionally, often no direct reference was made to baseline questionnaires preventing a clear assessment of the handling of continuous and categorical predictors (i.e., if data transformation was required between collection vs. input) unless stated in the text.

Tools tended to rate poorly for methods regarding handling of missing data. The main reasons for poor ratings included inappropriate assumptions, omitting predictors with missing data in general or for a particular predictor, and imputation of predictors with >50% missing participant data.

4. Discussion
4.1. Summary of Main Results

This systematic review of studies comparing multiple breast cancer risk assessment tools within general populations examined several metrics to evaluate risk assessment tools, namely: the ratio of the expected over observed number of breast cancer cases; evidence of miscalibration; the proportion of study group where E/O and 95%CI includes unity, and how these related to the observed cancer incidence rates across assigned risk groups. We found that no tool was consistently well-calibrated across multiple studies, and breast density or polygenic risk scores did not improve calibration. While most tools identified a risk group with higher rates of observed cancers, few tools identified lower-risk groups across different settings.

We did not apply a single metric to compare tools because the interpretation and value of each metric depends on how the risk assessment tool might be used. Where risk assessment tools are being used to advise an individual woman about her estimated breast cancer risk, specified as, for example, her 5-year or lifetime risk, the tool should have demonstrated very good calibration of E/O rates within her population to ensure a sufficiently accurate estimate. Communication of this information is also important, as these estimates are often misinterpreted as individual level risk so that, for example, an estimated 3% five-year risk is interpreted as the individual woman having a 3% risk of breast cancer in the next five years, when instead it indicates that 3% of women in the risk group to which she belongs would be expected to have a breast cancer diagnosed in the next five years [42].

The individual-level risk estimates generated by risk tools are also used in clinical practice to advise and manage women according to a risk group assignment based on their estimated risk of breast cancer, without necessarily reporting the estimated individual breast cancer risk for each woman. For example, the Royal Australian College of General Practitioners (RACGP) guidelines define women at 'moderately higher' risk as those with a 1.5 to 3 times higher than average risk, and women at 'potentially high' risk as more than 3 times the average population risk and recommend management based on these risk categories such as screening frequency and/or referral to specific breast imaging surveillance tests, or referral to specialist high-risk services [43]. These tools generally rely on individual risk estimation as the basis for risk group allocation. For example, the iPrevent tool draws on either the IBIS or BOADECIA risk tool depending on an assessment of initial factors such as family history, then assigns the individual to a risk group following the RACGP guidelines. Each woman's risk relative to the average is defined by the ratio of her estimated residual lifetime risk (to age 80) and the average residual lifetime population risk for women of her age. In a validation study of over 15,000 Australian women, iPrevent demonstrated good calibration for women under 50 years (E/O: 1.04; 95% CI = 0.93 to 1.16) but poor calibration for women aged 50 years and older (E/O: 1.24; 95% CI = 1.11 to 1.39), largely due to overestimation of risk in the highest study group decile [44]. These findings are concerning in terms of providing accurate risk estimation to individual women however, as noted by Phillips et al., "the extent of overestimation is unlikely to be of clinical importance because the actual 10-year [breast cancer] risks for these women substantially exceed thresholds for intensified screening and medical prevention (and for mutation carriers, risk-reducing mastectomy). Therefore, the overestimation would be unlikely to lead to an inappropriate change in their clinical management."

The issues mentioned above have potential consequences for how risk assessment tools should be evaluated in relation to risk-based population breast screening While GPs and specialists are (theoretically) able to refer an unlimited number of patients to services to which they are eligible, resource-constrained population risk-based screening programs would benefit from directing screening protocols for higher-risk (or lower-risk) clients to a priori proportions of the screening population. This could mean, for example, that a screening program would provide supplemental or alternative imaging tests to 10% of women deemed to be most likely to benefit from that imaging, based on their short-term breast cancer risk and the expected accuracy of their routine screening test (indicated by, for example, observed interval cancer rates). For this purpose, it should be sufficient to confirm that a risk tool can identify the 10% of screening clients for whom outcomes (observed rates of breast cancer and interval cancers) under the current approach to screening are significantly higher compared to clients with average outcomes in the screened population, even if that tool is not well calibrated in terms of expected and observed rates; this risk stratification could then be used to trial alternative approaches to screening.

This is an important consideration because requiring good E/O calibration of risk assessment tools across the risk spectrum is a difficult standard to reach. For example, a recent evaluation of six established risk models (IBIS, BOADICEA, BRCAPRO, BRCAPRO-BCRAT, BCRAT, and iCARE-lit) in over 52,000 Australian women concluded that only one model (BOADICEA) calibrated well across the spectrum of 15-year risk [26].

Even where good E/O calibration is achieved, this does not necessarily mean that observed rates are ranked well or that calibration is good across the risk spectrum. For example, in the study by McCarthy and colleagues [34], despite BRCAPRO exhibiting goodness-of-fit for the cohort, the observed rates fluctuated for women in the middle deciles, and the assessment of the KRKR tool by Jee et al. [37] on women aged 50 years or older demonstrated good calibration overall but was well-validated for only 30% of the risk groups (of note, this metric is more stringent for studies with a larger number of risk groups such as Jee et al., which had ten). Conversely, models with evidence of miscalibration can demonstrate good differentiation of a higher-risk group. For example, in the study by Hüsing et. al., although BCRmod recalibrated showed evidence of miscalibration to the study population, higher-risk groups (deciles 9–10) were well differentiated [36].

Overall, despite differences between risk assessment tools and study cohorts, most risk tools were able to identify a group of women with the highest risk of breast cancer, with only a few exceptions (Chen v1, ER-, KREA, KRKR and the original Korean model). For lower-risk women, some tools assessed consistently stratified women in the lowest categories of breast cancer risk across different settings (e.g., Tyrer-Cuzick version 8.0b; BRCAPRO version 2.1; iCARE tools). In the case of BCRAT, this depended on the version used; i.e., BCRAT version 3 was found to be consistent in distinguishing women in the lowest risk group whereas the same was not observed for versions 2 and 1. Of note, for some tools it was not possible to assess this feature across different settings as there was only one relevant study included (e.g., BCRmod [36], KREA and KRKR [37], ER+ tool [39]).

The BCRAT tool was the most evaluated risk assessment tool in the included articles, followed by the Tyrer-Cuzick tool, with increasing evaluation of iCARE tools in more recent publications. The number of risk factors considered by the different tools varied considerably. This is an important consideration for policy-makers and health services when selecting the most suitable tool for a specific application, as the number of predictors and the level of detail required for each one can be an impost for women and requires substantial resources to ensure complete and accurate risk information is provided and recorded.

The number of risk groups varied greatly between studies (4–10 groups). Reporting results for more groups provides more detail on how the tool performs as a graded association with increasing risk, which is informative for population-level applications where the availability of resources might be limited. For example, isolating smaller groups of women with very high risk may be more feasible for targeting more costly options (such as MRI) to higher-risk women as part of population breast screening.

We found that mammographic breast density has not been shown to improve the accuracy of breast cancer risk assessment tools based on self-reported information collected from questionnaires. We did not review evidence on the accuracy of breast density alone as a risk assessment tool, with an equivalent assessment of whether other risk predictors improved the accuracy of breast density as a risk assessment tool. However, this is a very active research area, and ongoing review of high-quality evidence is warranted.

Similarly, we found that the addition of a PRS score did not improve accuracy when added to self-reported information within the tools assessed, although this finding was based on a single study [29]. We did not review evidence on the accuracy of PRS alone as a risk assessment tool.

4.2. Comparison with other Published Work

A number of other systematic reviews have been published previously in this field [45–48]. These aimed to provide an overview of published risk assessment tools, basing their assessments on (i) calibration performance using the E/O ratio and (ii) discriminatory accuracy using the area under the receiver operating curve (AUC) and/or concordance statistic (C-statistic). In this review we focused on studies that assessed more than one risk assessment tool on one or more populations, how those tools compared to each other and what overall observations could be drawn by assessing these studies collectively. For this purpose, the AUC and C-statistic are not considered the appropriate metrics for assessing discrimination as they measure the ability of a tool to determine which women are at higher or lower risk of breast cancer than average, but not whether women within a study population have been stratified according to their level of risk, which is critical when evaluating these tools for the purpose of population-based risk-based screening. We recommend the use of observed rates of incident breast cancer according to tool-determined risk groups as it provides a better quantitative assessment of discrimination for this purpose, informing consideration of interventions that might target women at different thresholds of risk across the risk spectrum.

4.3. Applicability and Model Performance

We observed that tools that were recalibrated to the risk profiles of the population in which they were applied demonstrated an improvement in fit, as exemplified in the study by Chay and colleagues [32], which compared BCRAT to its Asian-American variant. This improvement in a risk assessment tool highlights the importance of making such adjustments when considering the application of any risk tool, especially on specific populations. Tools are usually developed using breast cancer incidence rates and risk factor data collected from one population and then applied to a different population without adjusting these parameters. This can lead to poorer model performance as the distribution of risk factors and breast cancer incidence can vary across populations. We need, however, to distinguish between recalibration and 'pre-calibration' as exemplified by the iCARE-based tools which uniquely incorporated calibration to population-based age-specific disease incidence rates before they were used [35]. As can be seen from Table 2 and associated graphs, these tools generally performed very well. They fell within the scope of this systematic review as they met the review's criterion of a tool calibrated to the study validation population of interest. This approach in the use of risk-prediction tools seems sensible given that population-based age-specific disease incidence is usually available and, as reinforced by this review, tools without calibration perform very differently in different settings.

Assessment of the studies included, revealed opportunities to improve standardisation of risk tool evaluations. Not all studies cited the specific version of the tool and package used. When these details were not provided, it was difficult for reviewers to deduce this information even if predictors were listed. For example, one study [36] provided a link to the BCRAT tool on the National Cancer Institute (NCI) website and a second study [35] using the same tool, also included the date and year accessed. However, the NCI provides the latest tool versions without detailed history of previous versions and updates; therefore, the version of the tool used by these studies at the time they were conducted had to be deduced. For studies that cited tool versions, these were often determined by the software used; e.g., BCRAT can be run on SAS Macro or R and these packages have their own tool-version numbers. For some models, the software was accessible through different sources. For example, BRCAPRO is accessible via the BayesMendel R package or within the CancerGene software program which now uses the code from BayesMendel. In the case of studies using the latter, even when the CancerGene software version was cited there was insufficient information available from the CancerGene website to deduce which version of the BayesMendel R package was used by that software. For full transparency it is recommended that authors provide the specific version of the risk assessment tools used including the software package, all predictors offered by that version and used in the study being reported.

4.4. Risk of Bias and Quality of the Evidence

Critical assessment of studies in terms of risk of bias is required to provide a comprehensive evaluation. We used the recently published PROBAST tool, specifically designed to thoroughly assess the risk of bias in relation to risk assessment tool studies. Only one previous systematic review identified from our searches had included a risk of bias assessment, although a tool for evaluating modelling studies was used instead of PROBAST [42]. All tools we evaluated across studies received an overall rating of 'high risk of bias'. Although this was driven mainly by rulings for the domain of analysis, there was also an evident lack of clarity in the reporting of key details contributing to ratings of 'unclear risk of bias' for 28–66% of tools for the predictor and outcomes domains.

One of the main areas of concern is the domain of predictors with respect to the collection and completeness of data on risk predictors, and the statistical methods used to deal with any data issues. One method that studies used to deal with missing predictors at the time of validation was multiple imputation (29, 35). Although this is a common method to deal with missing data, the reference dataset is simulated and thus possibly less reliable. This also limits our understanding of how missing data would be addressed at an individual level if the tool were utilised as part of health service provision. In other studies, researchers sometimes stated that missing data was handled according to the specifications of each software application (e.g., McCarthy et al. [34], Jantzen et al. [33]), however it was not always clear whether a predictor value was then classed as missing or whether the predictor was omitted from the tool (e.g., BRCAPRO version 2.1–3, Tyrer-Cuzick version 8.0b and BOADICEA v3 in Terry et al. [31]). In other cases, the approach to handling missing data was not reported. For example, Brentnall et al. [38] applied version 7.02 of the Tyrer-Cuzick model (developed in the UK) on a US cohort; this version included prior use of hormone replacement therapy (HRT) (yes/no) as a predictor without an option of selecting 'unknown' or 'missing' if these data were unavailable. The authors did not report any information regarding the collection of HRT data or how missing data was handled. Overall, it is not possible to evaluate the precise effect of missing predictor values on risk estimates unless provision of a 'missing' option has been made by tool providers, which may indeed be more reflective of actual use of tools in practice as sometimes information on predictors cannot be recalled. We recommend that future studies consider including information on how missing data are managed, as this would improve comparability between studies and help recognise the challenges of applying risk assessment tools to different settings and study populations. Overall, factors identified by our risk of bias analysis could potentially explain some of the observed differences in tool performance in different settings described throughout this review.

We also recommend more standardised and transparent reporting of risk assessment tools, using the 'Transparent Reporting of a multivariable prediction model for Individual Prognosis or Diagnosis' (TRIPOD) statement published in 2015 [49]. TRIPOD provides a 22-item checklist considered to be key for transparent reporting of risk assessment tool studies. The statement was created to increase the level of reporting standards as prior studies performing external validation of risk assessment tools were found to commonly lack clarity in reporting and tended not to present important details needed to understand how the tool might be applied or whether results reflected true performance of the tool [50]. This was reflected in a systematic review examining the methodological conduct and reporting of external validation studies for risk assessment tools that found that of 45 articles published in 2010, 16% did not report the number of outcome events when validating tools, 54% did not acknowledge missing data, and frequently, it was unclear as to whether the authors had applied a complete or an abridged version of the tool [50]. For our analysis, four studies [30,32,40,41] were published prior to the TRIPOD statement, however no studies published after 2015 refer to the TRIPOD statement or checklist.

4.5. Limitations

This systematic review has certain limitations. A number of studies that compared different risk assessment tools on the same population were not included due to the focus of this review to compare risk assessment tools generated from, or calibrated to, a different population to the study validation population of interest or tools specifically calibrated to the study population of interest. However, focusing on the selected studies in this review enabled a fairer comparison between tools and improvement in the quality of the evidence. Secondly, despite meeting the criteria for inclusion, some studies had to be excluded due to some required data being unavailable for full assessment. Nonetheless, efforts were made to contact the authors. Additionally, for studies which did not provide the number of women in each risk category, the calculated estimates may be inaccurate if numbers are distributed unequally between risk categories, as the number of women per category was estimated by dividing the numbers of participants equally among categories.

This review did not compare tools in terms of interval cancers (i.e., cancers diagnosed following a negative population screening test), breast cancer mortality, nor incidence of breast cancer defined by different tumour characteristics (e.g., sub-type, size, grade, nodal involvement). We did initially seek to assess these outcomes as this evidence is likely to be of interest for some applications, such as consideration of risk-based screening protocols, however insufficient evidence was available to make these comparisons between tools.

Finally, one of the methods used to assess risk assessment tools was based on E/O point estimates and their 95%CI including unity (E/O = 1). Studies where tools were applied on small cohorts of women have wider CIs and therefore be more likely to include this value compared to larger studies which have narrower CIs. Additionally, we characterised the functional form of observed cancer rates according to risk groups based on point estimates reported without uncertainty estimates (e.g., CIs). However, while we acknowledge these metrics have minor limitations, these were only two of the metrics employed; when evaluated collectively all metrics analysed provide sufficient information to enable a fair and balanced assessment of risk assessment tools.

5. Conclusions

This systematic review identified various questionnaire-based tools (sometimes incorporating mammographic density or genetic information) that are effective in assigning women to risk groups for incident breast cancer, for various metrics of tool performance. The most appropriate metrics to consider depend on how the risk tool is to be applied. While good calibration between expected and observed rates is essential for individual-level estimated breast cancer risk described as a rate over a specified period, tools demonstrating good differentiation of observed breast cancer incidence rates are potentially suitable for triaging women to population-level risk-based interventions such as risk-based breast cancer screening, even if they are not well calibrated in terms of expected versus observed outcomes across the risk spectrum. Current trials such as MyPeBS [51] and WISDOM [52] are allocating women to risk-based screening protocols based on their predicted risk of breast cancer as estimated by combining genetic information with scores from risk assessment tools which incorporate mammographic density (Tyrer-Cuzick and Breast Cancer Surveillance Consortium (BCSC) risk tools for MyPeBS [53]; BCSC risk tool for WISDOM [54]). Results from these studies will provide valuable information on the clinical utility of these detailed and resource-intensive risk assessment tools; in parallel, work is required to understand the relative utility of more parsimonious tools that may achieve similar outcomes while markedly reducing the impost of risk assessment on women and health services.

Supplementary Materials: The following supporting information can be downloaded at: https://www.mdpi.com/article/10.3390/cancers15041124/s1, Figure S1: additional graphs of risk calibration and observed rate of incident breast cancer for tools in included studies; Table S1: search strategy; Table S2: risk predictors within risk assessment tools compared in the studies included in the review; Table S3: detailed assessment of risk of bias of included risk assessment tools; List S1: articles excluded from the review at full text screening stage by reason for exclusion; Dataset S1: data extracted from included articles.

Author Contributions: Conceptualization, C.N.; Methodology, V.F., D.C., L.S.V. and C.N.; Formal analysis, C.N., V.F. and S.E.; Resources, C.N.; Data Curation, V.F. and D.C.; Writing—Original Draft Preparation, L.S.V., C.N., V.F. and D.C.; Writing—Review and Editing, all; Visualization, Q.L., L.S.V., V.F. and D.C.; Supervision: C.N., L.S.V., S.H., J.S. and S.E., Project Administration: V.F.; Funding Acquisition: C.N. All authors have read and agreed to the published version of the manuscript.

Funding: This research was conducted as part of the Roadmap to Optimising Screening in Australia for Breast (ROSA) project which received funding from the Australian Government Department of Health (contract reference 2000004049). The funder had no role in the study design, data collection and analysis, the decision to publish or the preparation of the manuscript. The funder had no role in the study design, data collection and analysis, the decision to publish or the preparation of the manuscript.

Informed Consent Statement: Written informed consent was not required as this review used data from previously published studies.

Data Availability Statement: The data supporting the findings of this work are available in the cited articles and in the manuscript's Supplementary Materials.

Acknowledgments: We would like to acknowledge Dianne O'Connell for her review and input to the umbrella protocol submitted to PROSPERO which included details on this systematic review.

Conflicts of Interest: LSV, VF and DC have received salary support via the grant from the Australian Government, Department of Health (see funding section) paid to their institution. CN leads the ROSA project which has received the above-named funding.

References

1. Schünemann, H.J.; Lerda, D.; Quinn, C.; Follmann, M.; Alonso-Coello, P.; Rossi, P.G.; Lebeau, A.; Nyström, L.; Broeders, M.; Ioannidou-Mouzaka, L.; et al. European Commission Initiative on Breast Cancer (ECIBC) Contributor Group. Breast Cancer Screening and Diagnosis: A Synopsis of the European Breast Guidelines. *Ann. Intern. Med.* **2020**, *172*, 46–56. [CrossRef] [PubMed]
2. Monticciolo, D.L.; Newell, M.S.; Hendrick, R.E.; Helvie, M.A.; Moy, L.; Monsees, B.; Kopans, D.B.; Eby, P.R.; Sickles, E.A. Breast Cancer Screening for Average-Risk Women: Recommendations from the ACR Commission on Breast Imaging. *J. Am. Coll. Radiol.* **2017**, *14*, 1137–1143. [PubMed]
3. Siu, A.L.; US Preventive Services Task Force. Screening for Breast Cancer: U.S. Preventive Services Task Force Recommendation Statement. *Ann. Intern. Med.* **2016**, *164*, 279–296.
4. Elder, K.; Nickson, C.; Pattanasri, M.; Cooke, S.; Machalek, D.; Rose, A.; Mou, A.; Collins, J.P.; Park, A.; De Boer, R.; et al. Treatment intensity differences after early-stage breast cancer (ESBC) diagnosis depending on participation in a screening program. *Ann. Surg. Oncol.* **2018**, *25*, 2563–2572. [CrossRef] [PubMed]
5. Nelson, H.D.; Pappas, M.; Cantor, A.; Griffin, J.; Daeges, M.; Humphrey, L. Harms of Breast Cancer Screening: Systematic Review to Update the 2009 U.S. Preventive Services Task Force Recommendation. *Ann. Intern. Med.* **2016**, *164*, 256–267. [PubMed]
6. BreastScreen Australia Program Website. Available online: https://www.health.gov.au/initiatives-and-programs/breastscreen-australia-program (accessed on 24 October 2022).
7. UK Breast Screening Program Website. Available online: https://www.nhs.uk/conditions/breast-screening-mammogram/when-youll-be-invited-and-who-should-go/ (accessed on 24 October 2022).
8. Canadian Breast Cancer Screening Program Information. Available online: https://www.partnershipagainstcancer.ca/topics/breast-cancer-screening-scan-2019-2020/ (accessed on 24 October 2022).
9. Sankatsing, V.D.V.; van Ravesteyn, N.T.; Heijnsdijk, E.A.M.; Broeders, M.J.M.; de Koning, H.J. Risk stratification in breast cancer screening: Cost-effectiveness and harm-benefit ratios for low-risk and high-risk women. *Int. J. Cancer.* **2020**, *147*, 3059–3067. [CrossRef] [PubMed]

10. Trentham-Dietz, A.; Kerlikowske, K.; Stout, N.K.; Miglioretti, D.L.; Schechter, C.B.; Ergun, M.A.; van den Broek, J.J.; Alagoz, O.; Sprague, B.L.; van Ravesteyn, N.T.; et al. Tailoring Breast Cancer Screening Intervals by Breast Density and Risk for Women Aged 50 Years or Older: Collaborative Modeling of Screening Outcomes. *Ann. Intern. Med.* 2016, *165*, 700–712. [CrossRef]
11. Gail, M.H. Twenty-five years of breast cancer risk models and their applications. *J. Natl. Cancer Inst.* 2015, *107*, djv042. [CrossRef]
12. Zhang, X.; Rice, M.; Tworoger, S.S.; Rosner, B.A.; Eliassen, A.H.; Tamimi, R.M.; Joshi, A.D.; Lindstrom, S.; Qian, J.; Colditz, G.A.; et al. Addition of a polygenic risk score, mammographic density, and endogenous hormones to existing breast cancer risk prediction models: A nested case-control study. *PLoS Med.* 2018, *15*, e1002644.
13. Shieh, Y.; Hu, D.; Ma, L.; Huntsman, S.; Gard, C.C.; Leung, J.W.; Tice, J.A.; Vachon, C.M.; Cummings, S.R.; Kerlikowske, K.; et al. Breast cancer risk prediction using a clinical risk model and polygenic risk score. *Breast Cancer Res Treat.* 2016, *159*, 513–525.
14. Nickson, C.; Procopio, P.; Velentzis, L.S.; Carr, S.; Devereux, L.; Mann, G.B.; James, P.; Lee, G.; Wellard, C.; Campbell, I. Prospective validation of the NCI Breast Cancer Risk Assessment Tool (Gail Model) on 40,000 Australian women. *Breast Cancer Res.* 2018, *20*, 155. [PubMed]
15. Brittain, H.K.; Scott, R.; Thomas, E. The rise of the genome and personalised medicine. *Clin. Med.* 2017, *17*, 545–551. [CrossRef] [PubMed]
16. Harkness, E.F.; Astley, S.M.; Evans, D.G. Risk-based breast cancer screening strategies in women. *Best Pract. Res. Clin. Obstet. Gynaecol.* 2020, *65*, 3–17. [PubMed]
17. Allman, R.; Spaeth, E.; Lai, J.; Gross, S.J.; Hopper, J.L. A streamlined model for use in clinical breast cancer risk assessment maintains predictive power and is further improved with inclusion of a polygenic risk score. *PLoS ONE* 2021, *16*, e0245375. [CrossRef]
18. Sherman, M.E.; Ichikawa, L.; Pfeiffer, R.M.; Miglioretti, D.L.; Kerlikowske, K.; Tice, J.; Vacek, P.M.; Gierach, G.L. Relationship of Predicted Risk of Developing Invasive Breast Cancer, as Assessed with Three Models, and and Breast Cancer Mortality among Breast Cancer Patients. *PLoS ONE* 2016, *11*, e0160966. [CrossRef]
19. Abdolell, M.; Payne, J.I.; Caines, J.; Tsuruda, K.; Barnes, P.J.; Talbot, P.J.; Tong, O.; Brown, P.; Rivers-Bowerman, M.; Iles, S. Assessing breast cancer risk within the general screening population: Developing a breast cancer risk model to identify higher risk women at mammographic screening. *Eur. Radiol.* 2020, *30*, 5417–5426. [CrossRef]
20. van Veen, E.M.; Brentnall, A.R.; Byers, H.; Harkness, E.F.; Astley, S.M.; Sampson, S.; Howell, A.; Newman, W.G.; Cuzick, J.; Evans, D.G.R. Use of Single-Nucleotide Polymorphisms and Mammographic Density Plus Classic Risk Factors for Breast Cancer Risk Prediction. *JAMA Oncol.* 2018, *4*, 476–482. [CrossRef]
21. Eriksson, M.; Czene, K.; Pawitan, Y.; Leifland, K.; Darabi, H.; Hall, P. A clinical model for identifying the short-term risk of breast cancer. *Breast Cancer Res.* 2017, *19*, 29.
22. Cancer Council Australia. Optimising Early Detection of Breast Cancer in Australia. Available online: https://www.cancer.org.au/about-us/policy-and-advocacy/early-detection-policy/breast-cancer-screening/optimising-early-detection (accessed on 24 October 2022).
23. Page, M.J.; McKenzie, J.E.; Bossuyt, P.M.; Boutron, I.; Hoffmann, T.C.; Mulrow, C.D.; Shamseer, L.; Tetzlaff, J.M.; Akl, E.A.; Brennan, S.E.; et al. The PRISMA 2020 statement: An updated guideline for reporting systematic reviews. *BMJ* 2021, *372*, n71.
24. Wolff, R.F.; Moons, K.G.M.; Riley, R.D.; Whiting, P.F.; Westwood, M.; Collins, G.S.; Reitsma, J.B.; Kleijnen, J.; Mallett, S.; PROBAST Group. PROBAST: A Tool to Assess the Risk of Bias and Applicability of Prediction Model Studies. *Ann. Intern. Med.* 2019, *170*, 51–58. [CrossRef]
25. Finazzi, S.; Poole, D.; Luciani, D.; Cogo, P.E.; Bertolini, G. Calibration belt for quality-of-care assessment based on dichotomous outcomes. *PLoS ONE* 2011, *6*, e16110. [CrossRef] [PubMed]
26. Li, S.X.; Milne, R.L.; Nguyen-Dumont, T.; English, D.R.; Giles, G.G.; Southey, M.C.; Antoniou, A.C.; Lee, A.; Winship, I.; Hopper, J.L.; et al. Prospective Evaluation over 15 Years of Six Breast Cancer Risk Models. *Cancers* 2021, *13*, 5194. [PubMed]
27. Marshall, A.; Altman, D.G.; Royston, P.; Holder, R.L. Comparison of techniques for handling missing covariate data within prognostic modelling studies: A simulation study. *BMC Med. Res. Methodol.* 2010, *10*, 7.
28. Sterne, J.A.C.; White, I.R.; Carlin, J.B.; Spratt, M.; Royston, P.; Kenward, M.G.; Wood, A.M.; Carpenter, J.R. Multiple imputation for missing data in epidemiological and clinical research: Potential and pitfalls. *BMJ* 2009, *338*, b2393.
29. Hurson, A.N.; Choudhury, P.P.; Gao, C.; Hüsing, A.; Eriksson, M.; Shi, M.; Jones, M.E.; Evans, D.G.R.; Milne, R.L.; Gaudet, M.M.; et al. Prospective evaluation of a breast-cancer risk model integrating classical risk factors and polygenic risk in 15 cohorts from six countries. *Int. J. Epidemiol.* 2021, *23*, dyab036. [CrossRef]
30. Powell, M.; Jamshidian, F.; Cheyne, K.; Nititham, J.; Prebil, L.A.; Ereman, R. Assessing breast cancer risk models in Marin County, a population with high rates of delayed childbirth. *Clin. Breast Cancer.* 2014, *14*, 212–220. [CrossRef]
31. Terry, M.B.; Liao, Y.; Whittemore, A.S.; Leoce, N.; Buchsbaum, R.; Zeinomar, N.; Dite, G.S.; Chung, W.K.; Knight, J.A.; Southey, M.C.; et al. 10-year performance of four models of breast cancer risk: A validation study. *Lancet Oncol.* 2019, *20*, 504–517.
32. Chay, W.Y.; Ong, W.S.; Tan, P.H.; Leo, N.Q.J.; Ho, G.H.; Wong, C.S.; Chia, K.S.; Chow, K.Y.; Tan, M.S.; Ang, P.S. Validation of the Gail model for predicting individual breast cancer risk in a prospective nationwide study of 28,104 Singapore women. *Breast Cancer Res.* 2012, *14*, R19. [CrossRef]
33. Jantzen, R.; Payette, Y.; de Malliard, T.; Labbe, C.; Noisel, N.; Broet, P. Validation of breast cancer risk assessment tools on a French-Canadian population-based cohort. *BMJ Open* 2021, *11*, e045078. [CrossRef]

34. McCarthy, A.M.; Guan, Z.; Welch, M.; Griffin, M.E.; Sippo, D.A.; Deng, Z.; Coopey, S.B.; Acar, A.; Semine, A.; Parmigiani, G.; et al. Performance of breast cancer risk assessment models in a large mammography cohort. *J. Nat. Cancer Inst.* **2020**, *112*, djz177.
35. Choudhury, P.P.; Wilcox, A.N.; Brook, M.N.; Zhang, Y.; Ahearn, T.; Orr, N.; Coulson, P.; Schoemaker, M.J.; Jones, M.E.; Gail, M.H.; et al. Comparative validation of breast cancer risk prediction models and projections for future risk stratification. *J. Nat. Cancer Inst.* **2020**, *112*, djz113. [CrossRef] [PubMed]
36. Hüsing, A.; Quante, A.S.; Chang-Claude, J.; Aleksandrova, K.; Kaaks, R.; Pfeiffer, R.M. Validation of two US breast cancer risk prediction models in German women. *Cancer Causes Control.* **2020**, *31*, 525–536. [CrossRef] [PubMed]
37. Jee, Y.H.; Gao, C.; Kim, J.; Park, S.; Jee, S.H.; Kraft, P. Validating breast cancer risk prediction models in the Korean Cancer Prevention Study-II Biobank. *Cancer Epidemiol. Biomark. Prev.* **2020**, *29*, 1271–1277.
38. Brentnall, A.R.; Cuzick, J.; Buist, D.S.M.; Bowles, E.J.A. Long-term Accuracy of Breast Cancer Risk Assessment Combining Classic Risk Factors and Breast Density. *JAMA Oncol.* **2018**, *4*, e180174. [CrossRef]
39. Li, K.; Anderson, G.; Viallon, V.; Arveux, P.; Kvaskoff, M.; Fournier, A.; Krogh, V.; Tumino, R.; Sánchez, M.J.; Ardanaz, E.; et al. Risk prediction for estrogen receptor-specific breast cancers in two large prospective cohorts. *Breast Cancer Res.* **2018**, *20*, 147. [PubMed]
40. Min, J.W.; Chang, M.C.; Lee, H.K.; Hur, M.H.; Noh, D.Y.; Yoon, J.H.; Jung, Y.; Yang, J.H.; Korean Breast Cancer Society. Validation of risk assessment models for predicting the incidence of breast cancer in Korean women. *J. Breast Cancer.* **2014**, *17*, 226–235. [CrossRef] [PubMed]
41. Arrospide, A.; Forne, C.; Rue, M.; Tora, N.; Mar, J.; Bare, M. An assessment of existing models for individualized breast cancer risk estimation in a screening program in Spain. *BMC Cancer* **2013**, *13*, 587. [CrossRef]
42. Keogh, L.A.; Steel, E.; Weideman, P.; Butow, P.; Collins, I.M.; Emery, J.D.; Mann, G.B.; Bickerstaffe, A.; Trainer, A.H.; Hopper, L.J.; et al. Consumer and clinician perspectives on personalising breast cancer prevention information. *Breast* **2019**, *43*, 39–47.
43. The Royal Australian College of General Practitioners. Guidelines for Preventive Activities in General Practice. 9th edn, updated. East Melbourne, Vic: RACGP. 2018. Available online: https://www.racgp.org.au/FSDEDEV/media/documents/Clinical%20Resources/Guidelines/Red%20Book/Guidelines-for-preventive-activities-in-general-practice.pdf (accessed on 28 October 2022).
44. Phillips, K.A.; Liao, Y.; Milne, R.L.; MacInnis, R.J.; Collins, I.M.; Buchsbaum, R.; Weideman, P.C.; Bickerstaffe, A.; Nesci, S.; Chung, W.K.; et al. Accuracy of Risk Estimates from the iPrevent Breast Cancer Risk Assessment and Management Tool. *JNCI Cancer Spectr.* **2019**, *3*, pkz066. [CrossRef]
45. Louro, J.; Posso, M.; Hilton Boon, M.; Román, M.; Domingo, L.; Castells, X.; Sala, M. A systematic review and quality assessment of individualised breast cancer risk prediction models. *Br. J. Cancer.* **2019**, *121*, 76–85.
46. Cintolo-Gonzalez, J.A.; Braun, D.; Blackford, A.L.; Mazzola, E.; Acar, A.; Plichta, J.K.; Griffin, M.; Hughes, K.S. Breast cancer risk models: A comprehensive overview of existing models, validation, and clinical applications. *Breast Cancer Res. Treat.* **2017**, *164*, 263–284. [PubMed]
47. Anothaisintawee, T.; Teerawattananon, Y.; Wiratkapun, C.; Kasamesup, V.; Thakkinstian, A. Risk prediction models of breast cancer: A systematic review of model performances. *Breast Cancer Res. Treat.* **2012**, *133*, 1–10. [PubMed]
48. Meads, C.; Ahmed, I.; Riley, R.D. A systematic review of breast cancer incidence risk prediction models with meta-analysis of their performance. *Breast Cancer Res. Treat.* **2012**, *132*, 365–377. [PubMed]
49. Moons, K.G.; Kengne, A.P.; Grobbee, D.E.; Royston, P.; Vergouwe, Y.; Altman, D.G.; Woodward, M. Risk prediction models: II. External validation, model updating, and impact assessment. *Heart* **2012**, *98*, 691–698. [PubMed]
50. Collins, G.S.; de Groot, J.A.; Dutton, S.; Omar, O.; Shanyinde, M.; Tajar, A.; Voysey, M.; Wharton, R.; Yu, L.M.; Moons, K.G.; et al. External validation of multivariable prediction models: A systematic review of methodological conduct and reporting. *BMC Med. Res. Methodol.* **2014**, *14*, 40.
51. MyPEBS. Available online: https://www.mypebs.eu/the-project/ (accessed on 24 October 2022).
52. WISDOM. Available online: https://www.thewisdomstudy.org/learn-more/ (accessed on 24 October 2022).
53. MyPeBS. Breast Cancer Risk Assessment Models. Available online: https://www.mypebs.eu/breast-cancer-screening/ (accessed on 27 October 2022).
54. The WISDOM Study. Fact Sheet for Healthcare Providers. Available online: https://thewisdomstudy.wpenginepowered.com/wp-content/uploads/2020/10/The-WISDOM-Study_Provider-Factsheet.pdf (accessed on 27 October 2022).

Disclaimer/Publisher's Note: The statements, opinions and data contained in all publications are solely those of the individual author(s) and contributor(s) and not of MDPI and/or the editor(s). MDPI and/or the editor(s) disclaim responsibility for any injury to people or property resulting from any ideas, methods, instructions or products referred to in the content.

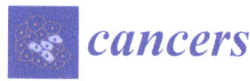

Review

Advanced Phytochemical-Based Nanocarrier Systems for the Treatment of Breast Cancer

Vivek P. Chavda [1,*], Lakshmi Vineela Nalla [2], Pankti Balar [3], Rajashri Bezbaruah [4], Vasso Apostolopoulos [5], Rajeev K. Singla [6,7], Avinash Khadela [8], Lalitkumar Vora [9] and Vladimir N. Uversky [10]

1. Department of Pharmaceutics and Pharmaceutical Technology, L. M. College of Pharmacy, Ahmedabad 380009, Gujarat, India
2. Department of Pharmacy, Koneru Lakshmaiah Education Foundation, Vaddeswaram, Guntur 522302, Andhra Pradesh, India
3. Pharmacy Section, L. M. College of Pharmacy, Ahmedabad 380009, Gujarat, India
4. Department of Pharmaceutical Sciences, Faculty of Science and Engineering, Dibrugarh University, Dibrugarh 786004, Assam, India
5. Institute for Health and Sport, Victoria University, Melbourne, VIC 3030, Australia
6. Institutes for Systems Genetics, Frontiers Science Center for Disease-Related Molecular Network, West China Hospital, Sichuan University, Xinchuan Road 2222, Chengdu 610064, China
7. School of Pharmaceutical Sciences, Lovely Professional University, Phagwara 144411, Punjab, India
8. Department of Pharmacology, L. M. College of Pharmacy, Ahmedabad 380009, Gujarat, India
9. School of Pharmacy, Queen's University Belfast, 97 Lisburn Road, Belfast BT9 7BL, UK
10. Department of Molecular Medicine, Byrd Alzheimer's Research Institute, Morsani College of Medicine, University of South Florida, Tampa, FL 33613, USA
* Correspondence: vivek.chavda@lmcp.ac.in

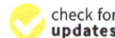

Citation: Chavda, V.P.; Nalla, L.V.; Balar, P.; Bezbaruah, R.; Apostolopoulos, V.; Singla, R.K.; Khadela, A.; Vora, L.; Uversky, V.N. Advanced Phytochemical-Based Nanocarrier Systems for the Treatment of Breast Cancer. *Cancers* 2023, *15*, 1023. https://doi.org/10.3390/cancers15041023

Academic Editor: Naiba Nabieva

Received: 30 December 2022
Revised: 2 February 2023
Accepted: 3 February 2023
Published: 6 February 2023

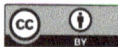

Copyright: © 2023 by the authors. Licensee MDPI, Basel, Switzerland. This article is an open access article distributed under the terms and conditions of the Creative Commons Attribution (CC BY) license (https://creativecommons.org/licenses/by/4.0/).

Simple Summary: Breast cancer is a concern for the healthcare system. Even with the advancement of science and technology, the current system for therapeutics and diagnostics seems to have numerous pitfalls. Phytochemical-mediated nanocarriers come into the picture to outrange the drawbacks of the conventional breast cancer management method. Phytochemicals have been a useful tool since time immemorial, and developing a sophisticated fusion of these chemicals with nanocarrier enhanced its effectiveness. This ensures targeted, time-controlled drug delivery. This article emphasizes the development of phytochemical-based nanocarriers corresponding to breast cancer. Moreover, the article presents the unhighlighted parts of the therapeutical industry to help patients. Enhancing patients' quality of life would uplift the healthcare system.

Abstract: As the world's most prevalent cancer, breast cancer imposes a significant societal health burden and is among the leading causes of cancer death in women worldwide. Despite the notable improvements in survival in countries with early detection programs, combined with different modes of treatment to eradicate invasive disease, the current chemotherapy regimen faces significant challenges associated with chemotherapy-induced side effects and the development of drug resistance. Therefore, serious concerns regarding current chemotherapeutics are pressuring researchers to develop alternative therapeutics with better efficacy and safety. Due to their extremely biocompatible nature and efficient destruction of cancer cells via numerous mechanisms, phytochemicals have emerged as one of the attractive alternative therapies for chemotherapeutics to treat breast cancer. Additionally, phytofabricated nanocarriers, whether used alone or in conjunction with other loaded phytotherapeutics or chemotherapeutics, showed promising results in treating breast cancer. In the current review, we emphasize the anticancer activity of phytochemical-instigated nanocarriers and phytochemical-loaded nanocarriers against breast cancer both in vitro and in vivo. Since diverse mechanisms are implicated in the anticancer activity of phytochemicals, a strong emphasis is placed on the anticancer pathways underlying their action. Furthermore, we discuss the selective targeted delivery of phytofabricated nanocarriers to cancer cells and consider research gaps, recent developments, and the druggability of phytoceuticals. Combining phytochemical and chemotherapeutic agents with nanotechnology might have far-reaching impacts in the future.

Keywords: phytochemicals; nanocarriers; breast cancer; chemotherapy; drug resistance

1. Introduction

One of the leading causes of fatality worldwide and a major barrier to extending life span is cancer, with breast cancer being among the most prevalent malignancies impacting women worldwide [1]. Women can develop breast cancer at any age after puberty, but the risk increases with age. According to the WHO, 2.3 million women worldwide had breast cancer in 2020, and 685,000 of them passed away from it [1]. Despite the notable improvements in survival in countries with early detection programs combined with the broad availability of different treatments, breast cancer continues to represent a significant societal health burden and has a large impact on the global number of cancer deaths due to the rapidly increasing rate of global aging [2]. According to a recent study, the number of new instances of breast cancer will reach more than 3 million cases annually by 2040 (an increase of 40%), and the number of deaths will reach more than 1 million cases annually (an increase of 50%) [3]. Currently, somewhere in the world, a woman is diagnosed with breast cancer every 14 s [4]. Various phytomedicines and nanotechnology-based interventions are under development [1–4].

Breast cancer, which originates from the epithelium of the milk ducts, is a highly heterogeneous neoplasm. It varies within each individual tumor, i.e., intratumor heterogeneity, and it significantly varies between patients, i.e., intertumor heterogeneity [5,6]. The histopathologic categorization of breast cancer is based on intertumor heterogeneity. The most prevalent (40–75%) histologic type of invasive breast cancer is invasive ductal carcinoma. Additionally, there are 21 more specific subtypes with distinct morphologic characteristics included in the WHO classification, among which the most common (5–15%) one is invasive lobular carcinoma [7]. According to the assessment of immunohistochemistry (IHC), the expression of estrogen receptor (ER), progesterone receptor (PR), and human epidermal growth factor receptor 2 (HER2) was found to be 80%, 60–70%, and 15–20%, respectively, in all invasive breast carcinomas [8–10]. Breast cancer is divided into four main intrinsic molecular subgroups with therapeutic and prognostic implications based on gene expression analysis: luminal A, luminal B, HER2-enriched, and basal-like [11]. The luminal A and B subtypes exhibit tumor heterogeneity among ER-positive breast tumors and seem to have higher rates of survival than the HER2-enriched and basal-like subtypes [12]. The HER2-enriched subtype, which comprises the $ER^-/PR^-/HER2^+$ and $ER^+/PR^+/HER2^+$ cancers, is characterized by elevated expression of the HER2 and proliferating genes. The basal-like subtype is triple-negative in 70% of cases and enriched for genes expressed in basal epithelial cells [11]. Breast tumors that do not express ER, PR, or HER2 are referred to as "triple-negative" breast carcinomas. Figure 1 represents the current state of the diagnosis, treatment, and theranostics of breast cancer. Breast imaging is frequently employed to assess the quality of breast implants, but it also plays a critical role in the detection, diagnosis, and clinical treatment of breast cancer [13]. Chemotherapy, surgical removal of the cancerous tissue, radiotherapy, immunotherapy, and a combination of any of these treatments have been the traditional methods of cancer treatment. Traditional chemotherapeutics are still the main type of treatment for many cancers that are in the late stages, despite obstacles such as systemic toxicity, limited selectivity, and a range of adverse effects [14]. Cancer treatment frequently involves drugs that specifically target cells that divide rapidly, which causes unwanted side effects on healthy, rapidly dividing cells, including hair follicles and the epithelium of the gastrointestinal tract (GIT). The fact that many cancer cells progressively gain resistance to standard kinds of therapy is also one of the exacerbating factors. The requirement for preoperative (neoadjuvant) systemic therapy is established based on the diagnosis and evaluation of the extent of breast cancer. Management for breast cancer requires targeted medicines that are efficient and have few unwanted side effects.

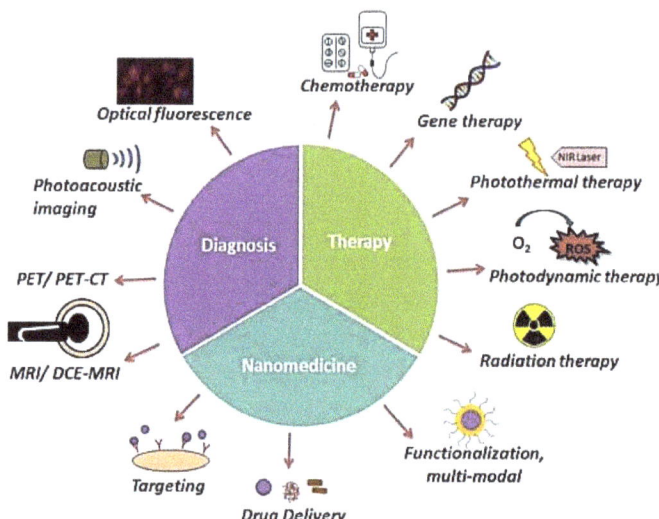

Figure 1. Current State of Breast Cancer Diagnosis, Treatment, and Theranostics. Adapted from [13] under CC BY license.

Major focus must be placed on reducing global gaps in access to diagnostics, multi-disciplinary therapy, and innovative drugs because breast cancer is a global concern. An increasing collection of credible research indicates that phytochemical components taken as nutraceuticals have chemo preventive action on several cancer types [15–17]. Figure 2 depicts examples of phytochemicals utilized for breast cancer treatment.

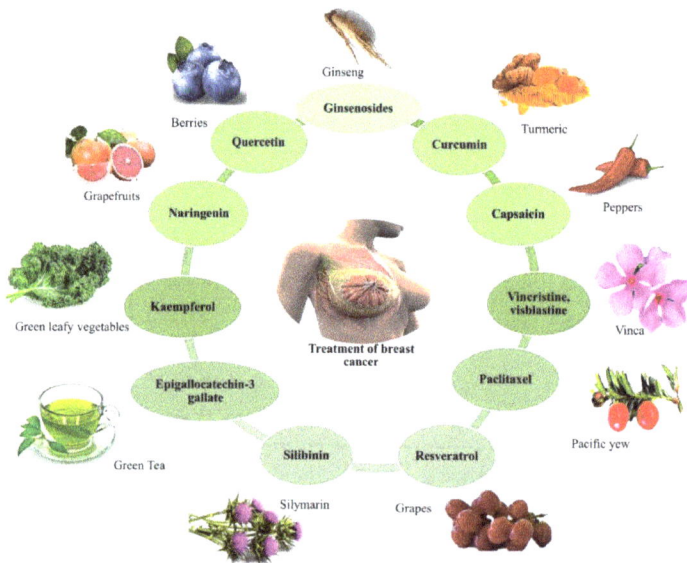

Figure 2. The role of various phytochemicals in the treatment of breast cancer.

It has been established that phytochemicals, the chemical substances (secondary plant metabolites) produced by plants in their various parts, are ideal candidates for the treatment. Various studies have revealed that such phytochemicals can act as chemo protectants that can control cellular and molecular processes such as DNA repair, apoptosis, cell proliferation, the cell cycle, and metastasis [18,19]. Many of these organic substances are also often comparatively less harmful and better tolerated by healthy cells. This is because many natural products are tolerated by normal cells, even at high dosages compared to chemotherapy medications.

Despite significant work in preclinical settings, there has been little progress in translating phytochemicals to humans [2,19]. One of the many causes of clinical failure may be the ineffective transport of promising natural substances to the target site. Therefore, it is crucial to develop novel efficient delivery methods that can minimize these drawbacks.

The use of nanoparticles (NPs) in medicine has made it possible to create medication delivery methods that are nanoformulated. Common drug carriers include micelles, polymeric dendrimers, quantum dots (QDs), microspheres, nanoemulsions, gold nanoparticles (GNPs), hydrogels, and liposomes. These drug carriers require different techniques for drug attachment, such as encapsulation, covalent binding, and adsorption [20].

Natural agent delivery methods based on nanotechnology have several benefits. One benefit of this nanotechnology is the ability to shield pharmaceuticals enclosed in nanoparticles from the damaging effects of external media, which provide prolonged systemic circulation [21]. Additionally, when compared to non-encapsulated free drugs, nanoparticles can augment the delivery of water-insoluble drugs, improve the passage of chemotherapeutic agents across cell membranes, allow the drugs to only be delivered to cancer cells, enhance drug distribution, offer sustained release of the drug, and assist in the delivery of two or more drugs for combined therapy [22].

1.1. Current Limitations of Breast Cancer Chemotherapy Regimens

Chemotherapy medications, which target rapidly proliferating cancer cells, can also harm rapidly proliferating healthy cells, including those in the bone marrow, digestive tract, and hair follicles [23]. However, after the course of treatment is complete or within a year of finishing chemotherapy, these side effects frequently fade away. They might last for a while in some instances. Hair loss, fatigue, loss of appetite, nausea and vomiting, constipation or diarrhea, mouth sores, changes to the skin or nails, neuropathy, chemo brain, and fatigue are among the more frequent short-term adverse effects. Although, infertility, bone thinning, heart damage, leukemia, and other long-term side effects of some chemotherapy medicines for breast cancer are also possible [24].

Due to its drug resistance and tendency to metastasize to distant organs such as the lymph nodes, bone, lung, and liver, breast cancer accounts for the majority of cancer-related fatalities in women [25]. The ATP-binding cassette (ABC) family protein, whose higher expression is correlated with higher resistance to chemotherapy, is widely established to have a significant role in drug resistance in a variety of malignancies. The excessive expression of proteins, such as P-GP1/ABCB1 (P-glycoprotein 1, also known as ATP-binding cassette subfamily B member 1 or ATP-dependent translocase ABCB1) and BCRP/ABCG2 (breast cancer resistance protein, also known as ATP-binding cassette subfamily G member 2 or broad substrate specificity ATP-binding cassette transporter ABCG2), causes multidrug resistance (MDR), which is a significant barrier to the diagnosis and treatment of breast cancer.

It is now recognized that the control of breast cancer and the spread of its metastasis involves a number of routes [26]. Understanding the biological activity of progesterone receptors (PRs), estrogen receptors (ERs), and human epidermal growth factor receptor 2 (also known as receptor tyrosine–protein kinase EGRB-2 or tyrosine kinase-type cell surface receptor HER2) for various subtypes of breast cancer has advanced. Despite recent developments in finding small molecules, proteins, and peptides for immunotherapy, controlled-release drug delivery and targeting are still not possible [27].

To aid in the detection and treatment of breast cancer, nanoparticles (NPs) bearing anticancer medicines can be actively or passively administered to the targeted tumor. NPs have numerous useful characteristics. To test drug effectiveness and overcome MDR, the controlled release of medicinal chemicals from NPs has been accomplished [28–30].

1.2. The Phytotherapeutics: Benefits and Their Delivery Challenges

Approximately 70% to 80% of the world population prefers herbal therapy as their primary type of treatment, making it one of the most significant forms of traditional medicine [31]. "Phyto pharmaceutical drug refers to an extract of a medicinal plant or a part of it that has been purified and standardized with defined minimum four bioactive or phytochemical compounds, for internal or external use by humans or animals for diagnosis, treatment, mitigation, or prevention of any disease or disorder" [32]. Due to the ineffectiveness of contemporary treatments for chronic diseases and because those treatments rarely show unfavorable serious side effects, the use of herbal medicines has become increasingly widespread in today's world. Many modern medications and their synthetic analogs have been developed based on the prototype compounds discovered in and isolated from plants. A few examples include vinblastine and vincristine from *Catharanthus roseus*, L-Dopa from *Mucuna prurita*, reserpine from *Rauvolfia serpentine*, and paclitaxel from *Taxus brevifolia* [33].

Notwithstanding the high worldwide breast cancer prevalence, the number of breast cancer patients who employ complementary and alternative therapies (CAMs) in addition to chemotherapy and radiation treatment is rising [34]. CAM is described as a group of methods, systems, and products from the medical and healthcare industries that are typically not included in the scope of mainstream medical care [35]. Herbal remedies or phytotherapy are the most widely utilized and oldest type of CAM practiced on cancer patients [36]. The biological effects of herbal medicines in the treatment of cancer can be wide-ranging and include enhancing the body's potential to fight cancer by increasing its ability to detoxify or clean itself, changing the way certain hormones and enzymes function, reducing the side effects and complications of chemotherapy and radiation treatment, and enhancing the body's immune system function, such as enhancing the synthesis of cytokines (interferon, interleukin, colony-stimulating factor, tumor necrosis factor, etc.) [37]. Moreover, it is clear that oxidative stress has a role in the development of cancer and that antioxidants play a role in both cancer prevention and cancer treatment, and the majority of plants are good providers of antioxidants. The majority of malignancies may be related to food, according to numerous research. Furthermore, dietary adjustments can lower the chances of the majority of malignancies [38]. The majority of herbal active ingredients are hydrophobic and have poor solubility. The restricted clinical usage of herbal medications is due to the poor solubility and hydrophobicity of their active ingredients, which results in poorer bioavailability and greater systemic clearance, necessitating repeated administration or an increased dose. Nano or micro formulations, however, can address these issues. Various types of polymer or lipid carriers are found in nanocarriers or sustained-release dosage forms, which are utilized to deliver drugs by a number of routes, such as transdermal, buccal, oral, and parenteral. They aid in greater therapeutic efficacy and localization at the desired target, which increases patient compliance [39]. For instance, oral polymeric nanoparticles can reduce the poor water solubility of *Cuscuta chinensis* [40]. Camptothecin's poor water solubility and harmful effects can be mitigated by intravenous injection, hydrogel of polymer conjugations, biodegradable implants, liposomes, polymeric nanoparticles, or solid lipid nanoparticles [41,42].

Although the use of herbal medicine has dramatically increased recently, there is still a dearth of research data in this area. The greatest hazard to consumer health is expected to result from the quality of herbal medicine being compromised as a result of adulteration and substitution caused by the rising demand for phytopharmaceutical medications on the worldwide market. The main problem for regulatory authorities is finding and identifying high-quality phytopharmaceuticals since interspecies diversity and uncertainty over vernacular nomenclature can lead to the adulteration and misidentification of raw materials for phytopharmaceutical drugs. In this review, we emphasize the recent advancements in understanding the mechanisms of action of phytochemical nanocarriers on various molecular pathways associated with breast cancer. We also discuss the phyto nanocarriers that are in clinical trials and their lacunas for commercialization.

2. Advanced Phytochemical Delivery Strategies

Many plant-derived secondary metabolites have low solubility and undesirable stability, restricting their use in therapeutic studies. For example, phenolic phytoconstituents have high antioxidant capability but are unstable under experimental settings. Furthermore, despite their great potential activity, bioactive compounds, such as paclitaxel and curcumin, have limited solubility and bioavailability, necessitating the use of hazardous solvents. The accompanying sections list the existing innovative delivery techniques for loading phytoconstituents for therapeutic effectiveness against breast cancer. Figure 3 depicts various types of nanocarriers with their properties.

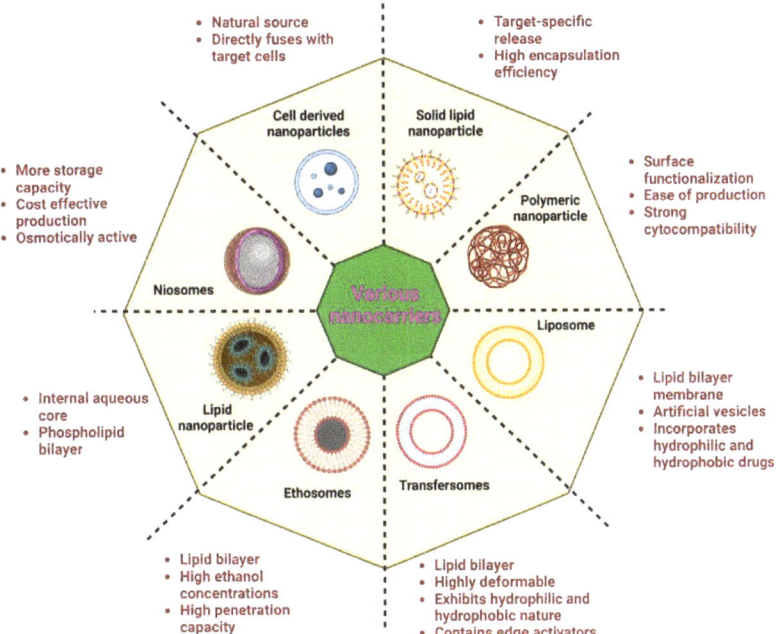

Figure 3. Types of nanocarriers with their characteristics. Created with BioRender.com accessed on 24 January 2023.

2.1. Phytochemical-Loaded Nanocarriers

2.1.1. Polymeric Nanoparticles (PNs)

Polymeric nanoparticles (PNs) have recently emerged as promising nanomaterials because of their desired characteristics, such as simplicity of surface functionalization, ease of production, strong cytocompatibility, and low toxicity. One of the most common methods of tailored drug delivery for treating breast cancer is the incorporation of phytonutrients into PNs. In this system, the phytochemical is either physically encapsulated into or covalently linked to the polymeric matrix.

PNs are globally classified as natural and synthetic PNs. Natural polymers, such as hyaluronic acid, chitosan, alginic acid, heparin, ethyl cellulose, and protein bovine serum albumin (BSA), are used for their excellent encapsulation efficiency and less intrusive nature, and they are strongly recommended. Synthetic polymers such as poly(lactic acid) (PLA), polyglycolic acid (PGA), poly(lactic-co-glycolic acid) (PLGA), poly anhydride (PLA), and poly(sulfobetaine methacrylate) (PSBMA) are also used for the fabrication of PNs. Phytochemical-loaded PNs are manufactured using conventional techniques, such as nanoprecipitation, layer-by-layer assembly, ionic gelation, and emulsion evaporation [43].

In a recent study, ginsenoside Rg5-loaded BSA NPs were developed using the desolvation process to increase the therapeutic effectiveness and tumor targetability of Rg5. The produced NPs were shown to disintegrate under acidic conditions but had good stability for eight weeks at 4 °C. Additionally, compared to free Rg5, the drug-loaded BSA NPs demonstrated better anticancer efficacy in MCF-7 cells, most likely by facilitating greater absorption of the drug and leading to more efficient cell death induction. Folic-modified drug-loaded BSA NPs outperformed free Rg5 and drug-loaded BSA NPs in an in vivo anticancer study using an MCF-7 xenograft mouse model for suppressing tumor growth. According to the in vivo real-time bioimaging analysis, the produced NPs had a better capacity for tumor accumulation [44] (Figure 4).

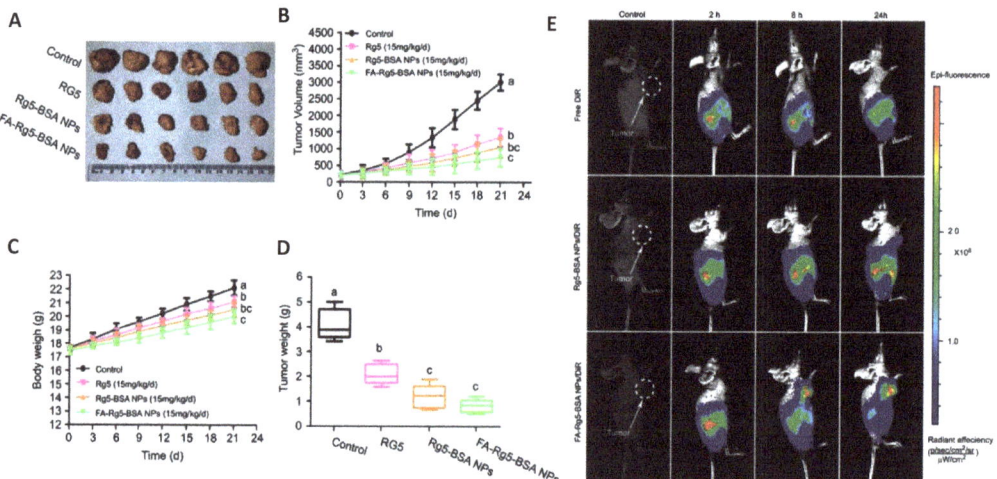

Figure 4. Ginsenoside-fabricated BSA NPs exhibited significant inhibition of breast cancer xenografts (**A**) tumor size, (**B**) tumor volume, (**C**) body weight, (**D**) tumor weight, and (**E**) in vivo bioluminescence after treatment for 21 days. Different letters (a,b,c) indicate significant differences between each group. Adapted with permission from [44] under (CC BY-NC 3.0).

Research on polymeric nanoparticles (both synthetic and natural) for administering phyto-derived therapeutic drugs, including curcumin, Epigallocatechin-3-gallate (EGCG), berberine, chrysin, and quercetin, is ongoing on a global scale. In brief, Kumari et al. developed a formulation based on curcumin nanoparticles and PGMD (poly-glycerol-malic acid-dodecanedioic acid) for anticancer efficacy against breast cancer cells. Both nanoparticles had entrapment effectiveness between 78% and 81%. The scratch assay and in vitro anticancer activities were performed on the breast cancer cell lines MCF-7 and MDA-MB-231. In the MCF-7 cell line, the IC50 of the nanoformulation was found to be 40.2 and 33.6 μM at 48 h; in the MDA-MB-231 cell line, it was 43.4 and 30.5 μM. This research revealed that the nanoparticles have more anticancer efficacy than curcumin alone [45].

Zeng et al. used nanotechnology that increased the capacity of EGCG to target MCF-7 cells. Two different types of EGCG nanoparticles (FA-NPS-PEG and FA-PEG-NPS) were developed, and their properties and effects on MCF-7 cells were investigated. The findings showed that I FA-NPS-PEG and FA-PEG-NPS both have great stability, and their particle sizes were 185.0 ± 13.5 nm and 142.7 ± 7.2 nm, respectively. Their encapsulation efficiencies of EGCG were $90.36 \pm 2.20\%$ and $39.79 \pm 7.54\%$, respectively. EGCG nanoparticles, specifically FA-NPS-PEG and FA-PEG-NPS, have been modified by folic acid and polyethylene glycol. These nanoparticles outperformed EGCG in terms of cellular uptake, the inhibition of MCF-7 cell proliferation, and the modification of the expression of several important PI3K-Akt pathway regulatory proteins [46]. Solanki et al. used the desolvation process to encapsulate berberine in BSA NPs, which are nanoparticles made of bovine serum albumin. For BSA NPs and berberine-BSA NPs, the average particle size of the produced nanoparticles was determined to be 116 and 166 nm, respectively. With a drug loading capacity of 7.78%, produced nanoparticles were shown to have an 85.65% drug entrapment efficiency. The BBR-BSA NPs were more cytotoxic to MDA-MB-231 breast cancer cells, according to an apoptotic and cellular uptake analysis. Still, increased intracellular uptake data suggest that berberine-BSA NPs could significantly boost anticancer activity at a lower dose of berberine [47].

In addition, Sulaiman et al. used a nano participation approach to develop nanochrysin or PLGA-PVA that was loaded with chrysin successfully. The current research demonstrated the cytocompatibility of the modified nanochrysin. The modified nanochrysin's in vitro anticancer activity toward the MCF-7 and SKOV-3 cell lines was examined. It was observed that the nanochrysin exerted dose-dependent cell growth arrest against both cancer cells. Compared to pure chrysin, the IC_{50} value of nanochrysin was substantially lower and promoted the apoptotic cell death pathway. As shown by the apoptotic assay techniques, it also exhibited anti-oxidant activity, a protective effect against DNA damage under H_2O_2 activity. The creation of a drug delivery system for the treatment of various cancers may benefit from the modified nanochrysin's high encapsulation efficacy, small particle size, and gradual release capabilities [48]. Furthermore, Zhou et al. developed PLGA-TPGS (D-α-tocopherol polyethylene glycol 1000 succinate)-based polymeric nanoparticulate systems for quercetin (Qu-NPs) oral delivery. They assessed the formulation's anticancer activity against triple-negative breast cancer both in vitro and in vivo. The average diameter of Qu-NPs is 198.4 ± 7.8 nm, with a high drug loading capacity of $8.1 \pm 0.4\%$. The Qu-NPs showed noticeably better inhibition of triple-negative breast cancer cell growth and metastasis. After oral gavage, 4T1-bearing mice showed a strong anticancer response to Qu-NPs, with a tumor inhibition ratio of 67.88% and fewer lung metastatic colonies. Additionally, quercetin's inhibitory effect on migrating MDA-MB231 cells with uPA knockdown was significantly reduced. Through the combined inhibition of urokinase-type plasminogen activator (uPA), Qu-NPs enhanced the anticancer and anti-metastatic effects that were already present [49].

2.1.2. Cell-Derived Nanovesicles (CDNs)

The ongoing worry about the biosafety of employing synthetic materials to transport natural products has accelerated the discovery and use of cell-derived nanovesicles (CDNs) [50]. Generally, CDNs are isolated from various natural sources (blood, milk, and cell culture media) and natural plants. Differential centrifugation, immunoaffinity separation, gel filtration chromatography, ultrafiltration, and polymer precipitation are used to separate or extract them. CDNs are created by isolation, biofabrication, and biolipid-based reconstruction. It was also shown that the exogenous stimulation (ultra-sonication and extrusion) of host cells increases the yield of CDNs [51,52].

There are two approaches to loading cargo (phytoconstituents) into CDNs: preloading and post-loading. Endogenous preloading is achieved by combining phytochemicals with host cells, after which spontaneously generated CDNs or biofabricated CDNs with bioactive cargo are collected. However, the preloading strategy is limited to CDNs generated from cell cultures or microorganisms, making it impracticable for plasma proteins or food. Post-loading entails the addition of phytochemicals to the preformed CDNs under various conditions. This approach includes passive incubation, sonication, surfactant permeabilization, and freeze—thaw cycles. Passive diffusion is the most widely used and safe technology for efficiently encapsulating bioactive compounds, such as curcumin and paclitaxel. However, it has poor encapsulation effectiveness [52,53].

Although active loading via electroporation improves the loading of nucleic acids and nanoparticles into CDNs, it can promote aggregation, alter the surface charge, induce instability, and potentially denature bioactive CDNs [54]. A recently proposed approach was the fusion of liposomes containing bioactive molecules with isolated CDNs to generate hybrid nanovesicles. By this approach, one can generate CDNs loaded with multiple bioactive molecules.

Furthermore, surface modification of the active target at specific sites can result in the increased targeting ability of CDNs with minimal toxicity and dosage reduction. CDN modification can be achieved either pre- or post-generation. In the first case, the host cells are incubated with phospholipids, such as DSPE-PEG-RGD and hyaluronic acid, resulting in the generation of functionalized CDNs [55]. In contrast, CDNs are enhanced in terms of membrane modification, protein derivatization, and lipid rectification in the post-modification technique [56]. Although active target modification enables specific targeting, the influence of ligand representation on the immune system, long-term stability, and loading capacity must be extensively investigated. Furthermore, CDNs may be functionalized by employing a variety of exogenous (temperature, photo responsive, and NIR) and endogenous (pH, enzyme overexpression) stimuli to create smart CDNs [52]. Bioactive phytochemicals, such as polyphenols, flavonoids, terpenoids, and alkaloids, have been exploited for CDN-based delivery. Table 1 lists the phytochemicals given against breast cancer via CDNs [53].

Table 1. List of the reported CDNs with phytochemicals for breast cancer treatment.

Cargo Loaded	CDNs Source	Preparation	Therapeutic Effect	References
Cucurbitacin B	MDA-MB-231 cells	Isolation, Bio fabrication	Metastasis inhibition	[57]
Paclitaxel	MDA-MB-231 cells	Isolation, Bio fabrication	Excellent antitumor activity	[58]
Withaferin A, anthocyanidins, and curcumin	Milk from Holstein and Jersey cows	Mixing	Inhibits inflammation	[59]
Black bean-derived phytoconstituents	Human mammary (MCF7), prostate (PC3), colon (Caco2), and liver (HepG2) cells	Electroporation	Induces cell death and cell cycle arrest	[60]
Berry-derived anthocyanidins	Raw milk from pasteurized Jersey cows	Simple mixing	Inhibits proliferation and inflammation	[61]
Honokiol (extracted from Magnolia plant)	Mesenchymal stem cells	Sonication	Inhibits cell cycle arrest and apoptosis	[62]

2.1.3. Lipid Nanoparticles

Lipid-based nanodrug delivery systems are among the most promising colloidal carriers for phytochemicals. Lipid-based nanoparticles, such as liposomes, solid lipid nanoparticles (SLNs), and nanostructured lipid carriers (NLCs), can transport hydrophobic and hydrophilic molecules utilizing the phospholipid bilayer or internal aqueous core.

Liposomes are biocompatible and biodegradable and exhibit quite low toxicity. In addition, integrating hydrophilic and lipophilic drugs, developing lipid domains, fluidity, polyvalent binding, fusion, longer retention of drugs, high drug loading capacity, site-specific targeting, and controlled drug release are further benefits of liposomes. Furthermore, they provide prolonged restorative effects, a reduced likelihood of probable adverse effects, and enhanced protection for drugs against physiological conditions [63]. Therefore, it is considered a smarter choice to incorporate anticancer phytochemicals into liposomes to overcome the constraints of the inability of traditional chemotherapy to suppress carcinogenesis and their ability to reduce lethal side effects completely.

These liposomes have a spherical shape, are composed of nontoxic phospholipids and cholesterol, and are surrounded by water (Figure 5A). They create vesicles in the presence of an aqueous solution that increases the stability and solubility of anticancer drugs while encapsulating them in liposomes. Various payloads with hydrophobic and hydrophilic molecules and charged molecules can be incorporated into liposomes (Figure 5B).

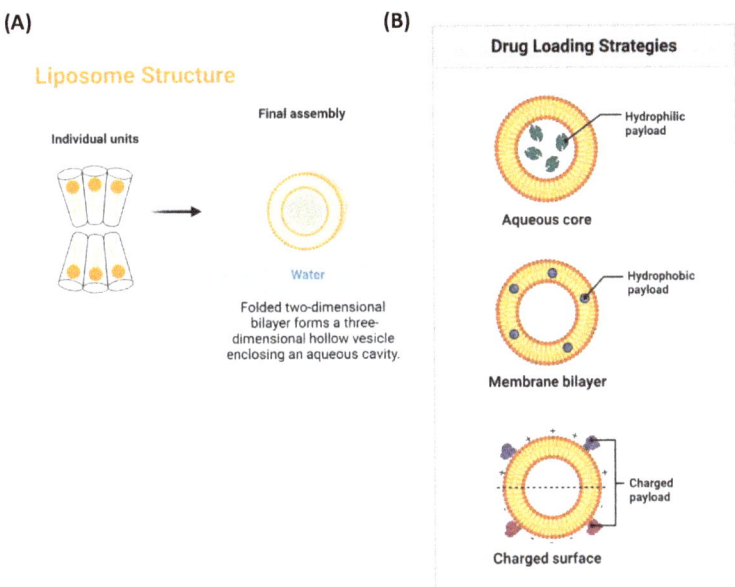

Figure 5. (**A**) Liposomal structure, (**B**) Various drug loading strategies with liposomes. Created with BioRender.com accessed on 24 January 2023.

In recent years, formulations of liposome-based phytochemicals have gained popularity. Chitosan and lecithin were used by Deshmukh et al. to create a liposomal nanosystem by an electrostatic deposition-assisted film hydration approach to safeguard chrysin (also known as 5,7-dihydroxyflavone, a flavone found in honey, propolis, passion flowers, *Passiflora caerulea* and *Passiflora incarnata*, and *Oroxylum indicum*) in the nanolipoidal shell [64]. Chrysin was encapsulated into liposomes and demonstrated increased anticancer efficiency in the MCF-7 cell line. After encapsulation in a liposome, chrysin's relative bioavailability increased five-fold, according to an in vivo pharmacokinetic study [64]. Quercetin and mycophenolic acid-loaded liposomes were independently synthesized by Patel et al., and both in vitro and in vivo experiments were then carried out [65]. Another study used a thin-layer hydration approach to develop thermosensitive betulinic acid-loaded magnetoliposomes. This study showed that MDA-MB-231 breast cancer cell lines and MCF 10A nontumor cell lines were more susceptible to the heightened effects of hyperthermia, as shown by in vitro experiments using the MTT assay, scratch assay, and LDH assay [66]. Furthermore, an in ovo study depicted the antiangiogenic effect of Lip + MIONPs + BA during hyperthermia treatment. In addition, resveratrol-containing liposomes that were coated with peptide and sucrose were used to treat breast cancer [67]. In vivo investigations on mice with breast cancer showed greater efficacy at lower dosages when compared to free resveratrol, with an IC_{50} of 20.89 mol^{-1} in MCF-7 breast cancer cell lines. The authors also demonstrated the downregulation of B-cell lymphoma-2 cells by increasing the expression of p53 [67]. Furthermore, pegylated liposomes were formulated with the combination of docetaxel and its 3-N-pentadecylphenol derivative. Due to the pegylated hydrogenated soy PC-3-N-pentadecylphenol derivative, docetaxel demonstrated improved stability over 30 days. MDA-MB-231 and MCF-7 breast cancer cell lines showed strong cytotoxic effects [68].

On the other hand, SLNs are a new class of safer and more effective gene/drug delivery systems. SLNs, which range in size from 50 nm to 1 μm, are submicron colloidal carriers made of physiological lipids distributed in an aqueous solution, and these physiological lipids remain solid at body and room temperature. SLNs provide several fascinating benefits, including physical stability, increased drug selectivity, protection of absorbed compounds from clearance and degradation, avoidance of organic solvent residue, simplicity in manufacture, low cost, and nontoxicity [69,70]. Therefore, SLNs have been widely employed to deliver phytochemicals, including curcumin, berberine, resveratrol, quercetin, and EGCG [70–74], to increase anticancer activities, protect labile molecules, increase oral bioavailability, and reduce adverse effects.

2.1.4. Transferosomes

Transfersomes are novel drug delivery systems that consist of phospholipids and a membrane-softening agent (such as Tween 80, Span 80, and sodium cholate), acting as edge activators (EAs) that facilitate the ultra deformable property of the transfersomes [75]. Due to their highly elastic nature, transfersomes can deform and squeeze themselves as intact vesicles through narrow pores, which are noticeably smaller than the diameter of transfersomes [75]. Transfersomes can pass through the intact stratum corneum along two intracellular lipid pathways distinct from one another in terms of their bilayer characteristics. High deformability and both hydrophilic and hydrophobic characteristics in transferosomes allow for improved intact vesicle penetration. This system is significantly more elastic and flexible than liposomal drug delivery, favoring effective skin penetration and, by extension, acting as an innovative drug delivery system [76]. Transferosomes avoid the obstacle of skin penetration by squeezing along the intracellular sealing lipid of the stratum corneum [77]. The transferome membrane is made flexible by combining a suitable surface-active agent in appropriate proportions [78]. In general, anionic surfactants are typically more successful at improving skin penetration than cationic surfactants, and the critical micelle concentration is likewise lower.

Nonionic surfactants with an uncharged polar head group are more tolerable than cationic and anionic surfactants [79]. Nonionic surfactants are thought to be less harmful, less hemolytic, and less irritating to cellular surfaces. They also tend to keep the pH of a solution close to physiological levels. Additionally, they serve various purposes, including their roles as solubilizing, emulsifying, and potent P-glycoprotein inhibitors, which are beneficial for increasing drug absorption and targeting particular tissues [80]. Transferosome delivery systems assure optimal distribution, increased bioavailability, and promising phytoactivity stability in herbal formulations [81]. These systems offer numerous advantages that include the accommodation of pharmaceuticals with various solubilities due to their hydrophobic and hydrophilic moieties, high entrapment efficiency, deformation and narrow pass-through constriction, biocompatibility and systemic as well as topical delivery of the drug [82–85].

Gadag et al. demonstrated the possibility of transpapillary transfer of resveratrol, a phytochemical, for treating breast cancer. In this study, the biomaterial soy phosphatidylcholine was used to encapsulate resveratrol into transfersomes (RVT-TRF) to provide sustained release of the drug. Iontophoresis accelerated RVT-TRF passage through the mammary papilla and into the breast tissue. In vitro transpapillary iontophoresis investigation on porcine mammary papilla revealed that RVT-TRF penetrated more readily than passive diffusion. Further evidence for transpapillary transport came from an in vitro fluorescence microscopy experiment with fluorescein-conjugated RVT-TRF. Compared to the oral administration of pure resveratrol, the optimized RVT-TRF demonstrated a greater maximum peak plasma concentration (C_{max}) and area under the curve (AUC) [86].

2.1.5. Ethosomes

Ethosomes are vesicles made of phospholipids, a high proportion of ethanol (20–50%), and water. The high ethanol concentrations in ethosomes alter the skin's lipid bilayer and increase the vesicles' capacity to penetrate the stratum corneum [87]. In terms of the proportion of ethanol, vesicular bilayer fluidity, mechanism of permeation through the skin, methods of preparation, and lack of adverse effects, ethosomes stand out from other lipid nanocarriers. The distribution of therapeutic drugs into a deeper epidermal layer and systemic circulation is made easy and successful by ethanol's efficient penetration enhancer function. Numerous compounds, including hydrophilic, lipophilic, and high molecular weight drugs, can be encapsulated by ethosomes [88]. Both occlusive and nonocclusive situations allow ethosomes to transfer the drugs over the skin successfully [89,90].

Ethosomes are vesicles that range in size from 30 nm to several microns. They are soft and flexible. It has been noted that when made using the same approach without any size-reduction steps, the size decreases with an increase in ethanol concentration from 20 to 45% and is caused by the high alcohol content. The vesicles obtain a net negative charge from ethanol, reducing their size [91,92]. Nasr et al. encapsulated thymoquinone (TQ), the main biologically active complex of black cumin seeds, in ethosomes by the response surface method. They applied it to in vitro breast cancer potential assessment. In this study, toxicity and release curves were established, and ethosomic TQ had higher cytotoxic activity than free TQ against MCF-7 cell lines. Free TQ and ethosomic TQ were found to have IC_{50} values of 1.10 μg/mL and 0.95 μg/mL, respectively [93].

2.1.6. Niosomes

Niosomes are novel drug delivery systems, nanometric lamellar vesicles created when a nonionic surfactant is combined with a cholesterol-like helper lipid. The nonionic surfactants use energy to produce a stable bilayer vesicle in hydrophilic situations (physical agitation and heating). While the hydrophilic heads in the bilayer structure remain in contact with the aqueous side, the hydrophobic sections are directed away from it. Niosome preparation requires the use of surfactants that are biocompatible, biodegradable, and nonimmunogenic. In vivo and in vitro, niosomes function similarly to liposomes by extending the circulation of the phytochemical that is encapsulated, modifying its organ distribution and enhancing bioavailability. Niosomes can improve the solubility and stability of phytochemicals, and targeting and regulating phytochemical release is their intended function.

Barani et al. developed niosomes of two distinct formulations that contained thymoquinone (TQ, a phytochemical compound found in *Carum carvil* seeds) and *C. carvil* extract (Carum) (Nio/TQ and Nio/Carum, respectively) and the properties of the resulting niosomes were investigated [94]. Compared to free TQ, both loaded formulations offered regulated release. The MTT assay demonstrated that loaded niosomes have more anticancer activity against the MCF-7 cancer cell line than free TQ and Carum. These findings were supported by a flow cytometric study. Cell cycle analysis revealed G2/M arrest in the formulations of TQ, Nio/TQ, and Carum. TQ, Nio/TQ, and Nio/Carum all significantly reduced the migration of MCF7 cells. These findings indicate that novel carriers with great effectiveness for encapsulating low soluble phytochemicals include TQ and Carum-loaded niosomes, which would also be advantageous systems for treating breast cancer [94].

In another study, neosomes containing Lawsone (2-hydroxy-1,4-naphthoquinone, also known as hennotannic acid, a major constituent of the henna plant (*Lawsonia inermis*)), nonionic surfactants, and cholesterol were prepared. An in vitro study showed that encapsulating Lawsone in niosomes significantly increased the anticancer activity of the formulation in the MCF-7 breast cancer cell line compared to the free Lawsone solution [95].

Recently, folate-targeted curcumin-loaded niosomes for site-specific delivery in breast cancer were investigated [96]. This study used folic acid (FA) and polyethylene glycol (PEG) to decorate synthesized curcumin-loaded niosomes to prevent breast cancer. Compared to the free drug and developed niosomes, it showed a significant increase in Bax and p53 gene expression levels. Bcl2 levels were lower with PEG-FA decorated niosomes than with undecorated niosomes and the free drug. The PEG-FA-modified niosomes showed the most preponderant endocytosis in the MCF7 and 4T1 cell uptake assays. The produced nanoformulations were taken up by breast cancer cells and sustained drug-release properties [96].

2.2. Phytochemical-Assisted Nanocarriers

Significant effort has recently been made toward synthesizing metal nanoparticles utilizing plant extracts as reducing agents to adhere to the general principles of green chemistry [97,98]. These methods have been shown to be economical and environmentally friendly ways to create different metal nanocomposites. Alkaloids, flavonoids, terpenoids, soluble carbohydrates, phenolic acids, and alkaloids are a few phytochemicals found in plants. They can act as reducing and stabilizing agents in the production of metal nanoparticles. Hence, this phytochemical-assisted synthesis of nanoparticles is a very promising technique for synthesizing nanoparticles, as the plant itself serves as a capping and reducing agent. Both intracellular and extracellular nanoparticle synthesis is possible in plant systems [99]. Growing the plant in organic media containing metal-rich elements, metal-rich soil, or metal-rich hydroponic solution are all examples of intracellular strategies for nanoparticle synthesis [100–102]. In addition, extracellular approaches use leaf extracts made by boiling and crushing leaves to create nanoparticles [103].

On the other hand, plant-derived edible NPs exhibit an economic advantage in scaling up for mass production [104]. The main obstacles between the laboratory and the clinic in nanomedicine, as is widely known, are biocompatibility and safety. Due to their high quantities of lipids, low levels of proteins, and abundance of RNAs, plant-derived edible NPs have a distinct advantage in these areas and are among the safest therapeutic NPs [105]. The formation of tumors in the leukemia mouse model is effectively inhibited by edible NPs derived from Citrus limon. It should be mentioned that extracting edible NPs with high yield and quality is challenging. The use of isosmotic buoyant density and isosmotic cushion ultracentrifugation, equilibrium density gradient ultracentrifugation, and differential ultracentrifugation combined with density gradient centrifugation have all recently emerged as promising extraction and purification methods [106]. In addition to their natural ingredients, edible plant-derived lipid nanoparticles can be employed as nanocarriers for chemical drugs. Phytochemicals or chemotherapeutic drugs can be encapsulated in nanostructures created from plant lipids using sonication [107]. Lipid nanoparticles, a unique and organic delivery technology, are easily biodegradable and free of environmental biohazards. These plant-derived lipid nanoparticles offer drug delivery to a particular site of the human body [108].

3. Evidence of the Role of Phytofabricated Nanocarriers against Breast Cancer

3.1. Anticancer Activity

3.1.1. Immunostimulation

Sijia et al. synthesized tea nanoparticles (TNPs) loaded with doxorubicin (DOX), and their in vitro immunostimulatory and anticancer activities were studied [109]. The TNPs significantly increased IL-6, TNF-α, and G-CSF in RAW264.7 macrophages and exhibited the ability to modulate macrophage immunostimulation. In addition, in comparison with free DOX, the DOX-loaded TNPs facilitated the intracellular delivery of DOX in sensitive (MCF-7) and resistant breast cancer cells (MCF-7/ADR) with enhanced in vitro cytotoxicity of IC50 (MCF-7-0.036 $\pm$ 0.012 and MCF-7/ADR-15.16 $\pm$ 7.05). The formulation exhibited pH-responsive release of doxorubicin, favoring in vivo antitumor applications [109]. Despite having an anticancer impact, there are only a few in vivo cancer investigations using TNPs, since it is unclear how exactly their toxicity is induced. TNPs may have several therapeutic benefits in cancer therapy if research continues to improve in this direction.

3.1.2. Apoptosis

The antitumor effects of quercetin have been thoroughly studied in a wide range of malignancies. Their potential was explored by Minaei et al. in the fabrication of mixed NPs by combining quercetin and lecithin for doxorubicin-induced apoptosis. The results of this investigation showed that the addition of nano-quercetin to doxorubicin enhanced its toxicity in the MCF-7 cell line [110]. In addition, a study from Kazi et al. with folate-decorated epigallocatechin-3-gallate loaded PLGA nanoparticles (FP-EGCG-NPs) evaluated the efficacy in breast cancer cells. Treatment with FP-EGCG-NPs in MDA-MB-231 and MCF-7 cells significantly induced cytotoxicity, high apoptotic potential, and high mitochondrial depolarization compared with EGCG alone. Furthermore, in a scintigraphic imaging study, the FP-EGCG-NPs labeled with technetium-99m (^{99m}Tc, a metastable nuclear isomer of technetium-99) exhibited tumor selectivity in MDA-MB-231 tumor-bearing nude mice. The US health agency, the National Institute of Health (NIH), recommended betulinic acid for its cell-specific toxicity for cancer chemotherapy.

Halder et al. synthesized lactoferrin (Lf)-attached betulinic acid nanoparticles (Lf-BAnp) for targeting aggressive triple-negative breast cancer (TNBC) cells by understanding the limiting capability of betulinic acid in terms of solubility and cell uptake. Lf-BAnp exhibits potential inhibitory activity against the proliferation and cell viability with cell cycle arrest [111]. The use of gold nanoparticles was significantly higher in nanotechnology due to their ease of production and biocompatibility with broad biomedical applications. Recent studies suggest that phytochemicals such as withanolide-A and Curcuma wenyujin, as natural active drugs in conjugation with AuNPs, can effectively overcome breast cancer drug resistance [112,113]. Additionally, Ruenraroengsak et al. examined the in vitro chemotherapeutic effectiveness of ZnONPs loaded through a mesoporous silica nanolayer (MSN) against drug-sensitive breast cancer cells (MCF-7: estrogen receptor-positive, CAL51: triple-negative) and their drug-resistant counterparts (MCF-7TX, CALDOX). Gold nanostars were coated with ZnO-MSNs (AuNSs). The mesoporous silica nanolayer (MSN)-ZnO-AuNSs decreased the viability of CAL51/CALDOX cells and MCF7/MCF-7-TX cells. In contrast, MSN-ZnO-AuNSs conjugated with Frizzled-7 (FZD-7) increased the toxicity by three times in resistant MCF-7TX cells.

3.1.3. Metastasis

Although medical advancements have significantly changed how BC patients are managed over the past few decades, metastases continue to be challenging to treat because of their resistance to therapeutic agents, molecular heterogeneity, and physiological barriers at different organ sites [114,115]. Systemic chemotherapy does not account for the enormous variations in tumor microenvironments due to the widely dispersed nature of metastasis [116,117]. Nanoformulations show definite benefits with the advancement of liposome or lipid nanoparticle technology, including improved therapeutic characteristics and pharmacokinetics and decreased drug toxicity. Additionally, they can be made to target cancer cells and the tumor microenvironment concurrently for improved targeting and therapy options.

Breast cancer-related mortality is mostly caused by tumor metastasis, which continues to be the main barrier to effective chemotherapy for the disease. α-Tocopherol polyethylene glycol (TPGS) and phosphatidylcholine (PC) were included in silibinin-loaded lipid nanoparticles (SLNs) developed using a thin-film hydration technique to prevent the metastasis of breast cancer. It was further shown that MDA-MB-231 breast cancer cells successfully absorbed the optimized SLNs, with particle sizes of approximately 45 nm and great serum stability. Notably, the SLNs could efficiently and significantly accumulate within tumor tissues. Through the downregulation of MMP-9 and Snail, SLNs had significantly higher inhibitory effects than free silibinin on the invasion and migration of MDA-MB-231 cells. In addition, in the spontaneous and blood vascular metastasis models, SLN treatment resulted in 67% and 39% less pulmonary metastasis formation than saline treatment, respectively. Additionally, TPGS and phosphatidylcholine-based blank lipid nanoparticles (BLNs) were the first to be discovered to have antimetastatic activity. Furthermore, neither of the mouse models treated with SLNs showed any clear signs of systemic toxicity. SLNs can potentially be a potent, low-toxicity tumor-targeted drug delivery system as a promising preventative therapeutic agent against breast cancer metastasis [118].

3.1.4. Angiogenesis

Cancer is a multifactorial disease influenced by genetic, epigenetic, and environmental factors. The culmination of numerous molecular changes causes the normal biological processes regulating cell proliferation, cell survival, genome stability, energy metabolism, and angiogenesis to become dysregulated. Angiogenesis, the quick rise in blood vessel development, is necessary for the availability of enough oxygen and nutrients for the growth of breast tumors. Like all human tissues, breast cancer cells require continuous hydration and oxygenation through the system's vascular network of capillaries. The angiogenic factors vascular endothelial growth factor (VEGF) A, B, and C, basic fibroblast growth factor (bFGF)/FGF-2, matrix metalloproteinases (MMPs), and IL-8, which are factors linked to breast cancer, are most frequently produced by adipose tissues [119,120]. Plant species contain ursolic acid (UA), a triterpene with anticancer action that its antiangiogenic properties may bring on. However, owing to its poor bioavailability and low water solubility, UA has a limited range of applications.

Rocha et al. created long-circulating, pH-sensitive liposomes containing ursolic acid to solve this problem (SpHL-UA). The authors used the relative tumor volume, dynamic contrast-enhanced magnetic resonance imaging (DCE-MRI), and histological analysis to study the antiangiogenic effects of free UA and SpHL-UA in mouse brain cancer and human breast tumor models. The actions of UA at different phases of tumor formation and its low toxicity have sparked interest in UA as a cancer therapeutic. To assess the antiangiogenic effect of UA in vivo, UA was liposome-encapsulated (SpHL-UA). The therapy with free UA or SpHL-UA utilizing proven tumor-bearing experimental animal models is also described. SpHL-UA did not show antiangiogenic activity in a gliosarcoma model and seemed to induce an antiangiogenic effect in the human breast tumor model [121].

3.1.5. Inhibition of Cancer Stem Cells

Luminal A is the most common breast cancer diagnosed frequently in female patients. Breast cancer stem cells (BCSCs) are a rare group of cells in breast cancer. They are responsible for aggressiveness, medication resistance, relapse, poor treatment response, and an overall decrease in the survival of these cancers. Enhancing the efficacy of breast cancer treatment requires focusing on BCSCs. In addition to expressing stemness markers, these cells can self-renew. A poor clinical outcome is caused by BCSCs, which play a significant role in developing drug resistance. To effectively prevent and cure breast cancer, researchers are working to identify and eliminate most of the tumor mass together with BCSCs. Because BCSCs have abnormal stemness-related gene expression, including CD44, SOX2, OCT4, c-MYC, KLF4, Nanog, and SALL4, they are crucial in the spread of cancer [122,123]. Of all breast cancer subtypes, triple-negative breast cancer (TNBC) has the highest rates of chemoresistance, metastases, and relapse. TNBC is a malignant condition resulting from a self-renewing cell subpopulation known as cancer stem cells (CSCs). They need to be eliminated because they are important limitations of TNBC treatment. In this regard, piperlongumine (PL) was investigated. It possesses extraordinary anticancer properties, but its application is constrained by poor pharmacokinetics. Therefore, a PLGA-based nanoformulation for PL (PL-NPs) was created to increase its biological activity, and the effects of PL and PL-NPs on CSCs in mammospheres were investigated. According to the findings, PL-NPs are more effectively absorbed by cells in mammospheres than PL. Additionally, this study showed that PL-NPs significantly reduce CSC expression of ALDH, self-renewability, chemoresistance, and EMT in mammospheres.

According to further investigation, the suppression of STAT3 may be the primary mechanism underlying these multimodal effects. This was confirmed when combined treatments with colivelin, a potent synthetic peptide STAT3 activator, revealed that the anti-CSC effects of PL and PL-NPs were reversed. All things considered, the data indicate that PL-NPs exhibit greater CSC suppression through the downregulation of STAT3 and shed light on the creation of PL-based nanomedicine for CSC targeting in TNBC [124].

3.1.6. Anti-Proliferative Activities

Most BC tumors have epithelial cell features and express HER-2 (a member of the epidermal growth factor receptor family) or estrogen receptors. Basal cells, which make up approximately one-fifth of BCs, do not fall under any one category of proliferation regulators. Regardless of the cell type, insulin-like growth factor (IGF) signaling is implicated in most BC cells. Cyclin-dependent kinases are activated by transcriptional and nontranscriptional processes in response to all cell proliferation inducers, leading to irreversible progression to the G1/S phase transition. A promising therapeutic approach that first concentrated on the metastatic disease was to disrupt this process. Since most phytochemicals have mechanisms that successfully reduce angiogenesis and cell proliferation, they are viewed as potential anticancer agents. By altering the Wnt/-catenin, PI3K/Akt/mTOR, and MAPK/ERK pathways, quercetin causes cell cycle arrest, which prevents cell proliferation, promotes apoptosis, affects autophagy, and decreases angiogenesis and metastasis in cancer cells [125,126]. In addition, EGCG, a polyphenolic flavonoid produced from green tea, suppresses cancer cell growth, angiogenesis, and migration while causing cell cycle arrest and apoptosis [127].

Furthermore, a limonoid triterpene called nimbolide is generated from Azadirachta indica leaves and flowers. Recent studies have shown that nimbolide inhibits proliferation by downregulating PI3K/AKT/mTOR and ERK signaling, induces ROS-mediated apoptosis and inhibits EMT, migration, and invasion in a variety of solid tumors, including pancreatic, breast, oral, and non-small cell lung cancer, in both in vitro and in vivo systems [128–130]. Balakrishnan et al. demonstrated that gold nanoparticle-conjugated quercetin inhibits epithelial–mesenchymal transition, angiogenesis, and invasiveness via the EGFR/VEGFR-2-mediated pathway in breast cancer. In response to AuNP-Qu-5 treatment, a significant decrease in the protein expression of vimentin, N-cadherin, Snail, Slug, Twist, MMP-2, MMP-9, p-EGFR, VEGFR-2, p-PI3K, Akt, and pGSK3 and an increase in the protein expression of E-cadherin were observed. Compared to free quercetin, AuNPs-Qu-5 prevented MCF-7 and MDA-MB-231 cells from migrating and invading. Human umbilical vein endothelial cells (HUVECs) treated with AuNPs-Qu-5 produced fewer capillary-like tubes and had worse cell survival. AuNPs-Qu-5 inhibited the creation of new blood vessels and tubes, according to in vitro and in vitro angiogenesis experiments. DMBA-induced mammary cancer in SD rats was treated with AuNPs-Qu-5, which inhibited tumor growth compared to free quercetin [131].

Various mechanisms of action of phytofabricated nanocarriers on breast cancer discussed in this article are depicted in Figure 6.

3.2. Theranostic Targeting

Theranostic approaches are accepted in the treatment of various diseases, including cancer, and incorporate both therapeutic and diagnostic approaches. BC is not overlooked, yet there are very limited studies and current therapeutic applications. Various nanoparticles (NPs), such as gold (Au), silver (Ag), metallic NPs, carbon-containing NPs, and polymers [132], are used in theranostic approaches, and with increasing technology, green synthesis is also justified [132]. Au NPs, when synthesized by chemical or physical means, tend to hold on to toxicity and eliminate excessive heat [133]. When derived from biological sources such as Olax scandens, it produces bearable toxicity, sufficient stability, and reduced immunogenicity [132]. Along with the therapeutic approach, it shows bright red fluorescence, providing an exact location of the MCF7 cell line (breast cell line) [134]. A phytochemical obtained from *Auxemma oncoclyx* named oncocalyxone has potent anticancer efficacy against MCF7 cells [135]. An in vitro study of sesamin showed its efficacy against BC by altering the G1 phase of cell division along with a reduction in cyclin D1, while sitosterol targets the G2/M phase to attain a similar response [136].

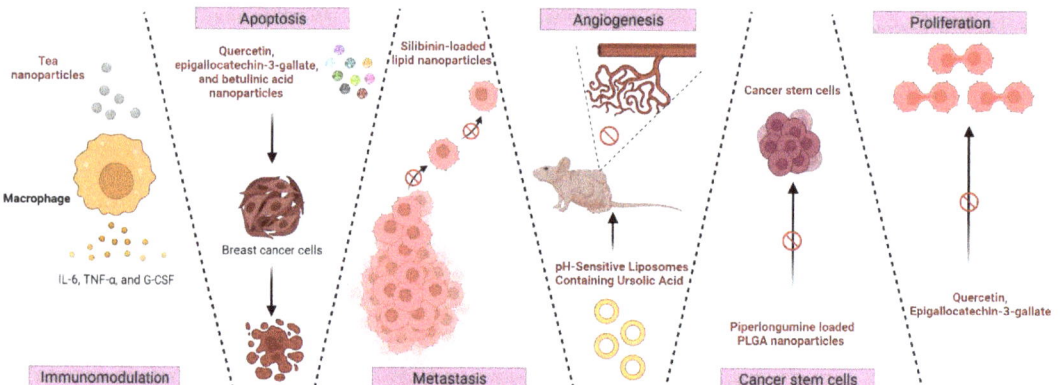

Figure 6. Illustration of the effect of phytofabricated nanocarriers on various mechanisms involved in the progression of cancer. Created with BioRender.com accessed on 21 December 2022.

Anacardic acid (AA) helps to arrest the cells in the cell cycle (G0/G1) and hence leads to apoptosis [137]. Kushwar et al. stated that when AA is associated covalently with docetaxel (DTX), bovine serum albumin and gemcitabine enhance apoptosis activity and enhance pharmacokinetics [138]. The therapeutic activity on MCF7 cells was higher than that of individual drugs used alone (AA and DTX) [138]. Emodin acts on 4TI breast tumors (a cell line) and suppresses macrophage infiltration, which is complementary to decreased tumor angiogenesis and enhanced T-cell activation [139]. Bimetallic nanostructures are receiving more attention in the developmental phase. A combination of Au–Ag bimetallic NPs proves itself as a better targeting entity [140]. Wu et al. concluded that this hybrid complex structure has a better tendency to absorb near-IR light and hence perform phototherapy in MCF-1 cells while leaving the surrounding cell undisturbed [141].

Theranostic-Related Patents

BC is a well-studied disease, yet extra efforts are needed to grasp its maximum effectiveness against this deadly disease. Scientists are attempting to develop innovative management techniques. A patent is a crucial human right provided to the inventor to enjoy the perks of his/her invention. To date, a total of 1,82,000 patents have been published on the topic "Breast Cancer". The patents filed on BC associated with theranostic approaches are described in Table 2.

Table 2. Patents dedicated to theranostic approaches in breast cancer.

Sr. No.	Patent	Nanoparticle	Remarks	Inventor(s)
1	US10201622B2	Magnetic core Gd-chelates	Target-Matrix metalloproteinases 14 (MMP-14) Imaging-MRI	Paul Loadman, Robert Falconer, Jason Gill, Jianghong Rao, Heike E. Daldrup-Link
2	WO2015014756A1	Magnetic core Gd-chelates	Target-Matrix metalloproteinases 14 (MMP-14) Imaging-MRI	Paul Loadman, Robert Falconer, Jason Gill, Jianghong Rao, Heike E. Daldrup-Link
3	CN104225595A	Aptamer (Cell SELEX)	Target-MDA-MB-231 breast cancer cell Imaging-near Infrared	Ju Yu Xiantian Jiang Wei Ding Lin Yu Junsheng Shen Zhen
4	US20150160222A1	Not clarified	Target-SET/KifC1	Ritu Aneja, Padmashree C.G. Rida
5	US9675714B1	Chitosan functionalized 2D graphene sheets Superparamagnetic iron oxide	Imaging-Nuclear magnetic resonance (NMR)	Subhra Mohapatra, Chunyan Wang
6	US20130323165A1	Magnetic cationic liposomal nanoparticles	Imaging-PET, MRI	Robert B. Campbell, Srinivas Sridhar

All the data are obtained from Wipo and Google patent.

4. Phytonanomedicines Approved by the FDA or in Preclinical and Clinical Trials

Breast cancer (BC) is the most prevailing cancer in women, and its prognosis has improved over the past few years. The mainstay of BC treatment is still chemoradiation therapy in the early and advanced stages [142]. However, poor selectivity, higher grades of systemic toxicities, and treatment resistance remain the major causes of therapeutic failure among these BC patients [143]. Novel drug delivery systems and drug combinations need to be designed to overcome these problems. Because of the inherent antineoplastic activity of numerous phytochemical components that are bioactive compounds obtained from natural fruits and vegetables, they can be incorporated into the management of various malignant conditions. However, the therapeutic potential of these phytochemical compounds is often hindered because of their poor pharmacokinetic parameters, such as poor solubility, stability, absorption, and quick metabolism. These constituents can be incorporated via nanocarriers, which help enhance their solubility and stability, to address these problems [21,143].

Doxorubicin is a conventionally used molecule for the management of breast cancer; however, it also produces reactive oxygen species (ROS). These ROS damage the different layers of the heart and are responsible for doxorubicin-mediated cardiotoxicity. This issue can be addressed by combining doxorubicin with quercetin, which is a plant-based flavonoid and has good antioxidant potential. The combination of quercetin–doxorubicin decreases the major adverse effect of cardiotoxicity mediated by doxorubicin, which has been observed in numerous in vitro studies. The results of numerous in vivo and in vitro studies show that quercetin dephosphorylates proto-oncogene tyrosine–protein kinase activity and inhibits inflammatory responses in cardiomyocytes. Thus, it protects cardiac myocytes against doxorubicin-mediated cardiotoxicity [144].

Another phytochemical constituent, 6-gingerol, along with paclitaxel, has been tested in vivo and in vitro for breast cancer treatment. Paclitaxel has numerous toxicities at its optimal dose, and therefore, its combination with 6-gingerol enhances its effectiveness at a lower dose. The combination of 5 nM paclitaxel with 10 μM 6-gingerol revealed the same viability as monotherapy with 20 nM paclitaxel [145].

The related in vivo, in vitro, and clinical studies have been mentioned in Tables 3 and 4 for the treatment of breast cancer.

Table 3. Preclinical studies utilizing phytochemical nanocarriers for breast cancer treatment.

Phytochemical Constituent	Anticancer Agent	Nanocarrier	Condition	Remarks	Reference
6-Gingerol	Paclitaxel	PEGylated naniosome	In vivo	Increased the effectiveness of paclitaxel, and lower dose of paclitaxel is needed for the anti-neoplastic activity.	[146]
Quercetin	Doxorubicin	Lecithin	In vivo	Prevents doxorubicin resistance in tumor cells and increases drug absorption and toxicities in malignant cells.	[110]
Quercetin	Doxorubicin	Au nanocages	In vitro	Gives synergistic effect by retaining the drug for longer period of time in malignant cells.	[147]

Table 4. Clinical studies utilizing phytochemical nanocarriers for breast cancer treatment.

Phytochemical Constituent-Based Drug	Nanocarrier	Phase of Clinical Trial	Condition	Remarks	References
Vinorelbine tartrate	Liposomal vinorelbine tartrate	Phase 1	Breast cancer	Inhibits microtubule polymerization and promotes cell apoptosis.	[148]
Paclitaxel	Albumin-stabilized paclitaxel	Phase 3	Metastatic breast cancer	Less exposure of toxic cremophor of the drug to non-cancerous cells thus enables higher dosing and improves paclitaxel penetration inside the cancer cells	[149]
Paclitaxel	Paclitaxel-loaded polymeric nanoparticles	Phase 4	Breast cancer	Increased blood stability and tumor-specific action by releasing drug inside tumor cells via a PH-sensitive action	[150]
Docetaxel	Nanosomal docetaxel lipid suspension	Phase 3	Breast cancer	Better stability, lower cytotoxicity to normal cells and easily pass-through leaky vasculature of tumor blood vessels	[151]

5. Lacunas of Phytofabricated Nanocarriers

Evidence is accumulating in support of an important notion that nanotechnology in general and phytofabricated nanocarriers, in particular, may represent an important solution for many existing challenges related to current breast cancer therapies. In fact, such phytofabricated nanoparticles, being advanced biomaterials characterized by the controllable and stimuli-responsive release of therapeutic agents, favorable biodistribution, great biocompatibility, excellent structural stability in serum, low level of side-effects, and prolonged half-life, clearly represent an exceptional way to noticeably increase the therapeutic efficiency combined with the considerable decrease in the potential toxic side-effects. Different carcinogenic metal ions can be reduced to nanoparticles via the natural antioxidant action of various phytoconstituents (primary and secondary metabolites), such as alkaloids, amino acids, flavonoids, polyphenols, proteins, sugars, tannic acids, and terpenoids [152]. The existing literature indicates that various metal nanoparticles with anticancer properties can be phytogenerated using different plants. Examples include green-synthesized silver nanoparticles (AgNPs) using Artemisia tournefortiana Rchb ethanol extract [153], Morus alba leaf extract [154], Annona muricata aqueous leaf extract [155], *Carissa carandas* aqueous extract [156], Leucophyllum frutescens and *Russelia equisetiformis* extracts [157], aqueous extracts of Acacia arabica (Arabic Gum) and *Opophytum forsskalii* (Samh) seeds [158], *Typha azerbaijanensis* aerial part and root extracts [159], and *Rubia cordifolia* L. leaf extract [160], as well as *Papaver somniferum* L. mediated green synthesis of lead oxide (PbO) and iron oxide (Fe_2O_3) nanoparticles [161] and alpha hematite nanoparticle (α-Fe_2O_3) production using *Rhus punjabensis* extracts [162], garlic extracts [163], extracts of the *Rheum emodi* root [164], and Salvadora persica aqueous extract [165]. Furthermore, tunable cobalt oxide nanoparticles (CoONPs) were generated using the phytochemicals present in the *Rhamnus virgata* leaf extract [166]; gold nanoparticles (AuNPs) were phytosynthesized using an aqueous extract of Ziziphus spina-christi leaves [167]; selenium nanoparticles (SeNPs) were phytofabricated from the *Carica papaya* extract [168] or using *Portulaca oleracea*-based green synthesis [169]; and gold (Au), iron (Fe), and selenium (Se) nanoparticles were fabricated using various natural plant extracts from the Fertile Crescent, where *Ephedra alata* and *Pistacia lentiscus* extracts were used to synthesize the Au-NPs, and the Fe-NPs and Se-NPs were generated using fruit, peel, and seed extracts of Punica granatum [4].

The listed examples, which likely represent the tip of the iceberg, clearly show that there are multiple options for the phytofabrication of different metal nanoparticles with anticancer properties. It is obvious that with so many possibilities for the phytoproduction of a variety of nanocarriers, one has a broad choice of both anticancer nanoparticles and means for their production. However, multiple questions need to be answered before moving into the commercial use of phytofabricated nanocarriers. Since the same metal nanoparticles can be phytofabricated using different extracts from different parts of different plants, careful comparative analysis of their therapeutic potential, lifetime and structural stability in serum, biodistribution, biocompatibility, and potential toxic side effects should be conducted to select the most promising candidate for commercialization. Among the various factors that must be taken into account at this stage, one should pay very serious attention to the global availability of the plants that are planned to be used for the phytofabrication of the nanoparticles. If the optimal plant is not naturally present at the required quantities in the wild, its plantation should be planned, which obviously will contribute to the cost of phytofabrication. Furthermore, facilities and protocols, which will be utilized for the phytofabrication of nanoparticles, should have a flexible design to allow for a rapid switch between different sources, if needed.

Therefore, although in comparison with traditional technologies for the synthesis of nanoparticles, green synthesis seems to be essentially more economical, the commercial viability of the processes for the mass production of phytofabricated nanocarriers requires careful evaluation.

6. Conclusions

Breast cancer is primarily treated by chemotherapy, radiotherapy, and surgical resection; however, the survival rate is still low because of adverse drug reactions, drug resistance, and tumor metastasis. As described in this review, an increasing amount of research has demonstrated the anti-tumorigenic effect of phytochemicals that can modulate cellular events and molecular pathways. However, their pharmacological capability is impeded by their low stability, low water solubility, poor absorption, and rapid metabolism. Nanotechnology-based approaches have shed some light on maximizing the potential use of phytochemicals to overcome formulation challenges. Nanocarriers can enhance the solubility and stability of phytochemicals. Apart from improving solubility and stability, nanocarriers could prolong their half-life and even accomplish site-targeting delivery.

However, the questions of nanotechnology are not yet fully answered in the case of real clinical translation. One of the major shortcomings is that, in general, these PNs can only encapsulate small amounts of actives. Tailor-made nanocarriers conjugated with specific ligands could enable loaded phytoconstituents to function at minimal doses. However, the manufacturing of functionalized nanomedicinal formulations for commercialization is a major obstacle. These shortcomings need to be technologically addressed to maximize the anticancer potential of natural medicines. In this sense, nanotechnology has emerged as a promising drug delivery system strategy in the long run.

Author Contributions: V.P.C. created the plot of the article. V.P.C., L.V.N., P.B., R.B., V.A., R.K.S., A.K., L.V. and V.N.U. All authors collected literature data and contributed to the writing of the article. V.P.C. and V.N.U. critically revised the article. All authors have read and agreed to the published version of the manuscript.

Funding: This research received no external funding.

Acknowledgments: VPC wants to dedicate this article to the 75th-year celebration of L. M. College of Pharmacy.

Conflicts of Interest: The authors declare no conflict of interest concerning the authorship and publication of this article.

References

1. Bray, F.; Ferlay, J.; Soerjomataram, I.; Siegel, L.; Torre, A.; Ahmedin, D. GLOBOCAN estimates of incidence and mortality worldwide for 36 cancers in 185 countries. *Glob. Cancer Stat.* **2021**, *73*, 209–249.
2. Greco, S.J. Breast cancer risk in a rapidly aging population: Advances and approaches to study the aging tissue microenvironment. *Breast Cancer Targets Ther.* **2019**, *11*, 111. [CrossRef]
3. Arnold, M.; Morgan, E.; Rumgay, H.; Mafra, A.; Singh, D.; Laversanne, M.; Vignat, J.; Gralow, J.R.; Cardoso, F.; Siesling, S. Current and future burden of breast cancer: Global statistics for 2020 and 2040. *Breast* **2022**, *66*, 15–23. [CrossRef]
4. Shnoudeh, A.J.; Qadumii, L.; Zihlif, M.; Al-Ameer, H.J.; Salou, R.A.; Jaber, A.Y.; Hamad, I. Green Synthesis of Gold, Iron and Selenium Nanoparticles Using Phytoconstituents: Preliminary Evaluation of Antioxidant and Biocompatibility Potential. *Molecules* **2022**, *27*, 1334. [CrossRef]
5. Turashvili, G.; Brogi, E. Tumor heterogeneity in breast cancer. *Front. Med.* **2017**, *4*, 227. [CrossRef] [PubMed]
6. Hawkins, R.; Killen, E.; Tesdale, A.; Sangster, K.; Thomson, M.; Steele, R.; Blackie, R. Oestrogen receptors, lactate dehydrogenase and cellularity in human breast cancer. *Clin. Chim. Acta* **1988**, *175*, 89–96. [CrossRef]
7. WHO Classification of Tumours of the Breast. Available online: https://espace.library.uq.edu.au/view/UQ:8984059 (accessed on 24 January 2023).
8. Dean-Colomb, W.; Esteva, F.J. Her2-positive breast cancer: Herceptin and beyond. *Eur. J. Cancer* **2008**, *44*, 2806–2812. [CrossRef] [PubMed]
9. Bardou, V.-J.; Arpino, G.; Elledge, R.M.; Osborne, C.K.; Clark, G.M. Progesterone receptor status significantly improves outcome prediction over estrogen receptor status alone for adjuvant endocrine therapy in two large breast cancer databases. *J. Clin. Oncol.* **2003**, *21*, 1973–1979. [CrossRef]
10. Harvey, J.M.; Clark, G.M.; Osborne, C.K.; Allred, D.C. Estrogen receptor status by immunohistochemistry is superior to the ligand-binding assay for predicting response to adjuvant endocrine therapy in breast cancer. *J. Clin. Oncol.* **1999**, *17*, 1474–1481. [CrossRef] [PubMed]
11. Sørlie, T.; Perou, C.M.; Tibshirani, R.; Aas, T.; Geisler, S.; Johnsen, H.; Hastie, T.; Eisen, M.B.; Van De Rijn, M.; Jeffrey, S.S. Gene expression patterns of breast carcinomas distinguish tumor subclasses with clinical implications. *Proc. Natl. Acad. Sci. USA* **2001**, *98*, 10869–10874. [CrossRef]
12. Sørlie, T.; Borgan, E.; Myhre, S.; Vollan, H.K.; Russnes, H.; Zhao, X.; Nilsen, G.; Lingjærde, O.C.; Børresen-Dale, A.-L.; Rødland, E. The importance of gene-centring microarray data. *Lancet Oncol.* **2010**, *11*, 719–720. [CrossRef]
13. Bhushan, A.; Gonsalves, A.; Menon, J.U. Current state of breast cancer diagnosis, treatment, and theranostics. *Pharmaceutics* **2021**, *13*, 723. [CrossRef]
14. Galmarini, D.; Galmarini, C.M.; Galmarini, F.C. Cancer chemotherapy: A critical analysis of its 60 years of history. *Crit. Rev. Oncol. Hematol.* **2012**, *84*, 181–199. [CrossRef]
15. Lall, R.K.; Syed, D.N.; Adhami, V.M.; Khan, M.I.; Mukhtar, H. Dietary polyphenols in prevention and treatment of prostate cancer. *Int. J. Mol. Sci.* **2015**, *16*, 3350–3376. [CrossRef]
16. Sawanny, R.; Pramanik, S.; Agarwal, U. Role of Phytochemicals in the Treatment of Breast Cancer: Natural Swords Battling Cancer Cells. *Curr. Cancer Ther. Rev.* **2021**, *17*, 179–196. [CrossRef]
17. Ranjan, A.; Ramachandran, S.; Gupta, N.; Kaushik, I.; Wright, S.; Srivastava, S.; Das, H.; Srivastava, S.; Prasad, S.; Srivastava, S.K. Role of phytochemicals in cancer prevention. *Int. J. Mol. Sci.* **2019**, *20*, 4981. [CrossRef] [PubMed]
18. DiMarco-Crook, C.; Xiao, H. Diet-based strategies for cancer chemoprevention: The role of combination regimens using dietary bioactive components. *Annu. Rev. Food Sci. Technol.* **2015**, *6*, 505–526. [CrossRef] [PubMed]
19. Ruiz, R.B.; Hernández, P.S. Cancer chemoprevention by dietary phytochemicals: Epidemiological evidence. *Maturitas* **2016**, *94*, 13–19. [CrossRef]
20. Bhattacharjee, H.; Balabathula, P.; Wood, G.C. Targeted nanoparticulate drug-delivery systems for treatment of solid tumors: A review. *Ther. Deliv.* **2010**, *1*, 713–734. [CrossRef]

21. Navya, P.; Kaphle, A.; Srinivas, S.; Bhargava, S.K.; Rotello, V.M.; Daima, H.K. Current trends and challenges in cancer management and therapy using designer nanomaterials. *Nano Converg.* **2019**, *6*, 23. [CrossRef] [PubMed]
22. Duan, X.; Li, Y. Physicochemical characteristics of nanoparticles affect circulation, biodistribution, cellular internalization, and trafficking. *Small* **2013**, *9*, 1521–1532. [CrossRef] [PubMed]
23. Pérez-Herrero, E.; Fernández-Medarde, A. Advanced targeted therapies in cancer: Drug nanocarriers, the future of chemotherapy. *Eur. J. Pharm. Biopharm.* **2015**, *93*, 52–79. [CrossRef] [PubMed]
24. Chemotherapy for Breast Cancer. Available online: https://www.mayoclinic.org/tests-procedures/chemotherapy-for-breast-cancer/about/pac-20384931 (accessed on 24 January 2023).
25. Grobmyer, S.R.; Zhou, G.; Gutwein, L.G.; Iwakuma, N.; Sharma, P.; Hochwald, S.N. Nanoparticle delivery for metastatic breast cancer. *Nanomed. Nanotechnol. Biol. Med.* **2012**, *8*, S21–S30. [CrossRef] [PubMed]
26. Davies, E.; Hiscox, S. New therapeutic approaches in breast cancer. *Maturitas* **2011**, *68*, 121–128. [CrossRef]
27. Singh, S.K.; Singh, S.; Lillard, J.W., Jr.; Singh, R. Drug delivery approaches for breast cancer. *Int. J. Nanomed.* **2017**, *12*, 6205. [CrossRef]
28. Eroles, P.; Bosch, A.; Pérez-Fidalgo, J.A.; Lluch, A. Molecular biology in breast cancer: Intrinsic subtypes and signaling pathways. *Cancer Treat. Rev.* **2012**, *38*, 698–707. [CrossRef] [PubMed]
29. Zhang, S.; Chu, Z.; Yin, C.; Zhang, C.; Lin, G.; Li, Q. Controllable drug release and simultaneously carrier decomposition of SiO_2-drug composite nanoparticles. *J. Am. Chem. Soc.* **2013**, *135*, 5709–5716. [CrossRef]
30. Beloqui, A.; Alhouayek, M.; Carradori, D.; Vanvarenberg, K.; Muccioli, G.G.; Cani, P.D.; Preat, V. A mechanistic study on nanoparticle-mediated glucagon-like peptide-1 (GLP-1) secretion from enteroendocrine L cells. *Mol. Pharm.* **2016**, *13*, 4222–4230. [CrossRef]
31. Yuan, H.; Ma, Q.; Ye, L.; Piao, G. The traditional medicine and modern medicine from natural products. *Molecules* **2016**, *21*, 559. [CrossRef]
32. India Regulatory Services > Phytopharmaceutical Drug—CliniExperts. Available online: https://cliniexperts.com/india-regulatory-services/phytopharmaceutical-drug/ (accessed on 24 December 2022).
33. Singh, B. *Herbal insecticides, Repellents Biomedicines: Effectiveness Commercialization*; Springer: New Delhi, India, 2016; pp. 127–145.
34. Boon, H.S.; Olatunde, F.; Zick, S.M. Trends in complementary/alternative medicine use by breast cancer survivors: Comparing survey data from 1998 and 2005. *BMC Women's Health* **2007**, *7*, 4. [CrossRef]
35. O'brien, K. Complementary and alternative medicine: The move into mainstream health care. *Clin. Exp. Optom.* **2004**, *87*, 110–120. [CrossRef] [PubMed]
36. Ma, H.; Carpenter, C.L.; Sullivan-Halley, J.; Bernstein, L. The roles of herbal remedies in survival and quality of life among long-term breast cancer survivors-results of a prospective study. *BMC Cancer* **2011**, *11*, 222. [CrossRef] [PubMed]
37. Ho, J.W.; Leung, Y.; Chan, C. Herbal medicine in the treatment of cancer. *Curr. Med. Chem.-Anti-Cancer Agents* **2002**, *2*, 209–214. [CrossRef]
38. Bahmani, M.; Shirzad, H.; Shahinfard, N.; Sheivandi, L.; Rafieian-Kopaei, M.J. Cancer phytotherapy: Recent views on the role of antioxidant and angiogenesis activities. *J. Evid.-Based Complement. Altern. Med.* **2017**, *22*, 299–309. [CrossRef] [PubMed]
39. Musthaba, S.M.; Baboota, S.; Ahmed, S.; Ahuja, A.; Ali, J. Status of novel drug delivery technology for phytotherapeutics. *Expert Opin. Drug Deliv.* **2009**, *6*, 625–637. [CrossRef]
40. Feng-Lin, Y.; Tzu-Hui, W.; Liang-Tzung, L.; Thau-Ming, C.; Chun-Ching, L. Preparation and characterization of *Cuscuta chinensis* nanoparticles. *Food Chem. Toxicol.* **2008**, *46*, 1771–1777.
41. Caiolfa, V.; Zamai, M.; Fiorino, A.; Frigerio, E.; Pellizzoni, C.; d'Argy, R.; Ghiglieri, A.; Castelli, M.; Farao, M.; Pesenti, E. Polymer-bound camptothecin: Initial biodistribution and antitumour activity studies. *J. Control. Release* **2000**, *65*, 105–119. [CrossRef]
42. Min, K.H.; Park, K.; Kim, Y.-S.; Bae, S.M.; Lee, S.; Jo, H.G.; Park, R.-W.; Kim, I.-S.; Jeong, S.Y.; Kim, K. Hydrophobically modified glycol chitosan nanoparticles-encapsulated camptothecin enhance the drug stability and tumor targeting in cancer therapy. *J. Control. Release* **2008**, *127*, 208–218. [CrossRef]
43. Sánchez, A.; Mejía, S.P.; Orozco, J. Recent advances in polymeric nanoparticle-encapsulated drugs against intracellular infections. *Molecules* **2020**, *25*, 3760. [CrossRef]
44. Dong, Y.; Fu, R.; Yang, J.; Ma, P.; Liang, L.; Mi, Y.; Fan, D. Folic acid-modified ginsenoside Rg5-loaded bovine serum albumin nanoparticles for targeted cancer therapy in vitro and in vivo. *Int. J. Nanomed.* **2019**, *14*, 6971. [CrossRef] [PubMed]
45. Kumari, M.; Sharma, N.; Manchanda, R.; Gupta, N.; Syed, A.; Bahkali, A.H.; Nimesh, S. PGMD/curcumin nanoparticles for the treatment of breast cancer. *Sci. Rep.* **2021**, *11*, 3824. [CrossRef] [PubMed]
46. Zeng, L.; Yan, J.; Luo, L.; Ma, M.; Zhu, H. Preparation and characterization of (−)-Epigallocatechin-3-gallate (EGCG)-loaded nanoparticles and their inhibitory effects on Human breast cancer MCF-7 cells. *Sci. Rep.* **2017**, *7*, 45521. [CrossRef] [PubMed]
47. Solanki, R.; Patel, K.; Patel, S.J.C.; Physicochemical, S.A.; Aspects, E. Bovine serum albumin nanoparticles for the efficient delivery of berberine: Preparation, characterization and in vitro biological studies. *Colloids Surf. A Physicochem. Eng. Asp.* **2021**, *608*, 125501. [CrossRef]
48. Sulaiman, G.M.; Jabir, M.S.; Hameed, A.H. Nanoscale modification of chrysin for improved of therapeutic efficiency and cytotoxicity. *Artif. Cells Nanomed. Biotechnol.* **2018**, *46*, 708–720. [CrossRef]

49. Zhou, Y.; Chen, D.; Xue, G.; Yu, S.; Yuan, C.; Huang, M.; Jiang, L. Improved therapeutic efficacy of quercetin-loaded polymeric nanoparticles on triple-negative breast cancer by inhibiting uPA. *RSC Adv.* **2020**, *10*, 34517–34526. [CrossRef]
50. Wu, P.; Zhang, B.; Ocansey, D.K.W.; Xu, W.; Qian, H. Extracellular vesicles: A bright star of nanomedicine. *Biomaterials* **2021**, *269*, 120467. [CrossRef]
51. Ortega, A.; Martinez-Arroyo, O.; Forner, M.J.; Cortes, R. Exosomes as drug delivery systems: Endogenous nanovehicles for treatment of systemic lupus erythematosus. *Pharmaceutics* **2020**, *13*, 3. [CrossRef]
52. Chen, C.; Wang, J.; Sun, M.; Li, J.; Wang, H.-M.D. Toward the next-generation phyto-nanomedicines: Cell-derived nanovesicles (CDNs) for natural product delivery. *Biomed. Pharmacother.* **2022**, *145*, 112416. [CrossRef]
53. Fuhrmann, G.; Serio, A.; Mazo, M.; Nair, R.; Stevens, M.M. Active loading into extracellular vesicles significantly improves the cellular uptake and photodynamic effect of porphyrins. *J. Control. Release* **2015**, *205*, 35–44. [CrossRef]
54. Zhang, X.; Zhang, H.; Gu, J.; Zhang, J.; Shi, H.; Qian, H.; Wang, D.; Xu, W.; Pan, J.; Santos, H.A. Engineered extracellular vesicles for cancer therapy. *Adv. Mater.* **2021**, *33*, 2005709. [CrossRef] [PubMed]
55. Wang, J.; Li, W.; Lu, Z.; Zhang, L.; Hu, Y.; Li, Q.; Du, W.; Feng, X.; Jia, H.; Liu, B.-F. The use of RGD-engineered exosomes for enhanced targeting ability and synergistic therapy toward angiogenesis. *Nanoscale* **2017**, *9*, 15598–15605. [CrossRef]
56. Herrmann, I.K.; Wood, M.J.A.; Fuhrmann, G. Extracellular vesicles as a next-generation drug delivery platform. *Nat. Nanotechnol.* **2021**, *16*, 748–759. [CrossRef] [PubMed]
57. Wang, K.; Ye, H.; Zhang, X.; Wang, X.; Yang, B.; Luo, C.; Zhao, Z.; Zhao, J.; Lu, Q.; Zhang, H. An exosome-like programmable-bioactivating paclitaxel prodrug nanoplatform for enhanced breast cancer metastasis inhibition. *Biomaterials* **2020**, *257*, 120224. [CrossRef] [PubMed]
58. Li, L.; Liang, N.; Wang, D.; Yan, P.; Kawashima, Y.; Cui, F.; Sun, S. Amphiphilic polymeric micelles based on deoxycholic acid and folic acid modified chitosan for the delivery of paclitaxel. *Int. J. Mol. Sci.* **2018**, *19*, 3132. [CrossRef] [PubMed]
59. Munagala, R.; Aqil, F.; Jeyabalan, J.; Gupta, R.C. Bovine milk-derived exosomes for drug delivery. *Cancer Lett.* **2016**, *371*, 48–61. [CrossRef] [PubMed]
60. Donoso-Quezada, J.; Guajardo-Flores, D.; González-Valdez, J. Enhanced exosome-mediated delivery of black bean phytochemicals (*Phaseolus vulgaris* L.) for cancer treatment applications. *Biomed. Pharmacother.* **2020**, *131*, 110771. [CrossRef]
61. Munagala, R.; Aqil, F.; Jeyabalan, J.; Agrawal, A.K.; Mudd, A.M.; Kyakulaga, A.H.; Singh, I.P.; Vadhanam, M.V.; Gupta, R.C. Exosomal formulation of anthocyanidins against multiple cancer types. *Cancer Lett.* **2017**, *393*, 94–102. [CrossRef]
62. Kanchanapally, R.; Khan, M.A.; Deshmukh, S.K.; Srivastava, S.K.; Khushman, M.; Singh, S.; Singh, A.P. Exosomal formulation escalates cellular uptake of honokiol leading to the enhancement of its antitumor efficacy. *ACS Omega* **2020**, *5*, 23299–23307. [CrossRef]
63. Antimisiaris, S.; Marazioti, A.; Kannavou, M.; Natsaridis, E.; Gkartziou, F.; Kogkos, G.; Mourtas, S. Overcoming barriers by local drug delivery with liposomes. *Adv. Drug Deliv. Rev.* **2021**, *174*, 53–86. [CrossRef] [PubMed]
64. Deshmukh, P.K.; Mutha, R.E.; Surana, S.J. Electrostatic deposition assisted preparation, characterization and evaluation of chrysin liposomes for breast cancer treatment. *Drug Dev. Ind. Pharm.* **2021**, *47*, 809–819. [CrossRef]
65. Patel, G.; Thakur, N.S.; Kushwah, V.; Patil, M.D.; Nile, S.H.; Jain, S.; Banerjee, U.C.; Kai, G. Liposomal delivery of mycophenolic acid with quercetin for improved breast cancer therapy in SD rats. *Front. Bioeng. Biotechnol.* **2020**, *8*, 631. [CrossRef]
66. Farcas, C.G.; Dehelean, C.; Pinzaru, I.A.; Mioc, M.; Socoliuc, V.; Moaca, E.-A.; Avram, S.; Ghiulai, R.; Coricovac, D.; Pavel, I. Thermosensitive betulinic acid-loaded magnetoliposomes: A promising antitumor potential for highly aggressive human breast adenocarcinoma cells under hyperthermic conditions. *Int. J. Nanomed.* **2020**, *15*, 8175. [CrossRef]
67. Zhao, Y.; Cao, Y.; Sun, J.; Liang, Z.; Wu, Q.; Cui, S.; Zhi, D.; Guo, S.; Zhen, Y.; Zhang, S. Anti-breast cancer activity of resveratrol encapsulated in liposomes. *J. Mater. Chem. B* **2020**, *8*, 27–37. [CrossRef] [PubMed]
68. Zawilska, P.; Machowska, M.; Wisniewski, K.; Grynkiewicz, G.; Hrynyk, R.; Rzepecki, R.; Gubernator, J. Novel pegylated liposomal formulation of docetaxel with 3-n-pentadecylphenol derivative for cancer therapy. *Eur. J. Pharm. Sci.* **2021**, *163*, 105838. [CrossRef] [PubMed]
69. García-Pinel, B.; Porras-Alcalá, C.; Ortega-Rodríguez, A.; Sarabia, F.; Prados, J.; Melguizo, C.; López-Romero, J.M. Lipid-based nanoparticles: Application and recent advances in cancer treatment. *Nanomaterials* **2019**, *9*, 638. [CrossRef]
70. Wang, L.; Li, H.; Wang, S.; Liu, R.; Wu, Z.; Wang, C.; Wang, Y.; Chen, M. Enhancing the antitumor activity of berberine hydrochloride by solid lipid nanoparticle encapsulation. *AAPS PharmSciTech* **2014**, *15*, 834–844. [CrossRef]
71. Wang, W.; Chen, T.; Xu, H.; Ren, B.; Cheng, X.; Qi, R.; Liu, H.; Wang, Y.; Yan, L.; Chen, S. Curcumin-loaded solid lipid nanoparticles enhanced anticancer efficiency in breast cancer. *Molecules* **2018**, *23*, 1578. [CrossRef]
72. Wang, W.; Zhang, L.; Chen, T.; Guo, W.; Bao, X.; Wang, D.; Ren, B.; Wang, H.; Li, Y.; Wang, Y. Anticancer effects of resveratrol-loaded solid lipid nanoparticles on human breast cancer cells. *Molecules* **2017**, *22*, 1814. [CrossRef] [PubMed]
73. Niazvand, F.; Orazizadeh, M.; Khorsandi, L.; Abbaspour, M.; Mansouri, E.; Khodadadi, A. Effects of quercetin-loaded nanoparticles on MCF-7 human breast cancer cells. *Medicina* **2019**, *55*, 114. [CrossRef]
74. Radhakrishnan, R.; Kulhari, H.; Pooja, D.; Gudem, S.; Bhargava, S.; Shukla, R.; Sistla, R. Encapsulation of biophenolic phytochemical EGCG within lipid nanoparticles enhances its stability and cytotoxicity against cancer. *Chem. Phys. Lipids* **2016**, *198*, 51–60. [CrossRef]
75. Opatha, S.A.T.; Titapiwatanakun, V.; Chutoprapat, R. Transfersomes: A promising nanoencapsulation technique for transdermal drug delivery. *Pharmaceutics* **2020**, *12*, 855. [CrossRef]

76. Rai, S.; Pandey, V.; Rai, G. Transfersomes as versatile and flexible nano-vesicular carriers in skin cancer therapy: The state of the art. *Nano Rev. Exp.* **2017**, *8*, 1325708. [CrossRef] [PubMed]
77. Sivannarayana, P.; Rani, A.P.; Saikishore, V.; VenuBabu, C.; SriRekha, V. Transfersomes: Ultra deformable vesicular carrier systems in transdermal drug delivery system. *Res. J. Pharm. Dos. Technol.* **2012**, *4*, 1.
78. Cevc, G.; Schätzlein, A.; Richardsen, H. Ultradeformable lipid vesicles can penetrate the skin and other semi-permeable barriers unfragmented. Evidence from double label CLSM experiments and direct size measurements. *Biochim. Biophys. Acta-Biomembr.* **2002**, *1564*, 21–30. [CrossRef]
79. Kim, B.; Cho, H.-E.; Moon, S.H.; Ahn, H.-J.; Bae, S.; Cho, H.-D.; An, S. Transdermal delivery systems in cosmetics. *Biomed. Dermatol.* **2020**, *4*, 10. [CrossRef]
80. Kumar, G.P.; Rajeshwarrao, P. Nonionic surfactant vesicular systems for effective drug delivery—An overview. *Acta Pharm. Sin. B* **2011**, *1*, 208–219. [CrossRef]
81. Chauhan, P.; Tyagi, B.K. Herbal novel drug delivery systems and transfersomes. *J. Drug Deliv. Ther.* **2018**, *8*, 162–168. [CrossRef]
82. Modi, C.; Bharadia, P. Transfersomes: New dominants for transdermal drug delivery. *Am. J. PharmTech Res. AJPTR* **2012**, *2*, 71–91.
83. Li, J.; Wang, X.; Zhang, T.; Wang, C.; Huang, Z.; Luo, X.; Deng, Y. A review on phospholipids and their main applications in drug delivery systems. *Asian J. Pharm. Sci.* **2015**, *10*, 81–98. [CrossRef]
84. Moawad, F.A.; Ali, A.A.; Salem, H.F. Nanotransfersomes-loaded thermosensitive in situ gel as a rectal delivery system of tizanidine HCl: Preparation, in vitro and in vivo performance. *Drug Deliv.* **2017**, *24*, 252–260. [CrossRef]
85. Bnyan, R.; Khan, I.; Ehtezazi, T.; Saleem, I.; Gordon, S.; O'Neill, F.; Roberts, M. Surfactant effects on lipid-based vesicles properties. *J. Pharm. Sci.* **2018**, *107*, 1237–1246. [CrossRef]
86. Gadag, S.; Narayan, R.; Sabhahit, J.N.; Hari, G.; Nayak, Y.; Pai, K.S.R.; Garg, S.; Nayak, U.Y. Transpapillary iontophoretic delivery of resveratrol loaded transfersomes for localized delivery to breast cancer. *Biomater. Adv.* **2022**, *140*, 213085. [CrossRef] [PubMed]
87. Touitou, E.; Dayan, N.; Bergelson, L.; Godin, B.; Eliaz, M.J. Ethosomes—Novel vesicular carriers for enhanced delivery: Characterization and skin penetration properties. *J. Control. Release* **2000**, *65*, 403–418. [CrossRef] [PubMed]
88. Godin, B.; Touitou, E. Ethosomes: New prospects in transdermal delivery. *Crit. Rev. Ther. Drug Carr. Syst.* **2003**, *20*, 63–102. [CrossRef]
89. Ainbinder, D.; Touitou, E. Testosterone ethosomes for enhanced transdermal delivery. *Drug Deliv.* **2005**, *12*, 297–303. [CrossRef]
90. Lopez-Pinto, J.; Gonzalez-Rodriguez, M.; Rabasco, A. Effect of cholesterol and ethanol on dermal delivery from DPPC liposomes. *Int. J. Pharm.* **2005**, *298*, 1–12. [CrossRef] [PubMed]
91. Touitou, E. Compositions for Applying Active Substances to or through the Skin. U.S. Patent US5540934A, 30 July 1996.
92. Touitou, E. Composition for Applying Active Substances to or through the Skin. U.S. Patent US5716638A, 10 February 1998.
93. Nasri, S.; Ebrahimi-Hosseinzadeh, B.; Rahaie, M.; Hatamian-Zarmi, A.; Sahraeian, R. Thymoquinone-loaded ethosome with breast cancer potential: Optimization, in vitro and biological assessment. *J. Nanostruct. Chem.* **2020**, *10*, 19–31. [CrossRef]
94. Barani, M.; Mirzaei, M.; Torkzadeh-Mahani, M.; Adeli-Sardou, M. Evaluation of carum-loaded niosomes on breast cancer cells: Physicochemical properties, in vitro cytotoxicity, flow cytometric, DNA fragmentation and cell migration assay. *Sci. Rep.* **2019**, *9*, 7139. [CrossRef]
95. Barani, M.; Mirzaei, M.; Torkzadeh-Mahani, M.; Nematollahi, M.H. Lawsone-loaded Niosome and its antitumor activity in MCF-7 breast Cancer cell line: A Nano-herbal treatment for Cancer. *DARU J. Pharm. Sci.* **2018**, *26*, 11–17. [CrossRef]
96. Honarvari, B.; Karimifard, S.; Akhtari, N.; Mehrarya, M.; Moghaddam, Z.S.; Ansari, M.J.; Jalil, A.T.; Matencio, A.; Trotta, F.; Yeganeh, F.E. Folate-targeted curcumin-loaded niosomes for site-specific delivery in breast cancer treatment: In silico and In vitro study. *Molecules* **2022**, *27*, 4634. [CrossRef]
97. Ahmed, S.; Ahmad, M.; Swami, B.L.; Ikram, S. A review on plants extract mediated synthesis of silver nanoparticles for antimicrobial applications: A green expertise. *J. Adv. Res.* **2016**, *7*, 17–28. [CrossRef]
98. Kuppusamy, P.; Yusoff, M.M.; Maniam, G.P.; Govindan, N. Biosynthesis of metallic nanoparticles using plant derivatives and their new avenues in pharmacological applications–An updated report. *Saudi Pharm. J.* **2016**, *24*, 473–484. [CrossRef]
99. Rai, M.; Yadav, A. Plants as potential synthesiser of precious metal nanoparticles: Progress and prospects. *IET Nanobiotechnol.* **2013**, *7*, 117–124. [CrossRef]
100. Gardea-Torresdey, J.L.; Parsons, J.; Gomez, E.; Peralta-Videa, J.; Troiani, H.; Santiago, P.; Yacaman, M.J. Formation and growth of Au nanoparticles inside live alfalfa plants. *Nano Lett.* **2002**, *2*, 397–401. [CrossRef]
101. Haverkamp, R.G.; Marshall, A.T.; van Agterveld, D. Pick your carats: Nanoparticles of gold–silver–copper alloy produced in vivo. *J. Nanopart. Res.* **2007**, *9*, 697–700. [CrossRef]
102. Harris, A.T.; Bali, R. On the formation and extent of uptake of silver nanoparticles by live plants. *J. Nanopart. Res.* **2008**, *10*, 691–695. [CrossRef]
103. Ankamwar, B. Biosynthesis of gold nanoparticles (green-gold) using leaf extract of *Terminalia catappa*. *E-J. Chem.* **2010**, *7*, 1334–1339. [CrossRef]
104. Zhang, M.; Viennois, E.; Xu, C.; Merlin, D. Plant derived edible nanoparticles as a new therapeutic approach against diseases. *Tissue Barriers* **2016**, *4*, e1134415. [CrossRef]
105. Zhuang, X.; Deng, Z.-B.; Mu, J.; Zhang, L.; Yan, J.; Miller, D.; Feng, W.; McClain, C.J.; Zhang, H.-G. Ginger-derived nanoparticles protect against alcohol-induced liver damage. *J. Extracell. Vesicles* **2015**, *4*, 28713. [CrossRef] [PubMed]

106. Li, Z.; Wang, H.; Yin, H.; Bennett, C.; Zhang, H.-G.; Guo, P. Arrowtail RNA for ligand display on ginger exosome-like nanovesicles to systemic deliver siRNA for cancer suppression. *Sci. Rep.* **2018**, *8*, 14644. [CrossRef]
107. Akuma, P.; Okagu, O.D.; Udenigwe, C.C. Naturally occurring exosome vesicles as potential delivery vehicle for bioactive compounds. *Front. Sustain. Food Syst.* **2019**, *3*, 23. [CrossRef]
108. Wang, Q.; Ren, Y.; Mu, J.; Egilmez, N.K.; Zhuang, X.; Deng, Z.; Zhang, L.; Yan, J.; Miller, D.; Zhang, H.-G. Grapefruit-Derived Nanovectors Use an Activated Leukocyte Trafficking Pathway to Deliver Therapeutic Agents to Inflammatory Tumor SitesHijacked Leukocyte Pathway for Targeted Delivery. *Cancer Res.* **2015**, *75*, 2520–2529. [CrossRef]
109. Yi, S.; Wang, Y.; Huang, Y.; Xia, L.; Sun, L.; Lenaghan, S.C.; Zhang, M. Tea nanoparticles for immunostimulation and chemo-drug delivery in cancer treatment. *J. Biomed. Nanotechnol.* **2014**, *10*, 1016–1029. [CrossRef] [PubMed]
110. Minaei, A.; Sabzichi, M.; Ramezani, F.; Hamishehkar, H.; Samadi, N. Co-delivery with nano-quercetin enhances doxorubicin-mediated cytotoxicity against MCF-7 cells. *Mol. Biol. Rep.* **2016**, *43*, 99–105. [CrossRef]
111. Halder, A.; Jethwa, M.; Mukherjee, P.; Ghosh, S.; Das, S.; Helal Uddin, A.; Mukherjee, A.; Chatterji, U.; Roy, P. Lactoferrin-tethered betulinic acid nanoparticles promote rapid delivery and cell death in triple negative breast and laryngeal cancer cells. *Artif. Cells Nanomed. Biotechnol.* **2020**, *48*, 1362–1371. [CrossRef]
112. Tabassam, Q.; Mehmood, T.; Raza, A.R.; Ullah, A.; Saeed, F.; Anjum, F.M. Synthesis, characterization and anti-cancer therapeutic potential of withanolide-A with 20nm sAuNPs conjugates against SKBR3 breast cancer cell line. *Int. J. Nanomed.* **2020**, *15*, 6649. [CrossRef]
113. Zhang, N.; Yu, J.; Liu, P.; Chang, J.; Ali, D.; Tian, X. Gold nanoparticles synthesized from *Curcuma wenyujin* inhibits HER-2/neu transcription in breast cancer cells (MDA-MB-231/HER2). *Arab. J. Chem.* **2020**, *13*, 7264–7273. [CrossRef]
114. Mu, Q.; Wang, H.; Zhang, M. Nanoparticles for imaging and treatment of metastatic breast cancer. *Expert Opin. Drug Deliv.* **2017**, *14*, 123–136. [CrossRef]
115. Al-Mahmood, S.; Sapiezynski, J.; Garbuzenko, O.B.; Minko, T. Metastatic and triple-negative breast cancer: Challenges and treatment options. *Drug Deliv. Transl. Res.* **2018**, *8*, 1483–1507. [CrossRef]
116. Bianchini, G.; Balko, J.M.; Mayer, I.A.; Sanders, M.E.; Gianni, L. Triple-negative breast cancer: Challenges and opportunities of a heterogeneous disease. *Nat. Rev. Clin. Oncol.* **2016**, *13*, 674–690. [CrossRef] [PubMed]
117. Covarrubias, G.; He, F.; Raghunathan, S.; Turan, O.; Peiris, P.M.; Schiemann, W.P.; Karathanasis, E. Effective treatment of cancer metastasis using a dual-ligand nanoparticle. *PLoS ONE* **2019**, *14*, e0220474. [CrossRef] [PubMed]
118. Xu, P.; Yin, Q.; Shen, J.; Chen, L.; Yu, H.; Zhang, Z.; Li, Y. Synergistic inhibition of breast cancer metastasis by silibinin-loaded lipid nanoparticles containing TPGS. *Int. J. Pharm.* **2013**, *454*, 21–30. [CrossRef] [PubMed]
119. Christiaens, V.; Lijnen, H.R. Angiogenesis and development of adipose tissue. *Mol. Cell. Endocrinol.* **2010**, *318*, 2–9. [CrossRef]
120. Yoshida, S.; Ono, M.; Shono, T.; Izumi, H.; Ishibashi, T.; Suzuki, H.; Kuwano, M. Involvement of interleukin-8, vascular endothelial growth factor, and basic fibroblast growth factor in tumor necrosis factor alpha-dependent angiogenesis. *Mol. Cell. Biol.* **1997**, *17*, 4015–4023. [CrossRef]
121. Rocha, T.G.R.; Lopes, S.C.D.A.; Cassali, G.D.; Ferreira, Ê.; Veloso, E.S.; Leite, E.A.; Braga, F.C.; Ferreira, L.A.M.; Balvay, D.; Garofalakis, A. Evaluation of antitumor activity of long-circulating and pH-sensitive liposomes containing ursolic acid in animal models of breast tumor and gliosarcoma. *Integr. Cancer Ther.* **2016**, *15*, 512–524. [CrossRef]
122. Abraham, B.K.; Fritz, P.; McClellan, M.; Hauptvogel, P.; Athelogou, M.; Brauch, H. Prevalence of CD44+/CD24−/low cells in breast cancer may not be associated with clinical outcome but may favor distant metastasis. *Clin. Cancer Res.* **2005**, *11*, 1154–1159. [CrossRef] [PubMed]
123. Charafe-Jauffret, E.; Ginestier, C.; Iovino, F.; Tarpin, C.; Diebel, M.; Esterni, B.; Houvenaeghel, G.; Extra, J.-M.; Bertucci, F.; Jacquemier, J. Aldehyde dehydrogenase 1–Positive cancer stem cells mediate metastasis and poor clinical outcome in inflammatory breast cancer. *Clin. Cancer Res.* **2010**, *16*, 45–55. [CrossRef]
124. Singh, P.; Sahoo, S.K. Piperlongumine loaded PLGA nanoparticles inhibit cancer stem-like cells through modulation of STAT3 in mammosphere model of triple negative breast cancer. *Int. J. Pharm.* **2022**, *616*, 121526. [CrossRef]
125. Tang, S.-M.; Deng, X.-T.; Zhou, J.; Li, Q.-P.; Ge, X.-X.; Miao, L. Pharmacological basis and new insights of quercetin action in respect to its anti-cancer effects. *Biomed. Pharmacother.* **2020**, *121*, 109604. [CrossRef]
126. Reyes-Farias, M.; Carrasco-Pozo, C. The anti-cancer effect of quercetin: Molecular implications in cancer metabolism. *Int. J. Mol. Sci.* **2019**, *20*, 3177. [CrossRef]
127. Aggarwal, V.; Tuli, H.S.; Tania, M.; Srivastava, S.; Ritzer, E.E.; Pandey, A.; Aggarwal, D.; Barwal, T.S.; Jain, A.; Kaur, G. Molecular mechanisms of action of epigallocatechin gallate in cancer: Recent trends and advancement. *Semin. Cancer Biol.* **2022**, *80*, 256–275. [CrossRef] [PubMed]
128. Subramani, R.; Gonzalez, E.; Arumugam, A.; Nandy, S.; Gonzalez, V.; Medel, J.; Camacho, F.; Ortega, A.; Bonkoungou, S.; Narayan, M. Nimbolide inhibits pancreatic cancer growth and metastasis through ROS-mediated apoptosis and inhibition of epithelial-to-mesenchymal transition. *Sci. Rep.* **2016**, *6*, 19819. [CrossRef] [PubMed]
129. Lin, H.; Qiu, S.; Xie, L.; Liu, C.; Sun, S. Nimbolide suppresses non-small cell lung cancer cell invasion and migration via manipulation of DUSP4 expression and ERK1/2 signaling. *Biomed. Pharmacother.* **2017**, *92*, 340–346. [CrossRef]
130. Sophia, J.; Kowshik, J.; Dwivedi, A.; Bhutia, S.K.; Manavathi, B.; Mishra, R.; Nagini, S. Nimbolide, a neem limonoid inhibits cytoprotective autophagy to activate apoptosis via modulation of the PI3K/Akt/GSK-3β signalling pathway in oral cancer. *Cell Death Dis.* **2018**, *9*, 1087. [CrossRef] [PubMed]

131. Balakrishnan, S.; Bhat, F.; Raja Singh, P.; Mukherjee, S.; Elumalai, P.; Das, S.; Patra, C.; Arunakaran, J. Gold nanoparticle–conjugated quercetin inhibits epithelial–mesenchymal transition, angiogenesis and invasiveness via EGFR/VEGFR-2-mediated pathway in breast cancer. *Cell Prolif.* **2016**, *49*, 678–697. [CrossRef]
132. Mukherjee, S.; Chowdhury, D.; Kotcherlakota, R.; Patra, S.; Vinothkumar, B.; Bhadra, M.P.; Sreedhar, B.; Patra, C.R. Potential theranostics application of bio-synthesized silver nanoparticles (4-in-1 system). *Theranostics* **2014**, *4*, 316. [CrossRef]
133. Gulia, K.; James, A.; Pandey, S.; Dev, K.; Kumar, D.; Sourirajan, A. Bio-Inspired Smart Nanoparticles in Enhanced Cancer Theranostics and Targeted Drug Delivery. *J. Funct. Biomater.* **2022**, *13*, 207. [CrossRef]
134. Dwivedi, A.D.; Gopal, K. Plant-mediated biosynthesis of silver and gold nanoparticles. *J. Biomed. Nanotechnol.* **2011**, *7*, 163–164. [CrossRef]
135. Cavalcanti, I.D.L.; Ximenes, R.M.; Pessoa, O.D.L.; Magalhães, N.S.S.; de Britto Lira-Nogueira, M.C. Fucoidan-coated PIBCA nanoparticles containing oncocalyxone A: Activity against metastatic breast cancer cells. *J. Drug Deliv. Sci. Technol.* **2021**, *65*, 102698. [CrossRef]
136. Awad, A.B.; Williams, H.; Fink, C.S. Phytosterols reduce in vitro metastatic ability of MDA-MB-231 human breast cancer cells. *Nutr. Cancer* **2001**, *40*, 157–164. [CrossRef]
137. Hamad, F.B.; Mubofu, E.B. Potential biological applications of bio-based anacardic acids and their derivatives. *Int. J. Mol. Sci.* **2015**, *16*, 8569–8590. [CrossRef]
138. Kushwah, V.; Katiyar, S.S.; Dora, C.P.; Agrawal, A.K.; Lamprou, D.A.; Gupta, R.C.; Jain, S. Co-delivery of docetaxel and gemcitabine by anacardic acid modified self-assembled albumin nanoparticles for effective breast cancer management. *Acta Biomater.* **2018**, *73*, 424–436. [CrossRef]
139. Iwanowycz, S.; Wang, J.; Hodge, J.; Wang, Y.; Yu, F.; Fan, D. Emodin Inhibits Breast Cancer Growth by Blocking the Tumor-Promoting Feedforward Loop between Cancer Cells and MacrophagesEmodin Blocks Cancer Cell–Macrophage Interaction. *Mol. Cancer Ther.* **2016**, *15*, 1931–1942. [CrossRef]
140. Roopan, S.M.; Surendra, T.V.; Elango, G.; Kumar, S.H.S. Biosynthetic trends and future aspects of bimetallic nanoparticles and its medicinal applications. *Appl. Microbiol. Biotechnol.* **2014**, *98*, 5289–5300. [CrossRef]
141. Wu, P.; Gao, Y.; Zhang, H.; Cai, C. Aptamer-guided silver–gold bimetallic nanostructures with highly active surface-enhanced raman scattering for specific detection and near-infrared photothermal therapy of human breast cancer cells. *Anal. Chem.* **2012**, *84*, 7692–7699. [CrossRef]
142. Przystupski, D.; Niemczura, M.J.; Górska, A.; Supplitt, S.; Kotowski, K.; Wawryka, P.; Rozborska, P.; Woźniak, K.; Michel, O.; Kiełbik, A. In search of Panacea—Review of recent studies concerning nature-derived anticancer agents. *Nutrients* **2019**, *11*, 1426. [CrossRef] [PubMed]
143. Wei, Q.-Y.; He, K.-M.; Chen, J.-L.; Xu, Y.-M.; Lau, A.T. Phytofabrication of nanoparticles as novel drugs for anticancer applications. *Molecules* **2019**, *24*, 4246. [CrossRef] [PubMed]
144. Lohiya, G.; Katti, D.S. A synergistic combination of niclosamide and doxorubicin as an efficacious therapy for all clinical subtypes of breast cancer. *Cancers* **2021**, *13*, 3299. [CrossRef] [PubMed]
145. Sartaj, A.; Baboota, S.; Ali, J. Assessment of Combination Approaches of Phytoconstituents with Chemotherapy for the Treatment of Breast Cancer: A Systematic Review. *Curr. Pharm. Des.* **2021**, *27*, 4630–4648. [CrossRef]
146. Wala, K.; Szlasa, W.; Sauer, N.; Kasperkiewicz-Wasilewska, P.; Szewczyk, A.; Saczko, J.; Rembiałkowska, N.; Kulbacka, J.; Baczyńska, D. Anticancer Efficacy of 6-Gingerol with Paclitaxel against Wild Type of Human Breast Adenocarcinoma. *Molecules* **2022**, *27*, 2693. [CrossRef]
147. Zhang, Z.; Xu, S.; Wang, Y.; Yu, Y.; Li, F.; Zhu, H.; Shen, Y.; Huang, S.; Guo, S. Near-infrared triggered co-delivery of doxorubicin and quercetin by using gold nanocages with tetradecanol to maximize anti-tumor effects on MCF-7/ADR cells. *J. Colloid Interface Sci.* **2018**, *509*, 47–57. [CrossRef] [PubMed]
148. A Bioequivalence Study of Vinorelbine Tartrate Injectable Emulsion in Patients with Advanced Cancer. 2012. Available online: https://clinicaltrials.gov/ct2/show/NCT00432562?term=NCT00432562&draw=2&rank=1 (accessed on 27 December 2022).
149. Gradishar, W.J.; Tjulandin, S.; Davidson, N.; Shaw, H.; Desai, N.; Bhar, P.; Hawkins, M.; O'Shaughnessy, J. Phase III trial of nanoparticle albumin-bound paclitaxel compared with polyethylated castor oil–based paclitaxel in women with breast cancer. *J. Clin. Oncol.* **2005**, *23*, 7794–7803. [CrossRef]
150. Park, I.H.; Sohn, J.H.; Kim, S.B.; Lee, K.S.; Chung, J.S.; Lee, S.H.; Kim, T.Y.; Jung, K.H.; Cho, E.K.; Kim, Y.S. An open-label, randomized, parallel, phase III trial evaluating the efficacy and safety of polymeric micelle-formulated paclitaxel compared to conventional cremophor EL-based paclitaxel for recurrent or metastatic HER2-negative breast cancer. *Cancer Res. Treat. Off. J. Korean Cancer Assoc.* **2017**, *49*, 569–577. [CrossRef] [PubMed]
151. Subramanian, S.; Prasanna, R.; Biswas, G.; Das Majumdar, S.K.; Joshi, N.; Bunger, D.; Khan, M.A.; Ahmad, I. Nanosomal docetaxel lipid suspension-based chemotherapy in breast cancer: Results from a multicenter retrospective study. *Breast Cancer Targets Ther.* **2020**, *12*, 77–85. [CrossRef]
152. Al-Hakkani, M.F.; Gouda, G.A.; Hassan, S.H. A review of green methods for phyto-fabrication of hematite (α-Fe$_2$O$_3$) nanoparticles and their characterization, properties, and applications. *Heliyon* **2021**, *7*, e05806. [CrossRef]
153. Baghbani-Arani, F.; Movagharnia, R.; Sharifian, A.; Salehi, S.; Shandiz, S.A.S. Photo-catalytic, anti-bacterial, and anti-cancer properties of phyto-mediated synthesis of silver nanoparticles from Artemisia tournefortiana Rchb extract. *J. Photochem. Photobiol. B Biol.* **2017**, *173*, 640–649. [CrossRef]

154. Singh, A.; Dar, M.Y.; Joshi, B.; Sharma, B.; Shrivastava, S.; Shukla, S. Phytofabrication of silver nanoparticles: Novel drug to overcome hepatocellular ailments. *Toxicol. Rep.* **2018**, *5*, 333–342. [CrossRef]
155. Meenakshisundaram, S.; Krishnamoorthy, V.; Jagadeesan, Y.; Vilwanathan, R.; Balaiah, A. Annona muricata assisted biogenic synthesis of silver nanoparticles regulates cell cycle arrest in NSCLC cell lines. *Bioorg. Chem.* **2020**, *95*, 103451. [CrossRef] [PubMed]
156. Singh, D.; Chaudhary, D.; Kumar, V.; Verma, A. Amelioration of diethylnitrosamine (DEN) induced renal oxidative stress and inflammation by *Carissa carandas* embedded silver nanoparticles in rodents. *Toxicol. Rep.* **2021**, *8*, 636–645. [CrossRef]
157. Mohammed, A.E.; Al-Megrin, W.A. Biological Potential of Silver Nanoparticles Mediated by *Leucophyllum frutescens* and *Russelia equisetiformis* Extracts. *Nanomaterials* **2021**, *11*, 2098. [CrossRef] [PubMed]
158. Aabed, K.; Mohammed, A.E. Phytoproduct, Arabic Gum and *Opophytum forsskalii* Seeds for Bio-Fabrication of Silver Nanoparticles: Antimicrobial and Cytotoxic Capabilities. *Nanomaterials* **2021**, *11*, 2573. [CrossRef]
159. Mirzaie, A.; Badmasti, F.; Dibah, H.; Hajrasouliha, S.; Yousefi, F.; Andalibi, R.; Kashtali, A.B.; Rezaei, A.H.; Bakhtiatri, R. Phyto-Fabrication of Silver Nanoparticles Using *Typha azerbaijanensis* Aerial Part and Root Extracts. *Iran. J. Public Health* **2022**, *51*, 1097. [CrossRef] [PubMed]
160. Chandraker, S.K.; Lal, M.; Khanam, F.; Dhruve, P.; Singh, R.P.; Shukla, R. Therapeutic potential of biogenic and optimized silver nanoparticles using *Rubia cordifolia* L. leaf extract. *Sci. Rep.* **2022**, *12*, 1–15.
161. Muhammad, W.; Khan, M.A.; Nazir, M.; Siddiquah, A.; Mushtaq, S.; Hashmi, S.S.; Abbasi, B.H. *Papaver somniferum* L. mediated novel bioinspired lead oxide (PbO) and iron oxide (Fe_2O_3) nanoparticles: In-vitro biological applications, biocompatibility and their potential towards HepG2 cell line. *Mater. Sci. Eng. C* **2019**, *103*, 109740. [CrossRef] [PubMed]
162. Naz, S.; Islam, M.; Tabassum, S.; Fernandes, N.F.; de Blanco, E.J.C.; Zia, M. Green synthesis of hematite (α-Fe_2O_3) nanoparticles using *Rhus punjabensis* extract and their biomedical prospect in pathogenic diseases and cancer. *J. Mol. Struct.* **2019**, *1185*, 1–7. [CrossRef]
163. Rath, K.; Sen, S. Garlic extract based preparation of size controlled superparamagnetic hematite nanoparticles and their cytotoxic applications. *Indian J. Biotechnol.* **2019**, *18*, 108–118.
164. Sharma, D.; Ledwani, L.; Mehrotra, T.; Kumar, N.; Pervaiz, N.; Kumar, R. Biosynthesis of hematite nanoparticles using *Rheum emodi* and their antimicrobial and anticancerous effects in vitro. *J. Photochem. Photobiol. B Biol.* **2020**, *206*, 111841. [CrossRef]
165. Miri, A.; Khatami, M.; Sarani, M. Biosynthesis, magnetic and cytotoxic studies of hematite nanoparticles. *J. Inorg. Organomet. Polym. Mater.* **2020**, *30*, 767–774. [CrossRef]
166. Abbasi, B.A.; Iqbal, J.; Khan, Z.; Ahmad, R.; Uddin, S.; Shahbaz, A.; Zahra, S.A.; Shaukat, M.; Kiran, F.; Kanwal, S. Phytofabrication of cobalt oxide nanoparticles from *Rhamnus virgata* leaves extract and investigation of different bioactivities. *Microsc. Res. Tech.* **2021**, *84*, 192–201. [CrossRef]
167. Hosny, M.; Eltaweil, A.S.; Mostafa, M.; El-Badry, Y.A.; Hussein, E.E.; Omer, A.M.; Fawzy, M. Facile synthesis of gold nanoparticles for anticancer, antioxidant applications, and photocatalytic degradation of toxic organic pollutants. *ACS Omega* **2022**, *7*, 3121–3133. [CrossRef]
168. Vundela, S.R.; Kalagatur, N.K.; Nagaraj, A.; Kadirvelu, K.; Chandranayaka, S.; Kondapalli, K.; Hashem, A.; Abd Allah, E.F.; Poda, S. Multi-biofunctional properties of phytofabricated selenium nanoparticles from Carica papaya fruit extract: Antioxidant, antimicrobial, antimycotoxin, anticancer, and biocompatibility. *Front. Microbiol.* **2021**, *12*, 769891. [CrossRef] [PubMed]
169. Fouda, A.; Al-Otaibi, W.A.; Saber, T.; AlMotwaa, S.M.; Alshallash, K.S.; Elhady, M.; Badr, N.F.; Abdel-Rahman, M.A. Antimicrobial, antiviral, and in-vitro cytotoxicity and mosquitocidal activities of *Portulaca oleracea*-based green synthesis of selenium nanoparticles. *J. Funct. Biomater.* **2022**, *13*, 157. [CrossRef] [PubMed]

Disclaimer/Publisher's Note: The statements, opinions and data contained in all publications are solely those of the individual author(s) and contributor(s) and not of MDPI and/or the editor(s). MDPI and/or the editor(s) disclaim responsibility for any injury to people or property resulting from any ideas, methods, instructions or products referred to in the content.

Article

Protective Factors against Fear of Cancer Recurrence in Breast Cancer Patients: A Latent Growth Model

Gabriella Bentley [1,*], Osnat Zamir [1], Rawan Dahabre [1], Shlomit Perry [1], Evangelos C. Karademas [2], Paula Poikonen-Saksela [3], Ketti Mazzocco [4,5], Berta Sousa [6] and Ruth Pat-Horenczyk [1,*] on behalf of the BOUNCE Consortium

1. School of Social Work and Social Welfare, Hebrew University of Jerusalem, Jerusalem 9190500, Israel
2. Department of Psychology, University of Crete and Foundation for Research and Technology, 70013 Heraklion, Greece
3. Helsinki University Hospital Comprehensive Cancer Center, University of Helsinki, 00100 Helsinki, Finland
4. Department of Oncology and Hemato-Oncology, University of Milan, 20139 Milan, Italy
5. Applied Research Division for Cognitive and Psychological Science, European Institute of Oncology IRCCS, 20139 Milan, Italy
6. Breast Unit, Champalimaud Clinical Centre, Champalimaud Foundation, 1400-038 Lisboa, Portugal
* Correspondence: gabriell.bentley@mail.huji.ac.il (G.B.); ruth.pat-horenczyk@mail.huji.ac.il (R.P.-H.)

Simple Summary: The present study's objective was to examine the protective factors of fear of cancer recurrence (FCR) as well as its trajectory. The study encompassed a sample of 494 women participating in an international longitudinal research project named "Predicting Effective Adaptation to Breast Cancer to Help Women to BOUNCE Back" (BOUNCE). The participants had recently been diagnosed with breast cancer (BC), ranging from tumor stage I to III, and were undergoing BC treatments. The study underscores the stability observed in the FCR levels and highlights the influence of coping self-efficacy on the initial FCR levels. However, greater positive cognitive–emotion regulation did not appear to contribute to the level or reduction of FCR. These findings bear significant implications, emphasizing the necessity of targeted coping strategies for BC patients during a critical timeframe, to mitigate the impact of FCR, a factor that is liable to undermine the quality of life and mental well-being of BC survivors.

Abstract: The current study aimed to examine the fear of cancer recurrence (FCR) trajectory and protective predictors in women coping with breast cancer (BC). The study's model investigated whether a higher coping self-efficacy and positive cognitive–emotion regulation at the time of the BC diagnosis would lead to reduced levels of FCR at six months and in later stages (12 and 18 months) post-diagnosis. The sample included 494 women with stages I to III BC from Finland, Italy, Portugal, and Israel. They completed self-report questionnaires, including the Fear of Cancer Recurrence Inventory (FCRI-SF), the Cancer Behavior Inventory-Brief Version (CBI-B), the Cognitive–Emotion Regulation Questionnaire (CERQ short), and medical–social-demographic data. Findings revealed that a higher coping self-efficacy at diagnosis predicted lower FCR levels after six months but did not impact the FCR trajectory over time. Surprisingly, positive cognitive–emotion regulation did not predict FCR levels or changes over 18 months. FCR levels remained stable from six to 18 months post-diagnosis. This study emphasizes the importance of developing specific cancer coping skills, such as coping self-efficacy. Enhancing coping self-efficacy in the first six months after BC diagnosis may lead to lower FCR levels later, as FCR tends to persist in the following year.

Keywords: BOUNCE; breast cancer; coping self-efficacy; fear of cancer recurrence; latent growth modeling; trajectories

1. Introduction

Breast cancer (BC) is the most prevalent type of cancer diagnosed among women [1] and involves a range of physical and psychological long-term issues, one of which is fear of cancer recurrence (FCR). FCR refers to the "worry or concern relating to the possibility that cancer will come back or progress" [2] (p. 3265). Such fears have been recognized as the most common concern of cancer patients [3–5] and as a central unmet need of women coping with BC [6]. Breast cancer patients often undergo significant changes in their identity and physical appearance, such as scars, fluctuations in weight, and other treatment-related side effects, which may be perceived as sources of danger and fear that may develop into FCR [7,8]. FCR manifests through cancer-related thoughts and feelings, such as about death, loneliness, and uncertainty [9], and it is likely to impair the quality of life and mental health [10,11].

FCR is present through the time of active disease, after completion of treatment [12], and along the survivorship trajectory [12–14]. Even years after the initial diagnosis, most survivors will still feel stressed about cancer progression or recurrence [13]. As such, for many cancer patients, surviving cancer means living with ongoing apprehension of the cancer recurring [12]. Several studies have indicated that FCR levels typically exhibit a relatively stable pattern throughout the survivorship cycle. For example, the initial FCR levels in BC patients obtained on the first day of radiation treatment were found as a strong predictor for the levels of FCR 2 months later [15] and throughout 18 months after completing treatment [16]. In addition, while some studies indicated that clinical levels of FCR at baseline tend to remain stable even 18 months after surgery [17,18], other studies have shown that FCR levels may be higher before surgery, but they tend to mildly decline, and then plateau [19,20]. Significant changes in FCR occurred during the month of pre-mammogram to the month post-mammogram assessment in another study [21]. Thus, the inconsistent evidence regarding the FCR trajectory among BC patients demands further examination of this issue.

While extensive research shows that FCR is a constant difficulty in the lives of cancer survivors, not much is known about protective factors against FCR. Previous studies have presented factors correlated with FCR, such as psychological distress, intrusive thoughts [11], female gender, and younger age [22]. A recent meta-analysis of a large heterogeneous cancer sample (N = 13,000) aimed to detect factors correlated with FCR, such as anxiety, depression, chemotherapy, and fatigue, which were positively associated with FCR, whereas optimism, social support, and quality of life were negatively associated with FCR [23]. Nevertheless, most of these studies showed correlations with FCR, but it is difficult to infer from them a protective and moderating role against FCR. For example, the study by McGinty et al. [21] found that reporting lower perceived risk and reassuring behaviors in BC patients had a protective role in FCR. Considering the increasing and relatively high survival rate of BC [24,25], it is imperative to identify initial protective factors in BC patients, especially at the crucial time of diagnosis, that can protect against FCR and its progression during cancer treatment and survival.

The Common-Sense Model (CSM) [26,27] postulated that coping with illness depends on two central representations of the illness, cognitive and emotional. The cognitive representation refers to the perceived health threat [27,28], including the evaluation of the duration and chronicity of the disease, the consequences of cancer, the perceived control, and the potential for a cure. These perceptions depend on the individual's history, knowledge, and beliefs about the illness. The perceived health threat may further induce emotional representations [26,27]. For instance, it may provoke worry and anxiety about cancer, or remorse over not receiving more aggressive treatments [29]. Relying on the CSM, the FCR Cognitive Formulation model [29] posits that the level of FCR varies depending on the cognitive and emotional representations of cancer, including the level of the perceived threat of cancer, which may provoke negative emotional representation (e.g., depression, horror, anger). The cognitive and emotional representations of cancer ultimately inform FCR levels.

In addition, the Conservation of Resources theory (COR) [30] posits a mechanism by which promotive and protective factors operate to strengthen coping with stressful experiences. When coping with a stressful condition, such as cancer, individuals tend to protect and acquire new resources to handle it [31]. Resources can include objects, states, and conditions that people value (e.g., personal-psychological competence, family relations) [30]. Individuals invest resources for the sake of defending against resource loss, recovering from losses, and gaining resources [32]. The number of resources determines a spiraling process of resource gain or loss, which determines the perceived capacity to handle the situation [33]. Hence, according to the COR theory, women diagnosed with BC who have greater resources may be able to preserve and acquire new resources to cope with BC, which may influence their perceived stress [34] and their FCR levels [29]. Further, having more resources may lead to resource gain and better adaptation over time [34]. Therefore, in this study, we focused on two resources against FCR growth, following a BC diagnosis. One resource pertains to a specific coping ability with cancer, namely coping self-efficacy, while the other refers to a general coping ability, i.e., positive cognitive–emotion regulation.

Protective Factors against FCR

One of the personal characteristics that can contribute to lower FCR levels is self-efficacy. Self-efficacy refers to an individual's perception of their ability to successfully perform actions that can lead to overcoming challenges and achieving goals [35]. Perceived self-efficacy is formed through evaluating one's behaviors and coping skills in dealing with a certain situation [36,37]. Individuals with high self-efficacy tend to perceive themselves as more capable of dealing with threats [37] such as illness and, therefore, will perceive greater control and adaptive health behaviors [38].

Furthermore, specifically, self-efficacy in coping with cancer (or coping self-efficacy) refers to the confidence one has in managing symptoms and emotions related to BC and it includes behaviors directed to benefit the process of recovery [39], such as seeking help, informing and reporting about symptoms, and adhering to follow-ups upon completion of the treatments [40]. Studies have demonstrated that BC patients with higher levels of coping self-efficacy achieve more favorable psychosocial and medical outcomes, such as experiencing fewer side effects, compared to those with lower coping self-efficacy [41]. Consequently, it is possible that BC patients with greater coping self-efficacy perceive their condition as more controllable [26], resulting in lower levels of FCR.

Consistent evidence indicates a link between higher levels of coping self-efficacy and lower levels of FCR, including in BC patients [21,42]. This finding has been observed in various studies conducted at different stages of the treatment and survivorship journey. For instance, a prospective longitudinal study demonstrated an association between greater coping self-efficacy and reduced FCR levels following cancer treatment completion [21] and among young BC survivors [43]. Greater coping self-efficacy also predicted lower FCR six to 24 months after the completion of the primary treatment [42,44]. In addition, coping self-efficacy mediated the effects of risk factors (e.g., anxiety and younger age) on FCR among survivors who were three to eight years post-diagnosis [40]. Lastly, clinically, in a four-week online intervention study, focusing on BC survivors with moderate to high FCR levels, greater coping self-efficacy predicted a significant decrease in FCR from baseline to post-intervention [45].

Moreover, cognitive–emotion regulation has been recognized as a significant predictor of better mental health in oncological patients [46], and thus may also protect against the development of FCR. Cognitive–emotion regulation is a cognitive process by which individuals manage emotionally arousing information, through monitoring, evaluating, and modifying responses to an event [47]. Individuals vary in their capacity to regulate emotions [48] by using thoughts to manage their emotions [49]. Cognitive–emotion regulation includes maladaptive and adaptive strategies. Adaptive cognitive emotion–regulation strategies include positive refocusing, positive reappraisal, putting the issues into perspective, acceptance, and planning [48,49]. These cognitive–emotion regulation strategies result in better well-being and psychological functioning [47]. The CSM [26,27] posits that personal characteristics, such as cognitive–emotion regulation, may affect the way women cope with BC. More specifically, it may impact the way women perceive and evaluate the severity of their illness, which informs their cognitive and emotional representations of cancer [26]. Finally, these representations can eventually mitigate FCR levels [26,29].

Indeed, former studies have demonstrated the correlation between positive cognitive–emotion regulation strategies and a lower FCR. Two clinical studies, including a 12-week emotion regulation group intervention [50] and emotion-focused therapy [51], showed a decrease in FCR levels after treatment. Similarly, a qualitative focus group study found that using acceptance and positive reappraisal were effective in coping with FCR [52]. Additionally, a prospective study that examined FCR levels, before and after radiation therapy, indicated that emotion regulation strategies, including reappraisal, are linked with lower levels of FCR [53].

The extant research suggests that coping self-efficacy [40] and positive cognitive–emotion regulation can play a protective role against FCR among BC survivors [53]. However, evidence regarding this association from the crucial times of diagnosis, treatment, and early recovery is lacking. Moreover, the predictive-moderating role of coping self-efficacy and positive cognitive–emotion regulation, as well as the exploration of individual differences in FCR over time, have not yet been studied. These gaps are addressed in this study.

Relying on the CSM [26,27] and the COR theory [30], the present study aimed to examine a longitudinal model, among an international sample of women coping with BC, by which two main protective factors would predict FCR and the development of the FCR trajectory. Specifically, we tested whether higher levels of coping self-efficacy and positive cognitive–emotion regulation, assessed at the time of BC diagnosis, would show a steeper decline in FCR levels at six months after diagnosis, and in the development of the FCR trajectory 12 and 18 months after diagnosis (see Figure 1). This period constitutes the approximate timeframe for managing both acute survivorship and the transitional stage of survivorship—meaning, the experience of diagnosis and receiving medical treatment—followed by the end of active treatment and the efforts to readjust to life [54,55]. Identifying individual differences in growth trends of FCR may foster the development of interventions designed to prevent FCR.

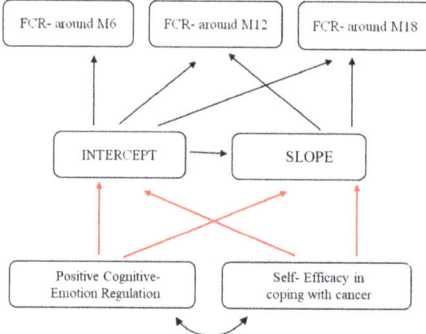

Figure 1. A conceptual model. A latent growth modeling analysis of positive cognitive–emotion regulation and self-efficacy in coping with cancer, predicting the fear of cancer recurrence trajectories. Note. Red darts = represent predicted negative correlations; black darts = represent predicted positive correlations.

Based on the lack of consensus in the literature regarding the change patterns of FCR over time, the first research question aimed to explore whether FCR levels (six months post-diagnosis) predict the trajectory of FCR levels later at 12 and 18 months post-diagnosis. Next, the following hypotheses addressed the two protective factors, such that greater coping self-efficacy measured at the time of diagnosis of BC will predict: (H1.a) a lower level of FCR at six months, and (H1.b) a steeper decline in FCR levels at 12 and 18 months since the diagnosis. Similarly, greater positive cognitive–emotion regulation measured at the time of diagnosis of BC will predict: (H2.a) a lower level of FCR at six months, and (H2.b) a steeper decline in FCR levels at 12 and 18 months since the diagnosis.

2. Materials and Methods

2.1. Procedure

Data for the current study were obtained through an international longitudinal research project named "Predicting Effective Adaptation to Breast Cancer to Help Women to BOUNCE Back" (BOUNCE). The BOUNCE study was conducted as part of a consortium project that promoted collaboration among countries and European oncology centers. Researchers, doctors, and therapists worked together in a multidisciplinary study, involving a multicultural sample from four oncology centers, each with extensive experience in the holistic treatment of many BC patients. These centers were in Italy, Finland, Israel, and Portugal. Participants enrolled for the study had to be: women between 40 and 70 years of age, with a recent diagnosis of histologically confirmed invasive early or locally advanced operable BC, tumor defined as stage I to III, receiving any type of systemic and local treatment according to local guidelines for BC, and capable of understanding the study protocol and providing informed consent. Women diagnosed with distant metastases, a history of another malignancy within the last five years (except cured basal cell skin carcinoma or in situ carcinoma of the uterine cervix), a history of severe mental, neurologic, or another chronic disease, and pregnant or breast-feeding at the time of recruitment, did not much the study's criteria. Ethical certifications were approved for the study by the ethical committee of the European Institute of Oncology (IEO; Approval No. R868/IEO916) and through ethical committees at each medical center.

Baseline assessments were conducted following the cancer diagnosis and before receiving medical treatment. The participating women were recruited for the study during their first hospital appointments or through a phone call initiated by a research assistant. A brief description of the study and its goals was presented. Following the signing of an informed consent form, they filled out a battery of self-report questionnaires in their local native language. After the initial assessment, the subsequent phases (six-month, 12-month, and 18-month follow-ups) were carried out by the research assistants from each medical center. At each time point, the participants were given the questionnaires in the form of printed or online surveys using the Noona survey software or the Qualtrics platform. The translation process of the questionnaires was obtained from the original tool developer or conducted by translation experts through a back-translation process. The medical data needed were assembled through the hospitals' medical record files.

2.2. Participants

The baseline assessment included 690 women, from whom 574 completed the six-month follow-up, 525 completed the 12-month follow-up, and 494 completed the 18-month follow-up, yielding an 83.18%, 74.4%, and 70% retention rate, respectively. Relevant tests were conducted to examine distinctions between participants who dropped out and participants who completed the study. Women retained at the six-month follow-up differed from the women who dropped out in the factors of country of origin ($\chi^2(3, N = 706) = 95.25, p = 0.000$), income level ($\chi^2(1, N = 663) = 6.80, p = 0.009$), and education level ($\chi^2(1, N = 702) = 7.52, p = 0.006$). Significant differences also emerged at the 12-month follow-up, in the country of origin ($\chi^2(3, N = 706) = 98.41, p = 0.000$), marital status ($\chi^2(1, N = 696) = 5.13, p < 0.05$), income level ($\chi^2(1, N = 663) = 5.36, p < 0.05$), and education level ($\chi^2(1, N = 702) = 13.64, p = 0.000$). Finally, women who completed the 18-month follow up differed from the women who dropped out based on their country of origin ($\chi^2(3, N = 706) = 122.96, p = 0.000$), income level ($\chi^2(1, N = 663) = 11.62, p = 0.001$), and education level ($\chi^2(1, N = 702) = 34.03, p = 0.000$). At all three time points, the women dropping out were more often Italian participants, and with lower income and educational levels. There were no significant differences in age, number of children, and disease stage between participants who dropped out and those who remained. Most relevant, there were no statistical differences in the levels of FCR at six months between participants that completed the study and those who dropped out.

Finally, the study sample comprised 494 women diagnosed with BC, ranging from tumor stage I to III and receiving BC treatments. Most of the women were diagnosed with stage I (47.9%) and II (41%), and a minority with stage III (11.1%). Participants ranged in age from 40 to 70 years, with an average age of 54.93 years (SD = 8.21). The largest group of participants were from Finland (31.9%), then from Italy (27.5%), Portugal (20.8%), and the least from Israel (19.8%). Majority of the women were married or were involved in an intimate relationship (73.7%), with a mean of 1.95 (SD = 1.46) children. At least 76% reported an average or higher-than-average family income level and majority of participants had earned at least a bachelor's degree (68.1%).

2.3. Measures

Socio-demographic data. A socio-demographic questionnaire assessed age, number of children, marital status (i.e., 0 = "married, common law partner, engaged"; 1 = "separated, divorced, single, widowed"), income level (i.e., 0 = "very low"; 1 = "average/high"), and education (i.e., 0 = "primary, secondary, high school"; 1 = "bachelor, postgraduate education, vocational non-academic diploma").

Fear of cancer recurrence. FCR was assessed using the Fear of Cancer Recurrence Inventory-Short Form (FCRI-SF) [56], a nine-item, self-report measure derived from the full 42-item form, assessing the presence and severity of intrusive thoughts associated with FCR (e.g., "How much time per day do you spend thinking about the possibility of cancer recurrence?"). The items are rated on a five-point Likert scale ranging from 0 ("not at all") to 4 ("a great deal"). A higher total mean score indicates higher levels of FCR [56]. In the current sample, the reliability coefficients of the scale at all three time points were high, with Cronbach's $\alpha = 0.86$, $\alpha = 0.85$, and $\alpha = 0.87$, at 6, 12, and 18 months, respectively.

Self-efficacy in coping with cancer. Self-efficacy in coping with cancer was measured with the Cancer Behavior Inventory-Brief Version (CBI-B) [57], which is a 12-item scale assessing self-efficacy for coping with cancer, including 4 aspects: maintaining independence and a positive attitude, participating in medical care, coping and stress management, and managing effect (e.g., "actively participating in treatment decisions"). The short version was derived from the full 33-item questionnaire (CBI-L) [58]. The items are rated on a 9-point Likert scale, ranging from 1 ("not at all confident") to 9 ("totally confident"). A higher total mean score indicates greater self-efficacy beliefs for engaging with the resources needed to cope with cancer. Internal consistency for the scale was high ($\alpha = 0.89$).

Positive cognitive–emotion regulation. The positive cognitive–emotion regulation scale was measured using the Cognitive–Emotion Regulation Questionnaire (CERQ short) [59], an 18-item, self-report measure for positive and negative cognitive–emotion self-regulation strategies. The short version was derived from the full 36-item questionnaire, comprising nine domains of emotion regulation strategies to cope with a stressful situation. The current study focused on 10 items, assessing the positive cognitive–emotion regulation strategies (e.g., "I think that I have to accept that this has happened"). The positive scale assesses putting the issues into perspective, positive refocusing, positive reappraisal, acceptance, and planning. Each domain is represented by two items in the short form. The items are rated on a five-point Likert scale, ranging from 1 ("almost never") to 5 ("almost always"). A higher mean score indicates higher positive cognitive–emotion regulation [59]. In our data, the reliability coefficient of the CERQ positive subscale was high (Cronbach's $\alpha = 0.81$).

2.4. Data Analysis

Preliminary analysis was conducted using SPSS version 25. The study hypotheses were tested using Structural Equation Modeling with AMOS, version 25 [60]. We utilized a latent growth model (LGMs) [61,62] to assess the growth trajectory of FCR levels and their predictors. This analysis estimated the change in repeated measures of FCR levels at six, 12, and 18 months after BC diagnosis. It also tested for the associations between the intercept (i.e., the initial level of FCR) and the slope (i.e., indicates the average rate of change of mean FCR) of the FCR levels. The hypotheses regarding the predictors of FCR growth were tested using a conditional model that included coping self-efficacy and positive cognitive–emotion regulation as predictors of the intercept and the slope of FCR. Model fit was evaluated by standard criteria, including a non-significant ($p > 0.05$) chi-squared statistic, a comparative fit index (CFI) and normed fit index (NFI) of more than 0.95, and a root mean square error of approximation (RMSEA) of less than 0.08 [63].

Since the preliminary analysis showed that some demographic variables were associated with missing data in FCR, including education, income, marital status, and country of origin, they were included as covariates in the model. We also included age as a covariate because it was found as a predictor of FCR in other studies [12,64,65]. We controlled for the nominal variable, country of origin, by converting it to three dummy variables and the quantitative variable age. Finally, we used the full information maximum likelihood (FIML) to handle missing data. FIML uses all available information from the observed data in the SEM analyses and is preferable to mean imputation and listwise or pairwise deletion [66].

3. Results

3.1. Preliminary Analysis

The Skewness and Kurtosis values indicated that the variables in the study did not present a significant bias to normal distribution (Skewness varied between -0.83 and 0.14, and Kurtosis between -0.42 and 0.21). The descriptive statistics and zero-order correlations of the study variables are displayed in Table 1.

Table 1. Means, standard deviations, and zero-order correlations of the study variables.

	1	2	3	4	5	M	SD
1. PCER	-					2.53	0.47
2. CSE	0.11 **	-				7.14	1.18
3. FCR-M6	0.03	−0.32 **	-			1.68	0.69
4. FCR-M12	−0.02	−0.34 **	0.69 **	-		1.65	0.70
5. FCR-M18	0.01	−0.34 **	0.69 **	0.73 **	-	1.64	0.74

Note. ** $p < 0.01$. PCER, positive cognitive–emotion regulation; CSE, coping self-efficacy; FCR, fear of cancer recurrence (M6/M12/M18: six, 12, and 18 months post-diagnosis).

The two protective factors against FCR—coping self-efficacy and positive cognitive–emotion regulation—were positively associated. Coping self-efficacy was negatively associated with FCR at all three time points. Positive cognitive–emotion regulation was not linked to FCR levels at any time point. The FCR levels at the three time points were positively associated with each other.

3.2. FCR Change from Six to Eighteen Months after BC Diagnosis

First, an unconditional LGM was run to assess the change along the trajectory of FCR levels between six, 12, and 18 months after BC diagnosis. The model adequately fit to the data ($\chi^2(df = 1) = 0.140$, $p = 0.71$; NFI = 1.00, CFI = 1.00, RMSEA = 0.000). Although baseline levels of FCR presented significant individual differences between participants (b = 0.33; SE = 0.03; Z = 9.94; $p < 0.001$) around a mean level of FCR (b = 1.68; SE = 0.03; Z = 60.27; $p < 0.001$), there were no significant changes over time, as indicated by the non-significant estimate of the slope's mean (b = −0.40; SE = 0.03; Z = −1.57; $p = 0.117$). In other words, the growth rate of FCR was homogeneous among participants considering the non-significant variance around the mean growth (b = 0.03; SE = 0.06; Z = 0.350; $p = 0.727$). The correlation between the intercept and the slope was not found to be significant (r = 0.035, $p = 0.300$).

Further, a conditional model was used to examine the effect of coping self-efficacy and positive cognitive–emotion regulation on the change in FCR levels (see Figure 2). First, this model was examined with all covariates, including marital status, income level, education, age, and country of origin. However, only age and country of origin emerged as significant predictors of intercept FCR levels; therefore, all other covariates were excluded from the final model.

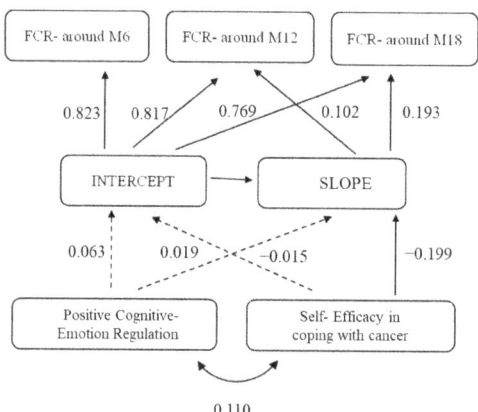

Figure 2. Latent growth modeling: coping self-efficacy predicts initial FCR levels. Note. Full dart = significant correlation; broken dart = non-significant correlation.

The model fit the data very well (χ^2(df = 9) = 16.42, p = 0.06; NFI = 0.99, CFI = 99.05, RMSEA = 0.03). Results showed that coping self-efficacy (at baseline) significantly predicted FCR at six months (β = −0.199; p < 0.001), indicating that women reporting greater coping self-efficacy at baseline reported lower levels of FCR after six months. No significant variance was found; thus, coping self-efficacy did not predict the growth rate of FCR later (β = −0.015; p = 0.508). In addition, positive cognitive–emotion regulation did not predict either the baseline levels (β = 0.063; p = 0.278) or the growth (β = 0.019; p = 0.735) of FCR over 18 months.

Finally, younger age was found as a significant covariate to a greater initial FCR level (β = −0.015; p < 0.001) but not the growth of FCR (β = 0.002; p = 0.526). Additionally, living in Israel (β = 0.338; SE = 0.084; p < 0.001) and Finland (β = 0.276; SE = 0.075; p < 0.001) were linked to higher FCR levels at baseline; further, living in Israel also predicted a sharper decline in FCR (β = −0.210; SE = 0.082; p < 0.05).

4. Discussion

The current study aimed to explore the trajectory of FCR levels between six and 18 months post-diagnosis. Additionally, the objective of this study was to examine two protective factors, namely coping self-efficacy and positive cognitive–emotion regulation, against FCR levels and their trajectories over six, 12, and 18 months following the initial diagnosis of BC. The findings partially supported our hypotheses and have implications for early interventions to improve and mitigate FCR among women with BC.

We identified relatively stable levels of FCR over one year, from six to 18 months after BC diagnosis. Our findings resemble previous studies, showing that FCR levels tend to remain steady over time [15–18] and have been found to be determined by the baseline levels [18,67]. Still, it should be noted that the FCR trajectory was measured in previous studies using diverse timeframes and intervals compared to the present study (e.g., two months after completing treatment, 18 months after surgery). Thus, it could be that the immutability of FCR in the current results is related to the timeframe of our study, during which women were dealing with intense treatments. The relative stability in FCR might change once survivors move on to a long-term follow-up phase, which includes less frequent visits and communication with the oncological team, as well as decreased family support to address arising fears, in comparison to the active treatment period [18]. The importance of recognizing the changes versus the stability of FCR along the survivorship trajectory is emphasized while concluding that the first six months post-diagnosis represent a window of opportunity to effectively impact the initial levels of FCR, that may not significantly change thereafter.

The current results suggest that the initial levels of FCR may develop through coping self-efficacy; however, it may not further promote a later decrease in FCR. Specifically, a higher coping self-efficacy at the time of diagnosis predicted lower FCR levels after six months. These findings align with previous studies that have linked a higher self-efficacy to a lower FCR [21,40,42–44]. Nonetheless, the current study expands the scope of existing literature by examining the effect of coping self-efficacy on FCR among an international sample of women, starting from BC diagnosis and continuing over time.

This study contributes to the theoretical literature by the notion that belief in one's capacity to manage cancer is crucial for successful coping with FCR [29]. These findings support the Common-Sense Model [27], which posits that the response to BC diagnosis and treatment is a subjective process involving mutual influences between exposure to a health threat and cognitive and emotional representations and responses [27,28]. The results of this study stress the significance of the beliefs of patients in their ability to influence their thoughts, emotions, and behaviors [37], specifically regarding coping with BC and its requirements, such that coping self-efficacy promotes a perception of competence to manage the illness [37], provides a higher sense of control [68,69], and ameliorates cancer-related stress [68,70]. Therefore, a higher coping self-efficacy can lead to a lower FCR [18,71–73].

Nonetheless, in the current study, greater coping self-efficacy measured at the time of diagnosis of BC did not predict a decline in FCR levels at 12 and 18 months since diagnosis. Even though a woman with coping self-efficacy may invest this resource initially, it has been found that over time, she may need additional and diverse resources [32] to cope with FCR and the demands that arise at each stage of receiving and completing treatment [54,55]. This suggests that as women may lose resources (e.g., coping with FCR), they will strive to protect their remaining resources (e.g., their initial ability of coping self-efficacy), such that managing FCR over time is a dynamic and ongoing demand. In addition to the bio-psychological aspects assessed in the current study, social perspectives such as the crucial role of social support [74] should be considered in the model examining protective factors that could alleviate FCR. The complexity of FCR is further evident in studies among BC survivors, who reported FCR as an intense, difficult, multi-dimensional experience [75], including dealing with feelings of being trapped in insecurity, experiencing suffering alone [76], a lack of control, and fear of death [77]. Thus, it seems that coping with FCR over time requires a wide range of resources. Hence, it is important to further explore protective resources and their ability to address FCR throughout the survivor's journey.

In contrast to our prediction, we found that greater positive cognitive–emotion regulation did not contribute to the level or reduction of FCR. This unexpected outcome may be explained by the need for specific and unique coping strategies when dealing with a BC diagnosis and FCR. For example, acquiring knowledge about BC [5], utilizing tools to manage uncertainty [78], and practicing mindfulness [79] are important, in addition to general positive cognitive–emotion regulation strategies. Specifically, although enhancing positive cognitive–emotion regulation strategies has been found effective for managing FCR among cancer patients in clinical studies [50,51], this connection is not evident when considering it as an inherent personal tendency. Furthermore, the negative impact of BC on psychological well-being might diminish over time, allowing for greater positive psychological changes to occur in the years following diagnosis [80]. Therefore, while positive cognitive–emotion regulation may not alleviate FCR at the time of receiving a BC diagnosis and undergoing active treatments, its role in later stages of survival warrants long-term assessments.

Finally, we found that younger age and country of origin predict FCR levels. Prior research indicated that younger women expressed higher FCR levels [65], but no change in

FCR over time. Understandably, worries regarding health, womanhood, parenting, and death worsen FCR [40], especially at a younger age [65].

This international sample has shown some cross-cultural differences. Patients from Israel and Finland reported greater initial FCR levels compared to patients from Portugal. The finding of higher FCR levels in Finland and Israel may be attributed to a combination of the level of diagnosis services, the quality of the medical system, options for effective treatments, and mortality rates [81,82]. However, as the study progressed, patients from Israel exhibited a decline in FCR over time, which can be associated with the high survival rate of BC patients in Israel compared to the OECD [83]. This decline may also be related to the effective universal public free health services that address the needs of cancer patients and their families, providing social security benefits and supportive psychosocial interventions [84]. Perhaps becoming more familiar with the system and receiving comprehensive support may ease patients' FCR.

4.1. Limitations and Future Directions

Several limitations of the current study need to be considered. First, the use of self-report measures can attract potential biases and statistical artifacts (i.e., memory and recall issues, social desirability bias), suggesting caution while interpreting the study's findings. Hence, future studies should consider varied type of tools for data collection, such as objective measures and behavioral observation measures. Second, the model was examined in a limited timeframe of 18 months since diagnosis, raising the need for further examination of the FCR trajectory, which may persist many years later [85,86]. Third, the study sample represents women with early-stage BC, middle age, and living in European countries; therefore, it might not be able to fully represent the BC and cancer patients' population. Despite the advantage of an international sample, intercultural differences were found that were not the focus of the article but indicate an important need to examine the differences in cultural influence and its effect on FCR. Further research should replicate the model, in various populations previously linked with FCR, such as different stages of cancer and cancer types, ages, and cultures, where the concepts of coping and a fear of cancer recurrence can differ.

4.2. Clinical Implications

Considering the evidence that FCR tends to be stable over the first 18 months post-diagnosis of BC, it is imperative to find effective ways to combat and mitigate this fear as early as possible. Especially during the first six months after diagnosis, it may be crucial to intervene to try to influence the FCR levels. Moreover, our study highlights the centrality of specific cancer coping skills, namely coping self-efficacy, rather than general skills, which can play a protective role against FCR during this time. The results suggest that strengthening coping self-efficacy during the time of diagnosis and the first six months following it may be an effective tool in fostering healthy disease perceptions [37] and a lower FCR [29]. Several interventions have been shown to be effective in improving self-efficacy among general cancer patients [87] and BC patients [41]; however, it is important to adapt them for women managing BC at the time of diagnosis, with a specific focus on FCR management.

In addition, there is a need to search for more relevant and amendable protective factors that can be implemented in prevention and intervention programs to reduce FCR and enhance the well-being of BC patients. Such programs may contribute to better adjustment among BC patients to the disease and its treatments, ultimately leading to reduced FCR [40,43,44].

5. Conclusions

The current study examined predictors of FCR and its trajectory. In line with the CSM and COR theory, the study emphasized the stability found in FCR levels over time and the impact of coping self-efficacy on the initial levels of FCR. However, enhanced positive cognitive–emotion regulation did not contribute to the level or reduction of FCR. These findings hold significance as they suggest the importance of specific coping skills for cancer patients, within a critical timeframe to impact the level of FCR, which is likely to impair the quality of life and mental health of BC survivors.

Author Contributions: Conceptualization, G.B., O.Z., S.P. and R.P.-H.; data curation, G.B., R.D., E.C.K., P.P.-S., K.M., B.S. and R.P.-H.; formal analysis, G.B. and O.Z.; investigation, R.D., P.P.-S., K.M., B.S. and R.P.-H.; methodology, G.B., O.Z., S.P. and R.P.-H.; resources, G.B. and P.P.-S.; software, G.B., O.Z. and P.P.-S.; supervision, O.Z. and R.P.-H.; validation, G.B., O.Z., P.P.-S. and R.P.-H.; visualization, R.P.-H.; writing—original draft, G.B., O.Z. and R.P.-H.; writing—review and editing, R.D., S.P., E.C.K., P.P.-S., K.M. and B.S. All authors have read and agreed to the published version of the manuscript.

Funding: This work was supported by the European Union's Horizon 2020 Research and Innovation Programme under Grant Agreement No. 777167. Gabriella Bentley is supported by the Canadian Friends of the Hebrew University (CFHU) Fellowship Fund.

Institutional Review Board Statement: Ethical certifications were held for the entire study through the ethical committee of the European Institute of Oncology (IEO; Approval No. R868/IEO916) and by the ethical committees required at each medical center.

Informed Consent Statement: Informed consent was obtained from all subjects involved in the study. All clinical centers obtained informed consent according to the local ethical committee in line with the European Institute of Oncology, Approval No. R868/IEO916.

Data Availability Statement: The anonymized data that support the findings of this study are available upon request from the corresponding author. The data are not publicly available due to privacy and ethical restrictions.

Conflicts of Interest: The authors declare no conflict of interest.

References

1. WHO. Breast Cancer. Available online: https://www.who.int/news-room/fact-sheets/detail/breast-cancer (accessed on 16 July 2023).
2. Lebel, S.; Ozakinci, G.; Humphris, G.; Mutsaers, B.; Thewes, B.; Prins, J.; Dinkel, A.; Butow, P. From Normal Response to Clinical Problem: Definition and Clinical Features of Fear of Cancer Recurrence. *Support. Care Cancer* **2016**, *24*, 3265–3268. [CrossRef] [PubMed]
3. Hodgkinson, K.; Butow, P.; Fuchs, A.; Hunt, G.E.; Stenlake, A.; Hobbs, K.M.; Brand, A.; Wain, G. Long-Term Survival from Gynecologic Cancer: Psychosocial Outcomes, Supportive Care Needs and Positive Outcomes. *Gynecol. Oncol.* **2007**, *104*, 381–389. [CrossRef] [PubMed]
4. Oxlad, M.; Wade, T.D.; Hallsworth, L.; Koczwara, B. 'I'm Living with a Chronic Illness, Not... Dying with Cancer': A Qualitative Study of Australian Women's Self-Identified Concerns and Needs Following Primary Treatment for Breast Cancer. *Eur. J. Cancer Care* **2008**, *17*, 157–166. [CrossRef]
5. Simonelli, L.E.; Siegel, S.D.; Duffy, N.M. Fear of Cancer Recurrence: A Theoretical Review and Its Relevance for Clinical Presentation and Management. *Psychooncology* **2017**, *26*, 1444–1454. [CrossRef]
6. Armes, J.; Oakley, C.; Ream, E. Patients' Supportive Care Needs Beyond the End of Cancer Treatment: A Prospective, Longitudinal Survey Symptomatic Care-Chemotherapy View Project. *Artic. J. Clin. Oncol.* **2009**, *27*, 6172–6179. [CrossRef]
7. Lewis-Smith, H.; Diedrichs, P.C.; Harcourt, D. A Pilot Study of a Body Image Intervention for Breast Cancer Survivors. *Body Image* **2018**, *27*, 21–31. [CrossRef] [PubMed]
8. Sebri, V.; Durosini, I.; Mazzoni, D.; Pravettoni, G. The Body after Cancer: A Qualitative Study on Breast Cancer Survivors' Body Representation. *Int. J. Environ. Res. Public Health* **2022**, *19*, 12515. [CrossRef]
9. Mutsaers, B.; Jones, G.; Rutkowski, N.; Tomei, C.; Séguin Leclair, C.; Petricone-Westwood, D.; Simard, S.; Lebel, S. When Fear of Cancer Recurrence Becomes a Clinical Issue: A Qualitative Analysis of Features Associated with Clinical Fear of Cancer Recurrence. *Support. Care Cancer* **2016**, *24*, 4207–4218. [CrossRef]
10. Mahendran, R.; Liu, J.; Kuparasundram, S.; Simard, S.; Chan, Y.H.; Kua, E.H.; Griva, K. Fear of Cancer Recurrence among Cancer Survivors in Singapore. *Singapore Med. J.* **2021**, *62*, 305. [CrossRef]
11. Crist, J.V.; Grunfeld, E.A. Factors Reported to Influence Fear of Recurrence in Cancer Patients: A Systematic Review. *Psychooncology* **2013**, *22*, 978–986. [CrossRef]
12. Simard, S.; Thewes, B.; Humphris, G.; Dixon, M.; Hayden, C.; Mireskandari, S.; Ozakinci, G. Fear of Cancer Recurrence in Adult Cancer Survivors: A Systematic Review of Quantitative Studies. *J. Cancer Surviv.* **2013**, *7*, 300–322. [CrossRef] [PubMed]
13. Koch, L.; Jansen, L.; Brenner, H.; Arndt, V. Fear of Recurrence and Disease Progression in Long-Term (≥ 5 Years) Cancer Survivors-a Systematic Review of Quantitative Studies. *Psychooncology* **2013**, *22*, 1–11. [CrossRef] [PubMed]

14. Thewes, B.; Zachariae, R.; Christensen, S.; Nielsen, T.; Butow, P. The Concerns About Recurrence Questionnaire: Validation of a Brief Measure of Fear of Cancer Recurrence amongst Danish and Australian Breast Cancer Survivors. *J. Cancer Surviv.* **2015**, *9*, 68–79. [CrossRef] [PubMed]
15. Yang, Y.; Cameron, J.; Bedi, C.; Humphris, G. Fear of Cancer Recurrence Trajectory during Radiation Treatment and Follow-up into Survivorship of Patients with Breast Cancer 11 Medical and Health Sciences 1112 Oncology and Carcinogenesis. *BMC Cancer* **2018**, *18*, 1002. [CrossRef]
16. Yang, Y.; Qi, H.; Li, W.; Liu, T.; Xu, W.; Zhao, S.; Yang, F.; Humphris, G.; Chen, Y.; Sun, H. Predictors and Trajectories of Fear of Cancer Recurrence in Chinese Breast Cancer Patients. *J. Psychosom. Res.* **2023**, *166*, 111177. [CrossRef]
17. Savard, J.; Ivers, H. The Evolution of Fear of Cancer Recurrence during the Cancer Care Trajectory and Its Relationship with Cancer Characteristics. *J. Psychosom. Res.* **2013**, *74*, 354–360. [CrossRef]
18. Shim, E.J.; Jeong, D.; Lee, S.B.; Min, Y.H. Trajectory of Fear of Cancer Recurrence and Beliefs and Rates of Medication Adherence in Patients with Breast Cancer. *Psychooncology* **2020**, *29*, 1835–1841. [CrossRef]
19. Custers, J.A.E.; Kwakkenbos, L.; van der Graaf, W.T.A.; Prins, J.B.; Gielissen, M.F.M.; Thewes, B. Not as Stable as We Think: A Descriptive Study of 12 Monthly Assessments of Fear of Cancer Recurrence Among Curatively-Treated Breast Cancer Survivors 0–5 Years After Surgery. *Front. Psychol.* **2020**, *11*, 580979. [CrossRef]
20. Dunn, L.B.; Langford, D.J.; Paul, S.M.; Berman, M.B.; Shumay, D.M.; Kober, K.; Merriman, J.D.; West, C.; Neuhaus, J.M.; Miaskowski, C. Trajectories of Fear of Recurrence in Women with Breast Cancer. *Support. Care Cancer* **2015**, *23*, 2033–2043. [CrossRef]
21. McGinty, H.L.; Small, B.J.; Laronga, C.; Jacobsen, P.B. Predictors and Patterns of Fear of Cancer Recurrence in Breast Cancer Survivors. *Health Psychol.* **2016**, *35*, 1–9. [CrossRef]
22. Koch-Gallenkamp, L.; Bertram, H.; Eberle, A.; Holleczek, B.; Schmid-Höpfner, S.; Waldmann, A.; Zeissig, S.R.; Brenner, H.; Arndt, V. Fear of Recurrence in Long-Term Cancer Survivors-Do Cancer Type, Sex, Time since Diagnosis, and Social Support Matter? *Health Psychol.* **2016**, *35*, 1329–1333. [CrossRef] [PubMed]
23. Zhang, X.; Sun, D.; Qin, N.; Liu, M.; Jiang, N.; Li, X. Factors Correlated with Fear of Cancer Recurrence in Cancer Survivors: A Meta-Analysis. *Cancer Nurs.* **2022**, *45*, 406–415. [CrossRef] [PubMed]
24. Dafni, U.; Tsourti, Z.; Alatsathianos, I. Systematic Review Breast Cancer Statistics in the European Union: Incidence and Survival across European Countries. *Breast Care* **2017**, *14*, 344–353. [CrossRef] [PubMed]
25. Maajani, K.; Jalali, A.; Alipour, S.; Khodadost, M.; Tohidinik, H.R.; Yazdani, K. The Global and Regional Survival Rate of Women With Breast Cancer: A Systematic Review and Meta-Analysis. *Clin. Breast Cancer* **2019**, *19*, 165–177. [CrossRef] [PubMed]
26. Diefenbach, M.A.; Leventhal, H. The Common-Sense Model of Illness Representation: Theoretical and Practical Considerations. *J. Soc. Distress Homeless* **1996**, *5*, 11–38. [CrossRef]
27. Leventhal, H.; Meyer, D.; Nerenz, D. The Common-Sense Representation of Illness Danger. In *Contributions to Medical Psychology*; Rachman, S., Ed.; Pergamon Press: New York, NY, USA, 1980.
28. Hagger, M.S.; Orbell, S. A Meta-Analytic Review of the Common-Sense Model of Illness Representations. *Psychol. Health* **2003**, *18*, 141–184. [CrossRef]
29. Lee-Jones, C.; Humphris, G.; Dixon, R.; Hatcher, M.B. Fear of Cancer Recurrence—A Literature Review and Proposed Cognitive Formulation to Explain Exacerbation of Recurrence Fears. *Psychooncology* **1997**, *6*, 95–105. [CrossRef]
30. Hobfoll, S.E. Conservation of Resources: A New Attempt at Conceptualizing Stress. *Am. Psychol.* **1989**, *44*, 513–524. [CrossRef]
31. Hobfoll, S.E. Traumatic Stress: A Theory Based on Rapid Loss of Resources. *Anxiety Res.* **1991**, *4*, 187–197. [CrossRef]
32. Hobfoll, S.E. The Influence of Culture, Community, and the Nested-Self in the Stress Process: Advancing Conservation of Resources Theory. *Appl. Psychol.* **2001**, *50*, 337–421. [CrossRef]
33. Halbesleben, J.R.B.; Neveu, J.-P.; Westman, M. Getting to the "COR": Understanding the Role of Resources in Conservation of Resources Theory. *J. Manag.* **2014**, *40*, 1334–1364. [CrossRef]
34. Hobfoll, S.E. Conservation of Resources Theory: Its Implication for Stress, Health, and Resilience. In *The Oxford Handbook of Stress, Health, and Coping*; Oxford Academic: Oxford, UK, 2011; pp. 127–147. [CrossRef]
35. Bandura, A. Regulation of Cognitive Processes through Perceived Self-Efficacy. *Dev. Psychol.* **1989**, *25*, 729. [CrossRef]
36. Bandura, A. *Social Foundations of Thought and Action: A Social Cognitive Theory*; Prentice-Hall: Upper Saddle River, NJ, USA, 1986.
37. Bandura, A. *Self-Efficacy: The Exercise of Control*; APA: Washington, DC, USA, 1997.
38. Glanz, K.; Rimer, B.K.; Viswanath, K. Stress, Coping, and Health Behavior. In *Health Behavior and Health Education: Theory, Research, and Practice*; APA: Washington, DC, USA, 2008; pp. 211–236.
39. Chirico, A.; Lucidi, F.; Merluzzi, T.; Alivernini, F.; De Laurentiis, M.; Botti, G.; Giordano, A. A Meta-Analytic Review of the Relationship of Cancer Coping Selfefficacy with Distress and Quality of Life. *Oncotarget* **2017**, *8*, 36800–36811. [CrossRef] [PubMed]
40. Ziner, K.W.; Sledge, G.W.; Bell, C.J.; Johns, S.; Miller, K.D.; Champion, V.L. Predicting Fear of Breast Cancer Recurrence and Self-Efficacy in Survivors by Age at Diagnosis. *Oncol. Nurs. Forum* **2012**, *39*, 287–295. [CrossRef]
41. Lev, E.L.; Daley, K.M.; Conner, N.E.; Owen, S.V. An Intervention to Increase Quality of Life and Self-Care Self-Efficacy and Decrease Symptoms in Breast Cancer Patients. *Res. Theory Nurs. Pract.* **2014**, *15*, 277–294. Available online: https://www.researchgate.net/publication/11490007 (accessed on 28 June 2020).

42. McGinty, H.L.; Goldenberg, J.L.; Jacobsen, P.B. Relationship of Threat Appraisal with Coping Appraisal to Fear of Cancer Recurrence in Breast Cancer Survivors. *Psychooncology* **2012**, *21*, 203–210. [CrossRef]
43. Katapodi, M.C.; Ellis, K.R.; Schmidt, F.; Nikolaidis, C.; Northouse, L.L. Predictors and Interdependence of Family Support in a Random Sample of Long-Term Young Breast Cancer Survivors and Their Biological Relatives. *Cancer Med.* **2018**, *7*, 4980–4992. [CrossRef]
44. Chirico, A.; Vizza, D.; Valente, M.; Lo Iacono, M.; Campagna, M.R.; Palombi, T.; Alivernini, F.; Lucidi, F.; Bruno, F. Assessing the Fear of Recurrence Using the Cancer Worry Scale in a Sample of Italian Breast Cancer Survivors. *Support. Care Cancer* **2022**, *30*, 2829–2837. [CrossRef]
45. Wagner, L.I.; Tooze, J.A.; Hall, D.L.; Levine, B.J.; Beaumont, J.; Duffecy, J.; Victorson, D.; Gradishar, W.; Leach, J.; Saphner, T.; et al. Targeted EHealth Intervention to Reduce Breast Cancer Survivors' Fear of Recurrence: Results From the FoRtitude Randomized Trial. *J. Natl. Cancer Inst.* **2021**, *113*, 1495–1505. [CrossRef]
46. Hamama-Raz, Y.; Pat-Horenczyk, R.; Perry, S.; Ziv, Y.; Bar-Levav, R.; Stemmer, S.M. The Effectiveness of Group Intervention on Enhancing Cognitive Emotion Regulation Strategies in Breast Cancer Patients: A 2-Year Follow-Up. *Integr. Cancer Ther.* **2016**, *15*, 175–182. [CrossRef]
47. Thompson, R.A. Emotional Regulation and Emotional Development. *Educ. Psychol. Rev.* **1991**, *3*, 269–307. [CrossRef]
48. Garnefski, N.; Kraaij, V. Relationships between Cognitive Emotion Regulation Strategies and Depressive Symptoms: A Comparative Study of Five Specific Samples. *Pers. Individ. Dif.* **2006**, *40*, 1659–1669. [CrossRef]
49. Garnefski, N.; Kraaij, V.; Spinhoven, P. Negative Life Events, Cognitive Emotion Regulation and Emotional Problems. *Pers. Individ. Dif.* **2001**, *30*, 1311–1327. [CrossRef]
50. Cameron, L.D.; Booth, R.J.; Schlatter, M.; Ziginskas, D.; Harman, J.E. Changes in Emotion Regulation and Psychological Adjustment Following Use of a Group Psychosocial Support Program for Women Recently Diagnosed with Breast Cancer. *Psychooncology* **2007**, *16*, 171–180. [CrossRef] [PubMed]
51. Almeida, S.N.; Elliott, R.; Silva, E.R.; Sales, C.M.D. Emotion-Focused Therapy for Fear of Cancer Recurrence: A Hospital-Based Exploratory Outcome Study. *Psychotherapy* **2022**, *59*, 261–270. [CrossRef]
52. De Vries, J.; Den Oudsten, B.L.; Jacobs, P.M.E.P.; Roukema, J.A. How Breast Cancer Survivors Cope with Fear of Recurrence: A Focus Group Study. *Support. Care Cancer* **2014**, *22*, 705–712. [CrossRef]
53. Guimond, A.-J.; Ivers, H.; Savard, J. Is Emotion Regulation Associated with Cancer-Related Psychological Symptoms? *Psychol. Health* **2019**, *34*, 44–63. [CrossRef]
54. Allen, J.D.; Savadatti, S.; Levy, A.G. The Transition from Breast Cancer "patient" to "Survivor". *Psychooncology* **2009**, *18*, 71–78. [CrossRef]
55. Miller, K.; Merry, B.; Miller, J. Seasons of Survivorship Revisited. *Cancer J.* **2008**, *14*, 369. [CrossRef]
56. Simard, S.; Savard, J. Fear of Cancer Recurrence Inventory: Development and Initial Validation of a Multidimensional Measure of Fear of Cancer Recurrence. *Support. Care Cancer* **2009**, *17*, 241–251. [CrossRef]
57. Heitzmann, C.A.; Merluzzi, T.V.; Jean-Pierre, P.; Roscoe, J.A.; Kirsh, K.L.; Passik, S.D. Assessing Self-Efficacy for Coping with Cancer: Development and Psychometric Analysis of the Brief Version of the Cancer Behavior Inventory (CBI-B). *Psychooncology* **2011**, *20*, 302–312. [CrossRef] [PubMed]
58. Merluzzi, T.V.; Philip, E.J.; Heitzmann Ruhf, C.A.; Liu, H.; Yang, M.; Conley, C.C. Self-Efficacy for Coping with Cancer: Revision of the Cancer Behavior Inventory (Version 3.0). *Psychol. Assess.* **2001**, *30*, 486–499. [CrossRef] [PubMed]
59. Garnefski, N.; Kraaij, V.; Spinhoven, P. *Manual for the Use of the Cognitive Emotion Regulation Questionnaire*; DATEC: Leiderdorp, The Netherlands, 2002.
60. Arbuckle, J.L. *IBM ®SPSS ®Amos ™ 25 User's Guide*; IBM: Armonk, NY, USA, 2017.
61. Windle, M. Alternative Latent-Variable Approaches to Modeling Change in Adolescent Alcohol Involvement. In *The Science of Prevention: Methodological Advances from Alcohol and Substance Abuse Research*; Bryant, K.J., Windle, M., West, S.G., Eds.; American Psychological Association: Washington, DC, USA, 1997; pp. 43–78. [CrossRef]
62. Willett, J.B.; Sayer, A.G. Using Covariance Structure Analysis to Detect Correlates and Predictors of Individual Change over Time. *Psychol. Bull.* **1994**, *116*, 363–381. [CrossRef]
63. Kline, R.B. *Principles and Practice of Structural Equation Modeling*, 5th ed.; Guilford Publications: New York City, NY, USA, 2023. [CrossRef]
64. Luigjes-Huizer, Y.L.; Tauber, N.M.; Humphris, G.; Kasparian, N.A.; Lam, W.W.T.; Lebel, S.; Simard, S.; Smith, A.B.; Zachariae, R.; Afiyanti, Y.; et al. What Is the Prevalence of Fear of Cancer Recurrence in Cancer Survivors and Patients? A Systematic Review and Individual Participant Data Meta-Analysis. *Psychooncology* **2022**, *31*, 879–892. [CrossRef]
65. Starreveld, D.E.J.; Markovitz, S.E.; van Breukelen, G.; Peters, M.L. The Course of Fear of Cancer Recurrence: Different Patterns by Age in Breast Cancer Survivors. *Psychooncology* **2018**, *27*, 295–301. [CrossRef]
66. Baraldi, A.N.; Enders, C.K. An Introduction to Modern Missing Data Analyses. *J. Sch. Psychol.* **2010**, *48*, 5–37. [CrossRef]
67. Schapira, L.; Zheng, Y.; Gelber, S.I.; Poorvu, P.; Philip, E.J.; Ruddy, K.J.; Tamimi, R.M.; Peppercorn, J.; Come, S.E.; Borges, V.F.; et al. Trajectories of Fear of Cancer Recurrence in Young Breast Cancer Survivors. *Cancer* **2021**, *128*, 335–343. [CrossRef]
68. Kreitler, S.; Peleg, D.; Ehrenfeld, M. Stress, Self-Efficacy and Quality of Life in Cancer Patients. *Psychooncology* **2007**, *16*, 329–341. [CrossRef]

69. Karademas, E.C.; Simos, P.; Pat-Horenczyk, R.; Roziner, I.; Mazzocco, K.; Sousa, B.; Oliveira-Maia, A.J.; Stamatakos, G.; Cardoso, F.; Frasquilho, D.; et al. Cognitive, Emotional, and Behavioral Mediators of the Impact of Coping Self-Efficacy on Adaptation to Breast Cancer: An International Prospective Study. *Psychooncology* **2021**, *30*, 1555–1562. [CrossRef]
70. Curtis, R.; Groarke, A.; Sullivan, F.J. Stress and Self-Efficacy Predict Psychological Adjustment at Diagnosis of Prostate Cancer. *Sci. Rep.* **2014**, *4*, 5569. [CrossRef]
71. Séguin Leclair, C.; Lebel, S.; Westmaas, J.L. Can Physical Activity and Healthy Diet Help Long-Term Cancer Survivors Manage Their Fear of Recurrence? *Front. Psychol.* **2021**, *12*, 2210. [CrossRef] [PubMed]
72. Shin, J.; Shin, D.W.; Lee, J.; Hwang, J.H.; Lee, J.E.; Cho, B.L.; Song, Y.-M. Exploring Socio-Demographic, Physical, Psychological, and Quality of Life-Related Factors Related with Fear of Cancer Recurrence in Stomach Cancer Survivors: A Cross-Sectional Study. *BMC Cancer* **2022**, *22*, 414. [CrossRef] [PubMed]
73. Tran, T.X.M.; Jung, S.; Lee, E.-G.; Cho, H.; Kim, N.Y.; Shim, S.; Kim, H.Y.; Kang, D.; Cho, J.; Lee, E.; et al. Fear of Cancer Recurrence and Its Negative Impact on Health-Related Quality of Life in Long-Term Breast Cancer Survivors. *Cancer Res. Treat.* **2021**, *54*, 1065–1073. [CrossRef] [PubMed]
74. Zheng, W.; Hu, M.; Liu, Y. Social Support Can Alleviate the Fear of Cancer Recurrence in Postoperative Patients with Lung Carcinoma. *Am. J. Transl. Res.* **2022**, *14*, 4804.
75. Almeida, S.N.; Elliott, R.; Silva, E.R.; Sales, C.M.D. Fear of Cancer Recurrence: A Qualitative Systematic Review and Meta-Synthesis of Patients' Experiences. *Clin. Psychol. Rev.* **2019**, *68*, 13–24. [CrossRef]
76. Lai, W.S.; Shu, B.C.; Hou, W.L. A Qualitative Exploration of the Fear of Recurrence among Taiwanese Breast Cancer Survivors. *Eur. J. Cancer Care* **2019**, *28*, e13113. [CrossRef]
77. Şengün İnan, F.; Üstün, B. Fear of Recurrence in Turkish Breast Cancer Survivors: A Qualitative Study. *J. Transcult. Nurs.* **2019**, *30*, 146–153. [CrossRef]
78. Dawson, G.; Madsen, L.T.; Dains, J.E. Interventions to Manage Uncertainty and Fear of Recurrence in Female Breast Cancer Survivors: A Review of the Literature. *Clin. J. Oncol. Nurs.* **2016**, *20*, E155–E161. [CrossRef]
79. Park, S.; Sato, Y.; Takita, Y.; Tamura, N.; Ninomiya, A.; Kosugi, T.; Sado, M.; Nakagawa, A.; Takahashi, M.; Hayashida, T.; et al. Mindfulness-Based Cognitive Therapy for Psychological Distress, Fear of Cancer Recurrence, Fatigue, Spiritual Well-Being, and Quality of Life in Patients With Breast Cancer—A Randomized Controlled Trial. *J. Pain Symptom Manag.* **2020**, *60*, 381–389. [CrossRef]
80. Tu, P.C.; Yeh, D.C.; Hsieh, H.C. Positive Psychological Changes after Breast Cancer Diagnosis and Treatment: The Role of Trait Resilience and Coping Styles. *J. Psychosoc. Oncol.* **2020**, *38*, 156–170. [CrossRef]
81. OECD/EU. *Health at a Glance: Europe 2018: State of Health in the EU Cycle*; OECD: Paris, France, 2018. [CrossRef]
82. OECD. *Finland: Country Health Profile 2019*; State of Health in the EU; OECD Publishing, Paris/European Observatory on Health Systems and Policies: Brussels, Belgium, 2019. [CrossRef]
83. Ministry of Health-Israel. Breast Cancer among Women in Israel- Update of Incidence and Mortality Data. Available online: https://www.health.gov.il/PublicationsFiles/breast_cancer_SEPT2018.pdf (accessed on 18 March 2020).
84. Zamir, O.; Bentley, G.; He, Y. A Promotive Process of Resource Gain Against Harsh and Inconsistent Discipline in Mothers Coping With Breast Cancer: A Serial Mediation Model. *Front. Psychiatry* **2022**, *13*, 859604. [CrossRef] [PubMed]
85. Ellegaard, M.B.B.; Grau, C.; Zachariae, R.; Bonde Jensen, A. Fear of Cancer Recurrence and Unmet Needs among Breast Cancer Survivors in the First Five Years. A Cross-Sectional Study. *Acta Oncol.* **2017**, *56*, 314–320. [CrossRef] [PubMed]
86. Götze, H.; Taubenheim, S.; Dietz, A.; Lordick, F.; Mehnert-Theuerkauf, A. Fear of Cancer Recurrence across the Survivorship Trajectory: Results from a Survey of Adult Long-term Cancer Survivors. *Psychooncology* **2019**, *28*, 2033–2041. [CrossRef] [PubMed]
87. Merluzzi, T.V.; Pustejovsky, J.E.; Philip, E.J.; Sohl, S.J.; Berendsen, M.; Salsman, J.M. Interventions to Enhance Self-Efficacy in Cancer Patients: A Meta-Analysis of Randomized Controlled Trials. *Psychooncology* **2019**, *28*, 1781–1790. [CrossRef]

Disclaimer/Publisher's Note: The statements, opinions and data contained in all publications are solely those of the individual author(s) and contributor(s) and not of MDPI and/or the editor(s). MDPI and/or the editor(s) disclaim responsibility for any injury to people or property resulting from any ideas, methods, instructions or products referred to in the content.

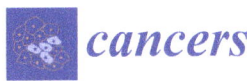

Article

LEM Domain Containing 1 Acts as a Novel Oncogene and Therapeutic Target for Triple-Negative Breast Cancer

Xiangling Li [1,2], Shilong Jiang [3], Ting Jiang [1], Xinyuan Sun [1], Yidi Guan [1], Songqing Fan [4] and Yan Cheng [1,2,5,*]

1. Department of Pharmacy, The Second Xiangya Hospital, Central South University, Changsha 410011, China
2. Hunan Provincial Engineering Research Centre of Translational Medicine and Innovative Drug, Changsha 410011, China
3. Department of Pharmacy, Xiangya Hospital, Central South University, Changsha 410008, China
4. Department of Pathology, The Second Xiangya Hospital, Central South University, Changsha 410011, China
5. Key Laboratory of Diabetes Immunology, Central South University, Ministry of Education, Changsha 410011, China
* Correspondence: yancheng@csu.edu.cn

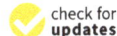

Citation: Li, X.; Jiang, S.; Jiang, T.; Sun, X.; Guan, Y.; Fan, S.; Cheng, Y. LEM Domain Containing 1 Acts as a Novel Oncogene and Therapeutic Target for Triple-Negative Breast Cancer. *Cancers* 2023, 15, 2924. https://doi.org/10.3390/cancers15112924

Academic Editor: Naiba Nabieva

Received: 12 April 2023
Revised: 17 May 2023
Accepted: 22 May 2023
Published: 26 May 2023

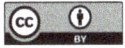

Copyright: © 2023 by the authors. Licensee MDPI, Basel, Switzerland. This article is an open access article distributed under the terms and conditions of the Creative Commons Attribution (CC BY) license (https://creativecommons.org/licenses/by/4.0/).

Simple Summary: Since TNBC shows the worst prognosis and limited treatment options, exploring novel molecular targets is urgently needed for effective treatment of TNBC. In this study, we demonstrated that LEMD1 is highly expressed in TNBC and contributes to poor prognosis of TNBC patients. LEMD1 silencing not only inhibited the proliferation and migration of TNBC cells in vitro, but also abolished tumor formation of TNBC cells in vivo. Mechanistically, LEMD1 promotes the progress of TNBC by activating the ERK signaling pathway. Knockdown of LEMD1 renders TNBC cells more sensitive to paclitaxel. Our results uncovered LEMD1 as a novel oncogene in TNBC, and targeting LEMD1 might be a promising therapeutic approach for the effective treatment of TNBC patients.

Abstract: Breast cancer is the most common deadly malignancy in women worldwide. In particular, triple-negative breast cancer (TNBC) exhibits the worst prognosis among four subtypes of breast cancer due to limited treatment options. Exploring novel therapeutic targets holds promise for developing effective treatments for TNBC. Here, we demonstrated for the first time that LEMD1 (LEM domain containing 1) is highly expressed in TNBC and contributes to reduced survival in TNBC patients, through analysis of both bioinformatic databases and collected patient samples. Furthermore, LEMD1 silencing not only inhibited the proliferation and migration of TNBC cells in vitro, but also abolished tumor formation of TNBC cells in vivo. Knockdown of LEMD1 enhanced the sensitivity of TNBC cells to paclitaxel. Mechanistically, LEMD1 promoted the progress of TNBC by activating the ERK signaling pathway. In summary, our study revealed that LEMD1 may act as a novel oncogene in TNBC, and targeting LEMD1 may be exploited as a promising therapeutic approach to enhance the efficacy of chemotherapy against TNBC.

Keywords: TNBC; LEMD1; ERK; therapeutic target

1. Introduction

Breast cancer is the most frequent female malignancy around the world, with high incidence and fatality [1]. Estrogen receptor (ER), progesterone receptor (PR) and epidermal growth factor receptor (Her2) on tumor cell surfaces are the main targets for therapeutic treatment of breast cancer. However, with the expression deficiency of these three key markers, triple negative breast cancer (TNBC) patients can benefit from neither endocrine therapy nor HER2-targeted therapy [2]. Chemotherapy still remains the mainstay systemic treatment for TNBC patients, despite its poor efficacy and severe toxic effect [3,4]. Moreover, TNBC patients share the clinical features of high invasiveness and metastatic potential, which also plagues the effectiveness of current treatment regimens [4]. Therefore, discovering effective targeted therapies for TNBC treatment is urgently needed.

LEM domain containing 1 (LEMD1) belongs to the cancer-testis antigen (CTA) family [5]. Since LEMD1 was first isolated from colorectal cancer in 2004, the role it plays during tumor progression has attracted widespread concern among researchers. It has been reported that LEMD1 is aberrantly overexpressed in a series of malignancies and is correlated with worse prognosis of tumor patients such as prostate cancer, colorectal cancer, gastric cancer and pancreatic cancer [5–9]. LEMD1 exerts oncogenic effects during tumorigenesis of various cancers. For example, the elevated expression of LEMD1 contributes to cell proliferation in gastric cancer [7]. LEMD1 also facilitates invasion and epithelial–mesenchymal transition (EMT) in oral squamous cell carcinoma, thyroid cancer and pancreatic cancer [8,10,11]. Transcriptome data has revealed that LEMD1 is highly expressed in cancer stem cells (CSCs)/cancer-initiating cells (CICs) and is important for the maintenance of CSCs/CICs in colorectal cancer [12]. Taken together, these studies demonstrate that LEMD1 plays a pivotal role in promoting tumor progression, suggesting its clinical value as a potential prognostic biomarker and therapeutic target in diverse tumors. Nevertheless, the biological function of LEMD1 in breast cancer has not been elucidated yet.

In this study, we innovatively explored the expression and the prognostic value of LEMD1 in TNBC. In addition, we elucidated the biological role and the clinical value of LEMD1 in the progress of TNBC, and also performed further analysis to clarify the underlying mechanism. In conclusion, our results revealed the biological function of LEMD1 during tumorigenesis of TNBC and provided a potential therapeutic strategy of targeting LEMD1 for TNBC treatment.

2. Materials and Methods

2.1. Bioinformatics Analysis

A series of genomic datasets in breast cancer, including GSE65216, GSE20713, GSE45827 and GSE76275, downloaded from Gene Expression Omnibus (GEO), provide gene expression profiles of tumor samples. In detail, GEPIA 2 (Gene Expression Profiling Interactive Analysis 2) was used to compare gene expressions between tumor and normal tissues of breast cancer samples, and to analyze the influence of LEMD1 expression on the survival outcome in multiple cancers. The association of LEMD1 and the overall survival of TNBC patients was completed by Kaplan–Meier Plotter. DNMIVD [13] was used to analyze LEMD1 methylation levels and its relationship with patients' survival. TIMER [14] is a web server providing data on LEMD1 expression in tumor tissues and corresponding normal tissues among various cancers. Additionally, we explored the influence of gene set expression on anti-cancer drug resistance by GSCALite server [15]. ROC plotter server [16] was utilized to analyze the correlation between the expression of LEMD1 and the therapeutic responses of TNBC patients to chemotherapy.

2.2. Cell Lines and Culture

The human breast cancer cell lines MDA-MB-468, BT549 and HCC1806 were cultured in RPMI-1640 medium. HEK-293T and MDA-MB-231 were cultured in DMEM medium. MDA-MB-436 was cultured in L-15 medium. These cells were all cultured in media supplemented with 10% fetal bovine serum (Gibco), penicillin (100 U/mL) and streptomycin (100 μg/mL). Additionally, all cell lines were maintained at 37 °C in a humidified atmosphere of 5% CO_2/95% air and identified via the STR method.

2.3. siRNA, shRNA, CRISPR/Cas9 Lentivirus and Plasmid Transfection

RiboBio (Guangzhou, China) supplied the siRNA targeting LEMD1. Cells in good growth condition were plated in 6-well plates and then transfected with siRNA according to the manufacturer's protocol. For the construction of stable silencing cells, the LEMD1 shRNA plasmids were transfected into HEK-293T cells and the supernatant of

HEK-293T cells was added into MDA-MB-231 cells, following by screening with 2 µg/mL of puromycin for a week. For the construction of LEMD1-KO cells, the CRISPER/CAS9 lentiviruses were transfected into MDA-MB-468 cells for 72 h, and then selected with 8 µg/mL of puromycin for a week. The plasmids involved in this study were transfected by Lipofectamine 8000 (Beyotime, Shanghai, China) reagent.

2.4. Western Blot

Cells were lysed with RIPA buffer containing protease inhibitor and phosphatase inhibitor at 4 °C for 30 min, and then centrifuged at $12,000\times g$ for 15 min at 4 °C. Proteins (20 µg) were run on SDS-PAGE gels and then transferred to PVDF membranes. After blocking with skim milk, the PVDF membranes were incubated in 5% BSA at 4 °C overnight with the corresponding primary antibodies as follows: LEMD1 (GTX16303, 1:1000, Genetex, Irvine, CA, USA), LEMD1 (ab201206, 1:1000, Abcam, Cambridge, UK), Lamin B1 (sc-377000, 1:500, Santa Cruz, Santa Cruz, CA, USA), E-cadherin (ET1607-75, 1:1000, Huabio, Hangzhou, China), N-cadherin (ET1607-37, 1:2000, Huabio, Hangzhou, China), vimentin (M1412-1, 1:1000, Huabio, Hangzhou, China), Bax (50599-2-lg, 1:1000, Proteintech, Chicago, IL, USA), Bcl-2 (#15071S, 1:1000, CST, Boston, MA, USA), ERK (#0102S, 1:1000, CST), p-ERK (#9101S, 1:1000, CST), Flag (M185-3L, 1:1000, MBL, Beijing, China), β-actin (20536, 1:7000, Proteintech), GAPDH (GB11002, 1:1000, Servicebio, Wuhan, China), following by treatment with the corresponding secondary antibody at room temperature for 1 h. Finally, the protein signals were visualized with ECL reagent.

2.5. RNA Isolation, Reverse Transcription (RT) and Real-Time PCR

Total RNA from cell lines was isolated using Trizol reagent (Invitrogen, Carlsbad, CA, USA). A total of 1 µg of RNA was reverse-transcribed using the PrimeScript RT Reagent Kit (Takara, Dalian, China). Real-time PCR was carried out using SYBR Green (Takara). The mRNA expression of all target genes was normalized to GAPDH.

2.6. Cell Viability Assays

The cells were plated in 96-well plates and treated with paclitaxel for 72 h. Then, cell viability was measured with CCK8 (Bimake, Shanghai, China) reagent. The cells were incubated at 37 °C for 2 h after adding CCK8. Additionally, the OD value at 450 nm was detected to determine cell viability.

2.7. Clonogenic Assay

Cells were plated in 6-well plates (500 cells/well) and treated with paclitaxel for 24 h. After the incubation of about 15 days, 4% paraformaldehyde and crystal violet were used to fix and stain the cell colonies.

2.8. 5-Ethynyl-2′-deoxyuridine Assay

According to the instruction, the cells were incubated with 5-Ethynyl-2′-deoxyuridine assay (EDU, RiboBio, Chengdu, China) for 2 h at 37 °C and fixed with 4% paraformaldehyde for 30 min, followed by permeating with 0.5% Triton X-100 for 10 min at room temperature. Then, cells were stained with 1× Apollo dye reaction solution for 30 min and treated with Hoechst for 30 min away from light at room temperature. Finally, a fluorescent microscope was needed to capture the images.

2.9. Wound Healing Assay

To measure cell migration, cells were plated in 6-well plates and maintained at 37 °C. A line was drawn with sterile 10 µL tips on the monolayer cells and rinsed with medium to remove any floating cell debris when the cells reached 100% confluence. Images were captured at the indicated time. The wound healing rate (%) was calculated and analyzed.

2.10. Cell Migration and Invasion

The cells' migration and invasion ability were examined using Matrigel and Transwell plates. The cells (3×10^4 cells/well) were inoculated into the upper chamber of the Transwell plate in serum-free medium. Particularly, the upper chambers were coated with Matrigel (BD, Biosciences, Chongqing, China) for the invasion assay. The medium containing 20% FBS was added to the lower chamber. After incubation for 24 h (migration) and 72 h (invasion), the cells on the submembrane surface were fixed with 4% paraformaldehyde and stained with crystal violet. The extra cells and the Matrigel were removed with cotton swabs, and then the invaded and migrated cells were photographed and counted.

2.11. Immunofluorescence Staining

MDA-MB-468 cells were seeded on a glass coverslip and fixed in 4% paraformaldehyde for 25 min at room temperature. Next, the cells were blocked in 5% bovine serum albumin (BSA) for 2 h and incubated with anti-LEMD1 antibody (GTX16303, 1:200, Genetex) at 4 °C overnight, followed by Alexa Fluor 594 dye-conjugated anti-rabbit IgG antibody. At the end of incubation, the cell nuclei were stained with DAPI for 2 min. The coverslip was washed with phosphate-buffered saline (PBS) and images were detected and captured using a confocal microscope.

2.12. Tissue Microarray (TMA) and Immunohistochemistry (IHC)

The Second Xiangya Hospital of Central South University (Changsha, China) provided the clinical specimens involved in this study. Additionally, all patients were given informed consent before the experiment. For TMA, samples embedded with paraffin were arranged by a tissue-arraying instrument; each sample was arranged in three 1-mmdiameter cores to reduce tissue loss and minimize tumor heterogeneity. IHC staining for LEMD1 (Abcam, ab201206, 1:100) was conducted by using the DAKO LSAB + System-HRP kit (DAKO, Copenhagen, Denmark) according to the protocols. The protein expression of LEMD1 was detected with a polyclonal antibody at a dilution of 1:200. IHC scores were evaluated by two independent pathologists in a blinded situation.

2.13. Semi-Quantitative Analysis of TMA and IHC Staining

Two independent pathologists, who were experienced in assessing IHC and were blinded to the clinical outcome of the involved patients, were invited to evaluate all of the samples. We determined the expression of LEMD1 by using two indicators: the intensity and the range of the staining. The percentage of immunoreactive cells was rated as follows: 0 points, <10% positive cells; 1 point, 10–40% positive cells; 2 points, 40–70% positive cells; 3 points, >70% positive cells. The staining intensity was rated as follows: 0 (no staining), 1 (weak staining), 2 (moderate staining), 3 (strong staining). The two scores were multiplied and used to divide the patients into a high expression group (score ≥ 3) and a low expression group (score < 3) of LEMD1. The final score is the mean of the scores assigned by the two pathologists [17,18].

2.14. RNA-Sequencing and Signaling Pathway Assays

Total RNA was extracted from MDA-MB-468 cell lines treated with LEMD1 siRNA or a negative control. After confirming the quality, purity and integrity of the RNA, a cDNA library was established from ~1 µg of total RNA. Then, the library was sequenced on an Illumina Novaseq6000 using 2×150 bp paired-end sequencing chemistry. The Kyoto Encyclopedia of Genes and Genomes (KEGG) pathway enrichment analysis was performed by analyzing the obtained genes. All services were provided by LC Biotech Corporation (Hangzhou, China).

2.15. Animal Studies

MDA-MB-231 cells with stable LEMD1 knockdown and control MDA-MB-231 cells were administered subcutaneously into 5-week-old female BALB/c nude mice (1×10^6 cells in 100 µL medium). Tumor sizes and body weights were measured every other day. Tumor volume was calculated as length × width^2 × (π/6). The subcutaneous tumors were excised, weighed and captured at the termination of the experiment.

2.16. Statistical Analysis

We analyzed the data using SPSS 22.0 and GraphPad Prism 8.0 software. Pearson's χ^2 test was used to analyze the association between LEMD1 expression and the clinicopathological features of breast cancer patients. A two-tailed unpaired Student *t* test was conducted to analyze the differences between two groups. $p < 0.05$ was considered statistically significant.

3. Results

3.1. The High Expression of LEMD1 Is Associated with Poor Prognosis in TNBC

In order to explore the genes involved in the progress of TNBC, we first screened 32 genes with specific high expressions in TNBC compared with other subtypes of breast cancer by analyzing GEO datasets including GSE65216, GSE20713 and GSE45827 ($\log_2 FC > 1.5$) (Figure 1A). The high expressions of these 32 genes in TNBC were also verified in the Cancer Genome Atlas Breast Invasive Carcinoma (TCGA-BRCA) (Figure 1B). We further analyzed the expressions of 32 genes in TNBC and normal breast tissue, and found that 8 genes (*LEMD1, ART3, EN1, UGT8, SHC4, HORMAD1, ZIC1, CT83*) showed higher expression in TNBC tissue compared to the normal breast tissue by GEPIA analysis (Figure 1C and Supplementary Figure S1). Considering the role of LEMD1 in breast cancer remains unknown, we further explored the biologic function and the clinical value of LEMD1 in TNBC.

Next, we confirmed LEMD1 expression in breast cancer tissues. Firstly, data from an independent breast cancer dataset consistently shows that LEMD1 is significantly upregulated in TNBC tumors compared to non-TNBC tumors (Figure 2A). Moreover, higher protein expressions of LEMD1 were observed in TNBC tissues compared to non-TNBC tissues in a tissue microarray (TMA) containing 80 breast cancer specimens we collected from the Second Xiangya Hospital (Figure 2B). In addition, we examined the protein expressions of LEMD1 in 63 TNBC patients from the Second Xiangya Hospital by immunohistochemistry (IHC) staining, and further analyzed the relationship between LEMD1 expressions and the clinicopathological features of TNBC patients. As shown in Figure 2C and Table 1, we found that high expression of LEMD1 was markedly associated with higher histology grade of TNBC patients, suggesting that LEMD1 may act as a cancer-promoting factor in TNBC. The survival curve, analyzed by Kaplan–Meier Plotter database, revealed that TNBC patients with higher LEMD1 expression showed worse overall survival (Figure 2D). In addition, the low expression of LEMD1 was positively correlated with improved survival in breast cancer patients, as shown by analysis of the clinical data of 85 patients we collected (Figure 2E). Since LEMD1 is one of the family members of cancer testis antigen that is often regulated by DNA demethylation, as reported [19–21], we analyzed the methylation level of LEMD1 in breast cancer. As shown in Supplementary Figure S2A,B, LEMD1 is hypomethylated in breast cancer tissues compared with normal tissues, and its hypomethylation was positively correlated with reduced disease-free interval (DFI) in breast cancer patients. These results indicated that LEMD1 is overexpressed and acts as a poor prognostic factor in TNBC.

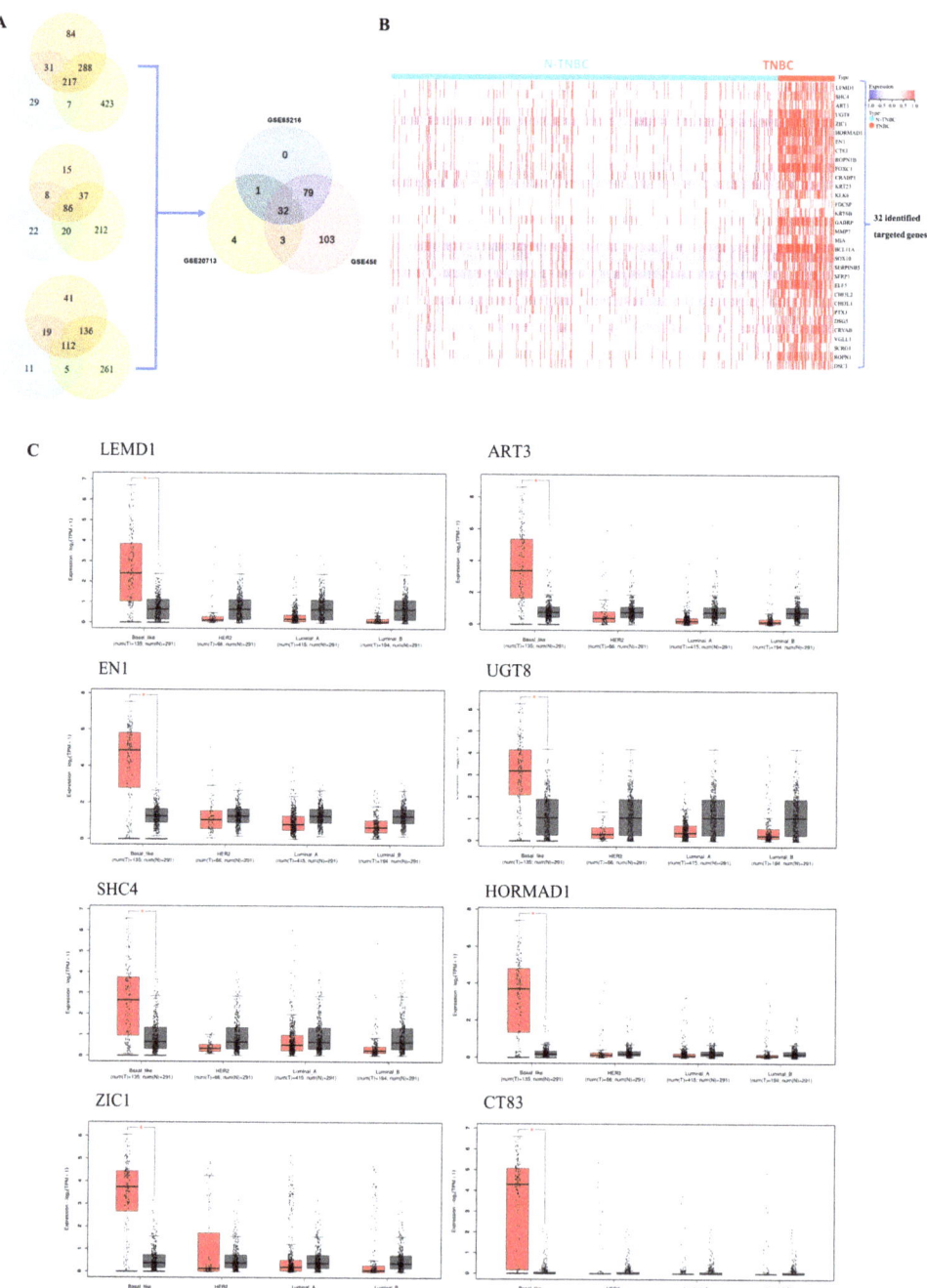

Figure 1. Screening of the high expression genes in TNBC. (**A**) Venn diagram of the differential genes between TNBC and non-TNBC samples in GEO datasets. (**B**) The expressions of 32 genes in TNBC and non-TNBC in the TCGA-BRCA cohort. Heat maps represent gene expression levels. (**C**) The GEPIA analysis of 8 genes with specific high expression in TNBC. Red represents tumor tissues and black represents corresponding normal tissues. * $p < 0.05$.

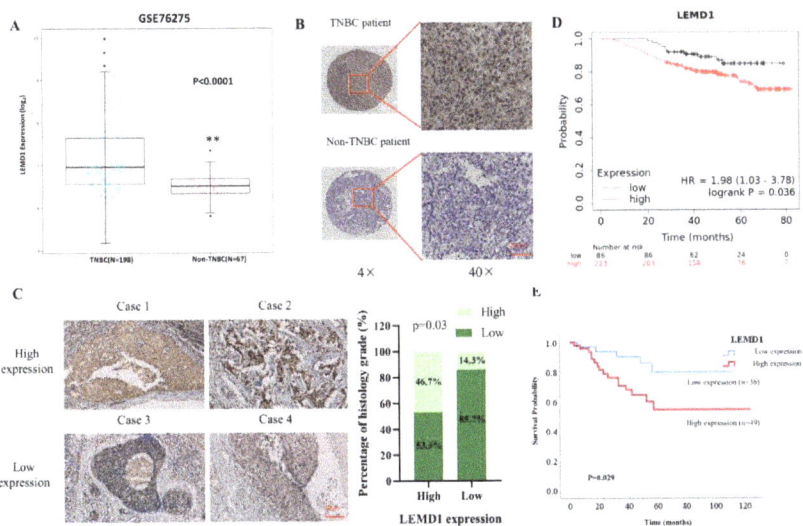

Figure 2. The relationship between LEMD1 and clinicopathological features of TNBC patients. (**A**) LEMD1 expressions of TNBC and non-TNBC patients in GSE76275 from GEO database. ** $p < 0.01$. (**B**) Representative images of LEMD1 from a tissue microarray containing 80 breast cancer patients. (**C**) Representative IHC images of LEMD1 in 63 clinical samples of TNBC patients. Scale bar, 50 μm. The positive correlation between LEMD1 expressions and the histology grade in TNBC patients. (**D**) Kaplan–Meier plot of the overall survival (OS) of TNBC patients from TCGA database. (**E**) Kaplan–Meier plots of the OS from a tissue microarray containing 85 breast cancer patients.

Table 1. The relationship between clinicopathological characteristics and LEMD1 expressions in 63 TNBC patients.

Characteristic	LEMD1		p Value
	Low	High	
Age, years			
<50	7	27	0.516
≥50	8	21	
Tumor size, cm			
<3	5	27	0.121
≥3	10	21	
Histology Grade			
Low	12	24	0.030
High	2	21	
Lymph node metastasis			
No	7	26	0.612
Yes	8	22	
TNM stage			
I/II	7	26	0.612
III/IV	8	22	

3.2. Pan-Cancer Analysis of LEMD1 Expression and Prognosis

In view of the critical role of LEMD1 in TNBC, we performed pan-cancer analysis to gain a more comprehensive understanding of LEMD1 in various cancers. Firstly, we analyzed LEMD1 expression in various cancers by comparing the transcriptome data between tumor tissues and corresponding adjacent normal tissues. The result shows that LEMD1 was highly expressed in various cancers, including bladder urothelial carcinoma (BLCA), invasive breast carcinoma (BRCA), cholangiocarcinoma (CHOL), colon adenocarcinoma (COAD), esophageal carcinoma (ESCA), glioblastoma multiforme (GBM), head and neck squamous cell carcinoma (HNSC), kidney chromophobe (KICH), kidney renal clear cell carcinoma (KIRC), kidney renal papillary cell carcinoma (KIRP), lung adenocarcinoma (LUAD), lung squamous cell carcinoma (LUSC), pancreatic adenocarcinoma (PAAD), prostate adenocarcinoma (PRAD), rectal adenocarcinoma (READ), stomach adenocarcinoma (STAD), thyroid carcinoma (THCA) and uterine corpus endometrial carcinoma (UCEC) (Supplementary Figure S3A), suggesting that LEMD1 may serve as a potential key regulator during tumorigenesis. Next, we analyzed the prognostic value of LEMD1 in pan-cancer and found that high expression of LEMD1 was significantly associated with worse OS rate in COAD ($p = 0.047$), KIRC ($p = 0.0065$), KIRP ($p = 0.023$) and PAAD ($p = 0.0027$) (Supplementary Figure S3B). These results revealed that LEMD1 is upregulated and may serve as a poor prognostic factor in multiple cancers.

3.3. LEMD1 Promotes the Progression of TNBC In Vitro and In Vivo

We next sought to investigate the biological functions of LEMD1 in TNBC. Firstly, we examined the subcellular location of LEMD1, and found that LEMD1 is located in the nucleus via immunofluorescence staining (Figure 3A). We further detected LEMD1 expressions in several TNBC cell lines and found that LEMD1 was highly expressed in MDA-MB-468 and MDA-MB-231 cells (Figure 3B). Therefore, we used siRNA/shRNA to knockdown LEMD1 expression in MDA-MB-468 cells and MDA-MB-231 cells, respectively (Figure 3C). Western blot analysis of LEMD1-knockdown cells also verified the nuclear localization of LEMD1 in TNBC cells (Supplementary Figure S4A). Importantly, we found that knockdown of LEMD1 significantly inhibited the cell viability in MDA-MB-468 and MDA-MB-231 cells (Figure 3D and Supplementary Figure S4B). The numbers of cells positive for EdU staining were also significantly decreased in TNBC cells with LEMD1 knockdown (Figure 3E and Supplementary Figure S4C). Furthermore, the inhibited proliferation induced by LEMD1 knockdown was also confirmed via a colony formation assay examining long-term survival (Figure 3F). These results indicated that LEMD1 silencing inhibited the proliferation of TNBC cells. We further explored whether LEMD1 could regulate the apoptosis of TNBC cells. As shown in Figure 3G and Supplementary Figure S4D, LEMD1 silencing increased cell apoptosis, as evidenced by the increased expression of Bax and the decreased expression of Bcl-2.

Moreover, we investigated the effect of LEMD1 knockdown on cell migration and invasion. Figure 3H and Supplementary Figure S4E,F show that the migration rates of TNBC cells in LEMD1-knockdown or knockout group were significantly decreased compared to those in control group. Transwell experiments demonstrated that migration and invasion were inhibited in TNBC cells with LEMD1 silencing (Figure 3I,J). We then tested the impact of LEMD1 knockdown on the epithelial–mesenchymal transition (EMT) process of TNBC cells. We found that LEMD1 silencing increased the expression of E-cadherin and decrease the expressions of N-cadherin and vimentin (Figure 3K and Supplementary Figure S4G), suggesting that LEMD1 promotes the EMT process of TNBC cells. Furthermore, we found that there is no significant change in the mRNA levels of Bax, Bcl-2, E-cadherin, N-cadherin and vimentin in cells with LEMD1 knockdown (Figure 3L and Supplementary Figure S4H), indicating that the regulation of LEMD1 on the expressions of the above proteins is a post-transcriptional modification. Taken together, these results demonstrated that LEMD1 functions as a promotive factor in the proliferation, migration and invasion of TNBC cells.

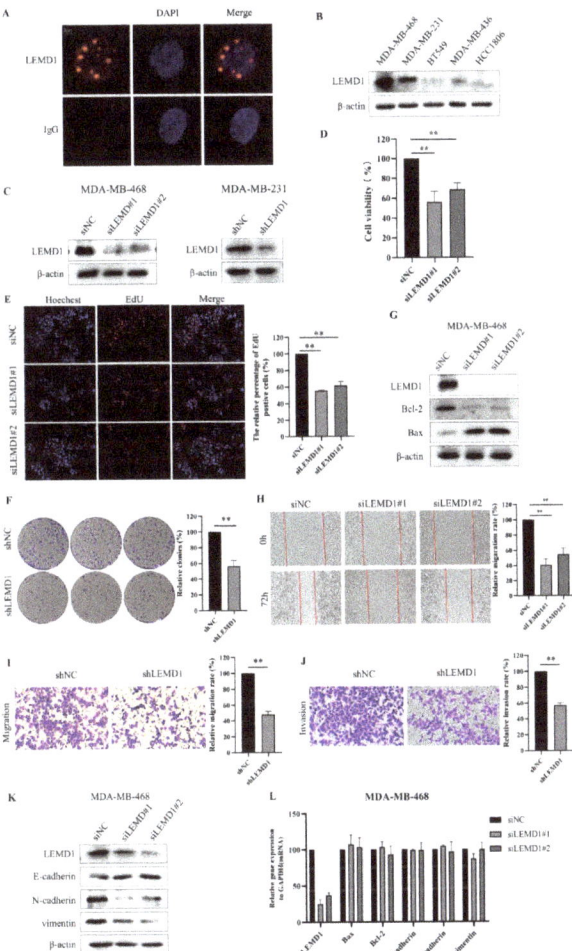

Figure 3. LEMD1 promotes the proliferation and migration of TNBC cells. (**A**) The subcellular location of LEMD1 was examined in MDA-MB-468 cells by immunofluorescence staining. IgG antibody was used for negative control. The location of the nucleus was indicated by DAPI. (**B**) The expressions of LEMD1 in TNBC cell lines were examined by Western blot, β-actin was used as a loading control. (**C**) The expressions of LEMD1 in MDA-MB-468 cells were knocked down by siRNA, and the expressions of LEMD1 in MDA-MB-231 cells were knocked down by shRNA. (**D**) CCK-8 reagent was applied to examine cell viability of MDA-MB-468 cells. ** $p < 0.01$, n = 3. (**E**) Cell proliferation of MDA-MB-468 cells was measured using EdU. Magnification ×100. ** $p < 0.01$, n = 3. (**F**) The colony formation assay in LEMD1-knockdown MDA-MB-231 and the corresponding negative control cells were used to examine cell proliferation. ** $p < 0.01$, n = 3. (**G**) Western blot analysis of the expressions of Bcl-2 and Bax in MDA-MB-468 cells, β-actin was used as a loading control. (**H**) Wound healing assays of MDA-MB-468 cells. Magnification ×100. ** $p < 0.01$, n = 3. Transwell migration assays (**I**) and Transwell invasion assays (**J**) in LEMD1-konckdown MDA-MB-231 cells and their corresponding negative control cells. Magnification ×200. ** $p < 0.01$, n = 3. (**K**) Western blot analysis of the expressions of E-cadherin, N-cadherin and vimentin in MDA-MB-468 cells, β-actin was used as a loading control. (**L**) qPCR analysis of the mRNA expressions of Bax, Bcl-2, E-cadherin, N-cadherin and vimentin in MDA-MB-468 cells. The original western blot figures could be found in Supplementary Figure S6A.

To extend the in vitro observations, we constructed a subcutaneous xenograft model in female nude mice to investigate the influence of LEMD1 silencing on tumor growth in vivo (Figure 4A). As shown in Figure 4B–D, no tumor formation was observed in MDA-MB-231 cells with knockdown of LEMD1 expression, indicating that LEMD1 silencing totally abolished tumor formation in vivo. There was no significant change in body weight in the mice of the two groups (Figure 4E). Collectively, these results confirmed that LEMD1 promotes the progression of TNBC.

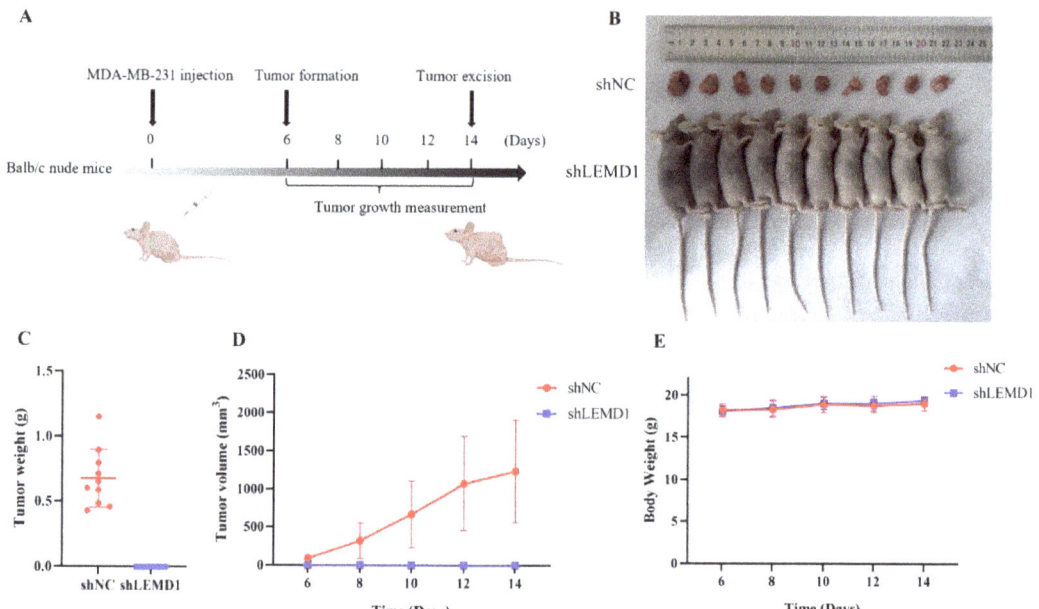

Figure 4. LEMD1 promotes tumor growth in vivo. shNC and shLEMD1 transfected MDA-MB-231 cells were administered subcutaneously into 5-week-old female Balb/c nude mice. (**A**) Diagram of the in vivo experiment. (**B–D**) The tumor sizes were monitored on the indicated days. After 2 weeks, the subcutaneous tumors were excised, weighed and photographed. (**E**) The body weight of the mice was recorded during the experiment.

3.4. LEMD1 Promotes the Cell Proliferation and Invasion by Activating ERK Signaling Pathway in TNBC

To explore the mechanism underlying the promotive effect of LEMD1 on the progression of TNBC, RNA-seq was conducted to detect the differentially expressed genes in LEMD1-silenced and control MDA-MB-468 cells. MAPK signaling pathway, an important oncogenic pathway regulating ubiquitous signal transduction process in cancers [22], showed significant differential expression in KEGG pathway enrichment analysis (Figure 5A). MAPK consists of ERK, p38, JNK and ERK5. Furthermore, protein–protein network analysis showed that there are close associations between ERK1/2 and the members of MAPK signaling pathway detected by RNA-seq (Supplementary Figure S5A), suggesting that ERK may mediate the carcinogenic role of LEMD1 in TNBC. To validate this hypothesis, we detected the protein expressions of ERK and p-ERK in LEMD1-knockout (KO) and LEMD1-knockdown (KD) cells. Figure 5B showed that LEMD1 knockout or knockdown remarkably down-regulated the expression of p-ERK, but did not change the expression of ERK, indicating that LEMD1 can activate ERK. Next, LEMD1-knockout and LEMD1-knockdown cells were transfected with ERK plasmid and then treated with the ERK inhibitor, U0126. Figure 5C showed that overexpression of ERK increased the expressions of

ERK and p-ERK, and the increased p-ERK induced by ERK overexpression can be reversed by U0126. To investigate whether ERK is involved in the regulation of LEMD1 on tumor progression, cell proliferation and migration were measured. As shown in Figure 5D–G and Supplementary Figure S5B,C, the inhibitory effects on the cell proliferation and migration induced by LEMD1-KD/KO were reversed by ERK overexpression in TNBC cells. It has been reported that ERK activation can promote EMT process in various cancers [23–25]. ERK activity can also inhibit cancer cell apoptosis by increasing Bcl-2 expression and decreasing Bax expression [26,27]. Consistently, we found that the regulation of E-cadherin, N-cadherin and vimentin expressions by LEMD1-KO/KD was significantly abolished by overexpression of ERK (Figure 5H and Supplementary Figure S5D). Moreover, the increase in Bax expression and the decrease in Bcl-2 expression induced by LEMD1-KO/KD were also rescued by ERK overexpression (Figure 5I and Supplementary Figure S5E). Moreover, cell viability assay also showed that the rescue effect of ERK overexpression in LEMD1-KO/KD cells could be canceled by U0126 treatment (Figure 5J and Supplementary Figure S5F), further confirming the crucial role of ERK activation in mediating the oncogenic role of LEMD1 in TNBC cells. Taken together, these data suggested that LEMD1 promotes the progression of TNBC by activation ERK signaling pathway.

3.5. LEMD1 Knockdown Enhances the Chemosensitivity of TNBC Cells to Paclitaxel

In the previous screening process of the target gene, we found that the high expression of LEMD1 was associated with anti-cancer drug resistance in breast cancer cell lines via genomic analysis (Figure 6A), which inspired us to explore the role of LEMD1 in chemotherapy resistance. Considering that chemotherapy remains the major means for TNBC treatment, we further investigated whether LEMD1 is involved in the regulation of the sensitivity of chemotherapeutic drugs in TNBC cells. Firstly, we evaluated the effect of LEMD1 on chemotherapeutic responses of TNBC patients by ROC plotter server. Figure 6B shows that TNBC patients with low LEMD1 expression benefited more from chemotherapies. Next, we further examined the impact of LEMD1 expression on the sensitivity of TNBC cells to paclitaxel, the main chemotherapeutic used for the treatment of TNBC. Figure 6C showed that BT549 and HCC1806 cells with lower LEMD1 expression were more sensitive to paclitaxel than MDA-MB-468 and MDA-MB-231 cells with higher LEMD1 expression, indicating the role of LEMD1 in promoting paclitaxel resistance of TNBC cells. Further experiments showed that LEMD1 knockdown markedly reduced the viability of MDA-MB-231 cells treated with paclitaxel (Figure 6D). The sensitization effect of LEMD1 knockdown on paclitaxel was also confirmed by colony formation assay and EdU assays (Figure 6E,F). LEMD1 knockdown further down-regulated the expression of Bcl-2, increased the expression of Bax compared to paclitaxel alone treatment (Figure 6G). These findings suggested that LEMD1 silencing enhances the efficacy of paclitaxel in TNBC cells.

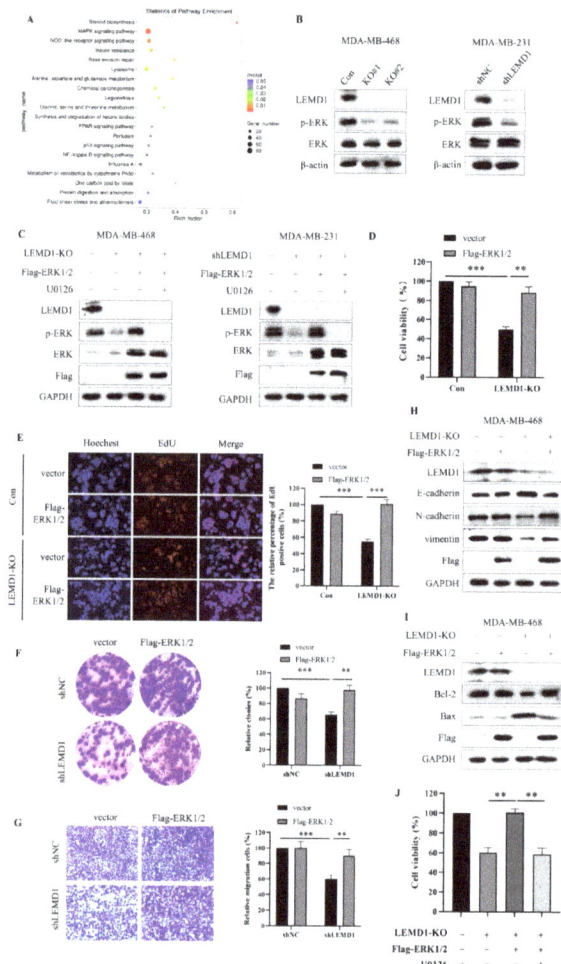

Figure 5. LEMD1 promotes cell proliferation and invasion by activating ERK in TNBC. (**A**) Signaling pathway enrichment analysis of siNC and siLEMD1 MDA-MB-468 cells by RNA-seq. (**B**) LEMD1 was knocked out by LEMD1-targeting CRISPER/CAS9 system in MDA-MB-468 cells and was knocked down by LEMD1 shRNA in MDA-MB-231 cells. The expressions of ERK, p-ERK were examined by Western blot. β-actin was used as a loading control. (**C**) LEMD1-knockout MDA-MB-468 cells and LEMD1-knockdown MDA-MB-231 cells were transfected with ERK plasmid and then treated with U0126, an ERK inhibitor. The expressions of ERK, p-ERK, Flag were examined by Western blot. GAPDH was used as a loading control. LEMD1-knockout MDA-MB-468 cells were transfected with ERK plasmid or empty vector plasmid. Cell viability was measured using the CCK8 assay (**D**) and EdU assay (**E**), magnification ×200. Additionally, LEMD1-knockdown MDA-MB-231 cells were transfected with ERK plasmid or empty vector plasmid. Cell proliferation was measured via colony formation assay (**F**). Cell migration ability was measured via Transwell migration assay (**G**). Magnification ×200. (**H**) The protein expressions of EMT markers including E-cadherin, N-cadherin, vimentin, and (**I**) The expressions of Bcl-2 and Bax in LEMD1-knockout MDA-MB-468 cells were measured via Western blot. GAPDH was used as a loading control. (**J**) LEMD1-knockout MDA-MB-468 cells were transfected with ERK plasmid and then treated with U0126 for 24 h. Cell viability was measured using the CCK8 assay. ** $p < 0.01$, *** $p < 0.001$, n = 3. The original western blot figures could be found in Supplementary Figure S6B.

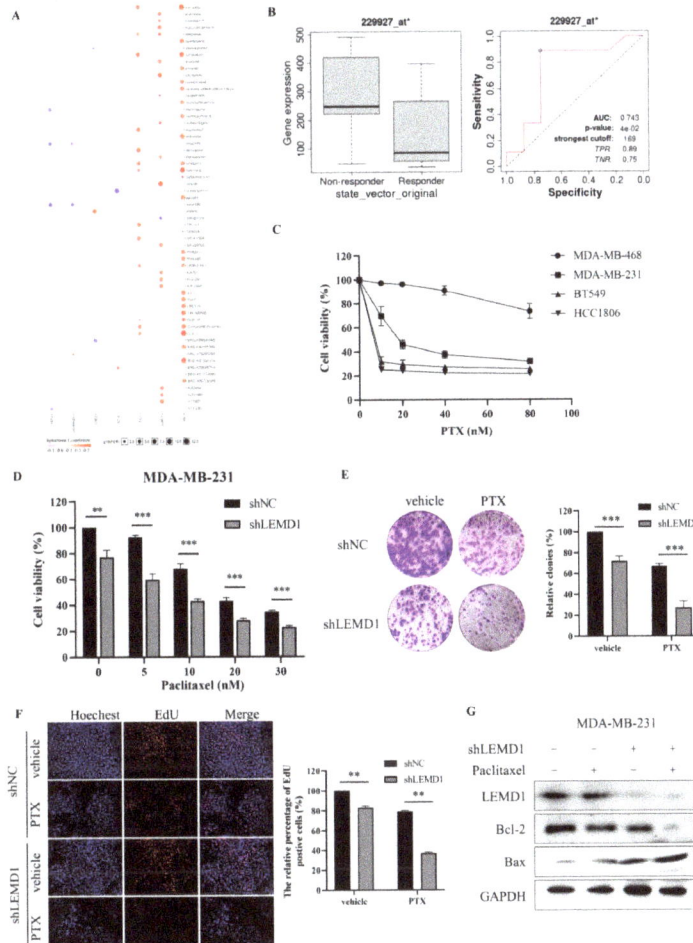

Figure 6. Knockdown of LEMD1 enhances the sensitivity of TNBC cells to paclitaxel. (**A**) Drug resistance analysis of LEMD1, ART3, UGT8, SHC4, HORMAD1, EN1, ZIC1 and CT83 in breast cancer patients by the GSCALite online tool. Red indicates positive relationship, while purple negative. (**B**) The receiver operating characteristic (ROC) curve between LEMD1 expression and therapeutic responses to chemotherapy in TNBC cohorts, * p = 0.04. (**C**) MDA-MB-468, MDA-MB-231, BT549 and HCC1806 cells were treated by paclitaxel with indicated concentration for 72 h. Cell viability was determined via CCK8 assay. (**D**) MDA-MB-231 cells were transfected with LEMD1 shRNA or a negative control, followed by treatment with paclitaxel for 72 h. Cell viability was determined via CCK8 assay. ** p < 0.01, *** p < 0.001, n = 3. (**E**) MDA-MB-231 cells were transfected with LEMD1 shRNA and treated with 10 nM paclitaxel. The colony formation assay was conducted. *** p < 0.001, n = 3. (**F**) MDA-MB-231 cells were transfected with LEMD1 shRNA or a negative control and were treated with 10 nM paclitaxel for 72 h. Then, the cells were subjected to an EdU assay. Magnification ×200. ** p < 0.01, n = 3. (**G**) MDA-MB-231 cells were transfected with LEMD1 shRNA and were treated with 10 nM paclitaxel for 72 h, the levels of Bcl-2 and Bax were analyzed by Western blot. GAPDH was used as a loading control. The original western blot figures could be found in Supplementary Figure S6C.

4. Discussion

Due to the clinical characteristics of lack of an appropriate target and rapid progression of patients, the treatment of TNBC still remains chiefly conventional chemotherapy up to now [4]. This dilemma drives researchers to explore novel molecular markers for targeted therapy. In this study, we demonstrated for the first time that LEMD1 is highly expressed in TNBC and is associated with poor prognosis in breast cancer patients. It has been reported that LEMD1 is upregulated in various kinds of malignancies and facilitates cancer progression [5–8]. Our pan-cancer analysis consistently showed that LEMD1 is overexpressed in various cancers and is associated with shorter survival of tumor patients. Importantly, knockdown of LEMD1 significantly inhibited the proliferation, migration and invasion of TNBC cells. Strikingly, the TNBC cells with LEMD1 knockdown did not form tumors in vivo. These results suggest that LEMD1 may be explored as a novel oncogene and potential therapeutic target for TNBC treatment.

Next, we aimed to figure out the underlying mechanism of LEMD1 promoting the progression of TNBC. We found that LEMD1 activates ERK, and the ERK-mediated signaling pathway is crucial for the regulation of cell proliferation and migration by LEMD1. Accumulating evidences have demonstrated that ERK/MAPK pathway is activated in about 40% of all human cancers, and ERK activation is indispensable for diverse fundamental cell functions including growth, survival and differentiation [22,28–30]. Besides, ERK activity also plays a crucial role in promoting the EMT process [23–25] and inhibiting apoptosis of tumor cells [26,27]. We found that the regulatory role in EMT protein, Bcl-2 and Bax, induced by LEMD1 knockdown, can be rescued by ERK overexpression, indicating that LEMD1 promotes cell proliferation and migration by activating ERK-mediated regulation of EMT proteins Bcl-2 and Bax. However, the precise mechanism of LEMD1 regulating ERK remains unclear. Dual-specificity phosphatases (DUSPs) can dephosphorylate many key signaling molecules, including MAPKs [31]. It was evidenced that ERK can be dephosphorylated by several DUSPs including DUSP5 [32], DUSP6 [33], DUSP9 [34] and DUSP15 [35]. Our transcriptome data showed that LEMD1 could downregulate the mRNA of DUSP5 and DUSP6, indicating that LEMD1 may increase ERK phosphorylation by downregulating DUSP5 and DUSP6.

In addition, we found that high expression of LEMD1 was significantly correlated with decreased responsiveness to chemotherapeutics in TNBC. LEMD1 knockdown combined with paclitaxel exhibited a stronger inhibitory effect on tumor cell proliferation compared to treatment with paclitaxel alone. These results revealed that high expression of LEMD1 may facilitate chemoresistance of TNBC cells, and targeting LEMD1 may provide an effective approach to increase the sensitivity of TNBC cells to chemotherapy.

In this study, we revealed for the first time that LEMD1 is overexpressed in TNBC through analysis of bioinformatic data and collected patient specimens. Silencing of LEMD1 not only inhibits the proliferation, migration and invasion abilities of TNBC cells in vitro, but also abolishes tumor formation of TNBC cells in vivo. Targeting of LEMD1 enhances the sensitivity of TNBC cells to paclitaxel. Mechanistically, we found that the ERK signaling pathway was involved in the regulation of LEMD1 on the proliferation and migration of TNBC cells. Our results revealed the promotive role of LEMD1 in the progress of TNBC and provided a potential therapeutic strategy of targeting LEMD1 for TNBC treatment.

5. Conclusions

In summary, our findings not only provided insight into understanding the mechanism underlying the regulation of cancer cell proliferation and migration by LEMD1, but also laid a solid foundation for the development of a novel oncogene and therapeutic target for TNBC treatment.

Supplementary Materials: The following supporting information can be downloaded at: https://www.mdpi.com/article/10.3390/cancers15112924/s1, Figure S1: The expressions of other 24 genes in breast cancer from GEPIA; Figure S2: The methylation analysis of LEMD1 in breast cancer.

(A) LEMD1 DNA methylation levels in normal and tumor samples of breast cancer patients. (B) The correlation between LEMD1 methylation levels and the disease-free interval (DFI) in breast cancer patients; Figure S3: Pan-cancer analysis of LEMD1 expression and the prognostic value. (A) The mRNA expressions of LEMD1 in cancers from TCGA. (B) GEPIA2 was used to perform the overall survival analysis by LEMD1 expression among various tumors by analyzing data from TCGA database. The survival map and the Kaplan-Meier curves with statistical significance were exhibited; Figure S4: The localization and the oncogenic function of LEMD1 in TNBC cells. (A) The expression of LEMD1 was detected in cytoplasm and nucleus by Western blot. β-actin was used as the cytoplasmic loading control, and Lamin B1 was used as the nuclear loading control. (B) MDA-MB-231 cells were transfected with shRNA or a negative control, CCK-8 reagent was applied to examine cell viability. ** p <0.01, n = 3. (C) Cell proliferation of MDA-MB-231 cells was measured using EdU. Magnification, ×100. ** p < 0.01, n = 3. (D) Western blot analysis of the expressions of Bcl-2 and Bax in MDA-MB-231 cells, β-actin was used as a loading control. (E) Wound healing assays of LEMD1-knockout MDA-MB-468 cells. Magnification, ×100. ** p <0.01, n = 3. (F) Wound healing assays of LEMD1-knockdown MDA-MB-231 cells. Magnification, ×100. ** p < 0.01, n = 3. (G) Western blot analysis of the expressions of E-cadherin, N-cadherin and vimentin in MDA-MB-231 cells, β-actin was used as a loading control. (H) qPCR analysis of the mRNA expressions of Bax, Bcl-2, E-cadherin, N-cadherin and vimentin in MDA-MB-231 cells; Figure S5: LEMD1 promotes the cell proliferation and invasion by activating ERK in TNBC. (A) The PPI network for ERK1 (MAPK3), ERK2 (MAPK1) and the 11 differential genes with significant variation in MAPK signaling pathway from RNA-seq. LEMD1-knockdown MDA-MB-231 cells were transfected with ERK plasmid or empty vector plasmid. (B) Cell viability was measured using the CCK8 assay. (C) Cell proliferation was measured by EdU assay. Magnification, ×200. (D) The protein expressions of EMT markers including E-cadherin, N-cadherin, vimentin, and (E) The expressions of Bcl-2 and Bax in LEMD1-knockdown MDA-MB-231 cells were measured by Western blot. GAPDH was used as a loading control. (F) LEMD1-knockdown MDA-MB-231 cells were transfected with ERK plasmid and then treated with U0126 for 24h. Cell viability was measured using the CCK8 assay; Figure S6: The original western blot figures.

Author Contributions: Y.C. and X.L. conceived and designed the study. X.L. performed the experiments. X.L., S.J., T.J., X.S. and Y.G. conducted the data analysis. S.F. provided the clinical samples. X.L. drafted the manuscript. Y.C. revised and approved the manuscript. All authors have read and agreed to the published version of the manuscript.

Funding: This research was funded by grants from the National Natural Science Foundation of China (No 81972480 to Y.C.), Natural Science Foundation of Hunan Province (No 2022JJ80106 to Y.C.), and Hunan Provincial Health Commission (No 202102080940 to Y.C.).

Institutional Review Board Statement: The animal study protocol was approved by the Ethics Committee of Central South University (Approved No: CSU-2022-0001-0007; date: 21 February 2022).

Informed Consent Statement: Informed consent was obtained from all subjects involved in the study.

Data Availability Statement: The datasets presented in this study can be found in online repositories. The names of the repository/repositories and accession number(s) can be found in the article.

Conflicts of Interest: The authors have declared that they have no conflict of interest.

References

1. Sung, H.; Ferlay, J.; Siegel, R.L.; Laversanne, M.; Soerjomataram, I.; Jemal, A.; Bray, F. Global Cancer Statistics 2020: GLOBOCAN Estimates of Incidence and Mortality Worldwide for 36 Cancers in 185 Countries. *CA Cancer J. Clin.* **2021**, *71*, 209–249. [CrossRef]
2. Harbeck, N.; Gnant, M. Breast cancer. *Lancet* **2017**, *389*, 1134–1150. [CrossRef]
3. Bianchini, G.; Balko, J.M.; Mayer, I.A.; Sanders, M.E.; Gianni, L. Triple-negative breast cancer: Challenges and opportunities of a heterogeneous disease. *Nat. Rev. Clin. Oncol.* **2016**, *13*, 674–690. [CrossRef]
4. Yin, L.; Duan, J.-J.; Bian, X.-W.; Yu, S.-C. Triple-negative breast cancer molecular subtyping and treatment progress. *Breast Cancer Res.* **2020**, *22*, 61. [CrossRef]
5. Yuki, D.; Lin, Y.-M.; Fujii, Y.; Nakamura, Y.; Furukawa, Y. Isolation of LEM domain-containing 1, a novel testis-specific gene expressed in colorectal cancers. *Oncol. Rep.* **2004**, *12*, 275–280. [CrossRef]
6. Ghafouri-Fard, S.; Ashtiani, Z.O.; Golian, B.S.; Hasheminasab, S.-M.; Modarressi, M.H. Expression of Two Testis-specific Genes, SPATA19 and LEMD1, in Prostate Cancer. *Arch. Med. Res.* **2010**, *41*, 195–200. [CrossRef]
7. Li, Q.; Ge, Y.; Chen, X.; Wang, L.; Xia, Y.; Xu, Z.; Li, Z.; Wang, W.; Yang, L.; Zhang, D.; et al. LEM domain containing 1 promotes proliferation via activating the PI3K/Akt signaling pathway in gastric cancer. *J. Cell. Biochem.* **2019**, *120*, 15190–15201. [CrossRef]

8. Cao, X.; Yao, N.; Zhao, Z.; Fu, Y.; Hu, Y.; Zhu, P.; Shi, W.; Tang, L. LEM domain containing 1 promotes pancreatic cancer growth and metastasis by p53 and mTORC1 signaling pathway. *Bioengineered* **2022**, *13*, 7771–7784. [CrossRef]
9. Martinez-Romero, J.; Bueno-Fortes, S.; Martín-Merino, M.; De Molina, A.R.; De Las Rivas, J. Survival marker genes of colorectal cancer derived from consistent transcriptomic profiling. *BMC Genom.* **2018**, *19* (Suppl. 8), 857. [CrossRef]
10. Sasahira, T.; Kurihara, M.; Nakashima, C.; Kirita, T.; Kuniyasu, H. LEM domain containing 1 promotes oral squamous cell carcinoma invasion and endothelial transmigration. *Br. J. Cancer* **2016**, *115*, 52–58. [CrossRef]
11. Xu, M.; Lin, B.; Zheng, D.; Wen, J.; Hu, W.; Li, C.; Zhang, X.; Zhang, X.; Qu, J. LEM domain containing 1 promotes thyroid cancer cell proliferation and migration by activating the Wnt/β-catenin signaling pathway and epithelial-mesenchymal transition. *Oncol. Lett.* **2021**, *21*, 442. [CrossRef]
12. Takeda, R.; Hirohashi, Y.; Shen, M.; Wang, L.; Ogawa, T.; Murai, A.; Yamamoto, E.; Kubo, T.; Nakatsugawa, M.; Kanaseki, T.; et al. Identification and functional analysis of variants of a cancer/testis antigen LEMD1 in colorectal cancer stem-like cells. *Biochem. Biophys. Res. Commun.* **2017**, *485*, 651–657. [CrossRef]
13. Ding, W.; Chen, J.; Feng, G.; Chen, G.; Wu, J.; Guo, Y.; Ni, X.; Shi, T. DNMIVD: DNA methylation interactive visualization database. *Nucleic Acids Res.* **2019**, *48*, D856–D862. [CrossRef]
14. Li, T.; Fu, J.; Zeng, Z.; Cohen, D.; Li, J.; Chen, Q.; Li, B.; Liu, X.S. TIMER2.0 for analysis of tumor-infiltrating immune cells. *Nucleic Acids Res.* **2020**, *48*, W509–W514. [CrossRef]
15. Liu, C.-J.; Hu, F.-F.; Xia, M.-X.; Han, L.; Zhang, Q.; Guo, A.-Y. GSCALite: A web server for gene set cancer analysis. *Bioinformatics* **2018**, *34*, 3771–3772. [CrossRef]
16. Fekete, J.T.; Győrffy, B. ROCplot.org: Validating predictive biomarkers of chemotherapy/hormonal therapy/anti-HER2 therapy using transcriptomic data of 3,104 breast cancer patients. *Int. J. Cancer* **2019**, *145*, 3140–3151. [CrossRef]
17. Qin, G.; Wang, X.; Ye, S.; Li, Y.; Chen, M.; Wang, S.; Qin, T.; Zhang, C.; Li, Y.; Long, Q.; et al. NPM1 upregulates the transcription of PD-L1 and suppresses T cell activity in triple-negative breast cancer. *Nat. Commun.* **2020**, *11*, 1669. [CrossRef]
18. Chen, X.; Wang, K.; Jiang, S.; Sun, H.; Che, X.; Zhang, M.; He, J.; Wen, Y.; Liao, M.; Li, X.; et al. eEF2K promotes PD-L1 stabilization through inactivating GSK3β in melanoma. *J. Immunother. Cancer* **2022**, *10*, e004026. [CrossRef]
19. Zhang, Y.; Zhang, Y.; Zhang, L. Expression of cancer–testis antigens in esophageal cancer and their progress in immunotherapy. *J. Cancer Res. Clin. Oncol.* **2019**, *145*, 281–291. [CrossRef]
20. Sharma, P.; Shen, Y.; Wen, S.; Bajorin, D.F.; Reuter, V.E.; Old, L.J.; Jungbluth, A.A. Cancer-Testis Antigens: Expression and Correlation with Survival in Human Urothelial Carcinoma. *Clin. Cancer Res.* **2006**, *12*, 5442–5447. [CrossRef]
21. Hemminger, J.A.; Toland, A.E.; Scharschmidt, T.J.; Mayerson, J.L.; Kraybill, W.G.; Guttridge, D.C.; Iwenofu, O.H. The cancer-testis antigen NY-ESO-1 is highly expressed in myxoid and round cell subset of liposarcomas. *Mod. Pathol.* **2013**, *26*, 282–288. [CrossRef]
22. Lee, S.; Rauch, J.; Kolch, W. Targeting MAPK Signaling in Cancer: Mechanisms of Drug Resistance and Sensitivity. *Int. J. Mol. Sci.* **2020**, *21*, 1102. [CrossRef]
23. Huang, L.; Chen, S.; Fan, H.; Ji, D.; Chen, C.; Sheng, W. GINS2 promotes EMT in pancreatic cancer via specifically stimulating ERK/MAPK signaling. *Cancer Gene Ther.* **2021**, *28*, 839–849. [CrossRef]
24. Wang, J.; Zhang, Z.; Li, R.; Mao, F.; Sun, W.; Chen, J.; Zhang, H.; Bartsch, J.-W.; Shu, K.; Lei, T. ADAM12 induces EMT and promotes cell migration, invasion and proliferation in pituitary adenomas via EGFR/ERK signaling pathway. *Biomed. Pharmacother.* **2018**, *97*, 1066–1077. [CrossRef]
25. Sheng, W.; Shi, X.; Lin, Y.; Tang, J.; Jia, C.; Cao, R.; Sun, J.; Wang, G.; Zhou, L.; Dong, M. Musashi2 promotes EGF-induced EMT in pancreatic cancer via ZEB1-ERK/MAPK signaling. *J. Exp. Clin. Cancer Res.* **2020**, *39*, 16. [CrossRef]
26. Wang, B.; Zhu, X.-X.; Pan, L.-Y.; Chen, H.-F.; Shen, X.-Y. PP4C facilitates lung cancer proliferation and inhibits apoptosis via activating MAPK/ERK pathway. *Pathol. Res. Pr.* **2020**, *216*, 152910. [CrossRef]
27. Castro, M.V.; Barbero, G.A.; Máscolo, P.; Ramos, R.; Quezada, M.J.; Lopez-Bergami, P. ROR2 increases the chemoresistance of melanoma by regulating p53 and Bcl2-family proteins via ERK hyperactivation. *Cell. Mol. Biol. Lett.* **2022**, *27*, 23. [CrossRef]
28. Degirmenci, U.; Wang, M.; Hu, J. Targeting Aberrant RAS/RAF/MEK/ERK Signaling for Cancer Therapy. *Cells* **2020**, *9*, 198. [CrossRef]
29. Chen, Y.; Nowak, I.; Huang, J.; Keng, P.C.; Sun, H.; Xu, H.; Wei, G.; Lee, S.O. Erk/MAP Kinase Signaling Pathway and Neuroendocrine Differentiation of Non–Small-Cell Lung Cancer. *J. Thorac. Oncol.* **2014**, *9*, 50–58. [CrossRef]
30. Setia, S.; Nehru, B.; Sanyal, S.N. Upregulation of MAPK/Erk and PI3K/Akt pathways in ulcerative colitis-associated colon cancer. *Biomed. Pharmacother.* **2014**, *68*, 1023–1029. [CrossRef]
31. Chen, H.-F.; Chuang, H.-C.; Tan, T.-H. Regulation of Dual-Specificity Phosphatase (DUSP) Ubiquitination and Protein Stability. *Int. J. Mol. Sci.* **2019**, *20*, 2668. [CrossRef] [PubMed]
32. Kidger, A.M.; Rushworth, L.K.; Stellzig, J.; Davidson, J.; Bryant, C.J.; Bayley, C.; Caddye, E.; Rogers, T.; Keyse, S.M.; Caunt, C.J. Dual-specificity phosphatase 5 controls the localized inhibition, propagation, and transforming potential of ERK signaling. *Proc. Natl. Acad. Sci. USA* **2017**, *114*, E317–E326. [CrossRef]
33. Domercq, M.; Alberdi, E.; Gomez, M.V.S.; Ariz, U.; Samartin, A.L.P.; Matute, C. Dual-specific Phosphatase-6 (Dusp6) and ERK Mediate AMPA Receptor-induced Oligodendrocyte Death. *J. Biol. Chem.* **2011**, *286*, 11825–11836. [CrossRef]

34. Li, Z.; Fei, T.; Zhang, J.; Zhu, G.; Wang, L.; Lu, D.; Chi, X.; Teng, Y.; Hou, N.; Yang, X.; et al. BMP4 Signaling Acts via Dual-Specificity Phosphatase 9 to Control ERK Activity in Mouse Embryonic Stem Cells. *Cell Stem Cell* **2012**, *10*, 171–182. [CrossRef]
35. Rodríguez-Molina, J.F.; Lopez-Anido, C.; Ma, K.H.; Zhang, C.; Olson, T.; Muth, K.N.; Weider, M.; Svaren, J. Dual specificity phosphatase 15 regulates Erk activation in Schwann cells. *J. Neurochem.* **2017**, *140*, 368–382. [CrossRef]

Disclaimer/Publisher's Note: The statements, opinions and data contained in all publications are solely those of the individual author(s) and contributor(s) and not of MDPI and/or the editor(s). MDPI and/or the editor(s) disclaim responsibility for any injury to people or property resulting from any ideas, methods, instructions or products referred to in the content.

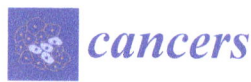

Article

Breast Digital Tomosynthesis versus Contrast-Enhanced Mammography: Comparison of Diagnostic Application and Radiation Dose in a Screening Setting

Luca Nicosia [1,*], Anna Carla Bozzini [1], Filippo Pesapane [1], Anna Rotili [1], Irene Marinucci [1], Giulia Signorelli [1], Samuele Frassoni [2], Vincenzo Bagnardi [2], Daniela Origgi [3], Paolo De Marco [3], Ida Abiuso [4], Claudia Sangalli [5], Nicola Balestreri [6], Giovanni Corso [7,8,9] and Enrico Cassano [1]

1 Breast Imaging Division, Radiology Department, IEO European Institute of Oncology IRCCS, 20141 Milan, Italy
2 Department of Statistics and Quantitative Methods, University of Milan-Bicocca, 20126 Milan, Italy
3 Medical Physics Unit, IEO European Institute of Oncology IRCCS, Via Ripamonti 435, 20141 Milan, Italy
4 Radiology Department, Università Degli Studi di Torino, 10124 Turin, Italy
5 Data Management, IEO European Institute of Oncology IRCCS, 20141 Milan, Italy
6 Department of Radiology, IEO European Institute of Oncology IRCCS, 20141 Milan, Italy
7 Division of Breast Surgery, IEO European Institute of Oncology IRCCS, 20141 Milan, Italy
8 Department of Oncology and Hemato-Oncology, University of Milan, 20122 Milan, Italy
9 European Cancer Prevention Organization, 20122 Milan, Italy
* Correspondence: luca.nicosia@ieo.it

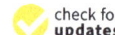

Citation: Nicosia, L.; Bozzini, A.C.; Pesapane, F.; Rotili, A.; Marinucci, I.; Signorelli, G.; Frassoni, S.; Bagnardi, V.; Origgi, D.; De Marco, P.; et al. Breast Digital Tomosynthesis versus Contrast-Enhanced Mammography: Comparison of Diagnostic Application and Radiation Dose in a Screening Setting. *Cancers* 2023, 15, 2413. https://doi.org/10.3390/cancers15092413

Academic Editor: Naiba Nabieva

Received: 28 February 2023
Revised: 15 April 2023
Accepted: 20 April 2023
Published: 22 April 2023

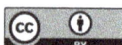

Copyright: © 2023 by the authors. Licensee MDPI, Basel, Switzerland. This article is an open access article distributed under the terms and conditions of the Creative Commons Attribution (CC BY) license (https://creativecommons.org/licenses/by/4.0/).

Simple Summary: Screening mammography reduces mortality from breast malignancy. However, breast cancer screening is, unfortunately, hindered due to the poor sensitivity of mammography in dense breasts: up to 15–30% of all cancers may be missed. Given the rapid development of Contrast-Enhanced Mammography (CEM) and its potential for diagnostic use, even in an asymptomatic population, it seems very important to correctly assess the Average Glandular Dose (AGD) for a single CEM examination. Few studies have compared the AGD of CEM versus Digital Mammography (DM) and protocols, including Digital Breast Tomosynthesis (DBT) plus DM, in the same group of patients. The additional role of tomosynthesis versus digital mammography in asymptomatic patients with dense breasts in screening examinations has been well investigated with encouraging results. In this study, we intend to compare the AGD and the diagnostic performance of CEM versus DM, and of CEM versus DM + DBT, performed in the same group of patients over the same period of time in a screening setting.

Abstract: This study aims to evaluate the Average Glandular Dose (AGD) and diagnostic performance of CEM versus Digital Mammography (DM) as well as versus DM plus one-view Digital Breast Tomosynthesis (DBT), which were performed in the same patients at short intervals of time. A preventive screening examination in high-risk asymptomatic patients between 2020 and 2022 was performed with two-view Digital Mammography (DM) projections (Cranio Caudal and Medio Lateral) plus one Digital Breast Tomosynthesis (DBT) projection (mediolateral oblique, MLO) in a single session examination. For all patients in whom we found a suspicious lesion by using DM + DBT, we performed (within two weeks) a CEM examination. AGD and compression force were compared between the diagnostic methods. All lesions identified by DM + DBT were biopsied; then, we assessed whether lesions found by DBT were also highlighted by DM alone and/or by CEM. We enrolled 49 patients with 49 lesions in the study. The median AGD was lower for DM alone than for CEM (3.41 mGy vs. 4.24 mGy, $p = 0.015$). The AGD for CEM was significantly lower than for the DM plus one single projection DBT protocol (4.24 mGy vs. 5.55 mGy, $p < 0.001$). We did not find a statistically significant difference in the median compression force between the CEM and DM + DBT. DM + DBT allows the identification of one more invasive neoplasm one in situ lesion and two high-risk lesions, compared to DM alone. The CEM, compared to DM + DBT, failed to identify only one of the high-risk lesions. According to these results, CEM could be used in the screening of asymptomatic high-risk patients.

Keywords: Contrast-Enhanced Mammography; Digital Breast Tomosynthesis; breast cancer screening; Average Glandular Dose

1. Introduction

About 12% of the world's diagnosed neoplasms are breast neoplasms, with about eight million women involved worldwide [1]. It has now been widely recognized that screening mammography reduces mortality from breast malignancy [2]: the mortality rate decreased by about 1.9% annually between 1998 and 2013.

A screening program aims to find small cancers before they become clinically evident; for example, European guidelines offer mammography every two years for the general female population from 50 to 70 years of age [3]. One of the main issues of mammographic screening is related to the poor sensitivity of mammography in dense breasts; up to 15–30% of all cancers may be missed [4].

Some studies have introduced Digital Breast Tomosynthesis (DBT) in mammography screening, especially in high-risk patients with dense breasts [5–7]. Those studies found increased cancer detection rates with DBT, from 1.9 to 4.1 per 1000 women screened with recall rates lower than or comparable to those with DM, and an increased cancer detection rate of up to 30–40% [8]. In accordance with the results of these studies, personalized screening based on breast density could be offered that would increase the cancer detection rate and reduce the number of recalls for benign conditions; in fact, DBT seems to be associated, in addition to an increased cancer detection rate, especially in dense breasts, with a higher positive predictive value of recalls [9,10].

In this context, moreover, many studies have confirmed the interesting performance of Contrast-Enhanced Mammography (CEM) when applied to the early detection of mammary neoplasms [11], and some preliminary studies have also evaluated the use of CEM in breast-screening programs, with encouraging results [12,13]. These preliminary studies show that CEM has a high negative predictive value in the evaluation of breast lesions and can significantly reduce the number of screening recalls for benign breast conditions, which suggests a potential for a reduction in screening recalls.

To our knowledge, however, the possible role of CEM as an alternative method to conventional screening mammography in some high-risk patient populations has not yet been prospectively investigated.

Given the rapid development of CEM and its potential for diagnostic use, even in an asymptomatic population (screening), it seems very important to correctly assess the Average Glandular Dose (AGD) for a single CEM examination. While many studies have evaluated the diagnostic performance of tomosynthesis and CEM, far fewer studies have compared the AGD of these two methods. In particular, as far as we know, only one study focused on the same group of patients undergoing both tomosynthesis and CEM at short intervals [14]. The dose can be affected by total breast thickness, breast density, and the age of patients [15–17].

The purpose of our study is to compare the AGD in the same group of patients undergoing two views of Digital Mammography (DM), plus one view of Digital Breast Tomosynthesis (DBT), followed by Contrast-Enhanced Mammography (CEM) within a short time (within two weeks). The execution of the diagnostic tests we performed on the same patients allowed us to reduce the variances that may occur in different patients (e.g., different breast density, total breast thickness, and age). AGD is a parameter that should be considered before proposing CEM in a screening setting in asymptomatic patients. As a secondary objective, we also wanted to evaluate whether the number of additional breast cancer lesions identified by tomosynthesis (compared with digital mammography alone) was also identified by CEM.

2. Materials and Methods

After the approval of our institutional review board and ethics committee, we started to enroll patients for a monocentric and prospective trial. All patients consented by signing a specific, informed consent for the study.

We performed preventive screening examinations in high-risk asymptomatic patients between 2020 and 2022. All participants were offered two-view Digital Mammography (DM) projections (Cranio Caudal and Medio Lateral) plus one projection with Digital Breast Tomosynthesis (DBT) (mediolateral oblique, MLO) in a single session examination; this protocol (DM plus one single projection DBT) reproduces what has already been investigated in the Malmö Breast Tomosynthesis Screening Trial with encouraging results [18].

For all patients in whom we found a suspicious lesion with DM + DBT (B.I.-RADS > 3), according to the Breast Imaging Reporting and Data System [19], a CEM examination (within two weeks) was performed. In each case, we used an AGD protocol in the range of international guidelines [20].

Protocol for CEM examination: two bilateral Cranio Caudal (CC) and mediolateral oblique (MLO) projection views were acquired after the intravenous injection of an iodinated contrast agent (Ioexolo) (300 mg/mL, 1.5 mL/kg, Omnipaque®, GE Healthcare, Chalfont St. Giles, UK). Two exposures were acquired, one with low energy (26–32 kVp) and one with high energy (45–49 kVp). The low- and high-energy images were then recombined to highlight the uptake of the contrast agent. In none of the cases in our study were late projections acquired.

Three mammography systems (GE® Healthcare, Senographe Pristina®, Chalfont St. Giles, UK, or the Amulet® Innovality® Fujifilm, Akasaka Minato-ku Tokyo, Japan or Selenia® Dimension® Hologic, Marlborough, MA, USA) were used for this study.

The device was equipped with these anode/filter combinations: Mo-Mo, Rh/Ag, W/Rh; W/Ag; W/Al; Mo/Cu; Rh/Cu; W/Cu (Mo: molybdenum; Rh: rhodium; Al: aluminum; W: tungsten; Cu: copper; Ag: silver) as we can see in Table 1.

Table 1. Systems used for this study with information of anode/filter combination for Digital Mammography (DM), Digital Breast Tomosynthesis (DBT), and Contrast-Enhanced Mammography (CEM).

System	Anode/Filter DM [1]	Anode/Filter DBT [2]	Anode/Filter CEM [3] LE [4]	Anode/Filter CEM HE [5]
General Electric Pristina	Mo/Mo [6] Rh [7]/Ag	Mo/Mo Rh/Ag	Mo/Mo Rh/Ag	Mo/Cu Rh/Cu
Hologic 3Dimensions	W [8]/Rh W/Ag [11]	W/Al [9]	W/Rh W/Ag	W/Cu [10]
Fuji Amulet Innovality	W/Rh	W/Al	W/Rh	W/Cu

[1] DM: Digital Mammography; [2] DBT: Digital Breast Tomosynthesis; [3] CEM: Contrast-Enhanced mammography; [4] LE: low energy; [5] HE: High energy; [6] Mo: molybdenum; [7] Rh: rhodium; [8] W: tungsten; [9] Al: aluminum; [10] Cu: copper; [11] Ag: silver.

We collected data regarding the age of enrolled patients, breast density, and average glandular dose in Milligray (mGy) of mammographic projections alone (DM), mammographic projections plus Digital Breast Tomosynthesis (DBT), and Contrast-Enhanced Mammography (CEM), respectively. AGD was then compared. We also measured and compared the compression force in Newton (N) and the total breast thickness in millimeters (mm) at the time of examination, both for the DM + DBT protocol and CEM protocol. Doses, in terms of average glandular doses, the compression force and the total breast thickness at the time of examination have been extracted from the DICOM header on images. Average glandular doses reported in the DICOM header were calculated with the Dance model for all the systems [21].

All lesions (BIRADS > 3) identified by DBT were biopsied; we assessed whether lesions found by DBT were also highlighted by DM alone and/or CEM. Two experienced radiologists evaluated all images with more than five years of experience in consensus. (L.N.: 5 years of experience in breast imaging and A.B.: more than 25 years of experience in breast imaging).

Image assessment was performed using the mammographic BIRADS [19] for DM + DBT and the new BIRADS for CEM [22]. In the case of enhancement at CEM, this was evaluated according to the lesion conspicuity descriptor (defined as the enhancement intensity relative to the surrounding background) [22,23].

According to the World Health Organization's classification of breast tumors, all lesions were categorized depending on the biopsy results [24].

In particular, we considered the following categorizations:
- B2: benign lesions.
- B3: high-risk lesions
- B5a: in situ lesions.
- B5b: invasive lesions.

2.1. Inclusion Criterion of the Study
- Asymptomatic patients undergoing mammography and tomosynthesis in which there is a dubious finding (BI-RADS > 3).
- Patients at high risk for the development of breast neoplasia (at least one first-degree relative with breast neoplasm).
- Patients with suspicious findings (BI-RADS > 3) undergoing CEM examination.
- Patients who have signed a specific, informed consent for the study.
- Patients with age > 18 years old.

2.2. Exclusion Criterion of the Study
- Patients with known allergy to iodinated contrast medium.
- Symptomatic patients with palpable breast lumps.
- Patients with breast implant(s).
- Patients with proven or supposed pregnancy.

2.3. Statistical Analysis

Continuous data were reported as medians and ranges, and categorical data were reported as counts and percentages. The paired t-test was used to compare the distribution of the AGD, the total breast thickness, and of the compression force between the examined techniques. A p-value less than 0.05 was considered statistically significant. All analyses were performed with the statistical software SAS 9.4 (SAS Institute, Cary, NC, USA).

3. Results

From a group of 125 high-risk and asymptomatic patients who have performed mammography plus tomosynthesis, we enrolled 49 patients in the study.

A flowchart diagram of the inclusion/exclusion criteria of the study is shown in Figure 1.

The median age of the patients was 52 years (range: 40–80). In 63% of cases, the lesion found was in microcalcifications, and in 29% of cases was in the form of mass. The breasts were dense in more than 70% of cases, according to the ACR classification [19]. In more than 50% of cases, the BI-RADS classification was 4a.

The descriptive characteristics of the patients are summarized in Table 2.

The median CEM AGD dose of our examinations was 4.24 mGy (range: 1.96–7.60), the median DM AGD was 3.41 mGy (range: 1.14–6.65), and the AGD of DM + one single projection DBT was 5.55 mGy (range: 2.07–10.06) (Figure 2).

The median AGD was lower for DM alone than for CEM ($p = 0.015$), and the AGD dose for CEM was significantly lower than for the DM plus one single projection DBT protocol ($p < 0.001$). The distribution of examinations performed per mammograph was as follows:

- CEM mammograph: 10 (20%) Fuji Amulet Innovality; 34 (69%) GE Pristina; 5 (10%) Hologic 3Dimensions.
- DM + DBT mammograph: 26 (53%) GE Pristina; 23 (47%) Hologic 3Dimensions.

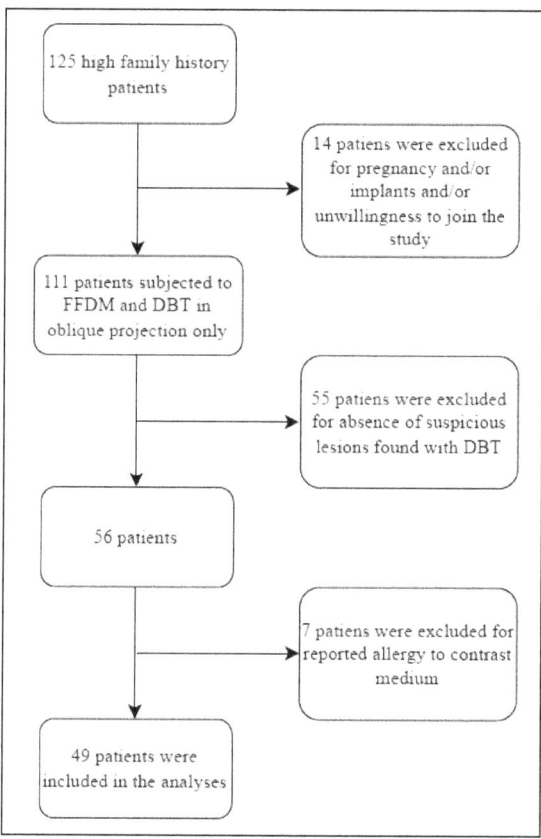

Figure 1. Flowchart diagram of the inclusion and exclusion criteria of the study.

Table 2. Descriptive characteristics of the patients.

Variable	Level	Overall (N = 49)
Age at CEM [1] (y [2]), median (min–max)		52 (40–80)
Type of lesion—DM [3] + DBT [4], N (%)	Microcalcifications	31 (63)
	Mass	14 (29)
	Mass with microcalcifications	1 (2)
	Architectural distortion	3 (6)
Density (ACR [5]), N (%)	B	12 (24)
	C	32 (65)
	D	5 (10)
BI-RADS–DBT, N (%)	3	7 (14)
	4a	25 (51)
	4b	8 (16)
	4c	9 (18)

[1] CEM: Contrast-Enhanced Mammography; [2] y: years; [3] DM: Digital Mammography; [4] DBT: Digital Breast Tomosynthesis; [5] ACR: American College of Radiology.

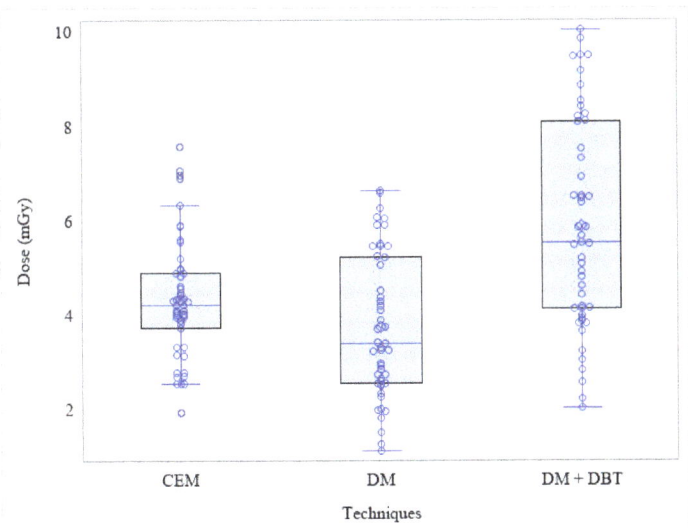

Figure 2. Average Glandular Dose (AGD) among different techniques. (CEM: Contrast-Enhanced Mammography; DM: Digital Mammography; DBT: Digital Breast Tomosynthesis).

Twenty-two patients had the same CEM and DM + DBT mammograph (18 GE Pristina and 4 Hologic 3Dimensions).

Among these 22 patients, the median CEM AGD was 4.51 mGy (range: 3.17–7.60), the median DM AGD alone was 4.31 mGy (range: 2.52–6.65), and the median AGD of DM + one single projection DBT was 6.52 mGy (range: 4.00–10.06) (Figure 3). The results of the paired *t*-test analyses were: CEM vs. DM + DBT: $p < 0.001$; DM vs. DM + DBT: $p < 0.001$; CEM vs. DM: $p = 0.27$.

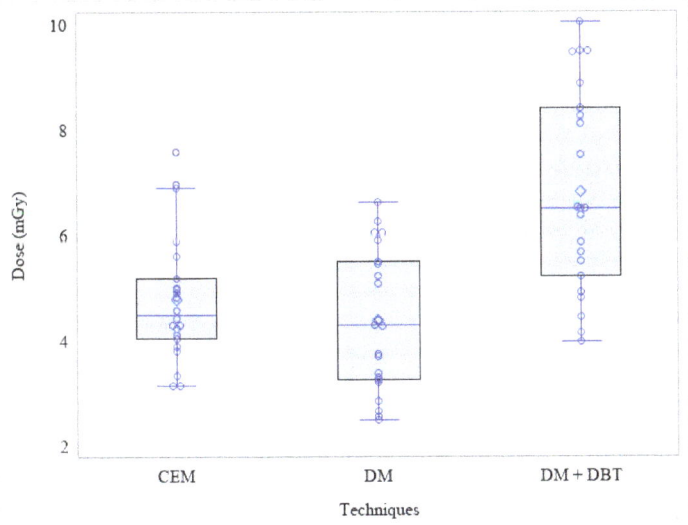

Figure 3. Average glandular dose among different techniques (CEM: Contrast-Enhanced Mammography; DM: Digital Mammography; DBT: Digital Breast Tomosynthesis) among the Twenty-two patients who performed CEM and DM + DBT with the same mammograph.

The median AGD for CEM was significantly lower than for the DM plus one single projection DBT protocol ($p < 0.001$).

The median CEM compression force (N) was 65 (range: 31–114), and the median DM + DBT compression force (N) was 69 (range: 28–116). We did not find a statistically significant difference in the median compression force between the CEM and DM + DBT examinations ($p = 0.79$).

In Figure 4, we can appreciate the similar distribution between compression force in CEM examinations and DM + DBT examinations.

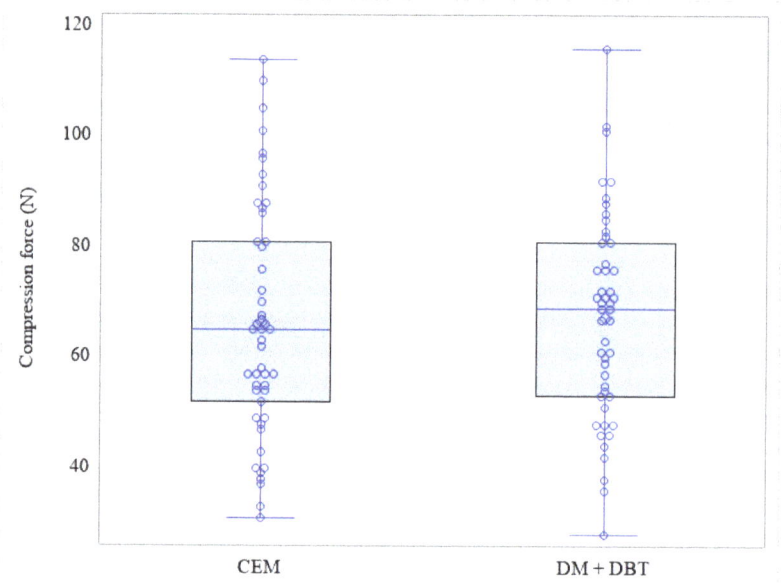

Figure 4. Distribution of CEM and DM + DBT compression force (N) (CEM: Contrast-Enhanced Mammography; DM: Digital Mammography; DBT: Digital Breast Tomosynthesis).

The median CEM breast thickness was 51mm (range: 29–79mm). The median DM + DBT breast thickness was 52 mm, (range: 31–79mm). The p-value of a paired t-test testing the difference in total breast thickness in the same patients was 0.009.

With the DM + DBT protocol, we identified 49 breast lesions deemed worthy of in-depth biopsy.

The overall histological results of the biopsy are summarized in Table 3. In particular, we obtained 30 (61%) B2 benign lesions, 9 (18%) high-risk B3 lesions, 7 (14%) B5a (in situ lesions), and 3 (6%) B5b (invasive lesions).

The analysis of DM images alone (without evaluating tomosynthesis projection) identified the presence of 38/49 lesions (78%). Of the 11 additional lesions found by DBT image analysis (10 of which were found in very dense breasts), 7 were benign lesions (B2), 2 were high-risk lesions (B3), 1 was an in-situ lesion (B5a), and 1 was an invasive lesion (B5b). In Figure 5, we can appreciate the example of a breast lesion studied with DM, DBT, and CEM.

Figure 5 shows a 41-year-old asymptomatic woman with grade I familiarity with breast neoplasm who performed a preventive oncologic screening examination with our study protocol (DM + DBT).

In (a), we show the left breast studied with DM in the mediolateral projection; here, a barely perceptible breast finding can be appreciated that could be easily interpreted as glandular tissue (arrow). In (b), the same breast is studied with a tomosynthesis acquisition

(DBT) that highlights the structural distortion associated with the breast finding (arrow). The recombined CEM image (c) highlights a nodule with suspicious enhancement (arrow).

Table 3. Histological results of the biopsy (N = 49).

	Histological Results of the Biopsy	Overall (N = 49)
B2	Adenosis	4
	Breast fibroadenoma	4
	Ductal hyperplasia without atypia	1
	Fibrocystic disease	18
	Fibrosis	1
	Flogosis	2
B3	Atypical ductal hyperplasia (Din1b)	2
	Atypical lobular hyperplasia (LIN1)	1
	Flat epithelial atypia (FEA)	1
	Intraductal papilloma	4
	Radial scar	1
B5a	High-grade ductal carcinoma in situ (DIN3)	3
	Intermediate-grade ductal carcinoma in situ (DIN2)	2
	Low-grade ductal carcinoma in situ (DIN1c)	2
B5b	Invasive ductal carcinoma	2
	Invasive lobular carcinoma	1

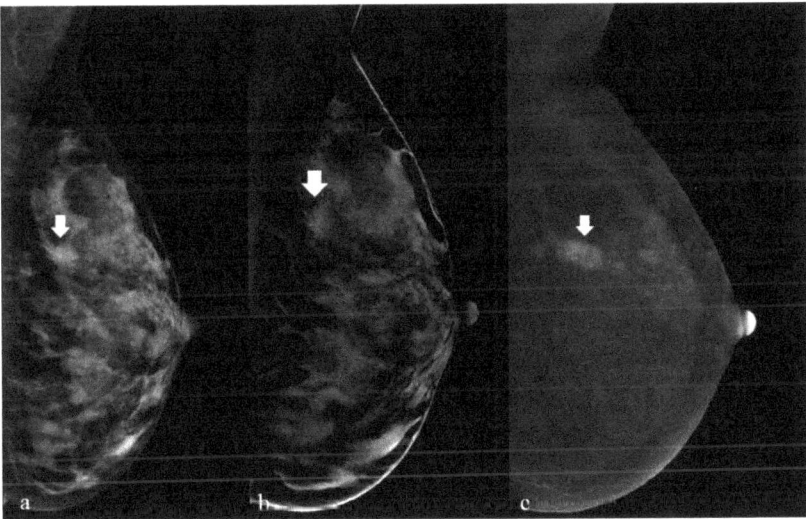

Figure 5. The appearance of a breast lesion with DM, DBT, and CEM.

The analysis of the low-energy CEM image alone, regarding the detection of breast lesions, showed very similar results to the DM analysis (See Table 4). The addition of recombined image analysis (as opposed to low energy analysis alone) allowed us to identify one more in situ lesion and two more invasive neoplasms. A schematic summary of lesion visibility by this method is shown in Table 4 (recombined image and low energy CEM are part of the same method and should therefore be considered together when considering whether there has been lesion detection or not).

Table 4. Histological results of the biopsy and visibility (N = 49).

Histological Results	Visibility									
	DM [1]		DM + DBT [2]		Recombined (CEM) [3]		Low Energy (CEM)		Recombined + Low Energy	
	No	Yes	No	Yes	No	Yes	No	Yes	No	Yes
B2 (N = 30)	7	23	0	30	25	5	8	22	6	24
B3 (N = 9)	2	7	0	9	6	3	2	7	2	7
B5a (N = 7)	1	6	0	7	2	5	1	6	0	7
B5b (N = 3)	1	2	0	3	0	3	2	1	0	3
Total	11	38	0	49	33	16	13	36	8	41

[1] DM: Digital Mammography; [2] DBT: Digital Breast Tomosynthesis; [3] CEM: Contrast-Enhanced mammography.

4. Discussion

Early diagnosis of breast cancer is the key to ensuring a better prognosis and management of patients with this disease [25]; mammography is the leading test in breast cancer screening examinations. It has been shown to reduce breast cancer-specific mortality [25]. The diagnostic performance of mammography in breasts with a predominantly adipose component is excellent. However, this performance declines dramatically in predominantly dense and highly dense breasts, representing about 50% of the population [26]. The sensitivity of mammography alone in identifying breast neoplasms in dense breasts may drop 50% below [27]. This value is too low to ensure early diagnosis and adequate management of life-threatening diseases [27,28].

The additional role of tomosynthesis in asymptomatic patients with predominantly dense breasts in screening examinations has been well investigated with encouraging results. DBT has demonstrated an increased cancer detection rate of 2.2 to 2.5 per 1000 screenings [5–8]. However, one of the main problems associated with the use of tomosynthesis in a screening setting is a non-negligible average glandular dose to which patients are subjected [29]. The possibility of screening examinations in high-risk patients with breast MRI has been investigated with excellent results [30,31]. However, even in this case, some issues must be solved, particularly the high cost, limited availability, and high false-positive rate [32].

Contrast-enhanced mammography has become increasingly popular in recent years, proving to be a technique with excellent diagnostic performance (even in the dense breast) that is relatively fast and cheap, with a low number of false positives [11]. As a result, its use in a screening context of high-risk patients could be a good compromise between cost and benefit. However, few studies have compared the AGD between CEM and tomosynthesis [14–17]. As far as we know, only one study has compared AGD in the same patients [14]. Our study presents results that are comparable to those of Philips et al. [14] in a group of 45 patients who underwent a CEM protocol and a tomosynthesis protocol at short intervals; in these results, CEM had a significantly lower average glandular dose than mammography protocols performed with tomosynthesis. Furthermore, as discussed in studies that have proposed MRI in high-risk patients [31,32], contrast agent exposure in screening seems to be acceptable for women at 20% or greater lifetime risk of breast cancer [33]. In our opinion, the conclusions reached in MRI on the contrast medium with Gadolinium can also be applied to the iodinated contrast agents used in CEM. One of the most comprehensive literature reviews published by Zanardo et al. [34], analyzed the adverse reactions to the use of contrast agents associated with CEM by evaluating more than 80 studies and using the fixed-effect model. A pooled rate of adverse reactions of 0.82% (0.64–1.05% 95% CI), with a total of 30 adverse reactions in 14,012 patients, was reported. Moreover, of these 30 adverse reactions, only 1 (3%) was found to be severe.

In our study, we reproduced the protocol with tomosynthesis in a single projection: tomosynthesis performed in a single projection lowers the AGD [18]. However, even in this case, according to our experience, CEM demonstrates a lower AGD. Promising results, in terms of the reduction of AGD in tomosynthesis screening protocols, could be obtained using the 2-D synthetic image of tomosynthesis as an alternative to digital mammography [35]. However, many doubts still need to be solved about the diagnostic quality of the 2-D synthetic image of tomosynthesis, which, right now, does not allow it to be considered a safe alternative to digital mammography [36,37].

One of the peculiar aspects of our study is that we performed DM + DBT and CEM in the same patients at short intervals.

The average glandular dose is, in fact, greatly influenced by the total breast thickness and breast density [20]. Comparing the methods performed on the same patients allowed us to minimize the confounding effect these variables could represent in the comparison. The AGD could be influenced by the different compression forces to which the breast was subjected during the examination; for example, in Figure 4, we can see no statistically significant difference between the average compressive forces to which the breasts were subjected during the examinations. This confounding effect was, therefore, also minimized.

Although a statistically significant difference was found with the paired t-test between breast thickness in the same patients and between the two types of examinations (DM + DBT and CEM), the difference was only a few mm (never approaching a centimeter). Therefore, in our opinion, it did not clinically significantly affect the average glandular dose. The variation of only a few millimeters of total breast thickness, in the same patients, between DM + DBT and CEM, can be appreciated in Supplementary Figure S1 (Matched Boxplot).

Finally, in our case history, we found that the CEM analysis identified all the cancerous lesions that tomosynthesis allowed us to identify more than the analysis of digital mammography alone. With the CEM, the two neoplasms would have been identified (one in situ and one infiltrating) that were "missed" with the DM. The results we obtained are therefore encouraging both in terms of AGD and diagnostic utility. In accordance with other preliminary retrospective studies performed on the same topic [38], CEM could be proposed as a screening test, especially in dense breasts, in patients at high risk for the development of neoplastic neoplasia.

One of the main limitations of our study is represented by its monocentric nature and the limited number of patients; therefore, our results should be considered as preliminary results to propose CEM in a screening protocol in asymptomatic, high-risk patients with predominantly dense breasts. Variable in AGD could also depend on system-specific equipment. Unfortunately, in our study, we had few examinations performed with mammograms to compare AGD between different vendors adequately. We recommend that efforts along these lines be made in subsequent studies. For example, based on results available in the literature [39,40], it seems that different vendors expose to different AGDs, depending on total breast thickness.

5. Conclusions

Contrast-enhanced mammography offers a lower AGD than digital mammography protocols with added tomosynthesis. Its diagnostic performance is no less than that of digital mammography plus tomosynthesis. Its use in screening settings in dense breasts and high-risk patients appears promising. This work may lay the basis for broader screening studies that confirm these results. CEM could improve detection in high-risk patients with dense breasts compared to conventional screening with a lower dose than protocols, including tomosynthesis. These results, if confirmed, could revolutionize the approach to preventive screening in high-risk patients, especially in cases of dense breasts.

Supplementary Materials: The following supporting information can be downloaded at: https://www.mdpi.com/article/10.3390/cancers15092413/s1, Figure S1: Matched BoxPlot of differences (in millimeters) in total breast thickness, in the same patients, between Contrast-Enhanced Mammography and Digital Mammography plus tomosynthesis.

Author Contributions: Conceptualization, L.N., N.B. and A.C.B.; methodology, F.P. and A.C.B.; software, D.O., P.D.M., N.B., V.B. and S.F.; validation, V.B., S.F. and E.C.; formal analysis, S.F. and V.B.; investigation, L.N., I.A., G.S. and A.R.; resources, E.C.; data curation, C.S.; writing—original draft preparation, L.N. and G.S.; writing—review and editing, I.M., G.C. and A.R.; visualization, A.R.; supervision, A.C.B. and E.C.; project administration L.N. and E.C. All authors have read and agreed to the published version of the manuscript.

Funding: This research received no external funding.

Institutional Review Board Statement: Institutional Review Board Statement: The study was conducted according to the guidelines of the Declaration of Helsinki and approved by the Ethics Committee of European Institute of Oncology (Protocol Number IEO 960, 7 September 2020).

Informed Consent Statement: Informed consent was obtained from all subjects involved in the study.

Data Availability Statement: The data presented in this study are available on request from the corresponding author. The data are not publicly available due to privacy concerns, in accordance with GDPR.

Conflicts of Interest: The authors declare no conflict of interest.

References

1. World Health Organization. Breast Cancer 2021. Available online: https://www.who.int/news-room/fact-sheets/detail/breast-cancer (accessed on 10 June 2022).
2. Independent UK Panel on Breast Cancer Screening. The benefits and harms of breast cancer screening: An independent review. *Lancet* **2012**, *380*, 1778–1786. [CrossRef]
3. Perry, N.; Broeders, M.; de Wolf, C.; Törnberg, S.; Holland, R.; von Karsa, L. European guidelines for quality assurance in breast cancer screening and diagnosis. Fourth edition—Summary document. *Ann. Oncol.* **2008**, *19*, 614–622. [CrossRef] [PubMed]
4. Bochud, F.O.; Valley, J.F.; Verdun, F.R.; Hessler, C.; Schnyder, P. Estimation of the noisy component of anatomical backgrounds. *Med. Phys.* **1999**, *26*, 1365–1370. [CrossRef]
5. Caumo, F.; Montemezzi, S.; Romanucci, G.; Brunelli, S.; Bricolo, P.; Cugola, L.; Gennaro, G. Repeat Screening Outcomes with Digital Breast Tomosynthesis Plus Synthetic Mammography for Breast Cancer Detection: Results from the Prospective Verona Pilot Study. *Radiology* **2021**, *298*, 49–57. [CrossRef]
6. Skaane, P. Breast cancer screening with digital breast tomosynthesis. *Breast Cancer* **2017**, *24*, 32–41. [CrossRef] [PubMed]
7. Pattacini, P.; Nitrosi, A.; Giorgi Rossi, P.; Iotti, V.; Ginocchi, V.; Ravaioli, S.; Vacondio, R.; Braglia, L.; Cavuto, S.; Campari, C.; et al. Digital Mammography versus Digital Mammography Plus Tomosynthesis for Breast Cancer Screening: The Reggio Emilia Tomosynthesis Randomized Trial. *Radiology* **2018**, *288*, 375–385. [CrossRef] [PubMed]
8. Ciatto, S.; Houssami, N.; Bernardi, D.; Caumo, F.; Pellegrini, M.; Brunelli, S.; Tuttobene, P.; Bricolo, P.; Fantò, C.; Valentini, M.; et al. Integration of 3D digital mammography with tomosynthesis for population breast-cancer screening (STORM): A prospective comparison study. *Lancet Oncol.* **2013**, *14*, 583–589. [CrossRef]
9. Li, T.; Houssami, N.; Noguchi, N.; Zeng, A.; Marinovich, M.L. Differential detection by breast density for digital breast tomosynthesis versus digital mammography population screening: A systematic review and meta-analysis. *Br. J. Cancer* **2022**, *127*, 116–125. [CrossRef]
10. Libesman, S.; Zackrisson, S.; Hofvind, S.; Seidler, A.L.; Bernardi, D.; Lång, K.; Robledo, K.P.; Houssami, N. An individual participant data meta-analysis of breast cancer detection and recall rates for digital breast tomosynthesis versus digital mammography population screening. *Clin. Breast Cancer* **2022**, *22*, e647–e654. [CrossRef]
11. Cozzi, A.; Magni, V.; Zanardo, M.; Schiaffino, S.; Sardanelli, F. Contrast-enhanced Mammography: A Systematic Review and Meta-Analysis of Diagnostic Performance. *Radiology* **2022**, *302*, 568–581. [CrossRef]
12. Lobbes, M.B.; Lalji, U.; Houwers, J.; Nijssen, E.C.; Nelemans, P.J.; van Roozendaal, L.; Smidt, M.L.; Heuts, E.; Wildberger, J.E. Contrast-enhanced spectral mammography in patients referred from the breast cancer screening programme. *Eur. Radiol.* **2014**, *24*, 1668–1676. [CrossRef] [PubMed]
13. Cozzi, A.; Schiaffino, S.; Fanizza, M.; Magni, V.; Menicagli, L.; Monaco, C.G.; Benedek, A.; Spinelli, D.; Di Leo, G.; Di Giulio, G.; et al. Contrast-enhanced mammography for the assessment of screening recalls: A two-centre study. *Eur. Radiol.* **2022**, *32*, 7388–7399. [CrossRef] [PubMed]
14. Phillips, J.; Mihai, G.; Hassonjee, S.E.; Raj, S.D.; Palmer, M.R.; Brook, A.; Zhang, D. Comparative Dose of Contrast-Enhanced Spectral Mammography (CESM), Digital Mammography, and Digital Breast Tomosynthesis. *AJR Am. J. Roentgenol.* **2018**, *211*, 839–846. [CrossRef] [PubMed]
15. James, J.R.; Pavlicek, W.; Hanson, J.A.; Boltz, T.F.; Patel, B.K. Breast Radiation Dose with CESM Compared with 2D FFDM and 3D Tomosynthesis Mammography. *AJR Am. J. Roentgenol.* **2017**, *208*, 362–372. [CrossRef] [PubMed]
16. Gennaro, G.; Cozzi, A.; Schiaffino, S.; Sardanelli, F.; Caumo, F. Radiation Dose of Contrast-Enhanced Mammography: A Two-Center Prospective Comparison. *Cancers* **2022**, *14*, 1774. [CrossRef] [PubMed]

17. Bicchierai, G.; Busoni, S.; Tortoli, P.; Bettarini, S.; Naro, F.D.; De Benedetto, D.; Savi, E.; Bellini, C.; Miele, V.; Nori, J. Single Center Evaluation of Comparative Breast Radiation dose of Contrast Enhanced Digital Mammography (CEDM), Digital Mammography (DM) and Digital Breast Tomosynthesis (DBT). *Acad. Radiol.* **2022**, *29*, 1342–1349. [CrossRef]
18. Lång, K.; Andersson, I.; Rosso, A.; Tingberg, A.; Timberg, P.; Zackrisson, S. Performance of one-view breast tomosynthesis as a stand-alone breast cancer screening modality: Results from the Malmö Breast Tomosynthesis Screening Trial, a population-based study. *Eur. Radiol.* **2016**, *26*, 184–190. [CrossRef]
19. D'Orsi, C.J.; Sickles, E.A.; Mendelson, E.B.; Morris, E.A. *ACR BI-RADS Atlas: Breast Imaging Re-Porting and Data System*; American College of Radiology: Reston, VA, USA, 2013.
20. International Atomic Energy Agency. *Dosimetry in Diagnostic Radiology: An International Code of Practice*; International Atomic Energy Agency: Vienna, Austria, 2007; Volume 457.
21. Dance, D.R.; Skinner, C.L.; Young, K.C.; Beckett, J.R.; Kotre, C.J. Additional factors for the estimation of mean glandular breast dose using the UK mammography dosimetry protocol. *Phys. Med. Biol.* **2000**, *45*, 3225–3240. [CrossRef]
22. Lee, C.H.; Phillips, J.; Sung, J.S.; Lewin, J.M.; Newell, M.S. *Contrast Enhanced Mammography (CEM) (A Supplement to ACR BI-RADS® Mammography 2013) Atlas, Breast Imaging Reporting and Data System*; American College of Radiology: Reston, VA, USA, 2022.
23. Nicosia, L.; Bozzini, A.C.; Palma, S.; Pesapane, F.; Meneghetti, L.; Pizzamiglio, M.; Abbate, F.; Latronico, A.; Bagnardi, V.; Frassoni, S.; et al. Breast Imaging Reporting and Data System and Contrast Enhancement Mammography: Lesion Conspicuity Likelihood of Malignancy and Relationship with Breast Tumor Receptor Status. *Acad. Radiol.* **2023**, *in press*. [CrossRef]
24. Hoon Tan, P.; Ellis, I.; Allison, K.; Brogi, E.; Fox, S.B.; Lakhani, S.; Lazar, A.J.; Morris, E.A.; Sahin, A.; Salgado, R.; et al. The 2019 World Health Organization classification of tumours of the breast. *Histopathology* **2020**, *77*, 181–185. [CrossRef]
25. Smith, R.A.; Duffy, S.W.; Gabe, R.; Tabar, L.; Yen, A.M.; Chen, T.H. The randomized trials of breast cancer screening: What have we learned? *Radiol. Clin. N. Am.* **2004**, *42*, 793–806. [CrossRef] [PubMed]
26. Kerlikowske, K.; Zhu, W.; Tosteson, A.N.; Sprague, B.L.; Tice, J.A.; Lehman, C.D.; Miglioretti, D.L.; Breast Cancer Surveillance Consortium. Identifying women with dense breasts at high risk for interval cancer: A cohort study. *Ann. Intern. Med.* **2015**, *162*, 673–681. [CrossRef]
27. Kolb, T.M.; Lichy, J.; Newhouse, J.H. Comparison of the performance of screening mammography, physical examination, and breast US and evaluation of factors that influence them: An analysis of 27,825 patient evaluations. *Radiology* **2002**, *225*, 165–175. [CrossRef]
28. Magnoni, F.; Corso, G. Progress in breast cancer surgical management. *Eur. J. Cancer Prev.* **2022**, *31*, 551–553. [CrossRef] [PubMed]
29. Svahn, T.M.; Houssami, N.; Sechopoulos, I.; Mattsson, S. Review of radiation dose estimates in digital breast tomosynthesis relative to those in two-view full-field digital mammography. *Breast* **2015**, *24*, 93–99. [CrossRef] [PubMed]
30. Hussein, H.; Abbas, E.; Keshavarzi, S.; Fazelzad, R.; Bukhanov, K.; Kulkarni, S.; Au, F.; Ghai, S.; Alabousi, A.; Freitas, V. Supplemental Breast Cancer Screening in Women with Dense Breasts and Negative Mammography: A Systematic Review and Meta-Analysis. *Radiology* **2023**, *306*, e221785. [CrossRef] [PubMed]
31. Kuhl, C.K.; Strobel, K.; Bieling, H.; Leutner, C.; Schild, H.H.; Schrading, S. Supplemental Breast MR Imaging Screening of Women with Average Risk of Breast Cancer. *Radiology* **2017**, *283*, 361–370. [CrossRef]
32. Li, F.Y.; Hollingsworth, A.; Lai, W.T.; Yang, T.L.; Chen, L.J.; Wang, W.T.; Wang, J.L.; Morse, A.N. Feasibility of Breast MRI as the Primary Imaging Modality in a Large Asian Cohort. *Cureus* **2021**, *13*, e15095. [CrossRef]
33. Sardanelli, F.; Cozzi, A.; Trimboli, R.M.; Schiaffino, S. Gadolinium Retention and Breast MRI Screening: More Harm Than Good? *AJR Am. J. Roentgenol.* **2020**, *214*, 324–327. [CrossRef]
34. Zanardo, M.; Cozzi, A.; Trimboli, R.M.; Labaj, O.; Monti, C.B.; Schiaffino, S.; Carbonaro, L.A.; Sardanelli, F. Technique, protocols and adverse reactions for contrast-enhanced spectral mammography (CESM): A systematic review. *Insights Imaging* **2019**, *10*, 76. [CrossRef]
35. Zuckerman, S.P.; Conant, E.F.; Keller, B.M.; Maidment, A.D.; Barufaldi, B.; Weinstein, S.P.; Synnestvedt, M.; McDonald, E.S. Implementation of Synthesized Two-dimensional Mammography in a Population-based Digital Breast Tomosynthesis Screening Program. *Radiology* **2016**, *281*, 730–736. [CrossRef] [PubMed]
36. Kleinknecht, J.H.; Ciurea, A.I.; Ciortea, C.A. Pros and cons for breast cancer screening with tomosynthesis—A review of the literature. *Med. Pharm. Rep.* **2020**, *93*, 335–341. [CrossRef] [PubMed]
37. Chikarmane, S. Synthetic Mammography: Review of Benefits and Drawbacks in Clinical Use. *J. Breast Imaging* **2022**, *4*, 124–134. [CrossRef]
38. Sorin, V.; Yagil, Y.; Yosepovich, A.; Shalmon, A.; Gotlieb, M.; Neiman, O.H.; Sklair-Levy, M. Contrast-Enhanced Spectral Mammography in Women With Intermediate Breast Cancer Risk and Dense Breasts. *AJR Am. J. Roentgenol.* **2018**, *211*, W267–W274. [CrossRef] [PubMed]
39. Kelly, M.; Tyler, N.; Mackenzie, A. Technical Evaluation of SenoBright HD Contrast-Enhanced Mammography Functions of Senographe GE Pristina System Technical Report 2004. December 2020. Available online: https://medphys.royalsurrey.nhs.uk/nccpm/files/other/Tech_Eval_CESMGE_Pristina_NCCPMformatFinalV2.pdf (accessed on 7 April 2023).
40. Kelly, M.; Rai, M.; Mackenzie, A. Technical Evaluation of Contrast Enhanced Mammography Functions Using Hologic I-View Software. Technical Report 2003. November 2020. Available online: https://medphys.royalsurrey.nhs.uk/nccpm/files/other/Tech_Eval_CESM_Hologic3Dimensions_Final.pdf (accessed on 7 April 2023).

Disclaimer/Publisher's Note: The statements, opinions and data contained in all publications are solely those of the individual author(s) and contributor(s) and not of MDPI and/or the editor(s). MDPI and/or the editor(s) disclaim responsibility for any injury to people or property resulting from any ideas, methods, instructions or products referred to in the content.

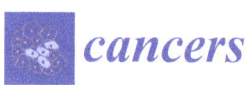

Article

Demographic and Clinical Features of Patients with Metastatic Breast Cancer: A Retrospective Multicenter Registry Study of the Turkish Oncology Group

Izzet Dogan [1], Sercan Aksoy [2], Burcu Cakar [3], Gul Basaran [4], Ozlem Ercelep [5], Nil Molinas Mandel [6], Taner Korkmaz [7], Erhan Gokmen [3], Cem Sener [8], Adnan Aydiner [1], Pinar Saip [1] and Yesim Eralp [9,*]

[1] Department of Medical Oncology, Institute of Oncology, Istanbul University, Istanbul 34093, Turkey; izzet.dogan@istanbul.edu.tr (I.D.)
[2] Department of Medical Oncology, Hacettepe University Cancer Institute, Ankara 06100, Turkey
[3] Department of Medical Oncology, Faculty of Medicine, Ege University, Izmir 35100, Turkey
[4] Department of Medical Oncology, Acibadem University, Altunizade Acibadem Hospital, Istanbul 34662, Turkey
[5] Department of Medical Oncology, Faculty of Medicine, Marmara University, Istanbul 34722, Turkey
[6] Department of Medical Oncology, Koç University Amerikan Hospital, Istanbul 34010, Turkey
[7] Department of Medical Oncology, Acibadem University, Maslak Acibadem Hospital, Istanbul 34457, Turkey
[8] Incidence Medical Research and Biostatistics Consultancy Services, Istanbul 34440, Turkey
[9] Research Institute of Senology, Acıbadem University, Maslak Acıbadem Hospital, Istanbul 34457, Turkey
* Correspondence: yesim.eralp@acibadem.com

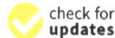

Citation: Dogan, I.; Aksoy, S.; Cakar, B.; Basaran, G.; Ercelep, O.; Molinas Mandel, N.; Korkmaz, T.; Gokmen, E.; Sener, C.; Aydiner, A.; et al. Demographic and Clinical Features of Patients with Metastatic Breast Cancer: A Retrospective Multicenter Registry Study of the Turkish Oncology Group. *Cancers* 2023, 15, 1667. https://doi.org/10.3390/cancers15061667

Academic Editor: Naiba Nabieva

Received: 16 February 2023
Revised: 4 March 2023
Accepted: 5 March 2023
Published: 8 March 2023

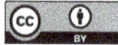

Copyright: © 2023 by the authors. Licensee MDPI, Basel, Switzerland. This article is an open access article distributed under the terms and conditions of the Creative Commons Attribution (CC BY) license (https://creativecommons.org/licenses/by/4.0/).

Simple Summary: Despite advances in treatment generated by clinical trials in metastatic breast cancer (MBC), their impact on routine daily practice and the reflection of the outcome within the community remains unclear. This study evaluates time-related differences in treatment patterns and outcome in a real-world patient population with MBC over a ten-year timeframe. Except for the HER2+ subgroup, which showed a significant survival benefit with the incorporation of novel agents, we failed to identify significant variations in outcomes for the remaining subgroups. A consistent feature we observed was the challenge in treating TNBC, which had the worst prognosis in both time-related cohorts. Elucidation of biologic characteristics to identify novel treatment options remains an unmet need to improve outcomes in TNBC. The favorable survival attained with routine endocrine agents in the luminal A subgroup suggests that barriers in access to CDK inhibitors may not have a negative impact on the outcome in subgroups of hormone receptor-positive patients, constituting an appealing strategy for communities with limited resources.

Abstract: This multicenter registry study aims to analyze time-related changes in the treatment patterns and outcome of patients with metastatic breast cancer (MBC) over a ten-year period. Correlations between demographic, prognostic variables and survival outcomes were carried out in database aggregates consisting of cohorts based on disease presentation (recurrent vs. de novo) and the diagnosis date of MBC (Cohort I: patient diagnosed between January 2010 and December 2014; and Cohort II: between January 2015 and December 2019). Out of 1382 patients analyzed, 52.3% patients had recurrent disease, with an increased frequency over time (47.9% in Cohort I vs. 56.1% in Cohort II, $p < 0.001$). In recurrent patients, 38.4% ($n = 277$) relapsed within two years from initial diagnosis, among which triple-negative BC (TNBC) was the most frequent (51.7%). Median overall survival (OS) was 51.0 (48.0–55.0) months for all patients, which was similar across both cohorts. HER2+ subtype had the highest OS among subgroups (HER2+ vs. HR+ vs. TNBC; 57 vs. 52 vs. 27 months, $p < 0.001$), and the dnMBC group showed a better outcome than recMBC (53 vs. 47 months, $p = 0.013$). Despite the lack of CDK inhibitors, luminal A patients receiving endocrine therapy had a favorable outcome (70 months), constituting an appealing approach with limited resources. The only survival improvement during the timeframe was observed in HER2+ dnMBC patients (3-year OS Cohort I: 62% vs. Cohort II: 84.7%, $p = 0.009$). The incorporation of targeted agents within standard treatment has improved the outcome in HER2+ MBC patients over time. Nevertheless, despite advances in early diagnosis and treatment, the prognosis of patients with TNBC remains poor, highlighting the need for more effective treatment options.

Keywords: breast cancer; metastasis; treatment; human epidermal growth factor receptor 2; hormone receptor; registries

---

1. Introduction

According to the Globocan registry, breast cancer (BC) is the most frequent cancer type among women in Turkey, with 24,175 new cases diagnosed in 2020, comprising 23.9% of all female cancers nationwide [1]. Based on the 2017 Turkish registry database, approximately 10% of all new patients present with metastatic disease annually, remaining relatively stable over the last decade [2]. Nevertheless, despite the similar incidence on a global scale, the estimated 5.7% mortality rate compares favorably with the global mortality rate reaching 15.5%, reflecting widespread adoption of modern diagnostic and therapeutic techniques in the management of patients diagnosed with breast cancer in Turkey [1,3]. Guidelines and reimbursement strategies for the diagnosis and treatment of oncology patients are determined through discussions held by the scientific and financial committees established under Order by the Turkish Ministry of Health. These national guidelines, consisting of evidence-based practice patterns and sequential treatment options, are implemented by the Social Security System to cover all healthcare expenses of Turkish citizens throughout the country. In accordance with these guidelines reflecting most of the modern treatment approaches in the higher Human Development Index countries, metastatic breast cancer patients have access to most targeted agents as well as cytotoxic and endocrine agents, which are updated regularly based on scientific evidence as well as fiscal and monetary policies of the time.

Although the prognosis of specific subtypes of metastatic BC (MBC) patients seems to have improved over the last decade, the outcome is highly variable based on differences in presentation, patient-related factors, genomic landscape of the disease, as well as disparities in healthcare and access to novel medications [4–7]. Advances in diagnostic techniques and increased awareness, especially in communities with a strong health infrastructure and high income, have resulted in a lower incidence of de novo metastatic presentation at initial diagnosis, with incidence rates declining from around 25–28% at the turn of the century to 6–9% in the past decade [8,9]. This shift in metastatic patterns may have affected prognosis over time, as metastatic disease following treatment for early-stage disease has been universally associated with a poor outcome. The shorter survival of recurrent MBC (recMBC) has been linked to several adverse prognostic factors, including a higher incidence of challenging subtypes such as triple-negative BC (TNBC) or the selection of resistant clones within histologic subgroups [10–12]. In fact, a retrospective U.S. cohort study encompassing a period of three decades extending from 1990 to 2020 has revealed a decrease in the incidence of metastatic progression from early-stage disease, whereas the incidence of de novo MBC (dnMBC) remained relatively constant. In concordance with the expected differences in outcomes, a reverse trend in 5-year cancer-specific survival (CSS) over time was noted, showing an approximately two-fold improvement in the de novo cohort from 28 to 55%, and a deterioration in recMBC from 23% to 13% [12].

Elucidating prognostic variances over time is critical for improving our understanding of the impact of modern treatment approaches in distinct pathologic subgroups and providing further insight into the evolving biology of metastatic patterns. Therefore, this large multicenter registry study was planned to examine survival differences in MBC over the last decade in a qualified real-life setting.

2. Materials and Methods

2.1. Study Design

The Turkish Oncology Group MBC was a multicenter retrospective registry study that aimed to collect the data of adult MBC patients diagnosed between 1 January 2010 and 31 December 2019 at seven tertiary oncology clinics in Turkey. The participating sites, which were identified based on patient volume, academic background, as well as dedication to breast cancer diagnosis and treatment, are academic-based public and private oncology centers known to deliver high-quality healthcare in accordance with globally accepted consensus guidelines. Since all investigators who were invited to participate agreed to contribute, there was no bias in regard to data collection among centers included in the study. Collectively, the database reflects real-world practice in both private and public-based comprehensive academic oncology centers from the three most populated cities comprising 28% of the Turkish population, providing a unique opportunity to evaluate changes in contemporary treatment patterns and outcomes over the analyzed period. Correlations between demographic, prognostic variables and survival outcomes were carried out in database aggregates consisting of cohorts based on disease presentation (recurrent vs. de novo) and the diagnosis date of MBC (Cohort I: patient diagnosed between January 2010 and December 2014; and Cohort II: between January 2015 and December 2019). The primary objective was to assess the impact of changes in utilization of modern treatment options on the outcome of various prognostic subgroups. Secondary endpoints included characterization of metastatic presentation patterns (recurrent vs. de novo) within the specified timeframe and outcomes. The study protocol was approved by the Acıbadem Mehmet Ali Aydınlar University Medical Research Ethics Committee (Approval no and date: 2020-23/35, 5 November 2020). Patients who had given consent for the use of medical records were included in the study.

2.2. Patients and Statistical Analysis

Adult patients aged 18 years or older who were diagnosed with MBC as reported by the investigators were included in this database. De novo disease was defined as MBC diagnosed concurrently or within 3 months of initial BC diagnosis. Initial pathologic diagnosis and treatment details of patients presenting with recMBC were collected from patient charts and reports provided by the investigator. Non-visceral disease was defined as skeletal, distant lymphatic or soft tissue metastasis. The number of metastatic sites were defined as the number of visceral systems involved, or in the case of non-visceral disease, as the number of distinct sites which were not in juxtaposition to an index lesion. Pathologic subgroups of recMBC were preferably based on metastatic site biopsies where available. Hormone-responsive (HR+) disease was defined as membranous estrogen (ER) or progesterone (PR) receptor expression in at least 1% of tumor cells. Luminal A was defined as ER $\geq 10\%$ (+), PR $\geq 20\%$ (+), Her2 (−) and Ki 67 < 20%. Patients were classified as luminal B disease if the tumors were PR < 20%, or Ki67 > 20%, or grade 3. Human epidermal growth factor receptor 2 (HER2) assessment was carried out according to the ASCO CAP 2018 guidelines by the pathology departments of each participating center. Tumors expressing ER or PR and HER2 were classified as luminal B-HER2+ tumors. TNBC was defined as tumors not expressing ER, PR or HER2.

Treatment details were recorded from patient charts, and first-line treatment was described as initial therapy following diagnosis of metastatic disease until progression. Endpoints were defined as: progression-free survival (PFS): time from metastatic diagnosis to first progression or death, whichever occurs first; overall survival (OS): time from metastatic diagnosis to death from any cause; and disease-free interval (DFI): defined as the time from initial diagnosis in the early disease setting to first recurrence.

Treatment patterns were compared descriptively between dnMBC and recMBC cohorts for the whole group and separately for each time period. Fisher's exact test or Chi-square test and the Mann–Whitney U-test were used to compare baseline patient and disease characteristics for categorical and continuous variables, respectively. Survival outcomes were estimated using the Kaplan–Meier product-limit method and compared within each subgroup by the log-rank test. Each endpoint was corrected for established prognostic factors. Hazard ratios (HRs) and their 95% confidence intervals (CIs) were estimated using the Cox regression analysis. Factors that were statistically significant in the univariate model were included in the multivariate model. Analyses were performed using SPSS version 23.0 (IBM Corp. Released 2015. IBM SPSS Statistics for Windows, Version 23.0. Armonk, NY, USA) and MedCalc statistical software version 12.7.0.0 (MedCalc Software, Ostend, Belgium). p values less than or equal to 5% were considered significant.

3. Results

The whole group recorded in the database included 1381 patients, with 641 and 740 patients analyzed in Cohorts I (January 2010–December 2014) and II (January 2015–December 2019), respectively. The median age of the whole patient group was 48 (range 17–91), comprising 755 (62.1%) HR+, 333 (27.4%) HER2+ and 128 (10.5%) TN patients. There were 342 patients (25%) younger than 40 years. Despite the significant shift towards private-based institutions after 2015 (17.6% vs. 30.3%, $p < 0.001$), significantly more patients were treated at community-based academic centers ($n = 1044$, 75%) as compared to private-based academic centers in the whole group ($n = 337$; 25%; $p < 0.001$). There was no difference in the distribution of relevant prognostic factors, including age ($p = 0.117$), stage at presentation (for recMBC only; $p = 0.84$), histology ($p = 0.42$), number of metastatic sites ($p = 0.21$) and use of ablative/local therapy in either cohort (17.5 vs. 15.5% in Cohort I vs. II; $p = 0.33$). At presentation, there were more patients with bone-only disease in the HR+ group ($n = 417$; 62.2%) as compared to HER2+ ($n = 122$; 18.2%) and TN ($n = 38$; 5.7%) subtypes ($p < 0.001$), with a similar distribution in each cohort. There was a numeric increase in the incidence of CNS involvement over time in the HER2+ (Cohort I: $n = 13$; 7.1%; Cohort II: $n = 18$; 12.0%) and the TN subgroups (Cohort I: $n = 8$; 11.8%; Cohort II: $n = 11$; 18.3%) as compared to the HR+ subtype (Cohort I: $n = 14$; 4.5% vs. Cohort II: $n = 19$; 4.2%) ($p = $ NS). Furthermore, there was a trend for a higher ratio of very young patients with MBC aged < 40 in Cohort II among HER2+ (32 vs. 20.2%, $p < 0.001$) and TN (23.3 vs. 19.1%, $p = $ NS) patients. Demographic characteristics in Cohorts I and II are summarized in Table 1.

3.1. Recurrent MBC

Out of 1381 patients analyzed, 52.3% ($n = 722$) of patients had recurrent disease, with an increased frequency over time (47.9% in Cohort I vs. 56.1% in Cohort II, $p < 0.001$). The median age of the patients was 46, ranging between 20 and 81. There was a higher incidence of premenopausal patients in the recMBC group as compared to de novo patients ($p < 0.001$). Forty six percent ($n = 337$) presented with bone-only disease, whereas 316 (43.8%) presented with visceral involvement and 69 (9.6%) with CNS metastasis. There were significantly more patients with HR+ disease ($n = 404$; 55.9%), as compared to HER2+ ($n = 144$; 19.9%) and TN groups ($n = 87$; 12.04%) ($p < 0.001$). Nevertheless, the majority of TN patients presented with recurrent disease as compared to dnMBC in the whole patient population ($n = 87$ vs. 41; 67.9% vs. 32.1%; $p = 0.109$). Time-dependent variations within the entire recMBC group regarding subgroups revealed a significant increase in the ratio of HR+ patients in Cohort II ($n = 251$; 60.5%) vs. Cohort I ($n = 153$; 49.8%) ($p = 0.004$), with an even distribution in luminal A (Cohort I: $n = 59$, 19.2% vs. Cohort II: $n = 99$, 23.9%; $p = 0.14$) vs. luminal B disease (Cohort I: $n = 94$, 30.6% vs. Cohort II: $n = 152$, 36.6%; $p = 0.09$). There was an opposite trend over time noted for HER2+ (Cohort II: $n = 77$, 18.6% vs. Cohort I: $n = 67$, 21.8%; $p = 0.277$), as well as TN patients (Cohort II: $n = 45$, 10.8% vs. Cohort I: $n = 42$, 13.7%; $p = 0.247$) (Table 2).

Table 1. Patient and treatment-related characteristics in all patients and subgroups.

Characteristics	All Patient (n = 1381)			HR+ (n = 755)			HER2+ (n = 333)			TNBC (n = 128)		
	Cohort I	Cohort II	p	Cohort I	Cohort II	p	Cohort I	Cohort II	p	Cohort I	Cohort II	p
n (%)	641 (46.4)	740 (53.6)		310 (41.1)	445 (58.9)		183 (55)	150 (45)		68 (53.1)	60 (46.9)	
Treatment center			<0.001			<0.001			0.002			0.021
Private-based	113 (17.6)	224 (30.3)		55 (17.7)	138 (31)		30 (16.4)	46 (30.7)		9 (13.2)	19 (31.7)	
Community-based	528 (82.4)	516 (69.7)		255 (82.3)	307 (69)		153 (83.6)	104 (69.3)		59 (86.8)	41 (68.3)	
Disease status			<0.001			0.056			0.007			0.158
Recurrent	307 (47.9)	415 (56.1)		153 (49.4)	251 (56.4)		67 (36.6)	77 (51.3)		42 (61.8)	45 (75)	
De novo	334 (52.1)	325 (43.9)		157 (50.6)	194 (43.6)		116 (63.4)	73 (48.7)		26 (38.2)	15 (25)	
Age group, median (range)	48 (17–84)	49 (20–91)	0.117	47 (17–84)	50 (23–82)	0.009	47 (20–80)	46 (25–91)	0.852	50 (24–83)	46 (29–81)	0.176
<40	167 (26.1)	175 (23.7)	0.010	99 (31.9)	100 (22.5)	<0.001	37 (20.2)	48 (32)	0.014	13 (19.1)	14 (23.3)	0.453
40–45	104 (16.2)	136 (18.4)		45 (14.5)	80 (18)		40 (21.9)	24 (16)		11 (16.2)	14 (23.3)	
45–50	104 (16.2)	81 (11.0)		45 (14.5)	47 (10.6)		32 (17.5)	12 (8)		12 (17.6)	11 (18.3)	
50–70	226 (35.3)	309 (41.8)		99 (31.9)	197 (44.3)		67 (36.6)	57 (38)		27 (39.7)	20 (33.3)	
>70	34 (6.1)	31 (4.7)		22 (7.1)	21 (4.7)		7 (3.8)	9 (6)		5 (7.4)	1 (1.7)	
Stage at diagnosis	n = 262	n = 357	0.844	n = 135	n = 226	0.740	n = 61	n = 65	0.542	n = 32	n = 37	0.793
I	29 (11.1)	45 (12.6)		14 (10.4)	28 (12.4)		6 (9.8)	10 (15.4)		2 (6.3)	4 (10.8)	
II	98 (37.4)	131 (36.7)		49 (36.3)	86 (38.1)		19 (31.1)	22 (33.8)		15 (46.9)	16 (43.2)	
III	135 (51.5)	181 (50.7)		72 (53.3)	112 (49.6)		36 (59)	33 (50.8)		15 (46.9)	17 (45.9)	
Histology [†]	n = 286	n = 381	0.416	n = 148	n = 242	0.014	n = 65	n = 74	0.368	n = 37	n = 40	0.117
IDC	243 (85.0)	305 (80.1)		126 (85.1)	185 (76.4)		56 (86.2)	66 (9.27)		33 (89.2)	33 (82.5)	
ILC	22 (7.7)	41 (10.8)		8 (5.4)	35 (14.5)		5 (7.7)	2 (2.7)		3 (8.1)	1 (2.5)	
Mixed	18 (6.3)	29 (7.6)		14 (9.5)	18 (7.4)		2 (3.1)	5 (6.8)		0 (0)	5 (12.5)	
Other	3 (1.0)	6 (1.6)		0 (0)	4 (1.7)		2 (3.1)	1 (1.4)		1 (2.7)	1 (2.5)	
ER receptor level	n = 516	n = 629	<0.001	n = 291	n = 436	0.043	n = 160	n = 137	0.012	n = 57	n = 51	NA
Negative	120 (23.3)	100 (15.9)		3 (1)	2 (0.5)		58 (36.3)	45 (32.8)		57 (100)	51 (100)	
1–9%	9 (1.7)	13 (2.1)		5 (1.7)	6 (1.4)		4 (2.5)	6 (4.4)		0 (0)	0 (0)	
10–20%	27 (5.2)	24 (3.8)		14 (4.8)	11 (2.5)		13 (8.1)	12 (8.8)		0 (0)	0 (0)	
21–50%	70 (13.6)	43 (6.8)		37 (12.7)	33 (7.6)		32 (20)	10 (7.3)		0 (0)	0 (0)	
>50%	290 (56.2)	449 (71.4)		232 (79.7)	384 (88.1)		53 (33.1)	64 (46.7)		0 (0)	0 (0)	

Table 1. Cont.

Characteristics	All Patient (n = 1381)			HR+ (n = 755)			HER2+ (n = 333)			TNBC (n = 128)		
	Cohort I	Cohort II	p	Cohort I	Cohort II	p	Cohort I	Cohort II	p	Cohort I	Cohort II	p
DFI from EBC diagnosis	n = 307	n = 415	0.022	n = 153	n = 251	0.049	n = 67	n = 77	0.775	n = 42	n = 45	0.459
<24 month	103 (33.6)	174 (41.9)		49 (32.0)	105 (41.8)		28 (41.8)	34 (44.2)		20 (47.6)	25 (55.6)	
≥24 month	204 (66.4)	241 (58.1)		104 (68.0)	146 (58.2)		39 (58.2)	43 (55.8)		22 (52.4)	20 (44.4)	
Number of metastatic sites at initial metastatic presentation	n = 641	n = 737	0.211	n = 310	n = 443	0.675			0.124			0.139
≤3	544 (84.9)	607 (82.4)		257 (82.9)	362 (81.7)		160 (87.4)	122 (81.3)		65 (95.6)	52 (86.7)	
>3	97 (15.1)	130 (17.6)		53 (17.1)	81 (18.3)		23 (12.6)	28 (18.7)		3 (4.4)	8 (13.3)	
Use local ablative treatment/surgery for oligometastatic disease			0.334			0.912			0.142			1.000
No	529 (82.5)	625 (84.5)		254 (81.9)	366 (82.2)		149 (81.4)	131 (87.3)		57 (83.8)	50 (83.3)	
Yes	112 (17.5)	115 (15.5)		56 (18.1)	79 (17.8)		34 (18.6)	19 (12.7)		11 (16.2)	10 (16.7)	
Sites of specific metastatic sites at initial metastatic presentation			0.090			0.708			0.066			0.037
Bone-only	292 (45.6)	378 (51.1)		168 (54.2)	249 (56)		67 (36.6)	55 (36.7)		16 (23.5)	22 (36.7)	
Visceral	310 (48.4)	312 (42.2)		128 (41.3)	177 (39.8)		103 (56.3)	77 (51.3)		44 (64.7)	27 (45)	
CNS	23 (3.6)	35 (4.7)		7 (2.3)	13 (2.9)		6 (3.3)	15 (10)		7 (10.3)	5 (8.3)	
Visceral + CNS	16 (2.5)	15 (2.0)		7 (2.3)	6 (1.3)		7 (3.8)	3 (2)		1 (1.5)	6 (10)	

[†] Data of 45 patients with unknown histology were excluded from the analysis. CNS = central nervous system; DFI = disease-free interval; EBC = early breast cancer; ER = estrogen receptor; HER2+ = human epidermal growth factor receptor 2 positive; HR+ = hormone-responsive disease; IDC = invasive ductal carcinoma; ILC = invasive lobular carcinoma; TNBC = triple-negative breast cancer.

Table 2. Patient characteristics by cohorts and metastatic pattern.

	Cohort I			Cohort II		
	Recurrent (n = 307)	De Novo (n = 334)	p-Value	Recurrent (n = 415)	De Novo (n = 325)	p-Value
Age, median (range)	46 (22–80)	49 (17–84)	<0.001	47 (20–81)	52 (23–91)	<0.001
Pathology subtypes, n (%)	n = 262	n = 299		n = 373	n = 282	
HR+	153 (58.4)	157 (52.5)	<0.001	251 (67.3)	194 (68.8)	0.007
HER2+	67 (25.6)	116 (38.8)		77 (20.6)	73 (25.9)	
TNBC	42 (16.0)	26 (8.7)		45 (12.1)	15 (5.3)	
HR+ subgroups, n (%)	n = 153	n = 157		n = 251	n = 194	
Luminal A	59 (38.6)	69 (43.9)	0.335	99 (39.4)	65 (33.5)	0.198
Luminal B	94 (61.4)	88 (56.1)		152 (60.6)	129 (66.5)	
Stage at early disease n (%)	n = 262			n = 357		
I	29 (11.1)	NA	NA	45 (12.6)	NA	NA
II	98 (37.4)	NA		131 (36.7)	NA	
III	135 (51.5)	NA		181 (50.7)	NA	
Metastatic Sites, n (%)	n:298	n:327		n:406	n:319	
Bone-only	137 (44.6)	155 (46.4)	<0.001	200 (48.2)	178 (54.8)	0.003
Visceral	140 (45.6)	170 (50.9)		176 (42.4)	136 (41.8)	
CNS	21 (6.8)	2 (0.6)		30 (7.2)	5 (1.5)	

CNS = central nervous system; HER2+ = human epidermal growth factor receptor 2 positive; HR+ = hormone-responsive disease; TNBC = triple-negative breast cancer.

In regard to DFI, 38.4% (n = 277) had relapsed within two years from initial diagnosis, comprising mostly the HR+ subtype (n = 154; 55.5%), followed by the HER2+ (n = 62, 22.4%) and TN (n = 45; 16.2%) subgroups. There were significantly more patients who relapsed within 24 months in Cohort II (n = 174; 62.8%) as compared to Cohort I (n = 103; 37.2%; p = 0.02). When analyzed separately within pathologic subtypes, the ratio of rapid progressors was the highest among the TNBC group (51.7%) (vs. the HER2+ (43.1%) and HR+ (38.1%; luminal A = 36.1% vs. luminal B = 39.4%) groups (p = 0.056)). Time-related changes in disease characteristics within each pathologic subgroup are summarized in Table 2.

3.2. De Novo MBC

There were 659 patients (47.7%) who presented with dnMBC in the entire cohort, consisting of 351 (53.2%) with HR+ disease, 189 (28.7%) with HER2+ and 41 (6.2%) with TN MBC. Despite a decreasing frequency over time (63.4% in Cohort I vs. 48.7% in Cohort II, p = 0.007), the HER2+ subtype was the largest group among all pathological subgroups presenting with de novo disease. The median age of the whole group was 50, ranging between 17 and 91. There was a higher ratio of patients with skeletal metastasis in the HR+ subgroup (56.4%) as compared to HER2+ (38.1%) and TN (24.4%) patients, and an opposite trend for visceral metastasis in each subgroup, respectively (40.7% vs. 58.7% vs. 68.3%; $p < 0.001$). The ratio of patients presenting with CNS involvement was highest in TN patients (7.3%) vs. HR+ (2.8%) and HER2+ (3.2%) subgroups (p = 0.313). Disease characteristics regarding metastatic presentation (recMBC vs. dnMBC) are summarized in Table 2.

3.3. Treatment Patterns

A significantly higher ratio of patients with HR+ disease received first-line chemotherapy (CT) in Cohort I (n = 148; 48.2%) vs. Cohort II (n = 172; 38.9%; p = 0.01), with an opposite trend for endocrine therapy (ET) (Cohort I (n = 118; 38.4%) vs. Cohort II (n = 194; 43.9%; p = 0.14)). Nevertheless, there was no change in trends to deliver CT as a first-line treatment to dnMBC in either cohort (Cohort I: $n = 79$; 50.3% vs. Cohort II: $n = 89$; 45.9%; $g = 0.41$) as compared to recMBC patients, who were less likely to receive front-line CT in Cohort II (Cohort I: $n = 69$; 46.0% vs. Cohort II: $n = 83$; 33.5%; $p = 0.013$). A minority of patients in Cohort II were treated with ET + CDK inhibitors as a first-line therapy following regulatory approval in 2019 ($n = 28$; 6.3%). In the HER2+ subgroup, there was a similar ratio of patients receiving standard first-line CT + HER2 blockade over time (Cohort I vs. Cohort II, 39.0% vs. 35.5%; respectively). In Cohort II, 27 (18.0%) patients were treated with CT + dual HER2 blockade with trastuzumab and pertuzumab, which was more frequently utilized in de novo ($n = 18$; 24.7%) vs. recurrent patients ($n = 9$; 11.7%; $p = 0.06$). There was a higher ratio of patients with TNBC who received platin-based front-line CT in Cohort II ($n = 19$; 32.8%) vs. Cohort I ($n = 14$; 22.2%; $p = 0.273$). Immunotherapy and CT combination was given to seven patients in Cohort II (12.1%) (dnMBC: $n = 3$; 20% vs. recMBC: $n = 4$; 9.3%; $p = NS$). A summary of front-line therapy for all subgroups within each cohort is given in Table 3.

Table 3. Time-related changes in first-line treatment patterns.

Subgroups	Cohort I				Cohort II			
	De Novo n (%)	Recurrent n (%)	p-Value		De Novo n (%)	Recurrent n (%)	p-Value	
HR+	157 (51.1)	150 (48.9)			194 (43.9)	248 (56.1)		
CT	79 (50.3)	69 (46.0)	0.449		89 (45.9)	83 (33.5)	**0.008**	
ET	62 (39.5)	56 (37.3)	0.698	0.363	84 (43.3)	110 (44.4)	0.824	0.014
ET + CDKi	1 (0.6)	0 (0)	1.000		8 (4.1)	20 (8.1)	0.136	
CT + ET	4 (2.5)	7 (4.7)	0.489		7 (3.6)	20 (8.1)	0.082	
Other	11 (7.0)	18 (12.0)	0.194		6 (3.1)	16 (6.0)	0.164	
HER2+	116 (63.4)	67 (36.6)			73 (48.7)	77 (51.3)		
CT + trastuzumab	50 (43.1)	21 (31.3)	0.116		12 (16.4)	15 (19.5)	0.786	
CT + dual blockade	1 (0.9)	0 (0)	1.000	0.349	18 (24.7)	9 (11.7)	0.064	0.131
ET + trastuzumab	10 (8.6)	8 (11.9)	0.639		1 (1.4)	6 (7.8)	0.117	
ET + dual blockade	0 (0)	0 (0)	NA		1 (1.4)	1 (1.3)	1.000	
Other	55 (47.4)	38 (56.7)	0.225		41 (56.2)	46 (59.7)	0.657	
TNBC	26 (41.3)	37 (58.7)			15 (24.2)	43 (75.8)		
CT (non-platin)	19 (73.1)	19 (51.4)	0.141		6 (40.0)	15 (34.9)	0.966	
CT (with platin)	3 (11.5)	11 (29.7)	0.161	0.167	3 (20.0)	16 (37.2)	0.340	0.542
CT + Immunotherapy	0 (0)	0 (0)	NA		3 (20.0)	4 (9.3)	0.360	
Other	4 (15.4)	7 (18.9)	1.000		3 (20.0)	8 (18.6)	1.000	

CDKi = cyclin-dependent kinase inhibitors; CT = chemotherapy; ET = endocrine therapy; HER2+ = human epidermal growth factor receptor 2 positive; HR+ = hormone-responsive disease; TNBC = triple-negative breast cancer.

3.4. Outcomes

Median PFS for all patients at initial treatment for metastatic disease was 18.0 (17.0–19.0) months, while significant variances were identified within pathologic subtypes (HR+ vs. HER2+ vs. TNBC; 19 vs. 18 vs. 10 months, $p < 0.001$). After a median follow-up period of 36 (0–142) months and 778 (56.3%) events, the median OS was 51.0 (48.0–55.0) months for all patients, with the TN subtype having the worst OS (HER2+ vs. HR+ vs. TNBC; 57 vs. 52 vs. 27 months, $p < 0.001$).

As for the primary endpoint, there was no significant difference in the outcome among patients in Cohorts I vs. II (51 vs. 51 months, $p = NS$) (Figure 1A,B). Nevertheless, time-related changes in outcomes were noted within HER2+ and HR+ subgroups dependent on metastatic presentation, as described in detail below.

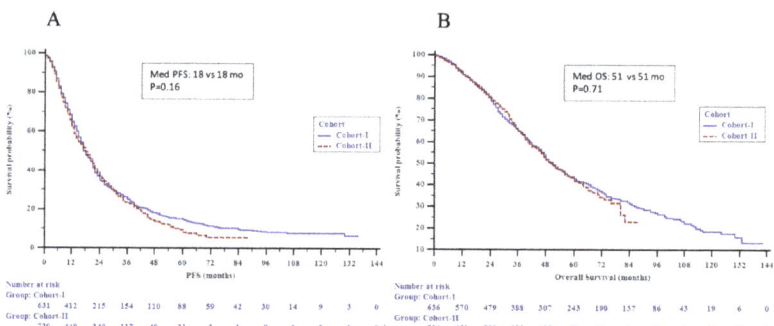

Figure 1. (**A**) Progression-free survival (PFS) by time cohorts and (**B**) overall survival (OS) by time cohorts in the patients.

We observed a significant difference in PFS (HR 1.16, 95% CI 1.04–1.31, p = 0.01) and OS (HR 1.20, 95% CI 1.04–1.38, p = 0.01) in dnMBC as compared to recMBC (Figure 2A,B). When recurrent patients were analyzed with respect to DFI, the TNBC subgroup showed a significantly higher OS in DFI $\geq$ 24 vs. DFI < 24 months (36 vs. 20 months; p = 0.043). Older age at presentation ($\geq$50), recurrent disease, visceral and CNS metastatic involvement, $\geq$3 metastatic sites at presentation and luminal B, and HER2+ and TNBC subtypes (vs. luminal A) were significantly associated with a poorer outcome by univariate analysis. Older age ($\geq$50), luminal B and TNBC subtypes (vs. luminal A), visceral and CNS metastatic involvement remained as independent predictors of poor OS by multivariate analysis (Table 4). When recurrent patients were analyzed separately, older age, luminal B and TNBC subtypes (vs. luminal A), stage III at initial diagnosis (vs. stage I and II), and visceral metastasis were identified as independent prognostic factors for a poorer overall survival (Table 5).

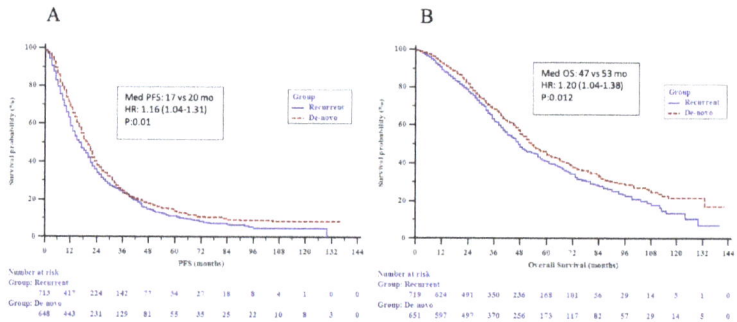

Figure 2. (**A**) Progression-free survival (PFS) by metastatic pattern and (**B**) overall survival (OS) by metastatic pattern in the patients.

Table 4. Univariate and multivariate analysis for overall survival in the whole cohort with metastatic breast cancer.

	Univariate Analysis		Multivariate Analysis	
	Hazard Ratio (CI 95%)	p Value	Hazard Ratio (CI 95%)	p Value
Age (<50 vs. ≥50)	1.25 (1.08–1.44)	**0.002**	1.25 (1.07–1.45)	**0.005**
Metastatic pattern (De novo vs. Recurrent)	1.19 (1.04–1.37)	**0.013**	1.14 (0.97–1.33)	0.100
Cohorts (Cohort II vs. Cohort I)	0.97 (0.84–1.13)	0.712		
Histopathological subtype				
Luminal A	Reference		Reference	
Luminal B	1.31 (1.08–1.61)	**0.007**	1.29 (1.06–1.58)	**0.013**
Luminal B-HER2+	0.89 (0.69–1.14)	0.343	0.85 (0.66–1.09)	0.188
HER2+	1.40 (1.04–1.89)	**0.029**	1.27 (0.94–1.73)	0.122
TNBC	2.26 (1.75–2.93)	**<0.001**	2.04 (1.57–2.66)	**<0.001**
Number of metastatic sites (≤3 vs. >3)	1.23 (1.03–1.49)	**0.023**	1.28 (1.05–1.59)	**0.013**
Visceral metastasis (No vs. Yes)	1.33 (1.15–1.53)	**<0.001**	1.37 (1.17–1.61)	**<0.001**
CNS metastasis (No vs. Yes)	1.56 (1.19–2.04)	**0.001**	1.95 (1.46–2.62)	**<0.001**
Use local ablative treatment/surgery (Yes vs. No.)	0.95 (0.79–1.15)	0.635		

CNS = central nervous system; HER2+ = human epidermal growth factor receptor 2 positive; TNBC = triple-negative breast cancer. Initial variants are analyzed as the referent variable. Multivariate analysis model p value ≤ 0.001.

Table 5. Univariate and multivariate analysis for overall survival in the recurrent patients with metastatic breast cancer.

	Univariate Analysis		Multivariate Analysis	
	Hazard Ratio (CI 95%)	p Value	Hazard Ratio (CI 95%)	p Value
Age (<50 vs. ≥50)	1.41 (1.16–1.72)	**<0.001**	1.38 (1.10–1.74)	**0.005**
Cohorts (Cohort II vs. Cohort I)	0.97 (0.79–1.19)	0.778		
Histopathological subtype				
Luminal A	Reference		Reference	
Luminal B	1.37 (1.04–1.80)	**0.027**	1.39 (1.04–1.87)	**0.026**
Luminal B-HER2+	0.86 (0.59–1.24)	0.412	0.97 (0.65–1.44)	0.865
HER2+	1.76 (1.15–2.70)	**0.010**	1.50 (0.96–2.34)	0.077
TNBC	2.13 (1.53–2.98)	**<0.001**	2.17 (1.49–3.15)	**<0.001**
DFI (≥24 months vs. <24 months)	1.05 (0.86–1.28)	0.608		
Stage at presentation (I + II vs. III)	1.36 (1.10–1.68)	**0.004**	1.52 (1.21–1.90)	**<0.001**
Number of metastatic sites (≤3 vs. >3)	1.32 (1.00–1.72)	0.054		
Visceral metastasis (No vs. Yes)	1.47 (1.21–1.78)	**<0.001**	1.53 (1.22–1.92)	**<0.001**
CNS metastasis (No vs. Yes)	1.35 (0.98–1.85)	0.068		
Use local ablative treatment/surgery (Yes vs. No)	0.81 (0.62–1.06)	0.126		

CNS = central nervous system; DFI = disease-free interval; HER2+ = human epidermal growth factor receptor 2 positive; TNBC = triple-negative breast cancer. Multivariate analysis model p value ≤ 0.001.

3.5. HER2+ Subgroup

Following conditional approval of use in visceral dnMBC in 2016, dual-HER2 blockade with trastuzumab and pertuzumab was more frequently used in Cohort II compared to Cohort I ($p < 0.001$), leading to substantial improvements in outcomes. Survival analysis revealed significant benefits in the de novo group in alignment with the approval indication for dual blockade (Cohort I vs. II; 3-year OS: 62.0% vs. 84.7%, $p = 0.009$), especially noted in those with visceral metastatic presentation (59.4% vs. 83.4%, $p = 0.03$), luminal B-HER2+ disease (61.2% vs. 89.2%, $p = 0.013$) and younger age < 40 years (40.0% vs. 94.7%, $p = 0.009$). The improvement in median OS in the de novo HER2+ group was linked to the favorable outcome in the luminal B-HER2+ subgroup, which showed a 3-year OS rate of 89.2% vs. 61.2% in Cohorts I and II, respectively ($p = 0.013$) (Table 6a,b and Figure 3A–C).

Table 6. Overall survival (OS) and progression-free survival (PFS) in recurrent and de novo patients within each time cohort.

a. In All Pathologic Subgroups

Pathology Subtypes		Recurrent MBC				De Novo MBC			
		N Events/Total N	Cohort I	Cohort II	p	N Events/Total N	Cohort I	Cohort II	p
HR+	OS	225/403	109/153	116/250	0.681	199/351	112/157	87/194	0.121
	Median (95% CI), months		49 (43–55)	48 (40–56)			57 (46–68)	52 (47–57)	
	PFS	352/404	141/153	211/251	0.308	298/351	144/157	154/194	0.424
	Median (95% CI), months		18 (15–21)	17 (13–21)			21 (18–24)	20 (18–22)	
Luminal A	OS	76/157	41/59	35/98	0.551	72/134	44/69	28/65	0.195
	Median (95% CI), months		53 (40–66)	76 (49–103)			70 (52–88)	53 (43–63)	
	PFS	139/158	54/59	85/99	0.710	110/134	62/69	48/65	0.551
	Median (95% CI), months		17 (14–20)	22 (16–28)			22 (15–29)	20 (17–23)	
Luminal B	OS	149/246	68/94	81/152	0.346	127/217	68/88	59/129	0.409
	Median (95% CI), months		48 (40–56)	44 (39–49)			52 (45–59)	49 (43–55)	
	PFS	213/246	87/94	126/152	0.255	188/217	82/88	106/129	0.668
	Median (95% CI), months		21 (16–26)	15 (11–19)			17 (14–20)	21 (18–24)	
HER2+	OS	73/144	43/67	30/77	0.340	95/189	74/116	21/73	0.009
	1-year survival %		86.4%	88.2%			89.6%	97.3%	
	2-year survival %		73.1%	79.8%			74.6%	91.4%	
	3-year survival %		54.3%	68.2%			62.0%	84.7%	
	PFS	84/136	40/64	44/72	0.671	63/186	42/114	21/72	0.037
	Median (95% CI), months		12 (9–15)	20 (16–24)			17 (15–19)	29 (19–39)	
TNBC	OS	64/87	31/42	33/45	0.005	31/40	21/26	10/14	0.731
	Median (95% CI), months		42 (32–52)	20 (14–26)			22 (11–33)	26 (13–39)	
	PFS	49/77	19/35	30/42	0.023	24/37	15/23	9/14	0.741
	Median (95% CI), months		15 (11–19)	7 (5–9)			9 (6–12)	8 (6–10)	

Table 6. Cont.

b. In HR+ and HER2+ subgroups									
		Recurrent MBC				De novo MBC			
Pathology Subtypes		N Events/Total N	Cohort I	Cohort II	p	N Events/Total N	Cohort I	Cohort II	p
Luminal A	OS Median (95% Cl), months	76/157	41/59 53 (40–66)	35/98 76 (49–103)	0.551	72/134	44/69 70 (52–88)	28/65 53 (43–63)	0.195
Luminal B	OS Median (95% Cl), months	149/246	68/94 48 (40–56) p = 0.444	81/152 44 (39–49) p = 0.012	0.346	127/217	68/88 52 (45–59) p = 0.104	59/129 49 (43–55) p = 0.591	0.409
Luminal B-HER2+	OS 3-year survival %	44/94	27/45 64.8%	17/49 75.9%	0.606	64/132	51/81 61.2%	13/51 89.2%	0.013
HR– /HER2+	OS Median (95% Cl), months or 3-year survival %	29/50	16/22 24 (13–35)	13/28 47 (32–62)	0.197	31/57	23/35 63.9%	8/22 74.2%	0.378

HR+ = hormone-responsive disease; HER2+ = human epidermal growth factor receptor 2 positive; MBC = metastatic breast cancer; OS = overall survival; PFS = progression-free survival; TNBC = triple-negative breast cancer.

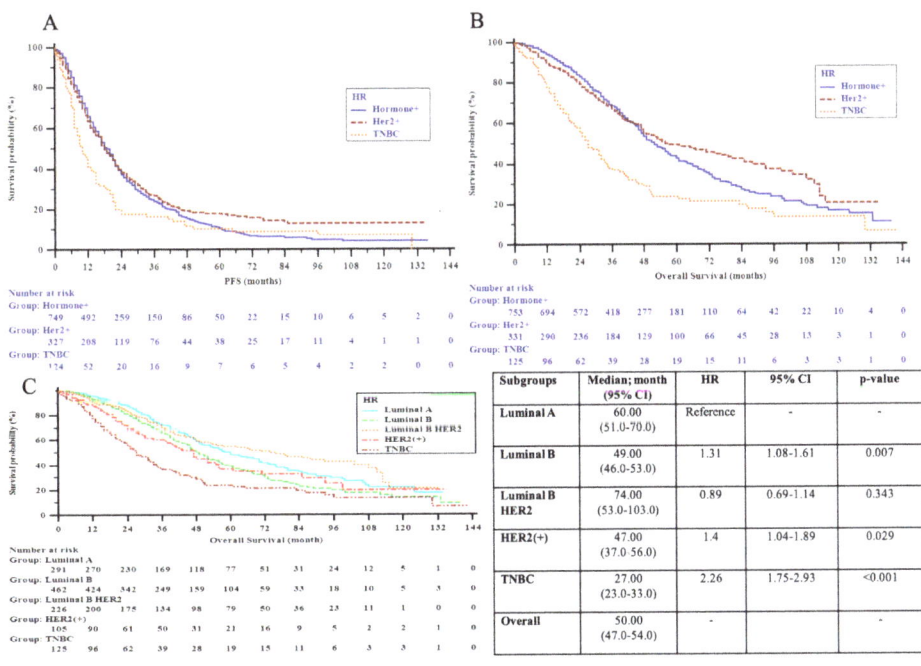

Figure 3. (**A**) Progression-free survival (PFS) by pathologic subgroups; (**B**) overall survival (OS) by pathologic subgroups; (**C**) overall survival (OS) by extended pathologic subgroups in the patients. HER2 = human epidermal growth factor receptor 2; TNBC = triple-negative breast cancer.

3.6. HR+ Subgroup

Despite the insignificant numeric improvement in PFS and OS in dnMBC patients, the outcomes of HR+ patients remained similar over the time points analyzed, reflecting the similar practice patterns in the use of first-line treatment and barriers to access CDK inhibitors. Patients in Cohort II with HR+ recMBC, who were more likely to receive first-line endocrine therapy than the previous 5-year period, showed similar OS and PFS, despite the higher incidence of unfavorable prognostic factors such as luminal B disease (60.6%) and a higher ratio of endocrine-resistant patients (Cohort I 32% vs. Cohort II 41.8%; $p = 0.049$). In Cohort II, the prognoses of recurrent luminal B patients were significantly worse as compared to recurrent luminal A patients (median OS: 44 vs. 76 months, $p = 0.012$).

When both time-related cohorts were combined, patients with luminal A who received ET as first-line treatment had a significant improvement in OS as compared to those who were treated with CT (70 months (95% CI 52–88) vs. 48 months (95%CI 35–61), respectively; $p = 0.008$). Luminal B patients had a numeric improvement in OS with first-line ET vs. CT (56 months (95% CI 46–66) vs. 46 months (95% CI 41–51); $p = 0.135$). There was no difference noted in PFS achieved with either treatment modality in both luminal A and B pathologic subtypes (Table 7).

Table 7. Treatment-related survival outcomes in luminal A and B subgroups.

	n (%)	PFS (Month)	p	OS (Month)	p
Overall					
Luminal A					
CT-ET	111 (45.5)	20	0.849	48	0.008
ET	133 (54.5)	20		70	
Luminal B					
CT-ET	209 (53.9)	17	0.711	46	0.135
ET	179 (46.1)	18		56	
Cohort I					
Luminal A					
CT-ET	60 (53.1)	19	0.293	49	0.052
ET	53 (46.9)	16		76	
Luminal B					
CT-ET	88 (57.5)	21	0.473	49	0.465
ET	65 (42.5)	19		58	
Cohort II					
Luminal A					
CT-ET	51 (38.9)	21	0.386	47	0.082
ET	80 (61.1)	21		57	
Luminal B					
CT-ET	121 (51.5)	16	0.208	45	0.093
ET	114 (48.5)	18		49	

CT = chemotherapy; ET = endocrine therapy; OS = overall survival; PFS = progression-free survival.

3.7. TN Subgroup

TN patients had the poorest outcome among all patients analyzed, with no significant improvement over time. Unexpectedly, recurrent patients in the latter cohort had a significantly worse PFS (7 vs. 15 months, $p = 0.023$) and OS (20 vs. 42 months, $p = 0.005$), most probably due to unfavorable prognostic factors such as a higher incidence of early progressors within two years after initial diagnosis (55.6% vs. 47.6%) and an increased ratio of CNS metastasis at presentation (18.3% vs. 11.8%).

There was a non-significant numeric increase in survival over time in the de novo group (26 vs. 22 months), 20% of whom had access to immunotherapy and 66.7% of whom received conventional non-platin-based chemotherapy in the first-line setting. When patients with ER < 10% (*n* = 11) were added to the de novo TN group, the outcomes remained similar (29 vs. 22 months, *p* = 0.421).

4. Discussion

In this retrospective multicenter cohort, we observed significant differences in metastatic presentation and outcome among histologic subgroups of MBC patients over the analyzed period. In contrast to existing data from large registry studies, our cohort included a high ratio of recurrent patients which increased over time from 48% to 56% [12,13]. Furthermore, we also observed a significant time-dependent increase in the incidence of refractory patients who developed metastatic disease within two years of early-stage BC treatment, consisting mainly of HR+ and TN subgroups. In fact, the proportion of TN patients showed an incremental increase among de novo (6.2%), recurrent patients with DFI > 24 months (9.4%) versus DFI < 24 months (16%), whereas the ratio of HR+ patients remained constant, accounting for the poor biologic behavior in refractory recurrent patients consistent with previous reports [13–15]. Nevertheless, the high incidence of dnMBC (43.9%) in Cohort II exceeds the previously reported ratios of de novo presentation, ranging between 28 and 30% among all MBC patients [16,17]. We also observed a higher proportion of de novo presentation among the entire HER2+ subgroup (48.7%), which is in line with existing data reporting that 37.5–49.8% of HER2+ MBC present with de novo disease [13,18–21].

Although there was no difference among both time-related cohorts based on age, 42% of patients diagnosed with MBC were premenopausal and there was a higher ratio of patients younger than 40 among HER2+ and TN subgroups. In fact, population-based studies have indicated a skewed age distribution towards a younger population with unfavorable prognosis over the last three decades. There has been a consistent increase noted in annual hazards of advanced stage at diagnosis in patients aged 25–39 among all race and ethnic groups analyzed, with a higher incidence of TN and HER2+ subgroups which were unaccounted for by clinical or genomic features [22,23]. Nevertheless, our findings suggested that younger age was independently associated with a favorable outcome, consistent with data from a recent study focusing on young patients with dnMBC. In this study, improved survival was noted in all subgroups except those with TNBC, indicating that variances in tumor biology might account for survival disparities [24]. In fact, a biomarker analysis of a retrospective case–control cohort has shown differential gene expression of de novo versus recurrent MBC, a finding which needs validation by further studies [19].

The median survival of the whole cohort over the analyzed period was 51 months. Although patients with de novo mBC had a significantly longer OS than those with recurrent disease by univariate analysis (53 vs. 47 mo; *p*: 0.013), the presentation pattern was not shown to be independently associated with the outcome (Table 4). Our findings compare favorably with previous registry studies which have reported median OS ranging between 22 and 37 months, with wide variations among pathologic subgroups [7,12,13,19,25–27]. Nevertheless, our findings indicate that de novo presentation may not be an independent prognostic factor per se. The favorable outcome may be associated with several confounders such as a lower tumor burden due to advances in diagnostic techniques, impact of age, histology, lack of resistance ensued by previous treatment pressure or a distinct biologic behavior independent of clinicopathologic factors as discussed by several studies [14,28,29]. Nevertheless, similar outcomes have been observed in recurrent patients with a long DFI. These observations suggest that there may be other contributing factors in the evolution of metastatic disease. In fact, outcomes of control arms from more recent phase III trials have repeatedly yielded superior results in comparison to data from registration studies, suggesting that time-related advances in diagnostic modalities and access to optimized health care systems could play a role in reported survival disparities [28,30–33]. With the caveat of making cross-trial comparisons, it is not possible to draw firm conclusions on time-related variances in survival. Although translational studies from large-scale prospective studies provide valuable information on spatial biologic characteristics of distinct subgroups, future prospects to address temporal variances in outcomes require a multi-faceted approach combining standardized modern health care with in-depth genomic monitoring of micrometastatic disease.

Although there was no difference noted in patient characteristics and outcomes between the two time-related cohorts, the only difference in survival over time was observed in the HER2+ subgroup, which reached significance in de novo luminal B-HER2+ patients treated over the last five-year period. Despite bearing an unfavorable patient profile enriched in a younger population with CNS involvement, the improvement in outcome in the HER2+ dnMBC most likely reflects the higher rates of access to combined trastuzumab and pertuzumab after 2015. Our results are in parallel with several registry data showing a significant outcome difference in patients with de novo as compared to recurrent HER2+ MBC which have reported superior survival rates only in the HER2+ subgroup [18,34–37]. A striking finding in our cohort was the favorable prognosis in the luminal B-HER2+ subgroup as compared to all pathologic subtypes, which has been consistently observed by others, reflecting the use of sequential endocrine therapy following chemotherapy and HER2 blockade in routine clinical practice [9,38,39]. In the absence of robust randomized data, clinical practice patterns favoring this approach have evolved through large-scale prospective registry data demonstrating improved outcomes with the addition of ET following completion of CT and HER2 blockade as compared to CT and HER2 targeting alone [40].

A consistent observation over the analyzed period was the poor survival in the TN subgroup, which has been determined as an independent prognostic factor on overall mortality in our cohort, as well as many others [8,20,26,27,41].

In concordance with contemporary community-based studies that have failed to reflect the significant survival benefits demonstrated by clinical trials, we did not observe significant variations in outcomes neither within the entire HR+ group (52 months), nor when broken down into luminal A (60 months) and luminal B (49 months) subgroups [27,35]. Although we collected data from private-based academic centers, a formal comparison of outcomes was not carried out, as this endpoint is not within the scope of the present analysis due to an inherent risk of potential bias. In general, the private sector is estimated to provide healthcare for approximately 30% of oncology patients nationwide, which is in line with our private-based cohort comprising 25% of the whole patient population. Although all centers included in this registry were chosen based on their ability to deliver optimal, standardized and high-quality healthcare, we have to acknowledge that there may be barriers in receipt of cancer care in academic-designated public centers which have been burdened by a growing patient volume, exceeding their capacity to provide timely and supportive care. Furthermore, a lack of optimized social and physical support, as well as difficulties in access to modern treatment options or enrollment in clinical trials, may account for disparities in health care in the general community setting. Therefore, it requires the countrywide collaboration of cancer centers with the Ministry of Health to identify barriers for accessible and value-based care, which will provide guidance in developing policies to implement equitable health care throughout the nation.

Nevertheless, recurrent luminal A patients had a significantly longer OS compared to luminal B patients in Cohort II (76 vs. 44 months, $p = 0.012$), which could be attributable to a time-related shift in first-line management of HR+ MBC from a higher ratio of CT use in Cohort I (CT 46% vs. ET 37%) to ET in Cohort II (ET 44% vs. CT 33%, $p = 0.008$). The inappropriate preference for CT as the initial therapy in our patient population contradicts recent guidelines and real-world experience that have reported more frequent use of ET for up to 70% of HR+ patients [13,26,27,35,42]. In fact, a contemporary Turkish observational study including 758 HR+ MBC patients treated between 2019 and 2020 reported a significant increase in ET use with 70% of patients receiving ET and CDK inhibitors as first-line therapy and a subsequent decline in first-line CT use from 49% to 20% following regulatory approval, which was associated with a significant improvement in PFS [43]. Nevertheless, despite strong evidence for improved OS with CDK inhibitors in the first-line setting reaching 64 months, the favorable OS ranging between 49 and 76 months in our luminal B and

A subgroups without access to contemporary endocrine targeted agents may provide an appealing option in limited resource settings [44].

Our study has many inherent limitations due to the retrospective nature of a registry database lacking information on comorbid conditions, menopausal status, family histories and genomic factors, all of which may have confounded the results. Data obtained from the heterogenous patient population cannot be extrapolated to the whole nation, especially in underserved areas. Most importantly, subtype classifications for most recurrent patients were based on initial pathology reports at initial diagnosis rather than repeated biopsies at metastatic presentation. This may have confounded outcomes in some histologic subgroups as they are more likely to include patients with poorer prognosis, especially in those with early recurrences. We were not able to assess the impact of novel therapies such as CDK inhibitors or immunotherapy since they were not approved for use at that time. Furthermore, data on time-on-treatment for switch maintenance ET or HER2 blockade could not be captured from patient files, which would provide valuable data on the impact of subsequent therapies for each prognostic subgroup.

Nevertheless, the main strengths of this study that should be mentioned are the collaborative efforts of tertiary academic centers providing high-quality pathologic data and standardized management within national limits. The data generated from this registry study reflects real-life practice patterns in both private and social security reimbursed systems while minimizing the impact of variances in routine diagnostic and management strategies. Furthermore, the patient population belongs to the three most populated cities with a high domestic migration rate, which represents national characteristics of MBC to a large extent.

5. Conclusions

In conclusion, our findings provide further proof that improved survival in MBC is associated with advances in treatment as observed especially in luminal B-HER2+ patients over the analyzed period. In fact, the unprecedented success of anti-HER2 therapies has affirmed that clinically relevant outcomes from trials adopted in routine practice can revolutionize the prognosis of a subgroup, highlighting the relevance of targeting biology. Furthermore, a consistent feature we observed was the challenge in treating TNBC, which was identified as the worst prognostic subgroup without any correlation with clinicopathologic confounders. Elucidation of biologic characteristics to identify novel treatment options remains an unmet need to improve outcomes in TNBC. Nevertheless, with increasing demand from the community to have access to newer-generation novel agents, the financial burden of cancer care has risen dramatically over the past decade. Emerging evidence suggests that real-world data provide relevant information on challenges to implement evolving therapeutic options in routine practice and the impact of increasing costs in widening social gaps and disparities in access to optimal health care [45]. Given the inherent heterogeneity of the analyzed cohort and complexities of decision making to treat MBC, we acknowledge the limitations of our data. However, the findings of this study may provide unique insights into the dynamics of practice patterns and outcomes, which may be used by healthcare authorities to identify whether the adoption of modern treatment options has improved survival and to shed light on future interventions to enhance quality of care.

Author Contributions: Conceptualization and methodology, Y.E., I.D., S.A., B.C., G.B., O.E., N.M.M., T.K., E.G., C.S., A.A. and P.S.; software, Y.E., I.D. and C.S.; validation, Y.E., I.D. and C.S.; formal analysis, Y.E., I.D. and C.S.; investigation, Y.E., I.D., S.A., B.C., G.B., O.E., N.M.M., T.K., E.G., C.S., A.A. and P.S.; resources, Y.E., I.D., S.A., B.C., G.B., O.E., N.M.M., T.K., E.G., C.S., A.A. and P.S.; data curation, Y.E., I.D. and C.S.; writing—original draft preparation, Y.E., I.D., B.C., O.E. and C.S.; writing—review and editing, Y.E., S.A., G.B., N.M.M., T.K., E.G., A.A. and P.S.; visualization, Y.E., S.A., G.B., N.M.M., T.K., E.G., A.A. and P.S.; supervision, Y.E.; project administration, Y.E.; funding acquisition, Y.E. All authors have read and agreed to the published version of the manuscript.

Funding: This study was supported by the Turkish Oncology Group with independent funding by Roche, Turkey.

Institutional Review Board Statement: The study was conducted in accordance with the Declaration of Helsinki and approved by the Acıbadem Mehmet Ali Aydınlar University Medical Research Ethics Committee (Approval no and date: 2020-23/35, 5 November 2020).

Informed Consent Statement: Patient consent was waived due to retrospective nature of the study.

Data Availability Statement: The data presented in this study are available on request from the corresponding author. This published paper contains all of the data produced or analyzed during this investigation.

Acknowledgments: We would like to thank Ayşe Esra Aydın, Gamze Alçı and Monitor CRO, İstanbul, Turkey, for all their support during the study process.

Conflicts of Interest: S.A.: consulting fees, honoraria from AstraZeneca, Bristol Myers Squibb, Lilly, Merck, Merck Sharpe & Dohme, Novartis, Pfizer. G.B.: consulting fees from Gilead. E.G.: consulting fees from Amgen, Astellas Pharma, AstraZeneca, Bristol Myers Squibb, Gilead, Janssen Turkiye, Novartis, Pfizer, Roche. Y.E.: Novartis Turkiye, Novartis Global, Gilead, Merck Sharpe & Dohme Global; educational honorarium from Novartis Turkiye, AstraZeneca Turkiye, GSK Turkiye, Gilead Turkiye; research support from Roche Turkiye; non-compensated mentorship for Boston Scientific; non-compensated educational meeting support for Roche Turkiye, AstraZeneca Turkiye. I.D., B.C., O.E., N.M.M., T.K., C.S., A.A. and P.S. declare no conflicts of interest.

References

1. Globocan 2020 Turkey. Available online: https://gco.iarc.fr/today/data/factsheets/populations/792-turkey-fact-sheets.pdf (accessed on 22 January 2023).
2. Turkish Ministry of Health, Cancer Statistics. Available online: https://hsgm.saglik.gov.tr/depo/birimler/kanser-db/istatistik/Turkiye_Kanser_Istatistikleri_2017.pdf (accessed on 22 January 2023).
3. Sung, H.; Ferlay, J.; Siegel, R.L.; Laversanne, M.; Soerjomataram, I.; Jemal, A.; Bray, F. Global Cancer Statistics 2020: GLOBOCAN Estimates of Incidence and Mortality Worldwide for 36 Cancers in 185 Countries. *CA Cancer J. Clin.* **2021**, *71*, 209–249. [CrossRef] [PubMed]
4. Allemani, C.; Matsuda, T.; Di Carlo, V.; Harewood, R.; Matz, M.; Nikšić, M.; Bonaventure, A.; Valkov, M.; Johnson, C.J.; Estève, J.; et al. CONCORD Working Group. Global surveillance of trends in cancer survival 2000-14 (CONCORD-3): Analysis of individual records for 37 513 025 patients diagnosed with one of 18 cancers from 322 population-based registries in 71 countries. *Lancet* **2018**, *391*, 1023–1075. [CrossRef] [PubMed]
5. Peto, R.; Boreham, J.; Clarke, M.; Davies, C.; Beral, V. UK and USA breast cancer deaths down 25% in year 2000 at ages 20–69 years. *Lancet* **2000**, *355*, 1822. [CrossRef] [PubMed]
6. Dawood, S.; Broglio, K.; Ensor, J.; Hortobagyi, G.N.; Giordano, S.H. Survival differences among women with de novo stage IV and relapsed breast cancer. *Ann. Oncol.* **2010**, *21*, 2169–2174. [CrossRef] [PubMed]
7. Lord, S.J.; Bahlmann, K.; O'Connell, D.L.; Kiely, B.E.; Daniels, B.; Pearson, S.A.; Beith, J.; Bulsara, M.K.; Houssami, N. De novo and recurrent metastatic breast cancer—A systematic review of population-level changes in survival since 1995. *EClinicalMedicine* **2022**, *44*, 101282. [CrossRef]
8. den Brok, W.D.; Speers, C.H.; Gondara, L.; Baxter, E.; Tyldesley, S.K.; Lohrisch, C.A. Survival with metastatic breast cancer based on initial presentation, de novo versus relapsed. *Breast Cancer Res. Treat.* **2017**, *161*, 549–556. [CrossRef]
9. Howlader, N.; Noone, A.M.; Krapcho, M.; Garshell, J.; Miller, D.; Altekruse, S.F.; Kosary, C.L.; Yu, M.; Ruhl, J.; Tatalovich, Z.; et al. *SEER Cancer Statistics Review, 1975–2012*; National Cancer Institute: Bethesda, MD, USA, 2015. Available online: https://seer.cancer.gov/archive/csr/1975_2012/ (accessed on 22 January 2023).
10. Ernst, M.F.; van de Poll-Franse, L.V.; Roukema, J.A.; Coebergh, J.W.; van Gestel, C.M.; Vreugdenhil, G.; Louwman, M.J.; Voogd, A.C. Trends in the prognosis of patients with primary metastatic breast cancer diagnosed between 1975 and 2002. *Breast* **2007**, *16*, 344–351. [CrossRef]
11. Hölzel, D.; Eckel, R.; Bauerfeind, I.; Baier, B.; Beck, T.; Braun, M.; Ettl, J.; Hamann, U.; Kiechle, M.; Mahner, S.; et al. Improved systemic treatment for early breast cancer improves cure rates, modifies metastatic pattern and shortens post-metastatic survival: 35-year results from the Munich Cancer Registry. *J. Cancer Res. Clin. Oncol.* **2017**, *143*, 1701–1712. [CrossRef]
12. Malmgren, J.A.; Mayer, M.; Atwood, M.K.; Kaplan, H.G. Differential presentation and survival of de novo and recurrent metastatic breast cancer over time: 1990-2010. *Breast Cancer Res. Treat.* **2018**, *167*, 579–590. [CrossRef]
13. File, D.M.; Pascual, T.; Deal, A.M.; Wheless, A.; Perou, C.M.; Claire Dees, E.; Carey, L.A. Clinical subtype, treatment response, and survival in De Novo and recurrent metastatic breast cancer. *Breast Cancer Res. Treat.* **2022**, *196*, 153–162. [CrossRef]

14. Lobbezoo, D.J.; van Kampen, R.J.; Voogd, A.C.; Dercksen, M.W.; van den Berkmortel, F.; Smilde, T.J.; van de Wouw, A.J.; Peters, F.P.; van Riel, J.M.; Peters, N.A.; et al. Prognosis of metastatic breast cancer: Are there differences between patients with de novo and recurrent metastatic breast cancer? *Br. J. Cancer* **2015**, *112*, 1445–1451. [CrossRef] [PubMed]
15. McKenzie, H.S.; Maishman, T.; Simmonds, P.; Durcan, L.; POSH Steering Group; Eccles, D.; Copson, E. Survival and disease characteristics of de novo versus recurrent metastatic breast cancer in a cohort of young patients. *Br. J. Cancer* **2020**, *122*, 1618–1629. [CrossRef] [PubMed]
16. Welch, H.G.; Gorski, D.H.; Albertsen, P.C. Trends in Metastatic Breast and Prostate Cancer–Lessons in Cancer Dynamics. *N. Engl. J. Med.* **2015**, *373*, 1685–1687. [CrossRef] [PubMed]
17. Heller, D.R.; Chiu, A.S.; Farrell, K.; Killelea, B.K.; Lannin, D.R. Why Has Breast Cancer Screening Failed to Decrease the Incidence of de Novo Stage IV Disease? *Cancers* **2019**, *11*, 500. [CrossRef] [PubMed]
18. Tripathy, D.; Brufsky, A.; Cobleigh, M.; Jahanzeb, M.; Kaufman, P.A.; Mason, G.; O'Shaughnessy, J.; Rugo, H.S.; Swain, S.M.; Yardley, D.A.; et al. De Novo Versus Recurrent HER2-Positive Metastatic Breast Cancer: Patient Characteristics, Treatment, and Survival from the SystHERs Registry. *Oncologist* **2020**, *25*, e214–e222. [CrossRef]
19. Seltzer, S.; Corrigan, M.; O'Reilly, S. The clinicomolecular landscape of de novo versus relapsed stage IV metastatic breast cancer. *Exp. Mol. Pathol.* **2020**, *114*, 104404. [CrossRef]
20. Barcenas, C.H.; Song, J.; Murthy, R.K.; Raghavendra, A.S.; Li, Y.; Hsu, L.; Carlson, R.W.; Tripathy, D.; Hortobagyi, G.N. Prognostic Model for De Novo and Recurrent Metastatic Breast Cancer. *JCO Clin. Cancer Inform.* **2021**, *5*, 789–804. [CrossRef]
21. Muller, K.; Jorns, J.M.; Tozbikian, G. What's new in breast pathology 2022: WHO 5th edition and biomarker updates. *J. Pathol. Transl. Med.* **2022**, *56*, 170–171. [CrossRef]
22. Johnson, R.H.; Chien, F.L.; Bleyer, A. Incidence of breast cancer with distant involvement among women in the United States, 1976 to 2009. *JAMA* **2013**, *309*, 800–805. [CrossRef]
23. Cathcart-Rake, E.J.; Ruddy, K.J.; Bleyer, A.; Johnson, R.H. Breast Cancer in Adolescent and Young Adult Women under the Age of 40 Years. *JCO Oncol. Pract.* **2021**, *17*, 305–313. [CrossRef]
24. Ogiya, R.; Sagara, Y.; Niikura, N.; Freedman, R.A. Impact of Subtype on Survival of Young Patients with Stage IV Breast Cancer. *Clin. Breast Cancer* **2019**, *19*, 200–207.e1. [CrossRef] [PubMed]
25. Kennecke, H.; Yerushalmi, R.; Woods, R.; Cheang, M.C.; Voduc, D.; Speers, C.H.; Nielsen, T.O.; Gelmon, K. Metastatic behavior of breast cancer subtypes. *J. Clin. Oncol.* **2010**, *28*, 3271–3277. [CrossRef] [PubMed]
26. Lindman, H.; Wiklund, F.; Andersen, K.K. Long-term treatment patterns and survival in metastatic breast cancer by intrinsic subtypes—An observational cohort study in Sweden. *BMC Cancer* **2022**, *22*, 1006. [CrossRef] [PubMed]
27. Deluche, E.; Antoine, A.; Bachelot, T.; Lardy-Claud, A.; Dieras, V.; Brain, E.; Debled, M.; Jacot, W.; Mouret-Reynier, M.A.; Goncalves, A.; et al. Contemporary outcomes of metastatic breast cancer among 22,000 women from the multicentre ESME cohort 2008–2016. *Eur. J. Cancer* **2020**, *129*, 60–70. [CrossRef]
28. Guo, F.; Kuo, Y.F.; Shih, Y.C.T.; Giordano, S.H.; Berenson, A.B. Trends in breast cancer mortality by stage at diagnosis among young women in the United States. *Cancer* **2018**, *124*, 3500–3509. [CrossRef]
29. Giaquinto, A.N.; Sung, H.; Miller, K.D.; Kramer, J.L.; Newman, L.A.; Minihan, A.; Jemal, A.; Siegel, R.L. Breast Cancer Statistics, 2022. *CA Cancer J. Clin.* **2022**, *72*, 524–541. [CrossRef]
30. Slamon, D.J.; Leyland-Jones, B.; Shak, S.; Fuchs, H.; Paton, V.; Bajamonde, A.; Fleming, T.; Eiermann, W.; Wolter, J.; Pegram, M.; et al. Use of chemotherapy plus a monoclonal antibody against HER2 for metastatic breast cancer that overexpresses HER2. *N. Engl. J. Med.* **2001**, *344*, 783–792. [CrossRef]
31. Swain, S.M.; Baselga, J.; Kim, S.B.; Ro, J.; Semiglazov, V.; Campone, M.; Ciruelos, E.; Ferrero, J.M.; Schneeweiss, A.; Heeson, S.; et al. Pertuzumab, trastuzumab, and docetaxel in HER2-positive metastatic breast cancer. *N. Engl. J. Med.* **2015**, *372*, 724–734. [CrossRef]
32. Jemal, A.; Robbins, A.S.; Lin, C.C.; Flanders, W.D.; DeSantis, C.E.; Ward, E.M.; Freedman, R.A. Factors That Contributed to Black-White Disparities in Survival Among Nonelderly Women with Breast Cancer Between 2004 and 2013. *J. Clin. Oncol.* **2018**, *36*, 14–24. [CrossRef]
33. Malinowski, C.; Lei, X.; Zhao, H.; Giordano, S.H.; Chavez-MacGregor, M. Association of Medicaid Expansion with Mortality Disparity by Race and Ethnicity Among Patients with De Novo Stage IV Breast Cancer. *JAMA Oncol.* **2022**, *8*, 863–870. [CrossRef]
34. Lambertini, M.; Di Maio, M.; Pagani, O.; Curigliano, G.; Poggio, F.; Del Mastro, L.; Paluch-Shimon, S.; Loibl, S.; Partridge, A.H.; Demeestere, I.; et al. The BCY3/BCC 2017 survey on physicians' knowledge, attitudes and practice towards fertility and pregnancy-related issues in young breast cancer patients. *Breast* **2018**, *42*, 41–49. [CrossRef] [PubMed]
35. Gobbini, E.; Ezzalfani, M.; Dieras, V.; Bachelot, T.; Brain, E.; Debled, M.; Jacot, W.; Mouret-Reynier, M.A.; Goncalves, A.; Dalenc, F.; et al. Time trends of overall survival among metastatic breast cancer patients in the real-life ESME cohort. *Eur. J. Cancer* **2018**, *96*, 17–24. [CrossRef] [PubMed]
36. Swain, S.M.; Miles, D.; Kim, S.B.; Im, Y.H.; Im, S.A.; Semiglazov, V.; Ciruelos, E.; Schneeweiss, A.; Loi, S.; Monturus, E.; et al. Pertuzumab, trastuzumab, and docetaxel for HER2-positive metastatic breast cancer (CLEOPATRA): End-of-study results from a double-blind, randomised, placebo-controlled, phase 3 study. *Lancet Oncol.* **2020**, *21*, 519–530. [CrossRef] [PubMed]
37. Zhang, X.; Leng, J.; Zhou, Y.; Mao, F.; Lin, Y.; Shen, S.; Sun, Q. Efficacy and Safety of Anti-HER2 Agents in Combination with Chemotherapy for Metastatic HER2-Positive Breast Cancer Patient: A Network Meta-Analysis. *Front. Oncol.* **2021**, *11*, 731210. [CrossRef]

38. Cobleigh, M.; Yardley, D.A.; Brufsky, A.M.; Rugo, H.S.; Swain, S.M.; Kaufman, P.A.; Tripathy, D.; Hurvitz, S.A.; O'Shaughnessy, J.; Mason, G.; et al. Baseline Characteristics, Treatment Patterns, and Outcomes in Patients with HER2-Positive Metastatic Breast Cancer by Hormone Receptor Status from SystHERs. *Clin. Cancer Res.* **2020**, *26*, 1105–1113. [CrossRef]
39. Tao, L.; Chu, L.; Wang, L.I.; Moy, L.; Brammer, M.; Song, C.; Green, M.; Kurian, A.W.; Gomez, S.L.; Clarke, C.A. Occurrence and outcome of de novo metastatic breast cancer by subtype in a large, diverse population. *Cancer Causes Control* **2016**, *27*, 1127–1138. [CrossRef]
40. Tripathy, D.; Kaufman, P.A.; Brufsky, A.M.; Mayer, M.; Yood, M.U.; Yoo, B.; Quah, C.; Yardley, D.; Rugo, H.S. First-line treatment patterns and clinical outcomes in patients with HER2-positive and hormone receptor-positive metastatic breast cancer from registHER. *Oncologist* **2013**, *18*, 501–510. [CrossRef]
41. Chavez-MacGregor, M.; Mittendorf, E.A.; Clarke, C.A.; Lichtensztajn, D.Y.; Hunt, K.K.; Giordano, S.H. Incorporating Tumor Characteristics to the American Joint Committee on Cancer Breast Cancer Staging System. *Oncologist* **2017**, *22*, 1292–1300. [CrossRef]
42. Cardoso, F.; Paluch-Shimon, S.; Senkus, E.; Curigliano, G.; Aapro, M.S.; André, F.; Barrios, C.H.; Bergh, J.; Bhattacharyya, G.S.; Biganzoli, L.; et al. 5th ESO-ESMO international consensus guidelines for advanced breast cancer (ABC 5). *Ann. Oncol.* **2020**, *31*, 1623–1649. [CrossRef]
43. Karadurmus, N.; Sendur, M.A.N.; Cil, T.; Cakmak Oksuzoglu, O.B.; Arslan, C.; Harputluoglu, H.; Sezgin Goksu, S.; Ozturk, B.; İnanç, M.; Cubukcu, E.; et al. Patient and treatment characteristics in HR+/HER2- metastatic breast cancer in a real-life setting. In Proceedings of the San Antonio Breast Cancer Symposium, San Antonio, TX, USA, 6–10 December 2022.
44. Hortobagyi, G.N.; Stemmer, S.M.; Burris, H.A.; Yap, Y.S.; Sonke, G.S.; Hart, L.; Campone, M.; Petrakova, K.; Winer, E.P.; Janni, W.; et al. Overall Survival with Ribociclib plus Letrozole in Advanced Breast Cancer. *N. Engl. J. Med.* **2022**, *386*, 942–950. [CrossRef]
45. Booth, C.M.; Karim, S.; Mackillop, W.J. Real-world data: Towards achieving the achievable in cancer care. *Nat. Rev. Clin. Oncol.* **2019**, *16*, 312–325. [CrossRef] [PubMed]

Disclaimer/Publisher's Note: The statements, opinions and data contained in all publications are solely those of the individual author(s) and contributor(s) and not of MDPI and/or the editor(s). MDPI and/or the editor(s) disclaim responsibility for any injury to people or property resulting from any ideas, methods, instructions or products referred to in the content.

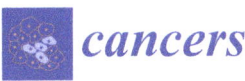

Article

Applying Explainable Machine Learning Models for Detection of Breast Cancer Lymph Node Metastasis in Patients Eligible for Neoadjuvant Treatment

Josip Vrdoljak [1], Zvonimir Boban [2], Domjan Barić [3], Darko Šegvić [4], Marko Kumrić [1], Manuela Avirović [5], Melita Perić Balja [6], Marija Milković Periša [7], Čedna Tomasović [8], Snježana Tomić [9], Eduard Vrdoljak [10,*] and Joško Božić [1,*]

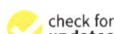

Citation: Vrdoljak, J.; Boban, Z.; Barić, D.; Šegvić, D.; Kumrić, M.; Avirović, M.; Perić Balja, M.; Periša, M.M.; Tomasović, Č.; Tomić, S.; et al. Applying Explainable Machine Learning Models for Detection of Breast Cancer Lymph Node Metastasis in Patients Eligible for Neoadjuvant Treatment. *Cancers* 2023, 15, 634. https://doi.org/10.3390/cancers15030634

Academic Editor: Naiba Nabieva

Received: 14 December 2022
Revised: 16 January 2023
Accepted: 17 January 2023
Published: 19 January 2023

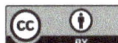

Copyright: © 2023 by the authors. Licensee MDPI, Basel, Switzerland. This article is an open access article distributed under the terms and conditions of the Creative Commons Attribution (CC BY) license (https://creativecommons.org/licenses/by/4.0/).

[1] Department of Pathophysiology, University of Split School of Medicine, 21000 Split, Croatia
[2] Department of Biophysics, University of Split School of Medicine, 21000 Split, Croatia
[3] Department of Physics, University of Zagreb Faculty of Science, 10000 Zagreb, Croatia
[4] Sigmoid Lab, Postindustria Group, 21000 Split, Croatia
[5] Department of Pathology, University Hospital of Rijeka, 51000 Rijeka, Croatia
[6] Department of Pathology, Clinical Hospital Sestre Milosrdnice, 10000 Zagreb, Croatia
[7] Department of Pathology, Clinical Hospital Zagreb, 10000 Zagreb, Croatia
[8] Department of Pathology, Clinical Hospital Dubrava, 10000 Zagreb, Croatia
[9] Department of Pathology, University Hospital of Split, 21000 Split, Croatia
[10] Department of Oncology, University Hospital of Split, 21000 Split, Croatia
* Correspondence: eduard.vrdoljak@mefst.hr (E.V.); josko.bozic@mefst.hr (J.B.)

Simple Summary: In this study, we trained and evaluated several machine-learning models with the aim of predicting breast cancer lymph node metastasis in patients eligible for neoadjuvant treatment. In neoadjuvantly treated patients, radiological and clinical methods are primary ways for determining axillary lymph node status, and radiological methods misdiagnose up to 30% of the patients. Hence, there is an unmet need for supplementary methods to aid oncologists and their multidisciplinary teams in assessing metastatic lymph node status and, consecutively, defining optimal treatment strategies. Good performance was achieved with a random forest algorithm (AUC: 0.79). We explored model explainability and, through it, exhibited how the models learned genuine relationships that were determined in previous studies. Such models can lead to more accurate disease stage prediction and consecutively better treatment selection, especially for NST patients, where radiological and clinical findings are often the only way of lymph node assessment.

Abstract: Background: Due to recent changes in breast cancer treatment strategy, significantly more patients are treated with neoadjuvant systemic therapy (NST). Radiological methods do not precisely determine axillary lymph node status, with up to 30% of patients being misdiagnosed. Hence, supplementary methods for lymph node status assessment are needed. This study aimed to apply and evaluate machine learning models on clinicopathological data, with a focus on patients meeting NST criteria, for lymph node metastasis prediction. Methods: From the total breast cancer patient data (n = 8381), 719 patients were identified as eligible for NST. Machine learning models were applied for the NST-criteria group and the total study population. Model explainability was obtained by calculating Shapley values. Results: In the NST-criteria group, random forest achieved the highest performance (AUC: 0.793 [0.713, 0.865]), while in the total study population, XGBoost performed the best (AUC: 0.762 [0.726, 0.795]). Shapley values identified tumor size, Ki-67, and patient age as the most important predictors. Conclusion: Tree-based models achieve a good performance in assessing lymph node status. Such models can lead to more accurate disease stage prediction and consecutively better treatment selection, especially for NST patients where radiological and clinical findings are often the only way of lymph node assessment.

Keywords: machine learning; breast cancer; neoadjuvant systemic treatment; lymph node metastasis

1. Introduction

Breast cancer is the most common cancer in women and contributes the most to women's cancer mortality, which defines its public health importance [1,2]. Notably, 95% of newly diagnosed breast cancer patients are diagnosed in an early, locoregional, non-metastatic stage of the disease, when a cure is a realistic goal [3].

After the introduction of adjuvant and neoadjuvant therapies in the treatment of early breast cancer, the probability of 5-year survival almost doubled in the last 50 years [4]. Prognostic and predictive factors, biomarkers, and, recently, genetic panels are crucial in defining an optimal treatment strategy [5]. Still, one of the most important prognostic and treatment decision-making factors is the positivity of metastatic axillary lymph nodes [6].

Due to a recent change in the treatment strategy, significantly more patients are treated with neoadjuvant systemic therapy (NST). The NST is assigned based on the tumor biology characteristics and radiological findings [7]. The neoadjuvant concept allows in vivo testing of treatment sensitivity, further personalization of the adjuvant part of systemic therapy, and provides the way to receive accelerated approval of new treatments. It is also valid for the development of predictive biomarkers and reduces patient numbers in clinical trials by the usage of new surrogate endpoints such as the pathological complete response (pCR) [8,9].

It is known that axillary lymph node status is not precisely determined by radiological tests, ending up with close to 30% of patients being misdiagnosed and potentially not directed to NST [10].

After NST, the initial status of axillary lymph nodes is often questionable due to metastases completely responding to the NST, which consequently highlights the problem in defining treatment intensity for HER2 positive patients, for example, to continue or not with dual antiHER2 blockade with pertuzumab and trastuzumab [11].

Despite all the breakthroughs in our understanding of breast tumor biology, adjuvant/neoadjuvant therapy in early breast cancer therapy is still significantly based on the stage of the disease, whereas lymph node positivity usually prevents de-escalation of systemic therapy or omittance of lymph node radiotherapy [7]. Therefore, our knowledge about the tumor's ability to metastasize and the actual status of lymph nodes is of paramount importance in our decision-making process.

Since NST is used more often and based on the rather limited accuracy of imaging methods applied in lymph node metastasis assessment, there is an unmet need for supplementary methods to aid oncologists and their multidisciplinary teams in the assessment of axillary lymph node status and consecutive definitions of optimal treatment strategies.

Due to exponential growth in oncology patient data, "Data Science" and machine learning techniques are extensively researched and applied as possible solutions to various clinical problems [12–14].

Machine learning, as a computational method that maps a mathematical function to a dataset in order to predict/classify the target variable, differs from traditional programming in that it directly learns from the data, without the need for explicit step-wise programming [15]. Traditional machine learning algorithms, such as support vector machines (SVM) and random forests (RF), have been successfully used to classify breast cancer into triple negative and non-triple negative types, predict the metastatic status of patients, and aid in detecting early disease recurrence [16,17]. Furthermore, more complicated models, such as the gradient-boosted trees and eXtreme Gradient Boosting (XGBoost), were used to predict survival outcomes in patients with epithelial ovarian cancer and the prediction of metastatic status in breast cancer, respectively [18,19]. The latest machine learning studies that focus on breast cancer achieved excellent performances, and are using deep learning techniques with radionics to classify breast cancer in radiological images or histopathological slides [20–23]. On the other hand, there are not many studies that utilize only clinicopathological features.

In this research, we trained and evaluated several machine learning models trained on multiple clinicopathological features obtained from the national-level breast cancer registry, with the goal of predicting patient axillary lymph node status accurately. By using a novel model explainability framework (SHAP), we presented how the model obtained its decision-making process. The study aims to evaluate explainable machine learning models for patients eligible for NST, as well as to assess how well the models can classify metastatic lymph nodes using only clinicopathological features.

This study's main contributions are:

- machine learning model training, optimization, and evaluation curated specifically for patients eligible for NST;
- exhibiting what the model learned and which predictors were the most important in its decision-making process through the use of Shapley values;
- presenting model results for our whole breast cancer population (n = 8381).

2. Materials and Methods

2.1. Data Source and Preparation

Data examined in this study were collected from all Croatian hospitals in which breast cancer patients are diagnosed and treated. The data were acquired by searching through the hospital information systems during a five-year period, from January 2017 to January 2022. Pathohistological and demographic data were obtained for all patients that contained MKB code 50 (code for breast cancer). Pathohistological data was in a standardized format that follows ASCO/CAP guidelines, which all Croatian hospitals use [24].

The Ethics Committee of the University Hospital of Split approved the study protocol (2181-147/01/06/M.S.-22-02). The study was performed in accordance with the World Health Organization Declaration of Helsinki of 1975 as revised in 2013, and the International Conference on Harmonization Guidelines on Good Clinical Practice [25,26]. We fully protected the patients' anonymity. The study was not preregistered.

The collected data consists of ten features: patient age at the time of diagnosis, tumor size (in cm), pathohistological type, immunophenotype, pathohistological grade, estrogen (ER) and progesterone (PR) receptor quantities (0–100), HER-2 levels (0–3), Ki-67 index (0–100), and lymph node metastasis status (0/1).

The case group was defined as patients with evidence of breast cancer axillary lymph node metastasis. Consequently, the control group was defined as patients without evidence of lymph node metastasis. Tumor samples were obtained via surgery and core needle biopsies, while the target variable ground truth (axillary lymph node positivity) was established by post-surgical lymph node pathohistological examination. While the tumor size was mostly obtained post-surgically, we argue how the model can also use radiologically determined tumor size (ultrasound, MRI, mammography, or CT), due to high concordance between the diagnostic methods and the final pathological measurement of tumor size (differences in tumor diameters <5 mm) [27,28].

Initial data set contained 13,580 entries, from which 3875 entries had various missing values, ranging from the target variable (lymph node metastasis status) to pathohistological type and grades. After we omitted the missing values, we were left with 9705 entries with complete data. From those 9705 entries, 1324 patients received neoadjuvant therapy, while 8381 received initial surgical treatment. We excluded 1324 neoadjuvantly treated patients from the analysis due to confounding effects of NST (NST would lead to lymph node negativity in up to 50% initially positive patients) [29].

Since the model's target population is patients who would potentially receive neoadjuvant therapy, we identified those patients from our study population (all patients that initially received surgical treatment) using the following criteria:

- all tumors with size >5 cm (irrespective to subtype),
- tumors with size $\geq$2 cm of triple-negative or HER-2 positive subtype,
- tumors of inflammatory subtype [30].

By applying the NST criteria stated above, 719 patients were identified for final analysis.

In addition to the model based only on patients who would potentially receive neoadjuvant treatment, we also trained a broader model that generalizes to our entire breast cancer population (n = 8381), to see if similar performances are obtained and to analyze feature importance. Study workflow with methods for model optimization and validation is presented in Figure 1.

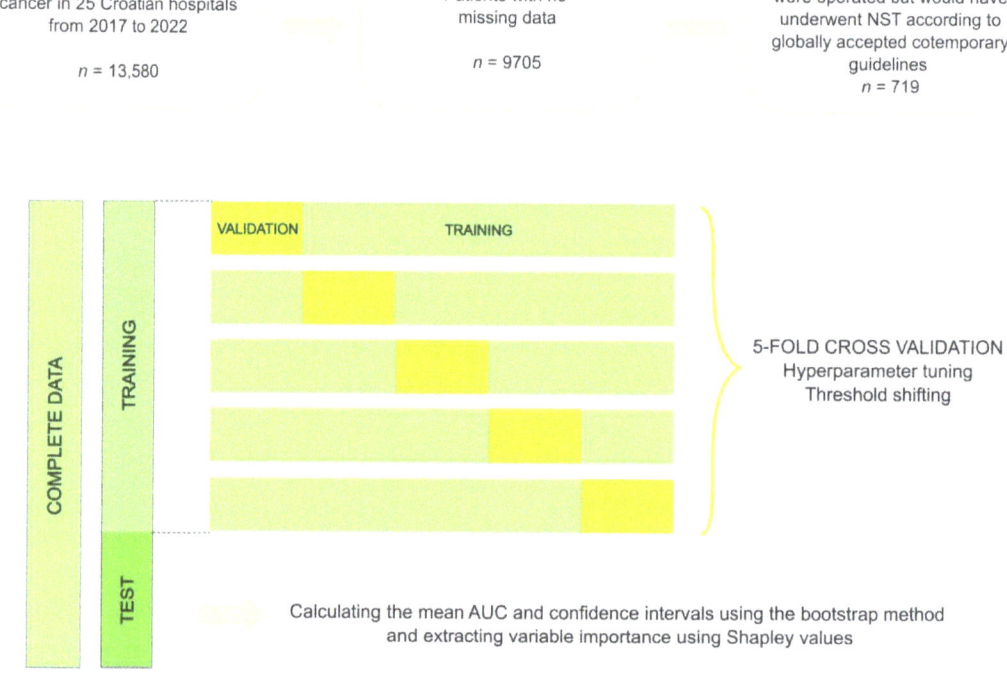

Figure 1. Study workflow.

2.2. Prediction Model Training, Optimization and Validation

We trained different models using three algorithms: logistic regression, random forest classifier, and eXtreme gradient boosting (XGBoost) classifier. Random forest and XGBoost were selected because of their high-ranking performances on tabular data, whereas logistic regression was chosen as a base classifier for comparison [31,32]. Furthermore, for evaluation purposes, univariate logistic regression was trained only on one feature (tumor size) as a baseline.

For all models, we first split the data into a training (80% of data) and test batch (20% of data). The NST-criteria dataset is fairly balanced when concerning the target variable (55% vs. 45%), whereas due to the unbalance in total study population (34% vs. 66%) the train-test split was stratified on the target variable. To further compensate for the unbalanced target variable, we used threshold shifting (by maximizing the f1-score), and balanced class weights were used for the random forest (where weights are automatically adjusted inversely proportional to class frequencies in the input data).

Categorical variables were "dummy encoded" (encoding the categorical variables to ones and zeroes). We then performed a stratified 5-fold cross-validation on the training sample to train and validate our model (Figure 1). The model's hyperparameters were optimized by performing a grid search (Figure 1). For the random forest we optimized the following hyperparameters: (1) maximal tree depth, (2) minimal number of samples required to split an internal node, (3) minimal number of samples required at a leaf node, (4) number of estimators. Whereas for XGBoost, the following hyperparameters were optimized: (1) maximal tree depth, (2) learning rate, (3) number of estimators, (4) minimum weight required to create a new node ("min_child_weight"), (5) gamma (pseudo-regularization parameter), (6) alpha (L1-regularization of leaf weights), (7) subsample (randomly selected training data prior to fitting to base learner), (8) subsample ratio of columns when constructing each tree ("colsample_bytree"), (9) subsample ratio of columns for each tree depth level ("colsample_bylevel"). Lastly, for logistic regression, we optimized for (1) solver (algorithm to use in the optimization problem), (2) regularization, and (3) regularization strength (C).

Additionally, since XGBoost can algorithmically deal with missing values, a subanalysis was performed on a dataset with missing values (after dropping the rows that miss the target variable; total $n = 10,540$, NST-criteria $n = 1389$).

Finally, the performance of the models was assessed on the test set, and the confidence intervals of the performance metrics were estimated using the bootstrap method of resampling with replacement (2000 bootstrapped samples). Modeling was performed using Python Programming Language (version 3.9.5, Python Software Foundation, Wilmington, DE, USA) using libraries "numpy", "pandas", "scikit-learn", and "xgboost", and with the R programming language (R Core Team, 2022, Vienna, Austria) using the "tidymodels", "ranger", "xgboost", "pROC", and "fastshap" packages.

2.3. Model Evaluation

Final evaluation and predictions were made on the test sample (20% of data). ROC curve was plotted, and areas under the curve (AUC) were obtained for each model with the following formula: $AUC = \int_0^1 TPR \, dFPR$, where $TPR = \frac{TP}{TP+FN}$ = sensitivity, and $FPR = \frac{FP}{TN+FP} = 1 - $ specificity.

2000 bootstrap samples obtained by resampling with replacement from the test set were used to determine the mean AUC values and calculate the 95% confidence intervals. F1-score (harmonic mean between sensitivity and positive predictive value), precision (positive predictive value), negative predictive value, sensitivity and specificity were also determined. The model with the highest AUC was selected for further investigation. The optimal cut-off points for sensitivity and specificity were based on the F1 score [33].

2.4. Feature Importance Analysis and Model Explainability

We assessed feature importance by using SHAP (SHapley Additive exPlanations), a unified framework for interpreting model predictions [34]. The method computes Shapley values from coalitional game theory. The baseline for these values is the mean of all predictions. Shapley values explain how much each of the features moves the estimate from the baseline in order to obtain the final probability. When conditioning on a selected feature (predictor), the Shapely values attribute the change in the expected model prediction to that feature [34]. Hence, Shapley values can be used to explain machine learning model predictions.

2.5. Statistical Analysis

Descriptive statistical analysis was performed to analyze the characteristics of the case (positive lymph node) and control (negative lymph node) groups. Concerning numerical data, Student's *t*-test was used to assess the comparison of means. Whereas for categorical variables, χ^2 test was used. Calculations were performed with Python Programming Language (version 3.9.5, Python Software Foundation) using the "scipy" library. Statistical significance was set at $p < 0.05$ for all comparisons.

3. Results
3.1. Patient Characteristics

In total, 5845 (69.7%) patients were identified as controls (no lymph node metastasis), while 2536 (30.3%) patients were identified as cases (positive lymph node/s) (Table 1). Statistically significant differences between cases and controls were observed in "Tumor size", "PR", "HER-2", and "Ki-67" features (Table 1).

Table 1. Patient characteristics (total population case/control comparison).

Variable	Cases, Lymph Node Metastasis Group (n = 2536)	Controls, Non-Lymph Node Metastasis Group (n = 5845)	Total (n = 8381)	p-Value
Age (range)	63.6 (21–92)	62.3 (25–89)	62.7 (12.6)	0.535 *
Tumor Size (cm)	2.7 (1.9)	1.7 (1.1)	2.01 (1.5)	<0.001 *
Ki-67	29.7 (18.7)	25.1 (18.4)	26.5 (18.7)	<0.001 *
ER	80.7 (33.7)	83.1 (32.2)	82.4 (32.7)	0.064 *
PR	50.8 (39.5)	54.3 (39.4)	53.2 (39.4)	<0.001 *
Tumor Grade (%)				<0.001 †
1	376 (14.8)	1638 (28)	2014 (24)	
2	1460 (57.6)	3148 (53.8)	4608 (54.9)	
3	700 (27.6)	1059 (18.2)	1759 (20.9)	
HER-2 (%)				<0.001 *
0	1092 (43.1)	2776 (47.5)	3868 (46.2)	
1	815 (32.1)	1953 (33.4)	2768 (33)	
2	344 (1.3)	629 (10.8)	914 (10.9)	
3	285 (11.2)	487 (8.3)	831 (9.9)	
Histological Type (%)				<0.001 †
NOS-invasive	2055 (81)	4586 (78.5)	6641 (79.2)	
Lobular Invasive	324 (12.8)	693 (11.9)	1017 (12.1)	
Ca with Medullary Characteristics	24 (0.9)	47 (0.8)	71 (0.8)	
Other (Rare Types)	133 (5.2)	519 (8.9)	652 (7.8)	
Immunophenotype (%)				<0.001 †
Luminal B	1517 (59.8)	3154 (53.9)	4671 (55.7)	
Luminal A	429 (16.9)	1628 (27.8)	2057 (24.6)	
Luminal B-her2	310 (12.3)	508 (8.7)	818 (9.8)	
Triple Negative	160 (6.3)	407 (6.9)	567 (6.7)	
HER2 Positive	120 (4.7)	148 (2.6)	268 (3.2)	

Data are presented as mean (standard deviation) and count (percentage); *—t-test for independent variables, †—χ^2 test; Ki-67—cellular proliferation index, ER—estrogen receptor index, PR—progesterone receptor index, HER-2—human epidermal growth factor receptor, NOS- not otherwise specified histological type. Other rare histological types include: mucinous invasive, micropapillary invasive, cribriform invasive, and inflammatory types).

In the NST criteria group, there were 426 (55%) patients with lymph node metastasis and 350 (45%) patients without metastasis. Since lymph node metastasis is present in 55% of the target population, we can see that our target variable is fairly balanced (55% vs. 45%), which differs from the total population where the ratio favors the non-metastasis group (34% vs. 66%).

Moreover, for the NST criteria group, while "Tumour size", "PR" and "Ki-67" also showed significant differences, there were also significant differences in "Age" and "ER" features and no significant difference in "HER-2" (Table 2).

Table 2. Patient characteristics (NST criteria group).

Variable	Cases, Lymph Node Metastasis Group (n = 392)	Controls, Non-Lymph Node Metastasis Group (n = 327)	Total (n = 719)	p-Value
Age (range)	66.9 (21–92)	64.2 (25–87)	65.7 (14.6)	0.016 *
Tumor Size (cm)	5.7 (3.02)	3.9 (2.5)	4.9 (2.9)	<0.001 *
Ki-67	43.4 (23.3)	50.6 (25.7)	46.7 (24.7)	<0.001 *
ER	40.01 (45.9)	13.7 (32.6)	28.1 (42.5)	<0.001 *
PR	21.8 (35.04)	7.51 (22.5)	15.2 (30.6)	<0.001 *

Table 2. Cont.

Variable	Cases, Lymph Node Metastasis Group (n = 392)	Controls, Non-Lymph Node Metastasis Group (n = 327)	Total (n = 719)	p-Value
Tumor Grade (%)				0.027 †
1	14 (3.6)	8 (2.4)	22 (3)	
2	133 (33.9)	97 (29.6)	230 (32)	
3	245 (62.5)	222 (68)	467 (65)	
HER-2 (%)				0.060 *
0	180 (46)	173 (53)	353 (49.1)	
1	79 (20.1)	55 (16.8)	134 (18.7)	
2	35 (8.9)	42 (12.8)	77 (10.7)	
3	98 (25)	57 (17.4)	155 (21.5)	
Histological Type (%)				<0.001 †
NOS-invasive	282 (71.9)	252 (77.2)	534 (74.3)	
Lobular Invasive	63 (16.1)	20 (6.1)	83 (11.5)	
Ca with Medullary Characteristics	15 (3.8)	12 (3.6)	27 (3.7)	
Other (Rare Types)	32 (8.2)	43 (13.1)	75 (10.4%)	
Immunophenotype (%)				<0.001 †
Luminal B	111 (28.4)	35 (10.7)	146 (20.3)	
Luminal A	26 (6.6)	7 (2.3)	33 (4.6)	
Luminal B-her2	35 (8.9)	8 (2.4)	43 (5.9)	
>Triple Negative	137 (34.9)	210 (64.2)	347 (48.4)	
HER-2 Positive	83 (21.2)	67 (20.4)	150 (20.8)	

Data are presented as mean (standard deviation) and count (percentage); *—t-test for independent variables; †—χ^2 test;).

3.2. Prediction Model Performance

3.2.1. Performance on NST Criteria Group

After training three different models on the NST-criteria group data (n = 621), validating and optimizing them via 5-fold cross-validation, and then evaluating them on the holdout test set (n = 155), the random forest classifier produced the highest result. (Table 3). Using default settings, the random forest classifier achieved an AUC of 0.76, whereas, after hyperparameter optimization, the score rose to 0.793 (95% CI 0.713–0.865) (Figure 2, Table 3). At the baseline decision threshold of 0.5, F1-score was 0.750 (95% CI: 0.690–0.812), sensitivity was 0.809 (95% CI 0.718–0.885), specificity 0.570 (95% CI 0.446–0.692), negative predictive value 0.714 (95% CI: 0.615–0.820) and the precision (positive predictive value) 0.694 (95% CI: 0.630–0.759). Another tree-based model, XGBoost, achieved an AUC of 0.783 (95% CI: 0.703–0.858) on the test set (Table 3). Finally, Logistic Regression has achieved an AUC of 0.763 (95% CI: 0.683–0.838), while univariate Logistic Regression (trained on "Tumor size") achieved an AUC of 0.688 (95% CI: 0.626–0.745) (Table 3).

Table 3. Model performances for predicting lymph node metastasis (NST criteria group).

Model	Mean AUC (95% CI)
Random Forest	0.793 (0.713–0.865)
XGBoost	0.783 (0.703–0.858)
Logistic Regression	0.763 (0.683–0.838)
Univariate Logistic Regression	0.645 (0.556–0.726)

Values are presented as mean (95% Confidence interval); AUC—area under the receiver operating characteristic curve.

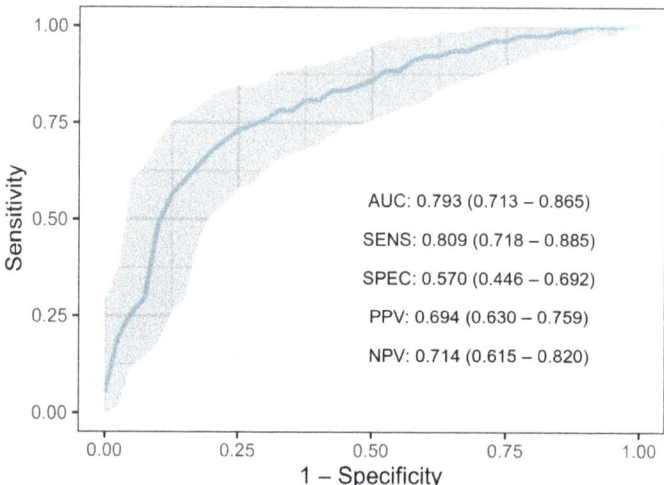

Figure 2. ROC-curve for Random Forest trained on NST-criteria group. (ROC—receiver operating characteristic curve, AUC—area under the curve, SENS—sensitivity, SPEC—specificity, PPV—positive predictive value, NPV—negative predictive value).

When evaluating XGBoost on the NST-criteria dataset that contained missing values (n = 1389), somewhat worse performances were obtained, with an AUC of 0.724 (95% CI: 0.654–0.785).

3.2.2. Performance on Entire Population

Due to a higher n, instead of 20%, we held out 10% of the data for the test set in the entire population. Therefore, 7543 rows of data were used for the training set, while 838 rows were held out in the test set. A 10-fold cross-validation scheme was performed on the training data to train and validate the models. Finally, their individual performances were assessed on the test set and standard deviations were obtained with the bootstrap method (Table 4). XGBoost ranked highest with a mean AUC of 0.762 (95% CI: 0.726–0.794), closely trailed by Random Forest with an AUC of 0.760 (95% CI: 0.71–0.78) (Table 4). Just like with Random Forest and XGBoost, Logistic Regression and Univariate Logistic Regression also scored lower than in the NST criteria group, with a mean AUC of 0.741 (95% CI: 0.706–0.775) and 0.589 (95% CI 0.577–0.614), respectively (Table 4). Concerning XGBoost's performance on other metrics at the baseline threshold, it achieved an F1 score of 0.448 (95% CI: 0.389–0.507), a sensitivity of 0.344 (95% CI: 0.289–0.403) and specificity of 0.903 (95%: 0.877–0.926), the positive predictive value of 0.607 (95% CI: 0.539–0.680), the negative predictive value of 0.761 (95% CI: 0.744–0.778) (Figure 3). To correct the class imbalance we changed the default threshold by maximizing the F1 score. Lowering the threshold to 0.28 increased the F1-score to 0.581 (95% CI: 0.545–0.618), sensitivity to 0.732 (95% CI: 0.676–0.787), and negative predictive value to 0.854 (95% CI: 0.827–0.881), while specificity decreased to 0.676 (95% CI: 0.637–0.714), and positive predictive value to 0.495 (95% CI: 0.461–0.531). When evaluating XGBoost on a total dataset that contained missing values (n = 10,540), somewhat worse performances were obtained, with an AUC of 0.731 (95% CI: 0.634–0.771).

Table 4. Model performances for predicting lymph node metastasis (entire population).

Model	Mean AUC (95% CI)
XGBoost	0.762 (0.726–0.795)
Random Forest	0.760 (0.724–0.794)
Logistic Regression	0.741 (0.706–0.775)
Univariate Logistic Regression	0.713 (0.686–0.739)

Values are presented as mean (95% Confidence interval); AUC—area under the receiver operating characteristic curve.

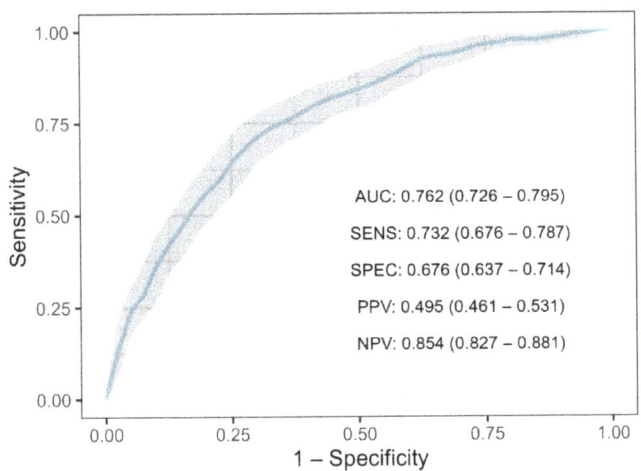

Figure 3. ROC-curve for XGBoost trained on total study population. (ROC—receiver operating characteristic curve, AUC—area under the curve, SENS—sensitivity, SPEC—specificity, PPV—positive predictive value, NPV—negative predictive value).

3.2.3. Feature Importance for Predicting Lymph Node Metastasis

After calculating Shapely values for the NST criteria group, tumor size was the most important feature, followed by ER, PR, and HER2 status (Figure 4).

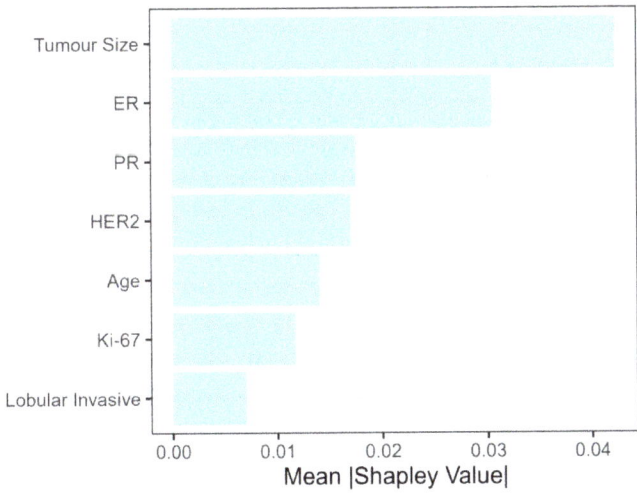

Figure 4. Shapley values (feature importance) for NST group.

Lymph node metastasis showed a linear dependence on tumor size up to 5 cm, after which a plateau is reached (Figure 5). Concerning age, there is a clear and sharp rise in dependency after the age of 75 (Figure 5). ER and PR status show a growing trend, with larger values more associated with nodal involvement, while hormone receptor negativity is associated with an absence of metastasis (Figure 5). Notably, this is highly correlated to tumor size, because most high ER and PR tumors were of luminal A and luminal B histological types, which have to be >5 cm in size to adhere to NST criteria.

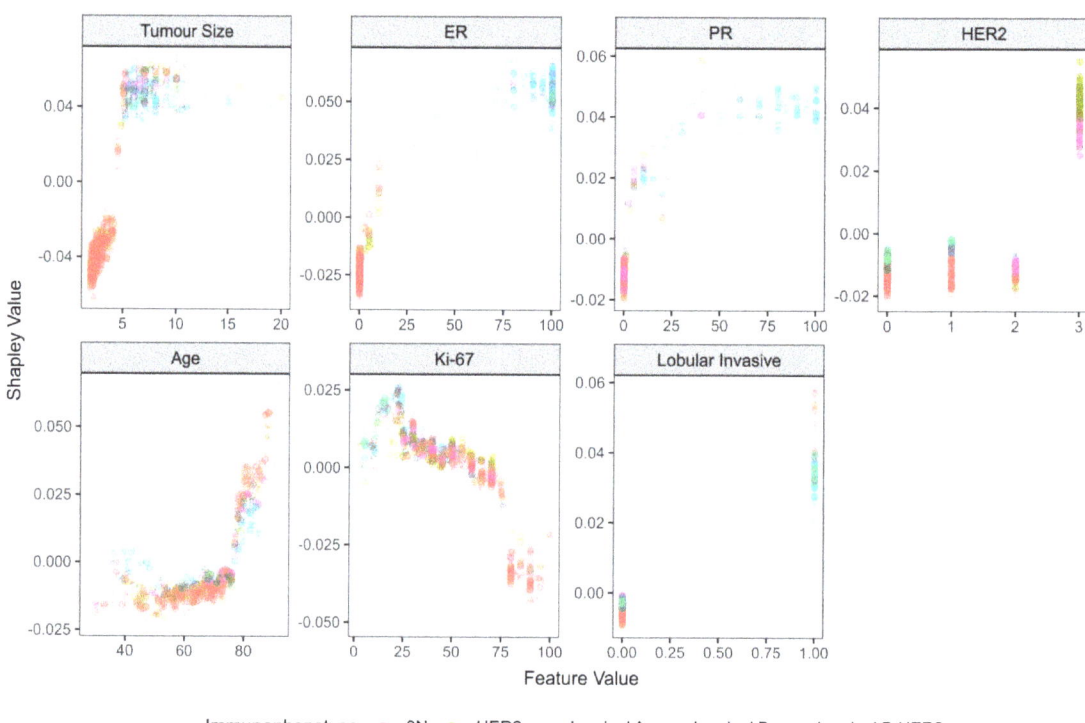

Figure 5. Dependency plot for Shapley values (NST criteria group).

For HER-2, the model associated HER-2 positivity with a higher chance of lymph node metastasis (Figure 5). Interestingly, Ki-67 exhibits an increase in Shapley values from 0 to 25%, after which it gradually decreases, with a sudden drop in values at around 75%. However, after a more detailed inspection, we can see that these values are predominantly associated with the triple-negative immunophenotype (Figure 5). Finally, the model associated lobular invasive histological type with a higher chance of lymph node metastasis (Figure 5).

While tumor size was also the most important feature when Shapley values were calculated on the total study population, the second most important feature was Ki-67, followed by age and tumor grade (Figure 6).

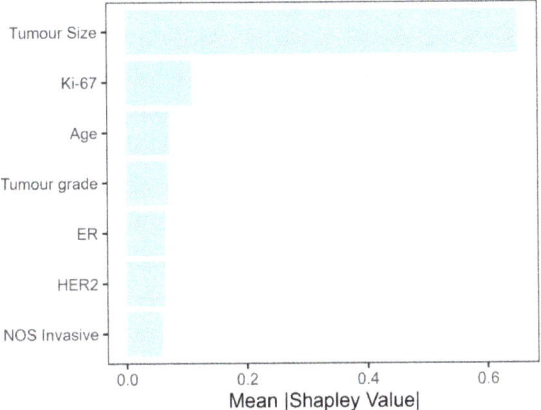

Figure 6. Shapley values (feature importance) for total study population.

For tumor size, the trend from the NST criteria group was confirmed on the total study population (growing dependency, with a plateau after 5 cm) (Figure 7). The same holds for HER-2 status, where HER-2 positivity is associated with lymph node metastasis (Figure 7). Tumor grade also shows a clear increasing trend (Figure 7). For Ki-67, there is a noticeable increase in Shapley values at index values of 25%, along with a decrease at around 75%. However, the Shapley values exhibit a high level of dispersion (Figure 7), indicating a dependence on the value of other variables. Age shows an interesting non-linear dependency, where patients younger than 40 and patients older than 75 were associated with a higher chance of metastasis (Figure 7).

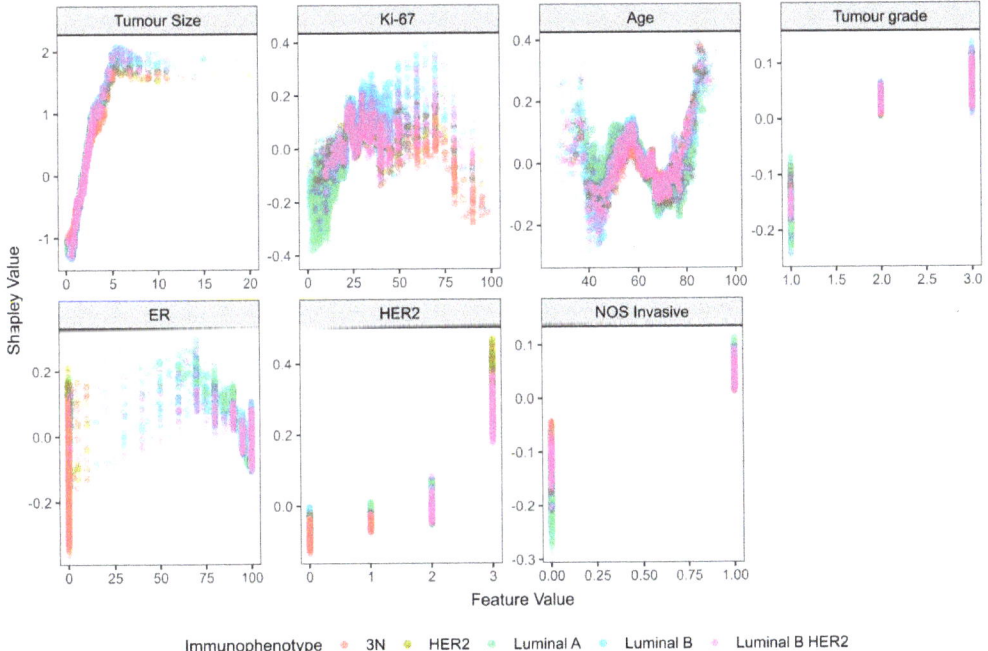

Figure 7. Dependency plot for Shapley values (total study population).

4. Discussion

In order to improve treatment outcomes, an increasing number of early breast cancer patients are treated with NST. To achieve optimal treatment strategy for every patient, and implement precision oncology, due to nonoptimal performance of existing diagnostic tools, there is a growing need for additional methods of axillary lymph node metastasis status evaluation. Additionally, to determine axillary lymph node status in patients with breast cancer who are initially treated with surgical therapy, sentinel lymph node dissection is recommended. It was reported that sentinel lymph node dissection has a usual false negative range of 7.5%, but can reach up to 27.3%, resulting in unradical axillary surgery and consequently suboptimal adjuvant therapy strategies based on wrong staging [35,36]. Therefore, other than patients receiving NST, patients receiving initial surgical therapy can also benefit from supplementary non-invasive methods for the determination of the lymph node status.

In this study, we trained, optimized, and validated multiple machine-learning models that can effectively help us predict axillary breast cancer lymph node metastasis. The random forest algorithm, an ensemble-based method, has produced the highest mean AUC score (0.793 for the NST criteria group, 0.760 for the total study population). Since the random forest algorithm consists of multiple decision trees and later combines their predictions, it reduces the risk of overfitting and thus provides a more robust model [37]. XGBoost, another robust ensemble tree-based model, produced a somewhat better result than random forest on the total study population. This is in line with previous studies showing that XGBoost and Random forest generally achieve comparable results, but based on the exact dataset, one will outperform the other [16,38]. Lastly, both models achieved improved performances when compared to the baseline univariate model that only used tumor size as a predictor.

When considering feature importance by Shapley values, the most important features in the NST criteria group were tumor size, ER, PR and HER2 status. Nodal involvement grew with tumor size up to 5 cm, and hence our findings corroborate the findings of Sopik and Narod, where a plateau in nodal metastasis was also reached after approximately 5 cm in tumor size [39]. For the NST-criteria group, Shapley values display a growing trend with an increase in ER and PR levels. Although this is surprising at first glance, this finding is probably an artifact of selection criteria. Namely, based on the selection criteria, tumors with high ER and/or PR values, corresponding to luminal A and B immunophenotypes, were only included if the tumor size was greater than 5 cm. This leads to an artificial correlation between high ER values and the probability of lymph node metastasis, which is actually based on the influence of tumor size. Consequently, the results concerning the effect of ER and PR were not confirmed when feature importance was examined in the total study population. The literature is also conflicted concerning the role of ER in predicting nodal involvement. For example, in a study by Alsumai et al., positive ER status was a significant predictor of nodal metastasis, whereas in another study ER and PR held no significant effect on axillary lymph node metastasis [40,41].

Furthermore, Shapley values for patient age showed that nodal involvement grows after 75 years of age. Similar results were reported by Wildiers et al., where nodal involvement grew after the age of 70 [42].

While tumor size was also the most important feature in the total study population, it was shown that the second most important feature was Ki-67, followed by tumor grade. Interestingly, when Shapley values for patient age were calculated on the total study population, a non-linear trend was observed, where both patients younger than 40 and patients older than 75 were associated with nodal involvement. This higher occurrence of lymph node metastasis in patients younger than 40 was also reported in previous studies [43,44]. Concerning Ki-67, higher values are generally associated with higher probabilities for metastasis. Interestingly, for Ki-67 values > 75%, Shapley values are mostly negative. However, when accounting for immunophenotype, this trend reversal is only visible for triple-negative carcinomas. Previous studies also showed that Ki-67 > 20% was positively correlated with lymph node metastasis, albeit they used pre-defined categories of <20% and >20% and did not account for differences in immunophenotype [45,46]. Hence, they potentially missed a more complex relationship that was explained through Shapley values.

Likewise, higher tumor grade is commonly associated with nodal metastasis [43]. Concerning HER-2, our model associates HER-2 positivity with nodal involvement. HER-2 was also a significant predictive factor for axillary nodal involvement (with a regression coefficient of 0.30) in another study where researchers developed a Lasso regression model to predict non-sentinel breast cancer lymph node metastasis [47]. Taken together, we can conclude that our model's decision-making process can be clinically explained because it has learned relationships whose importance was also confirmed by other studies.

Aside from the above observations, it is also worth noting that Shapley analysis has independently identified the commonly used cutoff points for ER, PR, Ki-67, and HER2 positivity.

Currently, we are witnessing a great interest in studies based on radiomics, combining radiological findings and deep learning methods to predict breast cancer lymph node status [48–51]. An interesting study by Zheng et al. joined deep learning radiomics of conventional ultrasound and shear wave elastography of breast cancer with clinicopathological data and obtained excellent results with an AUC of 0.902 (95% CI: 0.843–0.961) [52]. They also applied a model that was trained just with features from clinicopathological data, which produced a weaker AUC in comparison to ours (0.72 [95% CI: 0.63–0.82] vs. 0.79 [95% CI 0.72–0.87], respectively) [52]. This relatively poorer artificial neural networks (ANN) performance could potentially be explained by a relative underperformance of neural networks on tabular data [31]. It was shown that tree-based models (random forest and XGBoost) outperform deep learning methods on datasets with up to 10 000 training examples [31].

Similarly, another study that evaluated ANN trained on clinicopathological features for predicting breast cancer lymph node involvement achieved an AUC of 0.74 (95% CI: 0.72–0.76) [53]. However, one of their most predictive features was a lymphovascular invasion, a feature that is not always obtainable on core-needle biopsy and is not used by our model [54].

Random forest was also the best-performing algorithm in the study by Tseng et al., with performances similar to ours (mean AUC of 0.75) [17]. Another tree-based model (XGBoost), was shown to be the best-performing model in a study by Li et al., where the authors utilized tumor gene signatures to predict metastatic status in breast cancer [19]. Their optimized model achieved an AUC of 0.82 (SD ± 0.15) [19]. Likewise, in a study by Meng et al., a Lasso regression-based model achieved an AUC of 0.77 (95% CI 0.69–0.86) for the prediction of non-sentinel lymph node metastasis status [47]. Moreover, an older study that combined clinicopathological findings with diagnostic mammography and ultrasonography findings achieved an AUC of 0.77 (95% CI: 0.689–0.856) in breast cancer lymph node prediction with an alternating decision tree (ADTree) [55]. Therefore, our results are comparable with the results of other studies that predicted breast cancer lymph nodes and general metastasis [17,19,47,52,55] (Table 5).

Table 5. Comparison with other studies that used clinicopathological features for breast cancer lymph node classification.

Study (Algorithm Type)	Total Patients	Mean AUC (95% CI)
This study (XGBoost)	8381	0.76 (0.73–0.80)
Takada et al. [55] (ADTree)	467	0.77 (0.69–0.86)
Zheng et al. [52] (without radiomics, neural network)	1342	0.72 (0.63–0.82)
Dihge et al. [53] (neural network)	800	0.74 (0.72–0.76)
Meng et al. [47] (non-sentinel lymph node prediction, Lasso regression)	714	0.77 (0.69–0.86)

We believe that similar models could be locally optimized and validated to aid clinicians in their multidisciplinary workflow. Especially when dealing with patients who would receive NST, since lymph node status is an essential factor that affects optimal treatment selection and prognosis. Moreover, other beneficial tumor/patient data that can be obtained, such as gene expression and serum biomarkers, could lead to better model performances. Accordingly, future research can assess whether the addition of genetic and biomarker data increases the accuracy of machine-learning models.

Our study contains several limitations. Firstly, it was performed only on the Croatian population of early breast cancer patients. Thus, similar models should be validated on other population groups to provide better generalizability. Another limitation of this study is its retrospective nature, even though the data originated from a prospectively maintained database. Perhaps the most important limitation of the study was the relatively large number of patients who were excluded from the analysis due to incomplete data. Of course, we have no evidence that these data are missing completely at random (MCAR). Furthermore, a possible minor limitation of the generalizability of the results of this analysis could have been caused by the fact that part of the data was collected during the lockdown to control the COVID-19 pandemic.

Finally, this study offers novelty by presenting an explainable machine-learning framework with a clinically relevant decision-making process. A further strength of the present study is that it provides a unique perspective in which a multicenter dataset was obtained, and from subjects that were initially treated surgically, an additional subset was extracted by applying the NCCN criteria for NST [7]. In this way, the model was curated for NST-eligible patients, who could extract the greatest benefit from such a non-invasive method for determining axillary lymph node metastasis status.

5. Conclusions

We have shown that explainable tree-based machine learning methods trained on patient and tumor features obtained during regular pre-operative/pre-NST procedures achieve a good performance in predicting breast cancer axillary lymph node metastasis. Such models can lead to more accurate diagnosis and better treatment selection, especially for NST patients, where radiological and clinical findings are often the only way of lymph node assessment. Potential upstage of diagnosis based on machine learning models for some patients would result in NST and, consecutively, potentially more adjuvant therapy with non-cross resistant treatments and better patient outcomes. The addition of genetic and biomarker data and subsequent validation in multinational/multicenter studies is expected from future studies.

Author Contributions: Conceptualization, J.V., J.B. and E.V.; methodology, J.V., Z.B. and D.B.; software, J.V., Z.B., D.B. and D.Š.; validation, M.K., M.A., S.T. and Č.T.; formal analysis, J.V. and Z.B.; investigation, J.V.; resources, S.T., M.P.B., M.A., Č.T. and M.M.P.; data curation, S.T., M.P.B., Č.T., M.A. and M.M.P.; writing—original draft preparation, J.V.; writing—review and editing, Z.B., M.K., E.V. and J.B.; visualization, Z.B. and D.B.; supervision, J.B. and E.V.; project administration, J.B. All authors have read and agreed to the published version of the manuscript.

Funding: This research received no external funding.

Institutional Review Board Statement: The study was conducted in accordance with the Declaration of Helsinki, and approved by The Ethics Committee of University Hospital of Split (protocol code 2181-147/01/06/M.S.-22-02).

Informed Consent Statement: Not applicable.

Data Availability Statement: The dataset used and analyzed during the current study is available from the corresponding author upon reasonable request.

Acknowledgments: We thank Josipa Flam, Ingrid Belac Lovasić and Valerija Blažičević for their contribution in data collection. We thank Žarko Bajić for his advice and recommendations.

Conflicts of Interest: The authors declare no conflict of interest.

References

1. Siegel, R.L.; Miller, K.D.; Fuchs, H.E.; Jemal, A. Cancer statistics, 2022. *CA Cancer J. Clin.* **2022**, *72*, 7–33. [CrossRef] [PubMed]
2. Cancer Today. Available online: https://gco.iarc.fr/today/online-analysis-table?v=2020&mode=cancer&mode_population=continents&population=900&populations=900&key=asr&sex=2&cancer=39&type=1&statistic=5&prevalence=0&population_group=0&ages_group%5B%5D=0&ages_group%5B%5D=17&group_cancer=1&include_nmsc=0&include_nmsc_other=1 (accessed on 10 October 2022.).
3. Centers for Disease Control and Prevention. *Incidence and Relative Survival by Stage at Diagnosis for Common Cancers*; USCS Data Brief, n.A., GA: Centers for Disease Control and Prevention, US Department of Health and Human Services: Washington, DC, USA, 2021.
4. Nordenskjöld, A.E.; Fohlin, H.; Arnesson, L.G.; Einbeigi, Z.; Holmberg, E.; Albertsson, P.; Karlsson, P. Breast cancer survival trends in different stages and age groups—A population-based study 1989–2013. *Acta Oncol.* **2019**, *58*, 45–51. [CrossRef] [PubMed]
5. Walsh, M.F.; Nathanson, K.L.; Couch, F.J.; Offit, K. Genomic Biomarkers for Breast Cancer Risk. *Adv. Exp. Med. Biol.* **2016**, *882*, 1–32. [PubMed]
6. Kim, J.Y.; Ryu, M.R.; Choi, B.O.; Park, W.C.; Oh, S.J.; Won, J.M.; Chung, S.M. The prognostic significance of the lymph node ratio in axillary lymph node positive breast cancer. *J. Breast Cancer* **2011**, *14*, 204–212. [CrossRef] [PubMed]
7. Gradishar, W.J.; Moran, M.S.; Abraham, J.; Aft, R.; Agnese, D.; Allison, K.H.; Anderson, B.; Burstein, H.J.; Chew, H.; Dang, C.; et al. Breast Cancer, Version 3.2022, NCCN Clinical Practice Guidelines in Oncology. *J. Natl. Compr. Cancer Netw.* **2022**, *20*, 691–722. [CrossRef]
8. Cortazar, P.; Zhang, L.; Untch, M.; Mehta, K.; Costantino, J.P.; Wolmark, N.; Bonnefoi, H.; Cameron, D.; Gianni, L.; Valagussa, P.; et al. Pathological complete response and long-term clinical benefit in breast cancer: The CTNeoBC pooled analysis. *Lancet* **2014**, *384*, 164–172. [CrossRef]
9. Symmans, W.F.; Wei, C.; Gould, R.; Yu, X.; Zhang, Y.; Liu, M.; Walls, A.; Bousamra, A.; Ramineni, M.; Sinn, B.; et al. Long-Term Prognostic Risk After Neoadjuvant Chemotherapy Associated With Residual Cancer Burden and Breast Cancer Subtype. *J. Clin. Oncol.* **2017**, *35*, 1049–1060. [CrossRef]
10. Choi, H.Y.; Park, M.; Seo, M.; Song, E.; Shin, S.Y.; Sohn, Y.M. Preoperative Axillary Lymph Node Evaluation in Breast Cancer: Current Issues and Literature Review. *Ultrasound Q.* **2017**, *33*, 6–14. [CrossRef]
11. Piccart, M.; Procter, M.; Fumagalli, D.; Azambuja, E.d.; Clark, E.; Ewer, M.S.; Restuccia, E.; Jerusalem, G.; Dent, S.; Reaby, L.; et al. Adjuvant Pertuzumab and Trastuzumab in Early HER2-Positive Breast Cancer in the APHINITY Trial: 6 Years' Follow-Up. *J. Clin. Oncol.* **2021**, *39*, 1448–1457. [CrossRef]
12. Kann, B.H.; Hosny, A.; Aerts, H. Artificial intelligence for clinical oncology. *Cancer Cell* **2021**, *39*, 916–927. [CrossRef]
13. Boehm, K.M.; Khosravi, P.; Vanguri, R.; Gao, J.; Shah, S.P. Harnessing multimodal data integration to advance precision oncology. *Nat. Rev. Cancer* **2022**, *22*, 114–126. [CrossRef] [PubMed]
14. Iqbal, M.S.; Ahmad, W.; Alizadehsani, R.; Hussain, S.; Rehman, R. Breast Cancer Dataset, Classification and Detection Using Deep Learning. *Healthcare* **2022**, *10*, 2395. [CrossRef] [PubMed]
15. Sarker, I.H. Machine Learning: Algorithms, Real-World Applications and Research Directions. *SN Comput. Sci.* **2021**, *2*, 160. [CrossRef] [PubMed]
16. Kabiraj, S.; Raihan, M.; Alvi, N.; Afrin, M.; Akter, L.; Sohagi, S.A.; Podder, E. Breast Cancer Risk Prediction using XGBoost and Random Forest Algorithm. In Proceedings of the 2020 11th International Conference on Computing, Communication and Networking Technologies (ICCCNT), Kharagpur, India, 1–3 July 2020; pp. 1–4.
17. Tseng, Y.J.; Huang, C.E.; Wen, C.N.; Lai, P.Y.; Wu, M.H.; Sun, Y.C.; Wang, H.Y.; Lu, J.J. Predicting breast cancer metastasis by using serum biomarkers and clinicopathological data with machine learning technologies. *Int. J. Med. Inform.* **2019**, *128*, 79–86. [CrossRef]
18. Paik, E.S.; Lee, J.W.; Park, J.Y.; Kim, J.H.; Kim, M.; Kim, T.J.; Choi, C.H.; Kim, B.G.; Bae, D.S.; Seo, S.W. Prediction of survival outcomes in patients with epithelial ovarian cancer using machine learning methods. *J. Gynecol. Oncol.* **2019**, *30*, e65. [CrossRef]
19. Li, Q.; Yang, H.; Wang, P.; Liu, X.; Lv, K.; Ye, M. XGBoost-based and tumor-immune characterized gene signature for the prediction of metastatic status in breast cancer. *J. Transl. Med.* **2022**, *20*, 177. [CrossRef]
20. Altameem, A.; Mahanty, C.; Poonia, R.C.; Saudagar, A.K.J.; Kumar, R. Breast Cancer Detection in Mammography Images Using Deep Convolutional Neural Networks and Fuzzy Ensemble Modeling Techniques. *Diagnostics* **2022**, *12*, 1812. [CrossRef]
21. Muduli, D.; Dash, R.; Majhi, B. Automated diagnosis of breast cancer using multi-modal datasets: A deep convolution neural network based approach. *Biomed. Signal Process. Control* **2022**, *71*, 102825. [CrossRef]
22. Wakili, M.A.; Shehu, H.A.; Sharif, M.H.; Sharif, M.H.U.; Umar, A.; Kusetogullari, H.; Ince, I.F.; Uyaver, S. Classification of Breast Cancer Histopathological Images Using DenseNet and Transfer Learning. *Comput. Intell. Neurosci.* **2022**, *10*, 8904768. [CrossRef]
23. Heenaye-Mamode Khan, M.; Boodoo-Jahangeer, N.; Dullull, W.; Nathire, S.; Gao, X.; Sinha, G.R.; Nagwanshi, K.K. Multi-class classification of breast cancer abnormalities using Deep Convolutional Neural Network (CNN). *PLoS ONE* **2021**, *16*, e0256500. [CrossRef]
24. Hammond, M.E. ASCO-CAP guidelines for breast predictive factor testing: An update. *Appl. Immunohistochem. Mol. Morphol.* **2011**, *19*, 499–500. [CrossRef] [PubMed]
25. Dixon, J.R., Jr. The International Conference on Harmonization Good Clinical Practice guideline. *Qual. Assur.* **1998**, *6*, 65–74. [CrossRef]

26. World Medical Association Declaration of Helsinki: Ethical principles for medical research involving human subjects. *JAMA* **2013**, *310*, 2191–2194. [CrossRef] [PubMed]
27. Ahn, S.J.; Kim, Y.S.; Kim, E.Y.; Park, H.K.; Cho, E.K.; Kim, Y.K.; Sung, Y.M.; Choi, H.Y. The value of chest CT for prediction of breast tumor size: Comparison with pathology measurement. *World J. Surg. Oncol.* **2013**, *11*, 1477–7819. [CrossRef] [PubMed]
28. Cortadellas, T.; Argacha, P.; Acosta, J.; Rabasa, J.; Peiró, R.; Gomez, M.; Rodellar, L.; Gomez, S.; Navarro-Golobart, A.; Sanchez-Mendez, S.; et al. Estimation of tumor size in breast cancer comparing clinical examination, mammography, ultrasound and MRI—Correlation with the pathological analysis of the surgical specimen. *Gland. Surg.* **2017**, *6*, 330–335. [CrossRef]
29. Hyder, T.; Bhattacharya, S.; Gade, K.; Nasrazadani, A.; Brufsky, A.M. Approaching Neoadjuvant Therapy in the Management of Early-Stage Breast Cancer. *Breast Cancer* **2021**, *13*, 199–211. [CrossRef]
30. Korde, L.A.; Somerfield, M.R.; Carey, L.A.; Crews, J.R.; Denduluri, N.; Hwang, E.S.; Khan, S.A.; Loibl, S.; Morris, E.A.; Perez, A.; et al. Neoadjuvant Chemotherapy, Endocrine Therapy, and Targeted Therapy for Breast Cancer: ASCO Guideline. *J. Clin. Oncol.* **2021**, *39*, 1485–1505. [CrossRef]
31. Grinsztajn, L.; Oyallon, E.; Varoquaux, G. Why do tree-based models still outperform deep learning on tabular data? *arXiv* **2022**, arXiv:2207.08815.
32. Shwartz-Ziv, R.; Armon, A. Tabular data: Deep learning is not all you need. *Inf. Fusion* **2022**, *81*, 84–90. [CrossRef]
33. Blair, D.C. Information Retrieval, 2nd ed. C.J. Van Rijsbergen. London: Butterworths; 1979: 208 pp. Price: $32.50. *J. Am. Soc. Inf. Sci.* **1979**, *30*, 374–375. [CrossRef]
34. Lundberg, S.M.; Lee, S.-I. A unified approach to interpreting model predictions. In Proceedings of the 31st International Conference on Neural Information Processing Systems, Long Beach, CA, USA, 4–9 December 2017; pp. 4768–4777.
35. Pesek, S.; Ashikaga, T.; Krag, L.E.; Krag, D. The false-negative rate of sentinel node biopsy in patients with breast cancer: A meta-analysis. *World J. Surg.* **2012**, *36*, 2239–2251. [CrossRef] [PubMed]
36. Li, H.; Jun, Z.; Zhi-Cheng, G.; Xiang, Q. Factors that affect the false negative rate of sentinel lymph node mapping with methylene blue dye alone in breast cancer. *J. Int. Med. Res.* **2019**, *47*, 4841–4853. [CrossRef] [PubMed]
37. Breiman, L. Random Forests. *Mach. Learn.* **2001**, *45*, 5–32. [CrossRef]
38. Bentéjac, C.; Csörgő, A.; Martínez-Muñoz, G. A Comparative Analysis of XGBoost. *arXiv* **2019**, arXiv:1911.01914.
39. Sopik, V.; Narod, S.A. The relationship between tumour size, nodal status and distant metastases: On the origins of breast cancer. *Breast Cancer Res. Treat.* **2018**, *170*, 647–656. [CrossRef]
40. Alsumai, T.S.; Alhazzaa, N.; Alshamrani, A.; Assiri, S.; Alhefdhi, A. Factors Predicting Positive Sentinel Lymph Node Biopsy in Clinically Node-Negative Breast Cancer. *Breast Cancer* **2022**, *14*, 323–334. [CrossRef]
41. Yoshihara, E.; Smeets, A.; Laenen, A.; Reynders, A.; Soens, J.; Van Ongeval, C.; Moerman, P.; Paridaens, R.; Wildiers, H.; Neven, P.; et al. Predictors of axillary lymph node metastases in early breast cancer and their applicability in clinical practice. *Breast* **2013**, *22*, 357–361. [CrossRef]
42. Wildiers, H.; Van Calster, B.; van de Poll-Franse, L.V.; Hendrickx, W.; Røislien, J.; Smeets, A.; Paridaens, R.; Deraedt, K.; Leunen, K.; Weltens, C.; et al. Relationship between age and axillary lymph node involvement in women with breast cancer. *J. Clin. Oncol.* **2009**, *27*, 2931–2937. [CrossRef]
43. Rivadeneira, D.E.; Simmons, R.M.; Christos, P.J.; Hanna, K.; Daly, J.M.; Osborne, M.P. Predictive factors associated with axillary lymph node metastases in T1a and T1b breast carcinomas: Analysis in more than 900 patients. *J. Am. Coll. Surg.* **2000**, *191*, 1–6. [CrossRef]
44. Gajdos, C.; Tartter, P.I.; Bleiweiss, I.J. Lymphatic invasion, tumor size, and age are independent predictors of axillary lymph node metastases in women with T1 breast cancers. *Ann. Surg.* **1999**, *230*, 692–696. [CrossRef]
45. Yin, Y.; Zeng, K.; Wu, M.; Ding, Y.; Zhao, M.; Chen, Q. The levels of Ki-67 positive are positively associated with lymph node metastasis in invasive ductal breast cancer. *Cell Biochem. Biophys.* **2014**, *70*, 1145–1151. [CrossRef] [PubMed]
46. Jiang, Y.; Xu, H.; Zhang, H.; Ou, X.; Xu, Z.; Ai, L.; Sun, L.; Liu, C. Nomogram for prediction of level 2 axillary lymph node metastasis in proven level 1 node-positive breast cancer patients. *Oncotarget* **2017**, *8*, 72389–72399. [CrossRef] [PubMed]
47. Meng, L.; Zheng, T.; Wang, Y.; Li, Z.; Xiao, Q.; He, J.; Tan, J. Development of a prediction model based on LASSO regression to evaluate the risk of non-sentinel lymph node metastasis in Chinese breast cancer patients with 1-2 positive sentinel lymph nodes. *Sci. Rep.* **2021**, *11*, 19972. [CrossRef] [PubMed]
48. Yu, Y.; Tan, Y.; Xie, C.; Hu, Q.; Ouyang, J.; Chen, Y.; Gu, Y.; Li, A.; Lu, N.; He, Z.; et al. Development and Validation of a Preoperative Magnetic Resonance Imaging Radiomics-Based Signature to Predict Axillary Lymph Node Metastasis and Disease-Free Survival in Patients With Early-Stage Breast Cancer. *JAMA Netw. Open* **2020**, *3*, 28086. [CrossRef]
49. Pesapane, F.; Rotili, A.; Agazzi, G.M.; Botta, F.; Raimondi, S.; Penco, S.; Dominelli, V.; Cremonesi, M.; Jereczek-Fossa, B.A.; Carrafiello, G.; et al. Recent Radiomics Advancements in Breast Cancer: Lessons and Pitfalls for the Next Future. *Curr. Oncol.* **2021**, *28*, 2351–2372. [CrossRef]
50. Guo, X.; Liu, Z.; Sun, C.; Zhang, L.; Wang, Y.; Li, Z.; Shi, J.; Wu, T.; Cui, H.; Zhang, J.; et al. Deep learning radiomics of ultrasonography: Identifying the risk of axillary non-sentinel lymph node involvement in primary breast cancer. *EBioMedicine* **2020**, *60*, 24. [CrossRef]
51. Sannasi Chakravarthy, S.R.; Rajaguru, H. Automatic Detection and Classification of Mammograms Using Improved Extreme Learning Machine with Deep Learning. *IRBM* **2022**, *43*, 49–61. [CrossRef]

52. Zheng, X.; Yao, Z.; Huang, Y.; Yu, Y.; Wang, Y.; Liu, Y.; Mao, R.; Li, F.; Xiao, Y.; Hu, Y.; et al. Deep learning radiomics can predict axillary lymph node status in early-stage breast cancer. *Nat. Commun.* **2020**, *11*, 020–15027. [CrossRef]
53. Dihge, L.; Ohlsson, M.; Edén, P.; Bendahl, P.O.; Rydén, L. Artificial neural network models to predict nodal status in clinically node-negative breast cancer. *BMC Cancer* **2019**, *19*, 610. [CrossRef]
54. Harris, G.C.; Denley, H.E.; Pinder, S.E.; Lee, A.H.; Ellis, I.O.; Elston, C.W.; Evans, A. Correlation of histologic prognostic factors in core biopsies and therapeutic excisions of invasive breast carcinoma. *Am. J. Surg. Pathol.* **2003**, *27*, 11–15. [CrossRef]
55. Takada, M.; Sugimoto, M.; Naito, Y.; Moon, H.G.; Han, W.; Noh, D.Y.; Kondo, M.; Kuroi, K.; Sasano, H.; Inamoto, T.; et al. Prediction of axillary lymph node metastasis in primary breast cancer patients using a decision tree-based model. *BMC Med. Inform. Decis. Mak.* **2012**, *12*, 1472–6947. [CrossRef] [PubMed]

Disclaimer/Publisher's Note: The statements, opinions and data contained in all publications are solely those of the individual author(s) and contributor(s) and not of MDPI and/or the editor(s). MDPI and/or the editor(s) disclaim responsibility for any injury to people or property resulting from any ideas, methods, instructions or products referred to in the content.

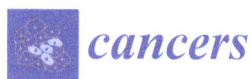

Article

BRCA1/2 Mutation Testing in Patients with HER2-Negative Advanced Breast Cancer: Real-World Data from the United States, Europe, and Israel

Reshma Mahtani [1,*], Alexander Niyazov [2], Bhakti Arondekar [3], Katie Lewis [4], Alex Rider [4], Lucy Massey [4] and Michael Patrick Lux [5]

[1] Miami Cancer Institute, 8900 Kendall Drive, Miami, FL 33176, USA
[2] Patient and Health Impact, Pfizer Inc., 235 42nd St., New York, NY 10017, USA
[3] Patient Health and Impact, Pfizer Inc., 500 Arcola Road, Collegeville, PA 19426, USA
[4] Oncology Franchise, Adelphi Real World, Adelphi Mill, Cheshire, Bollington SK10 5JB, UK
[5] Department of Gynecology and Obstetrics, Kooperatives Brustzentrum Paderborn, Frauenklinik St. Louise, Frauenklinik St. Josefs, Salzkotten Husener Straße 81, 33098 Paderborn, Germany
* Correspondence: rmahtani@baptisthealth.net; Tel.: +1-954-837-1490

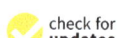

Citation: Mahtani, R.; Niyazov, A.; Arondekar, B.; Lewis, K.; Rider, A.; Massey, L.; Lux, M.P. *BRCA1/2* Mutation Testing in Patients with HER2-Negative Advanced Breast Cancer: Real-World Data from the United States, Europe, and Israel. *Cancers* **2022**, *14*, 5399. https://doi.org/10.3390/cancers14215399

Academic Editor: Naiba Nabieva

Received: 31 August 2022
Accepted: 22 October 2022
Published: 2 November 2022

Publisher's Note: MDPI stays neutral with regard to jurisdictional claims in published maps and institutional affiliations.

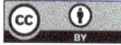

Copyright: © 2022 by the authors. Licensee MDPI, Basel, Switzerland. This article is an open access article distributed under the terms and conditions of the Creative Commons Attribution (CC BY) license (https:// creativecommons.org/licenses/by/ 4.0/).

Simple Summary: Poly(adenosine diphosphate-ribose) polymerase inhibitors have recently been shown to be effective for patients with human epidermal growth factor receptor 2—negative (HER2−) advanced breast cancer (ABC) who have a germline mutation in their breast cancer susceptibility gene 1 or 2 (*BRCA1/2*mut). This study evaluated differences in patient demographics, clinical characteristics, and *BRCA1/2*mut testing within the United States (US), European Union 4 (EU4; France, Germany, Italy, and Spain), and Israel in a real-world patient population with HER2− ABC. In the US, EU4, and Israel, 73%, 42%, and 99% of patients were tested for *BRCA1/2*mut, respectively. In the US and the EU4, patients who were not tested versus tested for *BRCA1/2*mut were more likely to have hormone receptor–positive (HR+)/HER2− ABC than triple-negative breast cancer, less likely to have a known family history of *BRCA1/2*-related cancer and were older. Efforts should be made to improve *BRCA1/2* testing rates in the US and Europe.

Abstract: Poly(adenosine diphosphate-ribose) polymerase inhibitors are approved to treat patients harboring a germline breast cancer susceptibility gene 1 or 2 mutation (*BRCA1/2*mut) with human epidermal growth factor receptor 2—negative (HER2−) advanced breast cancer (ABC). This study evaluated differences in patient demographics, clinical characteristics, and *BRCA1/2*mut testing within the United States (US), European Union 4 (EU4; France, Germany, Italy, and Spain), and Israel in a real-world population of patients with HER2− ABC. Oncologists provided chart data from eligible patients from October 2019 through March 2020. In the US, EU4, and Israel, 73%, 42%, and 99% of patients were tested for *BRCA1/2*mut, respectively. In the US and the EU4, patients who were not tested versus tested for *BRCA1/2*mut were more likely to have hormone receptor—positive (HR+)/HER2− ABC (US, 94% vs. 74%, $p < 0.001$; EU4, 96% vs. 78%, $p < 0.001$), less likely to have a known family history of *BRCA1/2*-related cancer (US, 6% vs. 19%, $p = 0.002$; EU4, 10% vs. 28%, $p < 0.001$), and were older (US, 68.9 vs. 62.5 years, $p < 0.001$; EU4, 66.9 vs. 58.0 years, $p < 0.001$). Among tested patients, genetic counseling was received by 45%, 53%, and 98% with triple-negative breast cancer, and 36%, 36%, and 98% with HR+/HER2− ABC in the US, EU4, and Israel, respectively. Efforts should be made to improve *BRCA1/2* testing rates in the US and Europe.

Keywords: advanced breast cancer; breast cancer susceptibility genes 1 and 2; genetic testing; human epidermal growth factor receptor 2—negative; poly(adenosine diphosphate-ribose) polymerase inhibitors; real-world

1. Introduction

An estimated 5% to 10% of breast cancers are caused by a genetic predisposition resulting from a mutation in a gene that increases the risk of breast cancer [1]. The genes most commonly affected in hereditary breast cancer and ovarian cancer are breast cancer susceptibility genes 1 and 2 (*BRCA1/2*) [2]. Approximately 3% to 6% of all breast cancer cases are caused by a *BRCA1/2* mutation (*BRCA1/2*mut) [3–5], and women with a genetic *BRCA1/2*mut have a cumulative 45% to 66% risk of developing breast cancer by 70 years of age [2]. Accordingly, genetic testing for breast cancer susceptibility has become an important part of disease management [1].

Tumors with a *BRCA1/2*mut are highly sensitive to inhibition of poly(ADP-ribose)polymerase (PARP) [6]. In 2018, the PARP inhibitors (PARPi) olaparib and talazoparib were approved by the US Food and Drug Administration (FDA) for treatment of patients with human epidermal growth factor receptor 2—negative (HER2−) advanced breast cancer (ABC) harboring a germline *BRCA1/2*mut (g*BRCA1/2*mut) and are now available in many countries for the treatment of g*BRCA1/2*mut HER2− ABC [7–9]. The approvals were based primarily on findings from the OlympiAD and EMBRACA randomized, open-label trials, which demonstrated a significantly improved progression-free survival, manageable adverse event profile, and improved patient-reported outcomes in patients with g*BRCA1/2*mut HER2− ABC who received olaparib or talazoparib compared with patients who received physician's choice of chemotherapy (OlympiAD: olaparib versus capecitabine, vinorelbine, or eribulin; EMBRACA: talazoparib versus capecitabine, vinorelbine, eribulin, or gemcitabine) [10–14]. These findings underscore that, in addition to hormone receptor (HR) status, HER2 status, and programmed death ligand 1 (PD-L1) status in triple-negative breast cancer (TNBC), information about *BRCA1/2*mut status is also an essential factor in determining choice of therapy.

With the approval of PARPi for germline (though not somatic) mutations, and the potential for effective therapeutic intervention in patients with a *BRCA1/2*mut, national and international guidelines have broadened eligibility criteria for g*BRCA1/2*mut testing [15,16]. The present analyses evaluated differences in patient demographics and clinical characteristics in a real-world population of patients with HER2− ABC to identify potential factors contributing to physicians' decisions to test for a *BRCA1/2*mut within the United States, European Union 4 (EU4; France, Germany, Italy, and Spain), and Israel. We also evaluated whether, and when, patients had undergone genetic counseling for *BRCA1/2*mut testing.

2. Methods

2.1. Data Source and Study Design

Data were obtained from the Adelphi Real World Disease Specific Programme (DSP^{TM}) for ABC, and the study was conducted from October 2019 through March 2020 in the United States, the EU4, and Israel. DSPs are large, multinational, point-in-time surveys of physicians and their patients presenting in a real-world clinical setting that assess disease management, disease-burden impact, and associated treatment effects [17].

Participating physicians were medical oncologists evaluating ≥5 patients with ABC per month, were actively involved in treating patients, and were recruited by local study teams. Physicians provided patient record forms (PRFs) for the next 8 eligible consulting patients: 4 patients receiving first-line advanced treatment and 4 receiving second- or later-line advanced treatment. Eligible patients were ≥18 years of age with stage IIIb to IV HER2− breast cancer and receiving therapy for ABC at the time of data collection; patients participating in a clinical trial were not eligible. Physicians reported on biomarker testing, including but not limited to homologous recombination repair genes, HER2, PD-L1, progesterone and estrogen receptor, PIK3CA, and *BRCA1/2*, and were asked the proportion of patients tested and the proportion of positive tests. Physicians were asked to report if testing was performed on blood, saliva, or buccal samples, and this information was used to confirm that *BRCA1/2*mut testing was germline. For US-based patients, this was also verified by inquiring the name of the laboratory where the testing was performed, whereas data for laboratory confirmation of test type were not available for the EU4 or Israel (Figure 1).

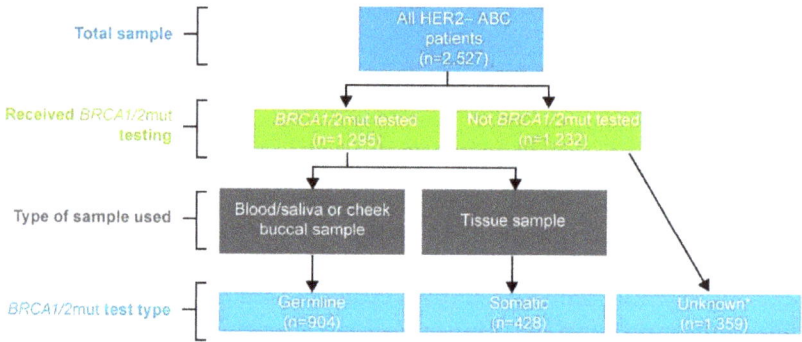

Figure 1. *BRCA1/2* mutation status testing. ABC = advanced breast cancer; *BRCA1/2* = breast cancer susceptibility gene 1 or 2; HER2− = human epidermal growth factor receptor 2 negative. * Includes not tested; not known to have a germline *BRCA1/2* mutation (*BRCA1/2*mut) test result; not known to have *BRCA1/2*mut germline and somatic wildtype test results.

The PRF included detailed questions on patient demographics, clinical assessments and outcomes, adverse events experienced at the time of data collection, treatment history, and physician-rated satisfaction with treatment. Physicians completed the PRFs using patient medical records as well as clinical judgment and diagnostic skills consistent with their decision-making process during routine clinical practice. Each patient with a PRF was invited to complete an optional patient form by pen and paper independently of their physician immediately after the consultation. The patient form included questions on their education, employment status, input to treatment decisions, and current disease status, as well as patient-reported outcome questionnaires that assessed their quality of life.

Patients provided informed consent for use of their anonymized and aggregated data for research and in scientific publications. Data were aggregated and de-identified before receipt by Adelphi Real World. The study was conducted in accordance with the Declaration of Helsinki and was approved by the Western Institutional Review Board (study protocol AG8643). Data collection was undertaken in line with European Pharmaceutical Market Research Association guidelines [18] and as such did not require ethics committee approval. Each survey was administered in full accordance with relevant legislation at the time of data collection, including the US Health Insurance Portability and Accountability Act of 1996 [19].

2.2. Outcomes and Measures

BRCA1/2 mutation testing rates and characteristics of patients undergoing testing were stratified by the type of test performed: any *BRCA1/2*mut, g*BRCA1/2*mut with or without a somatic *BRCA1/2*mut (g +/− s*BRCA1/2*mut), s*BRCA1/2*mut-only, unknown *BRCA1/2*mut (i.e., the physician was not aware of testing results, or it could not be verified if mutations were somatic or germline), and no *BRCA1/2*mut testing. Results were also stratified by HR status (i.e., HR+/HER2− or TNBC), practice setting, age, and family history of *BRCA1/2*-related cancer, and between-group comparisons were performed to identify possible factors that may have contributed to the decision to test patients within each region. Rates and timing of genetic counseling (i.e., before and/or after *BRCA1/2*mut testing) within each *BRCA1/2*mut testing group were also determined. Genetic counseling was performed by a geneticist or the treating physician.

2.3. Statistical Analysis

Descriptive summary statistics, including the mean, standard deviation, median, and range, were calculated for continuous variables. Frequency counts and percentages were calculated for categorical variables. Differences in demographics and clinical characteristics among *BRCA1/2*mut testing status groups were analyzed by Student's *t*-tests or Fisher exact tests. Values with $p < 0.05$ were considered statistically significant. A binomial exact test was performed to compare patients who received versus did not receive genetic counseling. Percentages and 95% CIs were reported; 95% CIs that did not cross 50%, or 0.50, indicated a significant difference ($p < 0.05$). Missing data were not imputed; thus, the sample size varied among variables assessed and is reported separately for each analysis. Analyses were performed with IBM® SPSS® Data Collection Survey Reporter Version 6 or later (International Business Machines Corp., Armonk, NY, USA) and STATA version 16.1 or later (StataCorp, College Station, TX, USA).

3. Results

3.1. BRCA1/2 Mutation Testing in the United States

Physicians completed PRFs for 407 US patients. Patients had a mean age of 64.2 years, 6% ($n = 26$) were premenopausal, 15% ($n = 63$) had a known family history of *BRCA1/2*-related cancer, 80% ($n = 325$) had HR+/HER2− disease, and 20% ($n = 82$) had TNBC. US patient characteristics stratified by *BRCA1/2*mut testing status are shown in Table 1. Overall, 73% ($n = 298$) of patients were tested for any type of *BRCA1/2*mut (germline, somatic, or unknown); among these, 47% ($n = 190$) received a g +/− s*BRCA1/2*mut test, 18% ($n = 75$) received an s*BRCA1/2*mut-only test, and 8% ($n = 33$) received an unknown type of *BRCA1/2*mut test. Those who were not tested for any *BRCA1/2*mut were significantly older than those who were tested (68.9 vs. 62.5 years; $p < 0.001$) and significantly less likely to be employed (18% vs. 33%; $p = 0.003$), premenopausal (2% vs. 8%; $p = 0.022$), have a family history of *BRCA1/2*-related cancer (6% vs. 19%; $p = 0.002$), have TNBC (6% vs. 26%; $p < 0.001$), or be tested in an academic setting (28% vs. 41%; $p = 0.021$) versus those who were tested.

Evaluating associations between *BRCA1/2*mut testing rates and HR+/HER2− and TNBC subtypes among US patients indicated that those with TNBC were tested for a g +/− s*BRCA1/2*mut at significantly higher rates compared with patients with HR+/HER2− disease (61% vs. 43%; $p = 0.004$; Table 2). s*BRCA1/2*mut-only testing rates were similar between patients with TNBC and those with HR+/HER2− disease (20% vs. 18%; $p = 0.75$).

Among patients with HR+/HER2− disease, fewer patients received any *BRCA1/2*mut testing in a community medical center compared with those in an academic medical center (64% vs. 75%, $p = 0.048$; Table 3). Those receiving treatment in an academic medical center were significantly more likely to receive g +/− s*BRCA1/2*mut testing but less likely to receive s*BRCA1/2*mut-only testing compared with those receiving care in a community medical center (g +/− s*BRCA1/2*mut, 54% vs. 37%, $p = 0.004$; s*BRCA1/2*mut-only, 12% vs. 22%, $p = 0.039$). Testing rates for each of the *BRCA1/2*mut testing groups among patients with TNBC were not significantly different across academic and community medical centers.

Among patients with HR+/HER2− ABC, overall *BRCA1/2*mut testing rates were lower for those who had no known family history of *BRCA1/2*-related cancer compared with those who did have a family history (67% vs. 84%, $p = 0.030$; Table 4). Among patients with TNBC, testing rates across all testing groups were not significantly different in patients with and without a known family history of *BRCA1/2*-related cancer.

Table 1. Patient demographics and clinical characteristics by *BRCA1/2*mut testing status among patients with HER2−ABC in the United States.

	Any BRCA1/2mut Testing (n = 298)	g +/− s BRCA1/2mut Testing (n = 190)	sBRCA1/2mut-Only Testing (n = 75)	Unknown BRCA1/2mut Testing (n = 33)	No BRCA1/2mut Testing (n = 109)	*p* Value (vs. Not Tested)			
						All Tested	g +/− s	s Only	Unknown
Mean patient age, y	62.5	62.9	60.7	64.5	68.9	<0.001	<0.001	<0.001	<0.001
Race									
White/Caucasian	200 (67)	126 (66)	50 (67)	24 (73)	66 (61)	0.240	0.320	0.439	0.223
African American	71 (24)	40 (21)	22 (29)	9 (27)	30 (28)	0.440	0.206	0.868	1.00
Employed	99 (33)	62 (33)	27 (36)	10 (30)	20 (18)	0.003	0.010	0.010	0.151
Premenopausal	24 (8)	13 (7)	10 (14)	1 (3)	2 (2)	0.022	0.095	0.004	0.560
Family history of *BRCA1/2*-related cancer *	56 (19)	36 (19)	15 (20)	5 (15)	7 (6)	0.002	0.003	0.010	0.150
HR status									
HR+/HER2−	222 (74)	140 (74)	59 (79)	23 (70)	103 (94)	<0.001	<0.001	0.002	<0.001
TNBC	76 (26)	50 (26)	16 (21)	10 (30)	6 (6)				
Academic medical center	122 (41)	89 (47)	19 (25)	14 (42)	31 (28)	0.021	0.002	0.737	0.140
Community-based center	176 (59)	101 (53)	56 (75)	19 (58)	78 (72)				

Values are n (%) unless noted otherwise. ABC = advanced breast cancer; *BRCA1/2*mut = breast cancer susceptibility gene 1 or 2 mutation; g = germline; HER2− = human epidermal growth factor receptor 2−negative; HR+ = hormone receptor-positive; s = somatic; TNBC = triple-negative breast cancer. * Defined as a family history of breast, ovarian, peritoneal, prostate, pancreatic, gastric, and/or fallopian tube cancer.

Table 2. *BRCA1/2*mut testing rates by HR status among patients with HER2− ABC in the United States, the EU4, and Israel.

	United States			EU4			Israel		
	HR+/HER2− (n = 325)	TNBC (n = 82)	*p* Value	HR+/HER2− (n = 1703)	TNBC (n = 223)	*p* Value	HR+/HER2− (n = 141)	TNBC (n = 53)	*p* Value
Any *BRCA1/2*mut testing	222 (68)	76 (93)	<0.001	631 (37)	174 (78)	<0.001	139 (99)	53 (100)	>0.99
g +/− s*BRCA1/2*mut testing	140 (43)	50 (61)	0.004	401 (24)	127 (57)	<0.001	135 (96)	51 (96)	>0.99
s*BRCA1/2*mut-only testing	59 (18)	16 (20)	0.752	155 (9)	31 (14)	0.029	1 (1)	2 (4)	0.182
Unknown *BRCA1/2*mut testing	23 (7)	10 (12)	0.171	75 (4)	16 (7)	0.090	3 (2)	0 (0)	0.563
No *BRCA1/2*mut testing	103 (32)	6 (7)		1072 (63)	49 (22)		2 (1)	0 (0)	

All values are n (%). ABC = advanced breast cancer; *BRCA1/2*mut = breast cancer susceptibility gene 1 or 2 mutation; EU4 = European Union 4 (France, Germany, Italy, and Spain); g = germline; HER2− = human epidermal growth factor receptor 2−negative; HR+ = hormone receptor-positive; s = somatic; TNBC = triple-negative breast cancer.

Table 3. BRCA1/2mut testing rates by practice setting among patients with HER2—ABC in the United States and the EU4.

	United States			EU4		
	Academic	Community	p Value	Academic	Community	p Value
HR+/HER2−	(n = 121)	(n = 204)		(n = 951)	(n = 752)	
Any BRCA1/2mut testing	91 (75)	131 (64)	0.048	386 (41)	245 (33)	0.001
g +/− sBRCA1/2mut testing	65 (54)	75 (37)	0.004	236 (25)	165 (22)	0.168
sBRCA1/2mut-only testing	15 (12)	44 (22)	0.039	109 (11)	46 (6)	<0.001
Unknown BRCA1/2mut testing	11 (9)	12 (6)	0.274	41 (4)	34 (5)	0.905
No BRCA1/2mut testing	30 (25)	73 (36)		565 (59)	507 (67)	
TNBC	(n = 32)	(n = 50)		(n = 123)	(n = 100)	
Any BRCA1/2mut testing	31 (97)	45 (90)	0.396	109 (89)	65 (65)	<0.001
g +/− sBRCA1/2mut testing	24 (75)	26 (52)	0.063	77 (63)	50 (50)	0.077
sBRCA1/2mut-only testing	4 (13)	12 (24)	0.259	25 (20)	6 (6)	0.003
Unknown BRCA1/2mut testing	3 (9)	7 (14)	0.733	7 (6)	9 (9)	0.436
No BRCA1/2mut testing	1 (3)	5 (10)		14 (11)	35 (35)	

All values are n (%). ABC = advanced breast cancer; BRCA1/2mut = breast cancer susceptibility gene 1 or 2 mutation; EU4 = European Union 4 (France, Germany, Italy, and Spain); g = germline; HER2− = human epidermal growth factor receptor 2–negative; HR+ = hormone receptor–positive; s = somatic; TNBC = triple-negative breast cancer.

Table 4. BRCA1/2mut testing rates by family history of BRCA1/2-related cancer * among patients with HER2− ABC in the United States, the EU4, and Israel.

	United States			EU4			Israel		
	Family History	No History	p Value	Family History	No History	p Value	Family History	No History	p Value
HR+/HER2−	(n = 43)	(n = 234)		(n = 280)	(n = 1356)		(n = 101)	(n = 39)	
Any BRCA1/2mut testing	36 (84)	156 (67)	0.030	173 (62)	437 (32)	<0.001	100 (99)	38 (97)	0.481
g +/− sBRCA1/2mut testing	22 (51)	99 (42)	0.317	120 (43)	274 (20)	<0.001	98 (97)	37 (95)	0.618
sBRCA1/2mut-only testing	11 (26)	45 (19)	0.408	33 (12)	111 (8)	0.063	1 (1)	0 (0)	1.00
Unknown BRCA1/2mut testing	3 (7)	12 (5)	0.711	20 (7)	52 (4)	0.024	1 (1)	1 (3)	0.481
No BRCA1/2mut testing	7 (16)	78 (33)		107 (38)	919 (68)		1 (1)	1 (3)	
TNBC	(n = 20)	(n = 57)		(n = 57)	(n = 157)		(n = 30)	(n = 20)	
Any BRCA1/2mut testing	20 (100)	53 (93)	0.568	51 (89)	118 (75)	0.023	30 (100)	20 (100)	1.00
g +/− sBRCA1/2mut testing	14 (70)	35 (61)	0.594	38 (67)	86 (55)	0.158	30 (100)	20 (100)	1.00
sBRCA1/2mut-only testing	4 (20)	12 (21)	1.00	6 (11)	24 (15)	0.505	0 (0)	0 (0)	1.00
Unknown BRCA1/2mut testing	2 (10)	6 (11)	1.00	7 (12)	8 (5)	0.125	0 (0)	0 (0)	1.00
No BRCA1/2mut testing	0 (0)	4 (7)		6 (11)	39 (25)		0 (0)	0 (0)	

All values are n (%). ABC = advanced breast cancer; BRCA1/2mut = breast cancer susceptibility gene 1 or 2 mutation; EU4 = European Union 4 (France, Germany, Italy, and Spain); g = germline; HER2− = human epidermal growth factor receptor 2–negative; HR+ = hormone receptor –positive; s = somatic; TNBC = triple-negative breast cancer. * Defined as a family history of breast, ovarian, peritoneal, prostate, pancreatic, gastric, and/or fallopian tube cancer.

When stratified by age group, BRCA1/2mut testing rates among patients with HR+/HER2− ABC declined with age, with 100%, 92%, 75%, and 60% of patients < 45, 45 to 54, 55 to 64, and ≥65 years of age, respectively, having any type of BRCA1/2mut test (Figure 2A). Among patients with TNBC, testing rates only slightly declined with age, with all patients < 55 years of age, 95% of patients 55 to 64 years of age, and 85% of patients ≥ 65 years of age having received a BRCA1/2mut test.

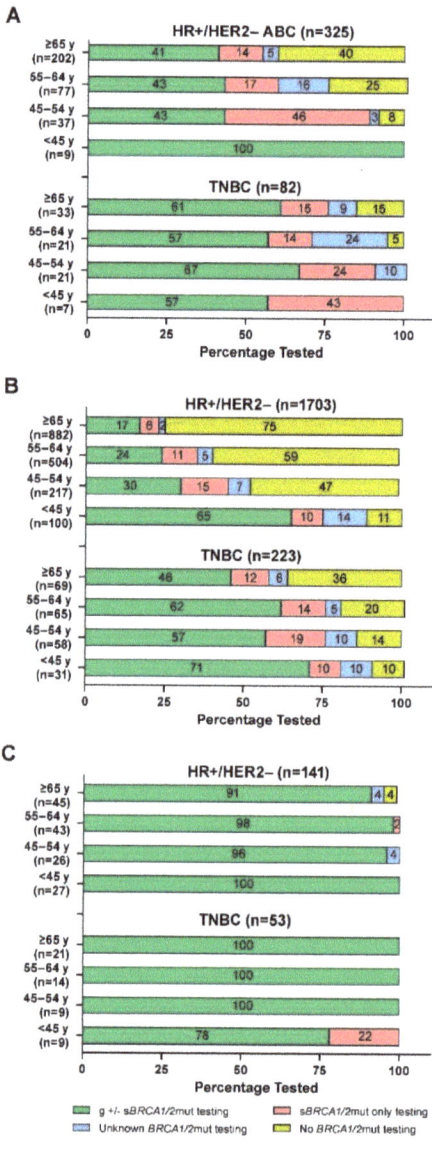

Figure 2. BRCA1/2mut testing rates by age group among patients with HER2− ABC in (**A**) the United States, (**B**) the EU4, and (**C**) Israel. Percentages may not add to exactly 100 because of rounding. ABC = advanced breast cancer; BRCA1/2mut = breast cancer susceptibility gene 1 or 2 mutation; g = germline; EU4 = European Union 4 (France, Germany, Italy, and Spain); HER2− = human epidermal growth factor receptor 2–negative; HR+ = hormone receptor–positive; s = somatic; TNBC = triple-negative breast cancer.

Among US patients with HR+/HER2− ABC tested for any BRCA1/2mut, 36% received genetic counseling (73 [91%] from a genetic counselor and 8 [10%] from the treating physician), 52% did not receive counseling (received vs. did not receive counseling: binomial test proportion 0.41 [95% CI, 0.34−0.48]), and, for 12% of patients, it was unknown if they received genetic counseling (Figure 3A). Approximately equal percentages of patients within this group received counseling before (13%), after (13%), or both before and after (9%) genetic testing; for 1% of patients, the timing of counseling was unknown (Figure 3A). The g +/− sBRCA1/2mut and sBRCA1/2mut-only testing subgroups had similar percentages of patients who received genetic counseling, 34% and 47%, respectively, but varied by the distribution of time points at which counseling was received. Among the patients with TNBC tested for any BRCA1/2mut, 45% received genetic counseling (88% from a genetic counselor and 12% from the treating physician), 37% did not receive counseling (received vs. did not receive counseling: binomial test proportion 0.54 [95% CI, 0.42−0.68]), and, for 18% of patients, it was unknown if they received genetic counseling (Figure 3A). As with the patients with HR+/HER2− ABC tested for any BRCA1/2mut, similar percentages of the patients with TNBC tested for any BRCA1/2mut received counseling before (16%), after (16%), or both before and after (13%) genetic testing (Figure 3A).

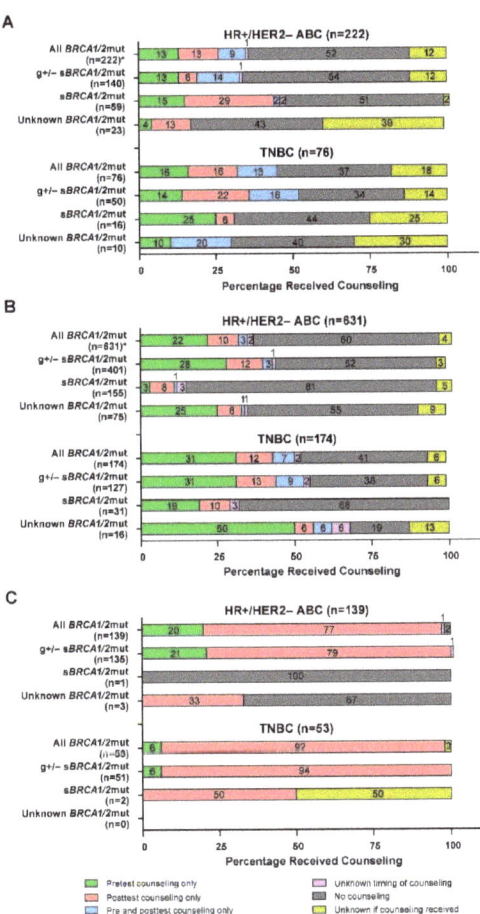

Figure 3. Receipt of genetic counseling by *BRCA1/2*mut testing type among patients with HER2− ABC in (**A**) the United States, (**B**) the EU4, and (**C**) Israel. Percentages may not add to exactly 100 because of rounding. * Indicates a statistically significant difference between those who had and did not have genetic counseling. ABC = advanced breast cancer; *BRCA1/2*mut = breast cancer susceptibility gene 1 or 2 mutation; g = germline; EU4 = European Union 4 (France, Germany, Italy, and Spain); HER2− = human epidermal growth factor receptor 2–negative; HR+ = hormone receptor–positive; s = somatic; TNBC = triple-negative breast cancer.

3.2. BRCA1/2 Mutation Testing in the European Union 4

Physicians completed PRFs for 1926 EU4 patients. Patients had a mean age of 63.1 years, 8% (n = 151) were premenopausal, 17% (n = 337) had a known family history of *BRCA1/2*-related cancer, 88% (n = 1703) had HR+/HER2− disease, and 12% (n = 223) had TNBC. EU4 patient characteristics stratified by *BRCA1/2*mut testing status are shown in Table 5. Overall, 42% (n = 805) of the patients were tested for any type of *BRCA1/2*mut; among these, 27% (n = 528) received a g +/− s*BRCA1/2*mut test, 10% (n = 186) received an s*BRCA1/2*mut-only test, and 5% (n = 91) received an unknown type of *BRCA1/2*mut test. Those who were not tested for a *BRCA1/2*mut were significantly older than those who were tested (66.7 vs. 58.0 years; $p < 0.001$) and significantly less likely to be employed (11% vs. 26%; $p < 0.001$), be premenopausal (3% vs. 15%; $p < 0.001$), have a family history of *BRCA1/2*-related cancer (10% vs. 28%; $p < 0.001$), have TNBC (4% vs. 22%; $p < 0.001$), or be tested in an academic setting (52% vs. 61%; $p < 0.001$).

Table 5. Patient demographics and clinical characteristics by *BRCA1/2*mut testing status among patients with HER2− ABC in the EU4.

	Any *BRCA1/2*mut Testing (n = 805)	g +/− s*BRCA1/2*mut Testing (n = 528)	s*BRCA1/2*mut-Only Testing (n = 186)	Unknown *BRCA1/2*mut Testing (n = 91)	No *BRCA1/2*mut Testing (n = 1121)	*p* Value (vs. Not Tested)			
						All Tested	g +/− s	s Only	Unknown
Mean patient age, y	58.0	57.9	59.7	55.3	66.7	<0.001	<0.001	<0.001	<0.001
Race									
White/Caucasian	752 (93)	489 (93)	180 (97)	83 (91)	1063 (95)	0.199	0.092	0.357	0.148
Employed	206 (26)	124 (23)	51 (27)	31 (34)	124 (11)	<0.001	<0.001	<0.001	<0.001
Premenopausal	118 (15)	75 (14)	25 (14)	18 (20)	33 (3)	<0.001	<0.001	<0.001	<0.001
Family history of *BRCA1/2*-related cancer *	224 (28)	158 (30)	39 (21)	27 (30)	113 (10)	<0.001	<0.001	<0.001	<0.001
HR status									
HR+/HER2−	631 (78)	401 (76)	155 (83)	75 (82)	1072 (96)	<0.001	<0.001	<0.001	<0.001
TNBC	174 (22)	127 (24)	31 (17)	16 (18)	49 (4)				
Academic medical center	495 (61)	313 (59)	134 (72)	48 (53)	579 (52)	<0.001	0.004	<0.001	0.913
Community-based center	310 (39)	215 (41)	52 (28)	43 (47)	542 (48)				

Values are *n* (%) unless noted otherwise. ABC = advanced breast cancer; *BRCA1/2*mut = breast cancer susceptibility gene 1 or 2 mutation; EU4 = European Union 4 (France, Germany, Italy, and Spain); g = germline; HER2− = human epidermal growth factor receptor 2–negative; HR+ = hormone receptor–positive; s = somatic; TNBC = triple-negative breast cancer. * Defined as a family history of breast, ovarian, peritoneal, prostate, pancreatic, gastric, and/or fallopian tube cancer.

Patients in the EU4 with TNBC were tested for a g +/− s*BRCA1/2*mut at significantly higher rates compared with patients with HR+/HER2− disease (57% vs. 24%; $p < 0.001$); the same was true for s*BRCA1/2*mut-only testing (14% vs. 9%; $p = 0.029$; Table 2). For patients with HR+/HER2− disease and those with TNBC, patients in academic medical centers were more likely to receive any *BRCA1/2*mut testing compared with those treated in community medical centers (HR+/HER2−, 41% vs. 33%; TNBC, 89% vs. 65%; both $p < 0.001$; Table 3). Considering family history, patients in the EU4 with HR+/HER2− ABC who had no known *BRCA1/2*-related family history were tested for any *BRCA1/2*mut at significantly lower rates than those who did have a family history (32% vs. 62%; $p < 0.001$; Table 4). For patients with TNBC, testing rates were only significantly lower for any *BRCA1/2*mut testing among those with no family history (75% vs. 89%; $p = 0.023$).

BRCA1/2 mutation testing rates among patients in the EU4 with HR+/HER2− ABC declined with age, with 89%, 53%, 41%, and 25% of patients < 45, 45 to 54, 55 to 64, and ≥65 years of age, respectively, receiving any type of *BRCA1/2*mut testing (Figure 2B). The same trend was observed among patients with TNBC, although, as noted, testing rates were generally lower among patients with HR+/HER2− disease compared with patients with TNBC.

Among EU4 patients with HR+/HER2− disease tested for any *BRCA1/2*mut, 36% received genetic counseling (177 [77%] from a genetic counselor and 57 [25%] from the treating physician), 60% did not receive counseling (received vs. did not receive counseling: binomial test proportion 0.38 [95% CI, 0.34–0.42]) and, for 4% of patients, it was unknown if they received counseling. Among the patients with TNBC tested for any *BRCA1/2*mut, 53% received genetic counseling (73 [79%] from a genetic counselor and 23 [25%] from the treating physician), 41% did not receive counseling (received vs. did not receive counseling: binomial test proportion 0.56 [95% CI, 0.48–0.64]) and, for 6% of patients, it was unknown if they received counseling. In patients with HR+/HER2− disease and those with TNBC, counseling was most often received before genetic testing (Figure 3B). Within each population, the percentage of patients who received genetic counseling was lowest among those tested for an s*BRCA1/2*mut only.

3.3. BRCA1/2 Mutation Testing in Israel

Physicians completed PRFs for 194 Israeli patients. Patients had a mean age of 56.7 years, 27% (n = 52) were premenopausal, 68% (n = 131) had a known family history of *BRCA1/2*-related cancer, 73% (n = 141) had HR+/HER2− disease, and 27% (n = 53) had TNBC. Overall, 99% (n = 192) of the patients were tested for any type of *BRCA1/2*mut; among these, 96% (n = 186) received a g +/− s*BRCA1/2*mut test, 2% (n = 3) received an s*BRCA1/2*mut-only test, and 2% (n = 3) received an unknown type of the *BRCA1/2*mut test. No significant differences in patient characteristics were observed among those who were tested for a *BRCA1/2*mut compared with those who were not. All patients received treatment at an academic medical center.

As expected, based on the nearly ubiquitous nature of *BRCA1/2*mut testing among Israeli patients, no significant differences were seen in testing rates by HR subtypes (Table 2) or *BRCA1/2*-related family history (Table 4). When stratified by HR subtype and age group, all patients received *BRCA1/2*mut testing, except for 2 with HR+/HER2− disease who were ≥65 years of age (Figure 2C). Nearly all Israeli patients who received *BRCA1/2*mut testing (98% for both HR+/HER2− and TNBC) also received genetic counseling, with most patients (77% of patients with HR+/HER2− and 92% of those with TNBC) receiving counseling after genetic testing (Figure 3C). All patients who received genetic counseling received it from a genetic counselor.

4. Discussion

Based on the efficacy of PARPi demonstrated in clinical trials and their subsequent approval for treatment of patients with g*BRCA1/2*mut HER2− ABC, guidelines on testing for g*BRCA1/2*mut have expanded to include new therapeutic indications in addition to clinical criteria such as patients diagnosed at an early age and patients with a strong family history (e.g., a first-degree relative diagnosed with breast cancer at an early age or with TNBC, two or more close relatives with breast cancer at any age, two or more close blood relatives with breast, pancreatic or prostate cancer at any age or a known *BRCA1/2* mutation in the family) [10,11,20]. The National Comprehensive Cancer Network Clinical Practice Guidelines in Oncology (NCCN Guidelines®) now recommend testing for a g*BRCA1/2*mut in all patients with recurrent or metastatic breast cancer to identify candidates for PARPi treatment [20]. The European Society for Medical Oncology (ESMO) international consensus guidelines recommend that patients with ABC be tested for a g*BRCA1/2*mut "as early as possible" [9].

This study used the Adelphi Real World DSP to evaluate *BRCA1/2*mut testing rates and related characteristics among patients with HER2− ABC in the United States, the EU4, and Israel during October 2019 to March 2020. We had previously assessed *BRCA1/2*mut testing rates in the United States and the EU5 (France, Germany, Italy, Spain, and the United Kingdom) in 2015 and 2017 to provide a historical baseline for *BRCA1/2*mut testing [21]. Average rates of testing for any *BRCA1/2*mut in 2015–2017 for patients with HR+/HER2− ABC and those with TNBC were 43% and 72%, respectively, in the United States and 18% and 33%, respectively, in the EU5. Testing rates were substantially higher in the current study; testing rates for any *BRCA1/2*mut in patients with HR+/HER2− ABC and those with

TNBC were 68% and 93%, respectively, in the United States and 37% and 78%, respectively, in the EU4. The FDA approval in 2018 and the subsequent European Medicines Agency authorization of PARPi for the treatment of patients with HER2− ABC likely contributed to the increase in BRCA1/2mut testing rates from 2015 and 2017 to 2019 and 2020. Despite the increased rates of BRCA1/2mut testing in the current study, gBRCA1/2mut testing rates were still relatively low among some patient groups. Testing rates for patients with HR+/HER2− ABC were lower in both the United States and the EU4 compared with patients with TNBC, with only 37% of patients with HR+/HER2− ABC in the EU4 being tested for any BRCA1/2mut. The relatively higher rates of testing in patients with TNBC likely reflects the increased awareness of the prevalence of gBRCA1/2mut among these patients [22]. However, a substantial percentage of patients with TNBC, particularly in the EU4 (49 of 223 [22%]), were not tested for any BRCA1/2mut, underscoring the need for testing to inform treatment decisions for patients with such limited options [22].

BRCA1/2 mutation testing rates in older patients were also relatively low in both the United States and the EU4, particularly for those with HR+/HER2− ABC. For example, among patients with HR+/HER2− ABC tested for any BRCA1/2mut in the United States, 60% of those who were ≥65 years of age and 100% of those <45 years of age were tested; in the EU4, only 25% of patients ≥ 65 years of age were tested, while 89% of those <45 years of age were tested. Testing rates in the United States and the EU4 were also generally lower among those who were postmenopausal, had no known BRCA1/2-related family history of cancer, and were treated in community medical centers (vs. academic medical centers). These findings highlight the need for increased gBRCA1/2mut testing, with efforts specifically concentrated among patients with these demographic or clinical characteristics, to aid in identification of patients eligible for PARPi treatment.

There were also appreciable numbers of patients in the United States (18%) and the EU4 (10%), but not Israel, who received sBRCA1/2mut-only testing. Although patients with metastatic breast cancer with an sBRCA1/2mut have been shown to respond to PARPi [23,24], PARPi have not been approved to treat this patient group. The ESMO international consensus guidelines indicate that the therapeutic implications of sBRCA1/2mut in patients with breast cancer need further evaluation and should not be used for decision-making in clinical practice [9]. Because patients who were enrolled in clinical trials were excluded from this study, the reason some patients received sBRCA1/2mut-only testing is uncertain, but it is possible that they provided tissue samples for experimental studies.

BRCA1/2 mutation testing rates were notably higher in Israel compared with the United States and the EU4. This is likely related to the high percentages of Israeli patients with Ashkenazi Jewish ethnicity, which is associated with an approximately 10-fold increase in the prevalence of BRCA1/2mut relative to the general population (approximately 2.0% vs. 0.2%) [25]. Possibly related to this risk factor, the percentage of patients with BRCA1/2-related family history was much higher in Israel (68%) compared with the United States or EU4 (15% and 17%, respectively), and the mean age among Israeli patients was lower compared with patients in the United States or EU4 (56.7 vs. 64.2 and 63.1 years, respectively). In addition, the proportion of patients who were premenopausal was much higher in Israel (27%) compared with the United States (6%) and EU4 (8%). An awareness that breast cancer incidence is higher in younger patients (i.e., premenopausal patients) who carry a BRCA1/2mut may have also contributed to the high rate of BRCA1/2mut testing in Israel. Although we did not identify patients of Ashkenazi Jewish ethnicity in the United States or EU4, rates of BRCA1/2mut testing among Ashkenazi Jews in the United States and the EU4 may be higher than the general population.

The study also identified considerable gaps in genetic counseling among patients tested for a BRCA1/2mut in the United States and the EU4, particularly in patients with HR+/HER2− ABC, where less than half of those who were tested received genetic counseling. Genetic counseling is important because it informs patients and their family members not only about genetic predisposition but also different therapeutic strategies for treatment of their cancer. The ESMO international consensus guidelines recommend that genetic counseling be provided to patients with ABC and their families if a pathogenic germline mutation is identified [9]. A rapidly increasing demand for genetic counseling resulting from the recent expansion of indications of PARPi among patients with ABC, as well as patients with ovarian and prostate cancer, with a deleterious *BRCA1/2*mut may be contributing to the relatively low rate of patients receiving genetic counseling observed in this study. Our findings indicate that improved awareness of and access to genetic counseling is needed in the United States and the EU4. In Israel, as with g*BRCA1/2*mut testing, essentially all patients received genetic counseling; most (up to 92%) received posttest counseling only. In Israel, as well as in Germany, genetic counseling is a legal requirement as a part of genetic testing [26]. Furthermore, Israel has one of the highest levels of genetic counselors per capita, second only to Cuba and the United States [27]. These factors, along with the high level of awareness and genetic testing, likely contribute to the high rate of genetic counseling in Israel.

The strengths of this study include the use of real-world data, which are important for informing patient care [28], across a large patient population spanning multiple countries. The generalizability of study results may be limited in that the DSP only includes data from physicians willing to take part; furthermore, patients may not be fully representative of the broader patient population because data were more likely to be collected from patients who frequently consulted their physicians. Data quality is also subject to accurate reporting by physicians and patients and may be subject to recall bias. Additionally, patient diagnosis was determined by physician judgment and diagnostic skills rather than a formalized checklist; however, this process is reflective of disease diagnosis in the real world. The high testing rate in Israel may also be due to tests occurring before the illness or during the initial breast cancer diagnosis. In addition, physician-reported mutation testing in blood was used as a proxy for g*BRCA1/2*mut testing. Because blood is used as source material for the testing of circulating tumor DNA, it cannot be verified that all testing conducted on blood samples was germline testing only.

5. Conclusions

Substantial percentages of patients with HER2− ABC in the United States and the EU4 do not undergo *BRCA1/2*mut testing, which is important for identifying patients who may benefit from PARPi treatment. Efforts should be made to increase testing rates, especially among older or postmenopausal patients and patients with HR+/HER2− ABC (vs. those with TNBC), without a known *BRCA1/2*-related family history, or who are treated in community medical centers.

Author Contributions: Conceptualization: R.M., A.N., B.A., A.R., K.L. and M.P.L.; Methodology: R.M., A.N., B.A., A.R., K.L. and M.P.L.; Formal Analysis: R.M., A.N., B.A., K.L., L.M. and M.P.L.; Investigation: R.M., A.N., B.A., K.L., L.M. and M.P.L.; Writing—Review and Editing: R.M., A.N., B.A., A.R., K.L., L.M. and M.P.L.; Visualization: A.N., B.A., A.R. and K.L.; Supervision: A.N., B.A., A.R. and K.L. All authors have read and agreed to the published version of the manuscript.

Funding: This study was sponsored by Pfizer Inc. Pfizer was involved in study design; interpretation of data; writing the report; and the decision to submit the report for publication.

Institutional Review Board Statement: The study was conducted in accordance with the Declaration of Helsinki and was approved by the Western Institutional Review Board (study protocol AG8643).

Informed Consent Statement: Patients provided informed consent for use of their anonymized and aggregated data for research and in scientific publications.

Data Availability Statement: Data collection was undertaken by Adelphi Real World as part of an Adelphi DSP independent survey sponsored by multiple pharmaceutical companies, of which one was Pfizer Inc. Publication of study results was not contingent on the sponsor's approval or censorship of the manuscript. All data that support the findings of this study are the intellectual property of Adelphi Real World. All requests for access should be addressed directly to Katie Lewis at katie.lewis@adelphigroup.com.

Acknowledgments: Medical writing support was provided by John Teiber of ICON (Blue Bell, PA) and funded by Pfizer.

Conflicts of Interest: R.M.: contracted research funding from Genentech; consultant for Pfizer, Eli Lilly, Merck, Novartis, Daiichi-Sankyo, Sanofi, Seattle Genetics, Gilead, Genentech, Hologic, Eisai, AstraZeneca, Puma, Agendia, and Amgen. A.N., B.A.: employees of and own stock in Pfizer Inc. K.L., A.R., L.M.: employees of Adelphi Real World. M.P.L.: honoraria for lectures, consulting or advisory role for Eli Lilly, AstraZeneca, M.S.D., Novartis, Pfizer, Eisai, Exact Sciences, Daiichi-Sankyo, Grünenthal, Gilead, Pierre Fabre, PharmaMar, Onkowissen, and Roche; fees for travel, accommodations, expenses from Roche and Pfizer; editorial board member of Medac; fees for non-CME services from Eli Lilly, Roche, M.S.D., Novartis, Pfizer, Exact Sciences, Daiichi-Sankyo, Gilead, Grünenthal, AstraZeneca, and Eisai.

References

1. Gadzicki, D.; Evans, D.G.; Harris, H.; Julian-Reynier, C.; Nippert, I.; Schmidtke, J.; Tibben, A.; van Asperen, C.J.; Schlegelberger, B. Genetic testing for familial/hereditary breast cancer—Comparison of guidelines and recommendations from the UK, France, the Netherlands and Germany. *J. Community Genet.* **2011**, *2*, 53–69. [CrossRef] [PubMed]
2. Pujol, P.; Barberis, M.; Beer, P.; Friedman, E.; Piulats, J.M.; Capoluongo, E.D.; Garcia Foncillas, J.; Ray-Coquard, I.; Penault-Llorca, F.; Foulkes, W.D.; et al. Clinical practice guidelines for BRCA1 and BRCA2 genetic testing. *Eur. J. Cancer* **2021**, *146*, 30–47. [CrossRef] [PubMed]
3. Fasching, P.A.; Yadav, S.; Hu, C.; Wunderle, M.; Haberle, L.; Hart, S.N.; Rubner, M.; Polley, E.C.; Lee, K.Y.; Gnanaolivu, R.D.; et al. Mutations in BRCA1/2 and other panel genes in patients with metastatic breast cancer—Association with patient and disease characteristics and effect on prognosis. *J. Clin. Oncol.* **2021**, *39*, 1619–1630. [CrossRef]
4. Tung, N.; Lin, N.U.; Kidd, J.; Allen, B.A.; Singh, N.; Wenstrup, R.J.; Hartman, A.R.; Winer, E.P.; Garber, J.E. Frequency of germline mutations in 25 cancer susceptibility genes in a sequential series of patients with breast cancer. *J. Clin. Oncol.* **2016**, *34*, 1460–1468. [CrossRef]
5. Meynard, G.; Villanueva, C.; Thiery-Vuillemin, A.; Mansi, L.; Montcuquet, P.; Meneveau, N.; Chaigneau, L.; Bazan, F.; Almotlak, H.; Dobi, E.; et al. Real-life study of BRCA genetic screening in metastatic breast cancer. *Ann. Oncol.* **2017**, *28*, V94. [CrossRef]
6. Neviere, Z.; De La Motte Rouge, T.; Floquet, A.; Johnson, A.; Berthet, P.; Joly, F. How and when to refer patients for oncogenetic counseling in the era of PARP inhibitors. *Ther. Adv. Med. Oncol.* **2020**, *12*, 1758835919897530. [CrossRef]
7. US Food and Drug Administration. FDA Approves Olaparib for Germline BRCA-Mutated Metastatic Breast Cancer. Available online: https://www.fda.gov/drugs/resources-information-approved-drugs/fda-approves-olaparib-germline-brca-mutated-metastatic-breast-cancer (accessed on 31 January 2022).
8. US Food and Drug Administration. FDA Approves Talazoparib for gBRCAm HER2-Negative Locally Advanced or Metastatic Breast Cancer. Available online: https://www.fda.gov/drugs/drug-approvals-and-databases/fda-approves-talazoparib-gbrcam-her2-negative-locally-advanced-or-metastatic-breast-cancer (accessed on 31 January 2022).
9. Cardoso, F.; Paluch-Shimon, S.; Senkus, E.; Curigliano, G.; Aapro, M.S.; Andre, F.; Barrios, C.H.; Bergh, J.; Bhattacharyya, G.S.; Biganzoli, L.; et al. 5th ESO-ESMO international consensus guidelines for advanced breast cancer (ABC 5). *Ann. Oncol.* **2020**, *31*, 1623–1649. [CrossRef]
10. Robson, M.; Im, S.A.; Senkus, E.; Xu, B.; Domchek, S.M.; Masuda, N.; Delaloge, S.; Li, W.; Tung, N.; Armstrong, A.; et al. Olaparib for metastatic breast cancer in patients with a germline BRCA mutation. *N. Engl. J. Med.* **2017**, *377*, 523–533. [CrossRef]
11. Litton, J.K.; Rugo, H.S.; Ettl, J.; Hurvitz, S.A.; Gonçalves, A.; Lee, K.-H.; Fehrenbacher, L.; Yerushalmi, R.; Mina, L.A.; Martin, M.; et al. Talazoparib in patients with advanced breast cancer and a germline BRCA mutation. *N. Engl. J. Med.* **2018**, *379*, 753–763. [CrossRef]
12. Robson, M.; Ruddy, K.J.; Im, S.A.; Senkus, E.; Xu, B.; Domchek, S.M.; Masuda, N.; Li, W.; Tung, N.; Armstrong, A.; et al. Patient-reported outcomes in patients with a germline BRCA mutation and HER2-negative metastatic breast cancer receiving olaparib versus chemotherapy in the OlympiAD trial. *Eur. J. Cancer* **2019**, *120*, 20–30. [CrossRef]
13. Hurvitz, S.A.; Goncalves, A.; Rugo, H.S.; Lee, K.H.; Fehrenbacher, L.; Mina, L.A.; Diab, S.; Blum, J.L.; Chakrabarti, J.; Elmeliegy, M.; et al. Talazoparib in patients with a germline BRCA-mutated advanced breast cancer: Detailed safety analyses from the phase III EMBRACA trial. *Oncologist* **2020**, *25*, e439–e450. [CrossRef] [PubMed]
14. Im, S.A.; Xu, B.; Li, W.; Robson, M.; Ouyang, Q.; Yeh, D.C.; Iwata, H.; Park, Y.H.; Sohn, J.H.; Tseng, L.M.; et al. Olaparib monotherapy for Asian patients with a germline BRCA mutation and HER2-negative metastatic breast cancer: OlympiAD randomized trial subgroup analysis. *Sci. Rep.* **2020**, *10*, 8753. [CrossRef] [PubMed]
15. Daly, M.B.; Pal, T.; Berry, M.P.; Buys, S.S.; Dickson, P.; Domchek, S.M.; Elkhanany, A.; Friedman, S.; Goggins, M.; Hutton, M.L.; et al. Genetic/familial high-risk assessment: Breast, ovarian, and pancreatic, version 2.2021, NCCN Clinical Practice Guidelines in Oncology. *J. Natl. Compr. Cancer Netw.* **2021**, *19*, 77–102. [CrossRef]
16. Gonzalez-Santiago, S.; Ramon, Y.C.T.; Aguirre, E.; Ales-Martinez, J.E.; Andres, R.; Balmana, J.; Grana, B.; Herrero, A.; Llort, G.; Gonzalez-Del-Alba, A.; et al. SEOM clinical guidelines in hereditary breast and ovarian cancer (2019). *Clin. Transl. Oncol.* **2020**, *22*, 193–200. [CrossRef] [PubMed]

17. Anderson, P.; Benford, M.; Harris, N.; Karavali, M.; Piercy, J. Real-world physician and patient behaviour across countries: Disease-Specific Programmes—A means to understand. *Curr. Med. Res. Opin.* **2008**, *24*, 3063–3072. [CrossRef] [PubMed]
18. European Pharmaceutical Market Research Association. EphMRA Code of Conduct. 2020. Available online: https://www.ephmra.org/sites/default/files/2022-08/EPHMRA%202022%20Code%20of%20Conduct.pdf (accessed on 1 September 2021).
19. US Department of Health & Human Services. Summary of the HIPAA Privacy Rule. Available online: https://www.hhs.gov/hipaa/for-professionals/privacy/laws-regulations/index.html (accessed on 26 May 2021).
20. Referenced with Permission from the NCCN Clinical Practice Guidelines in Oncology (NCCN Guidelines®) for Breast Cancer V.4.2022. © National Comprehensive Cancer Network, Inc. 2022. All Rights Reserved. Accessed July 5, 2022. To View the Most Recent and Complete Version of the Guideline, NCCN Makes No Warranties of Any Kind Whatsoever Regarding Their Content, Use or Application and Disclaims any Responsibility for Their Application or Use in any Way. Available online: NCCN.org (accessed on 1 September 2021).
21. Lux, M.P.; Lewis, K.; Rider, A.; Niyazov, A. Real-world multi-country study of *BRCA1/2* mutation testing among adult women with HER2-negative advanced breast cancer. *Future Oncol.* **2022**, *18*, 1089–1101. [CrossRef]
22. Bayraktar, S.; Gutierrez-Barrera, A.M.; Liu, D.; Tasbas, T.; Akar, U.; Litton, J.K.; Lin, E.; Albarracin, C.T.; Meric-Bernstam, F.; Gonzalez-Angulo, A.M.; et al. Outcome of triple-negative breast cancer in patients with or without deleterious *BRCA* mutations. *Breast Cancer Res. Treat.* **2011**, *130*, 145–153. [CrossRef]
23. Walsh, E.M.; Mangini, N.; Fetting, J.; Armstrong, D.; Chan, I.S.; Connolly, R.M.; Fiallos, K.; Lehman, J.; Nunes, R.; Petry, D.; et al. Olaparib use in patients with metastatic breast cancer harboring somatic *BRCA1/2* mutations or mutations in non-*BRCA1/2*, DNA damage repair genes. *Clin. Breast Cancer* **2022**, *22*, 319–325. [CrossRef]
24. Russo, A.; Incorvaia, L.; Capoluongo, E.; Tagliaferri, P.; Gori, S.; Cortesi, L.; Genuardi, M.; Turchetti, D.; De Giorgi, U.; Di Maio, M.; et al. Implementation of preventive and predictive *BRCA* testing in patients with breast, ovarian, pancreatic, and prostate cancer: A position paper of Italian Scientific Societies. *ESMO Open* **2022**, *7*, 100459. [CrossRef]
25. US National Institutes of Health. BRCA Gene Mutations: Cancer Risk and Genetic Testing. Available online: https://www.cancer.gov/about-cancer/causes-prevention/genetics/brca-fact-sheet#r18 (accessed on 27 April 2022).
26. The Health Policy Partnership. Genetic Testing for BRCA Mutations: A Policy Paper. Available online: https://www.healthpolicypartnership.com/app/uploads/Genetic-testing-for-BRCA-mutations-a-policy-paper.pdf (accessed on 23 May 2022).
27. Abacan, M.; Alsubaie, L.; Barlow-Stewart, K.; Caanen, B.; Cordier, C.; Courtney, E.; Davoine, E.; Edwards, J.; Elackatt, N.J.; Gardiner, K.; et al. The global state of the genetic counseling profession. *Eur. J. Hum. Genet.* **2019**, *27*, 183–197. [CrossRef]
28. Sherman, R.E.; Anderson, S.A.; Dal Pan, G.J.; Gray, G.W.; Gross, T.; Hunter, N.L.; LaVange, L.; Marinac-Dabic, D.; Marks, P.W.; Robb, M.A.; et al. Real-world evidence—What is it and what can it tell us? *N. Engl. J. Med.* **2016**, *375*, 2293–2297. [CrossRef] [PubMed]

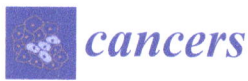

Article

Recurrence Score® Result Impacts Treatment Decisions in Hormone Receptor-Positive, HER2-Negative Patients with Early Breast Cancer in a Real-World Setting—Results of the IRMA Trial

Dominik Dannehl [1,*], Tobias Engler [1], Lea L. Volmer [1], Annette Staebler [2], Anna K. Fischer [2], Martin Weiss [1], Markus Hahn [1], Christina B. Walter [1], Eva-Maria Grischke [1], Falko Fend [2], Florin-Andrei Taran [3], Sara Y. Brucker [1] and Andreas D. Hartkopf [1,4]

[1] Department for Womens' Health, Tuebingen University, 72076 Tübingen, Germany
[2] Department for Pathology and Neuropathology, Tuebingen University, 72076 Tübingen, Germany
[3] Department for Gynecology and Obstetrics, Freiburg University, 79085 Freiburg im Breisgau, Germany
[4] Department for Gynecology and Obstetrics, Ulm University, 89081 Ulm, Germany
* Correspondence: dominik.dannehl@med.uni-tuebingen.de

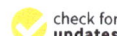

Citation: Dannehl, D.; Engler, T.; Volmer, L.L.; Staebler, A.; Fischer, A.K.; Weiss, M.; Hahn, M.; Walter, C.B.; Grischke, E.-M.; Fend, F.; et al. Recurrence Score® Result Impacts Treatment Decisions in Hormone Receptor-Positive, HER2-Negative Patients with Early Breast Cancer in a Real-World Setting—Results of the IRMA Trial. *Cancers* 2022, *14*, 5365. https://doi.org/10.3390/cancers14215365

Academic Editors: Naiba Nabieva and Javier Cortes

Received: 22 September 2022
Accepted: 22 October 2022
Published: 31 October 2022

Publisher's Note: MDPI stays neutral with regard to jurisdictional claims in published maps and institutional affiliations.

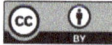

Copyright: © 2022 by the authors. Licensee MDPI, Basel, Switzerland. This article is an open access article distributed under the terms and conditions of the Creative Commons Attribution (CC BY) license (https://creativecommons.org/licenses/by/4.0/).

Simple Summary: Hormone receptor-positive (HR+), HER2-negative (HER2−) is the most common breast cancer subtype (approximately 75% of all breast cancer cases). Adjuvant chemotherapy can be administered to patients that undergo operative tumor removal with only few metastatic axillary lymph nodes (0–3). However, using classical risk biomarkers to guide adjuvant chemotherapy recommendation leads to overtreatment of patients including unnecessary possible chemotherapy-related toxicities. This prospective study assessed whether the multigene-expression assay Oncotype DX® that has been validated in two large clinical phase III trials, effectively reduces adjuvant chemotherapy recommendation in a real-world setting. This study could demonstrate that absolute adjuvant chemotherapy recommendation can be reduced by nearly 15% using Oncotype DX®. Furthermore, this study could show that the Oncotype DX® recurrence score correlates to classic biomarkers that are commonly used to classify the aggressiveness of breast cancer.

Abstract: Background: Patients with hormone receptor-positive (HR+), HER2-negative (HER2−) early breast cancer (eBC) with a high risk of relapse often undergo adjuvant chemotherapy. However, only a few patients will gain benefit from chemotherapy. Since classical tumor characteristics (grade, tumor size, lymph node involvement, and Ki67) are of limited value to predict chemotherapy efficacy, multigene expression assays such as the Oncotype DX® test were developed to reduce over- and undertreatment. The IRMA trial analyzed the impact of Recurrence Score® (RS) assessment on adjuvant treatment recommendations. Materials and methods: The RS result was assessed in patients with HR+/HER2− unilateral eBC with 0–3 pathologic lymph nodes who underwent primary surgical treatment at the Department for Women's Health of Tuebingen University, Germany. Therapy recommendations without knowledge of the RS result were compared to therapy recommendations with awareness of the RS result. Results: In total, 245 patients underwent RS assessment. Without knowledge of the RS result, 92/245 patients (37.6%) would have been advised to receive chemotherapy. After RS assessment, 56/245 patients (22.9%) were advised to undergo chemotherapy. Chemotherapy was waived in 47/92 patients (51.1%) that were initially recommended to receive it. Chemotherapy was added in 11/153 patients (7.2%) that were recommended to not receive it initially. Summary: Using the RS result to guide adjuvant treatment decisions in HR+/HER2− breast cancer led to a substantial reduction of chemotherapy. In view of the results achieved in prospective studies, the RS result is among other risk-factors suitable for the individualization of adjuvant systemic therapy.

Keywords: oncotype DX; recurrence score; breast cancer; individualized therapy

1. Introduction

Breast cancer is the most common cancer in women in Germany and worldwide [1,2]. The most frequent tumor subtype is hormone receptor-positive (HR+), HER2-negative (HER2−) early breast cancer (eBC). Patients with no or 1–3 involved pathologic lymph nodes account for approximately 70% of all breast cancer cases [3,4]. Patients with high clinicopathologic risk factors, such as large tumor size, high tumor grade, lymph node involvement, or a high proliferative index (Ki67) often undergo chemotherapy to reduce the risk of recurrence [5,6]. Yet, many of these patients may not benefit from chemotherapy. Hence, recent research has focused on biomarkers that can predict chemotherapy benefit in eBC, and several multigene-expression assays have been developed and validated in large prospective phase III trials [7–11].

One of the various commercially available multigene-expression assays is the Oncotype DX® test. It analyzes the expression pattern of 16 breast cancer-related genes and 5 reference genes to calculate a Recurrence Score® (RS) result, ranging from 1 to 100, to identify patients at a high risk of recurrence [12]. Retrospective analyses of biomaterial from the prospective NSABP B-20 (lymph node negative) and SWOG-8814 (lymph node positive) studies were able to demonstrate that patients with a high Recurrence Score (RS > 30) result are likely to benefit from chemotherapy [13–15]. The prospective randomized TAILORx clinical trial subsequently found that endocrine therapy is non-inferior to chemoendocrine therapy in node negative patients with an RS 11–25 [10]. In node-positive patients (RxPONDER trial), however, only postmenopausal women with an RS < 26 did not benefit from chemotherapy [11].

The IRMA (impact of Recurrence Score on adjuvant treatment decisions and tumor cell dissemination in estrogen receptor-positive and HER2-negative patients with early breast cancer) trial was designed to prospectively evaluate the impact of RS testing on adjuvant therapy recommendations in a clinical real-world setting. The primary endpoint was to evaluate the change in adjuvant chemotherapy recommendation after RS testing as compared to chemotherapy recommendation without knowledge of the RS result. Secondary endpoints were the influence of the RS result on tumor cell dissemination (which will be reported elsewhere), and to assess the association of the RS result with clinicopathologic factors.

2. Materials and Methods

IRMA is a prospective, single-center investigator-initiated registry study. It was conducted according to the guidelines of the Declaration of Helsinki and approved by the Ethics Committee of Tuebingen University (789/2018BO2). Furthermore, the study was registered under the ID NCT03961880. The study was supported by Exact Sciences.

All patients included in this analysis were treated for eBC at the Department for Women's Health of Tuebingen University Hospital, Germany. Only patients with HR+/HER2− unilateral eBC without extensive lymph-node involvement (0–3 positive lymph nodes) who underwent complete surgical resection at the Department for Women's Health of Tubingen University were eligible for this study. To facilitate decision making, enrollment into the IRMA study could be based on clinical lymph node status. Exclusion criteria were primary systemic therapy, recurrent or metastatic disease, bilateral breast cancer, or a previous history of secondary malignancy.

Tumors were counted as HR+ if they had a positive estrogen receptor (ER) and/or a positive progesterone receptor (PR) expression according to immunohistochemistry ($\geq$10% positive cells for ER, $\geq$10% positive cells for PR). The HER2-status was assessed to local standards by using the HERCEPT test (DAKO, Glostrup, Denmark). Expression of HER2 was scored on a 0 to +3 scale. Tumors with a score of +3 were considered HER2-positive. In case of a score of +2, HER2 amplification was determined by fluorescence in-situ hybridization using the Pathvysion® Kit (Vysis, Downers Grove, IL, USA). Ki67 was assessed using the M7240 monoclonal mouse anti-human Ki67 antibody MIB-1 (Agilent Dako, Santa Clara, CA, USA). The number of Ki67 positive cell nuclei was estimated for the entire core biopsy in a semiquantitative evaluation in steps of 10% by a board certified pathologist as part of the clinical routine workup. Based on St. Gallen consensus for breast cancer, Ki67 values were divided into two prognostic groups: 0–19% (Ki67 low) and $\geq 20\%$ (Ki67 high) [16]. For Oncotype DX analyses, paraffin-embedded tumor tissue samples were submitted to Exact Sciences (Redwood City, CA, USA), according to guidelines provided by the manufacturer. Based on the classification that was used in TAILORx, patients were divided into two prognostic groups: 0–25 (RS low) and ≥ 26 (RS high) [10,11].

Surgery and radiation therapy were administered according to national guidelines. Postoperative systemic treatment recommendation was assessed twice: first, an interdisciplinary tumor conference at Tuebingen University Hospital advised the receipt of chemotherapy or not without knowledge of the RS results. Subsequently, in a further tumor conference after receipt of the RS result, a new decision on adjuvant chemotherapy was made.

Data processing and statistical analysis were performed using Jupyter Notebook (Version 6.3.0, Project Jupyter, open-access and community developed) on Anaconda (Version 3.0, Anaconda Inc., Austin, TX, USA) with the Python extension packages pandas (Version 1.4.1, open-access and community developed), numeric Python (Version 1.22.2, open-access and community developed), and scientific Python (Version 1.8.0, open-access and community developed). Data visualization was achieved using the Python extension packages Matplotlib (Version 3.5.0, open-access and community developed) and Plotly (Version 3.5.0, open-access and community developed). Lucid® (Lucid Software Inc., South Jordan, UT, USA) was used for designing flow charts and data visualization.

Normality distribution was assessed using the Shapiro–Wilk test. Normally distributed data were tested for significance using two-sided Student's t-test with a significance level of $\alpha = 0.05$. Non-normally distributed data were analyzed using the Mann–Whitney-U test with a significance level of $\alpha = 0.05$ as well. The relationship between nominally scaled independent variables was assessed using the x^2-test.

3. Results

3.1. Patient Characteristics

In total, 245 patients were included in this study. Table 1 displays the main patient characteristics. Of all patients, 34.7% were premenopausal, whereas 65.3% were postmenopausal. Mean age ($\pm$SD) was 57.0 ± 11.3 years. The most common histology was no special type (76.7%). The most common grading was G2 (75.5%) while the most frequent tumor classifications were T1 (55.1%) and N0 (72.2%). Mean Ki67 values were $19.6 \pm 12.5\%$ and mean RS values were 16.9 ± 10.2.

Table 1. Overall patient characteristics.

Items	Overall	RS < 26	RS $\geq$ 26	p-Value
Patients	245	209	36	<0.0001
	100.0%	85.3%	14.7%	
Age	57.0 $\pm$ 11.3	57.5 $\pm$ 11.0	54.4 $\pm$ 12.8	0.1383
Menopausal status				
Premenopausal	85	70	15	0.4460
	34.7%	33.5%	41.7%	
Postmenopausal	160	139	21	
	65.3%	66.5%	58.3%	
Histology				
NST	188	158	30	0.5891
	76.7%	75.6%	83.3%	
ILC	49	44	5	
	20.0%	21.1%	13.9%	
Other	8	7	1	
	3.3%	3.4%	2.8%	

Table 1. Cont.

Items	Overall	RS < 26	RS ≥ 26	p-Value
Grading				<0.0001
G1	32	29	3	
	13.1%	13.9%	8.3%	
G2	185	170	15	
	75.5%	81.3%	41.7%	
G3	28	10	18	
	11.4%	4.8%	50.0%	
Tumor size				0.1156
pT1	135	120	15	
	55.1%	57.4%	41.7%	
pT2-4	110	89	21	
	44.9%	42.6%	58.3%	
Nodal involvement				0.5433
pN0	177	153	24	
	72.2%	73.2%	66.7%	
pN1	68	56	12	
	27.8%	26.8%	33.3%	
Ki67	19.6 ± 12.5%	16.3 ± 7.6%	31.5 ± 20.3%	<0.0001
RS	16.9 ± 10.2	13.8 ± 5.8	35.4 ± 10.6	<0.0001

NST = Non-special type, ILC = Invasive lobular carcinoma, RS = Recurrence Score.

3.2. Recurrence Score Results

A total of 14.7% of patients had an RS result ≥ 26 (Table 1). Tumor grade was associated with the RS result ($p < 0.0001$, x^2-test). The most frequent grade in the RS high group was G3 (50%) and G2 (81.3%) in the RS low group. There was no association between the RS result and age, menopausal status, histology, tumor size, or lymph node involvement.

Patients with an RS result ≥ 26 exhibited a significantly higher mean Ki67 proliferation index (RS high vs. RS low: 31.5 ± 20.3% vs. 16.3 ± 7.6%; $p < 0.0001$, Mann–Whitney U-test). Nevertheless, a concordant classification of Ki67 and RS result in the categories "high" and "low" was found in only 60.8% of the cases (49.4% concordant "low", 11.4% concordant "high"). In 39% of all cases a discordant classification can be observed. However, in 35.9% a low RS is associated with a high Ki67 and only in 3.3% a high RS result is associated with a low Ki67. Figure 1 displays the distribution of RS and Ki67.

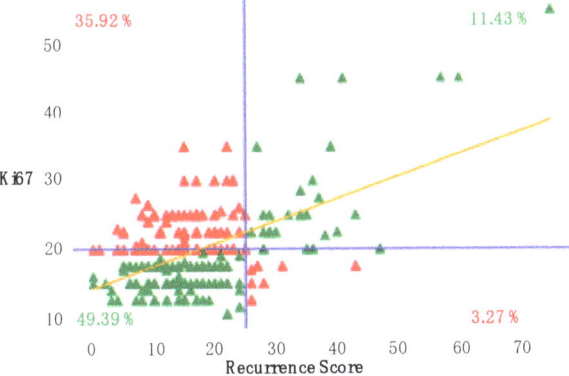

Figure 1. Correlation of Recurrence Score and Ki67: A clinical cut-off value for the Recurrence Score (RS) is ≥26 and for Ki67 is ≥20% (blue lines). Patients with concordant RS and Ki67 values are displayed in green. Discordant RS and Ki67 values are highlighted in red. The yellow line extrapolates the correlation coefficient (Rho = 0.54).

4. Chemotherapy Recommendation

Without knowledge of the RS result, 92/245 patients (37.6%) would have received chemotherapy (Figure 2). After RS assessment, 56/245 patients (22.9%) were advised to undergo chemotherapy. Chemotherapy was waived in 47/92 patients (51.1%) that were initially recommended to receive it. Chemotherapy was added in 11/153 patients (7.2%) that were initially recommended to not receive it. Furthermore, 62/245 patients (25.3%) actually started with adjuvant chemotherapy.

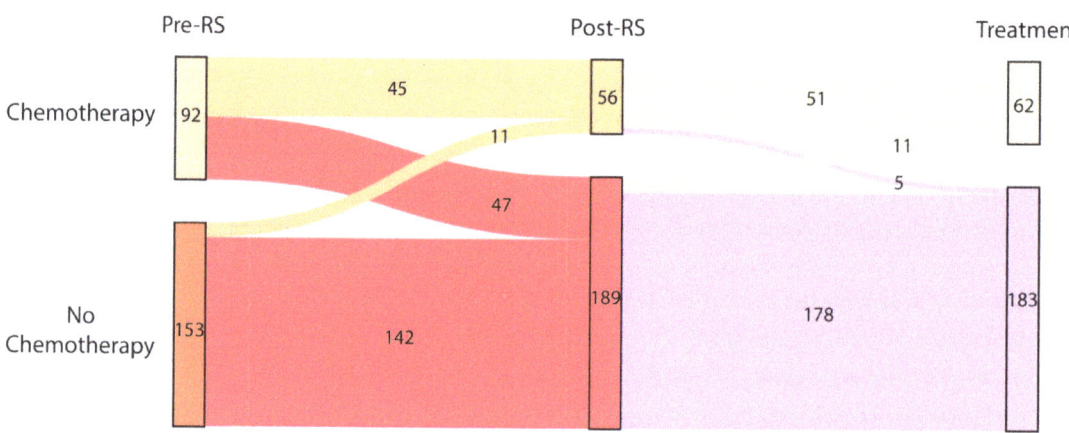

Figure 2. Changes in treatment recommendation due to Recurrence Score (RS) assessment and final treatment decision.

Without knowledge of the Recurrence Score, 92/245 patients were recommended chemotherapy and 153/245 patients were recommended to not undergo chemotherapy (left column). After knowledge of the RS result, chemotherapy recommendation was changed in 58 patients: 56/245 patients were recommended chemotherapy and 189/245 patients were recommended to not undergo chemotherapy (middle column). After patient informed consent, 62/245 patients eventually started chemotherapy (right column).

After awareness of the RS result, 22.9% of all patients were recommended chemotherapy. Mean age of patients in the chemotherapy group was 52.2 ± 11.9 years (Table 2). These patients were significantly younger compared to patients that were not recommended to receive chemotherapy (58.5 ± 10.8 years; $p = 0.0002$, t-test). There was an association between menopausal status and recommendation for chemotherapy. Whereas 29.1% of patients in the no chemotherapy group were premenopausal, 53.6% of patients that were recommended to receive chemotherapy were premenopausal ($p = 0.0013$, x^2-test). High tumor grade was also significantly associated with the recommendation to receive chemotherapy ($p < 0.0001$, x^2-test). 41.1% of all patients in the chemotherapy group had G3 compared to 2.7% in the no chemotherapy group. Furthermore, larger tumor size significantly correlates to chemotherapy recommendation ($p = 0.0106$, x^2-test). In the chemotherapy group, 60.7% of all patients had larger tumors (pT2-4) compared to 40.2% in the no chemotherapy group. Moreover, pathologic lymph node involvement was also correlated with chemotherapy recommendation ($p = 0.0454$, x^2-test). The Ki67 proliferation index was significantly higher in patients that were recommended to receive chemotherapy (chemo vs. no chemo: 29.3 ± 17.7% vs. 16.7 ± 8.6%; $p < 0.0001$, Mann–Whitney U-test). The RS result was also significantly higher in patients in the chemotherapy group (chemo vs. no chemo: 29.6 ± 11.9 vs. 13.2 ± 5.7; $p < 0.0001$, Mann–Whitney U-test). Consequently, significantly more patients in the chemotherapy group were classified in the RS high group (RS ≥ 26: 64.3%; $p < 0.0001$, x^2-test).

Table 2. Patient characteristics compared with chemotherapy recommendation in knowledge of Recurrence Score result.

Items	Overall	No Chemo	Chemo	p-Value
Patients	245 100.0%	189 77.1%	56 22.9%	
Age	57.0 ± 11.3	58.5 ± 10.8	52.2 ± 11.9	0.0002
Menopausal status				
Premenopausal	85 34.7%	55 29.1%	30 53.6%	0.0013
Postmenopausal	160 65.3%	134 70.9%	26 46.4%	
Histology				
NST	188 76.7%	158 75.1%	46 82.1%	0.5159
ILC	49 20.0%	40 21.2%	9 16.1%	
Other	8 3.3%	7 3.7%	1 1.8%	
Grading				
G1	32 13.1%	28 14.8%	4 7.1%	<0.0001
G2	185 75.5%	156 82.5%	29 41.8%	
G3	28 11.4%	5 2.7%	23 41.1%	
Tumor size				
pT1	135 55.1%	113 59.8%	22 39.3%	0.0106
pT2-4	110 44.9%	76 40.2%	34 60.7%	
Nodal involvement				
pN0	177 72.2%	142 75.7%	34 60.7%	0.0454
pN1	68 27.8%	46 24.3%	22 39.3%	
Ki67	19.6 ± 12.5%	16.7 ± 8.6%	29.3 ± 17.7%	<0.0001
RS	16.9 ± 10.2	13.2 ± 5.7	29.6 ± 11.9	<0.0001
RS Group				
Low	209 85.3%	189 100%	20 35.7%	<0.0001
High	36 14.7%	0 0%	36 64.3%	

NST = Non-special type, ILC = Invasive lobular carcinoma, RS = Recurrence Score.

5. Discussion

The IRMA trial is a prospective study that demonstrates how treatment recommendations in clinical routine are impacted using multigene-expression assays. Using the RS result, chemotherapy was spared in approximately half of the patients that were recommended to receive it by means of "classical" clinicopathologic risk factors. Conversely, RS result could identify a small group of patients who might benefit from chemotherapy, although they were initially recommended to not receive it. These findings are highly comparable with the REMAR trial, a multicentric prospective trial that also aimed at characterizing changes in treatment recommendation after the use of Oncotype DX assay [17]. Both the IRMA and the REMAR trials found that using the RS result leads to a meaningful reduction of chemotherapy use and, with respect to the results of TAILORx and RxPONDER trials, can reduce overtreatment [10,11].

Multiple studies aim at assessing the influence of classical clinicopathologic risk factors such as tumor size, tumor grade, Ki67, lymph node involvement, age, ER, and PR status on the results of multigene-expression assays [8,18,19]. This information can be used to select patients that mostly benefit from the use of multigene expression assays [20,21]. The MINDACT trial validated the use of the 70-gene signature to assess a low-risk group with an excellent prognosis [8]. Patients that either had a low genomic with a high clinical risk, or a low clinical with a high genomic risk did not benefit from adjuvant chemotherapy regarding distant recurrence or OS [8]. In contrast, the TAILORx and RxPONDER trials did not answer the question whether patients with a high RS result, but a low clinical risk, can safely omit chemotherapy or whether patients with a low RS result, but a high clinical risk, would have gained benefit from chemotherapy administration. In the IRMA trial, 29/62 patients (46.8%) actually received chemotherapy with an RS result < 26 while 3/183 patients (1.6%) did not receive chemotherapy although they had an RS > 26.

Moreover, statistical models that condense clinicopathologic and genetic risk factors were developed [22]. Whereas a secondary analysis of all patients (pre- and postmenopausal) of the TAILORx trial could demonstrate that patients with an RS < 16 do not gain additional prognostic information by including clinicopathologic risk factors, premenopausal lymph node-negative patients with an RS result between 16 and 25 and a high clinicopathologic risk have increased distant recurrence rates. In particular, women younger than 50 with an RS result between 16 and 25 seem to benefit from additional chemotherapy [10,18,23]. In the IRMA trial, 19/245 (7.8%) patients aged <50 years exhibited an RS result between 16 and 25, yet 12 of these (63.2%) did not receive chemotherapy. Moreover, in the RxPONDER trial, premenopausal patients with lymph-node involvement did benefit from chemotherapy regardless of the RS result and there was no statistical association between RS result and the efficacy of chemotherapy when considering a Recurrence Score of 0–25. [11]. In our current trial, 26/245 patients were premenopausal and displayed node-positive eBC. Prior to the publication of the RxPONDER results on 9 December 2020, 5/16 premenopausal node-positive patients (31.3%) were recommended to receive chemotherapy. Yet, after publication of the RxPONDER results, 8/10 premenopausal node-positive patients (80%) were advised to receive chemotherapy.

Further studies are required to elucidate why, in contrast to postmenopausal patients, premenopausal women with high clinicopathologic risk factors do benefit from chemotherapy administration even in case of a low-risk RS result. A popular hypothesis is that chemotherapy induces ovarian function suppression in premenopausal women [24]. Although there are emerging data that the addition of ovarian function suppression to endocrine treatment positively impacts prognosis, no study has investigated whether this approach can be used to replace adjuvant chemotherapy. Moreover, retrospective analyses may suggest that RS result partially depends on the menstrual cycle, since key genes that comprise the RS algorithm are expressed differently in the different menstrual cycle phases [25].

According to recent German guidelines, multigene-expression assays can be used in HR+/HER2− patients with 0–3 involved lymph nodes if established clinical and pathological factors do not allow therapy decisions regarding the use of chemotherapy [26]. However, the IRMA trial clearly shows that even highly experienced oncologists working in a large tertiary care center are not able to correctly classify the risk of recurrence in HR+/HER2− eBC by solely using "classical" clinicopathologic risk factors. In comparison, the recent national comprehensive cancer network (NCCN) guidelines recommend that the use of multigene-expression assays should be considered in patients with HR+/HER2− eBC based on lymph node involvement. Patients with no pathologic lymph nodes involved (pN0) should be recommended to assess RS if the tumor size is larger than 0.5 cm. Patients with one to three involved pathologic lymph nodes (pN1) should be considered to undergo RS testing if they are eligible for chemotherapy administration [27].

Since additional use of multigene-expression assays implies further financial burden for the health care system, models have been developed to describe the cost-effectiveness of these tests [28–30]. A recently published study demonstrated that the use of multigene-expression assays in Canada could significantly reduce chemotherapy prescription in the RS low group. Interestingly, they also highlighted that RS testing is associated with excess costs in 70- to 80-year-old patients. In this cohort, chemotherapy prescription is not concordant to RS testing result [30]. Thus, the authors underlined the importance of careful patient selection in these age groups. Moreover, another recently published study, evaluating the cost-effectiveness of different multigene-expression assays in Germany, showed that all available assays (Oncotype DX, Mammaprint, Prosigna, Endopredict) reduce overall treatment costs [29]. Several statistical models using clinicopathologic risk factors to identify patients that will most likely benefit from RS testing are currently available, which might help to further reduce overall treatment costs [20,21,31].

In the absence of multigene-expression assays, clinical decision-making regarding chemotherapy use is based on the presumed molecular subtype of the tumor [32]. To classify HR+/HER2− tumors into luminal A-like and luminal B-like, most clinicians are using the proliferation marker Ki67. The International Ki67 Working Group (IKWG) reported that very low (<5%) and high values (>30%) of Ki67 are well defined cut-off values to recommend chemotherapy or not [33]. A predefined secondary analysis of the monarchE trial recently found that Ki67 values $\geq$ 20% are prognostic of a worse prognosis [34]. However, Ki67 assessment is prone to a high interrater variability, pointing out the need for a more standardized Ki67 assessment [33]. In line with previous studies, we found a modest correlation between RS and Ki67 results [19,35]. Using a threshold of 20%, as recently validated in the monarchE trial [34], we found a concordance rate of 60.8% as compared to the RS low and high groups. The correlation was highest among high-risk patients (high Ki67 and high RS, Rho = 0.71). Nevertheless, in 35.2% of all cases high Ki67 values were associated with low RS values, highlighting that a high Ki67 value is not a valid surrogate for the RS result. Yet, a low Ki67 value correlates with low RS values in 93.8%, suggesting that Ki67 values should be partially implemented in preclinical risk scores to assess which patient needs to undergo RS testing.

The strength of this study is its prospective design, and that the IRMA trial was incorporated into the clinical routine. Thus, the IRMA trial was able to describe the influence of RS testing on therapy recommendation in a real-world situation. The reduced deviation from therapy recommendation after awareness of the RS result compared to similar studies may be attributed to the single center interdisciplinary tumor board at a tertiary care center of the highest standard [17]. However, some patients diverge from final therapy recommendation: 8/11 patients (72.7%) that were not recommended to undergo chemotherapy after RS result, but eventually received chemotherapy, were recommended to undergo chemotherapy based on clinicopathologic risk factors. The remainder stated they wanted to receive chemotherapy due to elevated security needs. All patients (100%) that did not undergo chemotherapy albeit a high RS also would have received a chemotherapy recommendation based on clinicopathologic risk factors. However, contraindications to chemotherapy were only reported in 1/5 (20%) patients. Although the results of IRMA were similar to comparable multicentric studies, the single center approach limits external validity of IRMA [17]. Another limitation of this study is that follow-up data are not available, and it is therefore not possible to assess how clinicopathologic factors, information on the RS result, and treatment recommendations will impact survival.

6. Conclusions

This prospective study, which was closely related to clinical practice, showed that the use of adjuvant chemotherapy was substantially reduced by determining the RS result. Only a few patients who would not have been recommended adjuvant chemotherapy if the RS result had not been determined were recommended to receive it after obtaining the RS result. In addition to other clinicopathologic risk factors, the RS result is useful for individualizing adjuvant therapy recommendations in patients with HR+/HER2− breast carcinoma.

Author Contributions: Conceptualization, F.-A.T. and A.D.H.; methodology, F.-A.T. and A.D.H.; software, D.D.; validation, T.E., L.L.V., M.W. and A.D.H.; formal analysis, D.D.; investigation, D.D. and A.D.H.; resources, A.S., A.K.F., F.F. and S.Y.B.; data curation, D.D.; writing—original draft preparation, D.D.; writing—review and editing, T.E., L.L.V., A.S., A.K.F., M.W., M.H., C.B.W., E.-M.G., F.-A.T., S.Y.B. and A.D.H.; visualization, D.D.; supervision, T.E., L.L.V., M.W., M.H., C.B.W., E.-M.G., S.Y.B. and A.D.H.; project administration, A.S., A.K.F., F.F. and A.D.H.; funding acquisition, F.-A.T., S.Y.B. and A.D.H. All authors have read and agreed to the published version of the manuscript.

Funding: This research was partly funded by Exact Sciences.

Institutional Review Board Statement: The study was conducted in accordance with the Declaration of Helsinki, and approved by the Institutional Ethics Committee of Tuebingen University, Germany (approval date: 8 January 2019; protocol code 789/2018BO2).

Informed Consent Statement: Informed consent was obtained from all subjects involved in the study.

Data Availability Statement: The data presented in this study are available on request from the corresponding author. The data are not publicly available due to the German data protection acts in respect to patient data.

Acknowledgments: We thank the patients and their families and caregivers for participating in this trial. The study was supported by Exact Sciences, Redwood City, CA, USA.

Conflicts of Interest: A.D.H. received honoraria from AstraZeneca, Exact Sciences, Gilead, GSK, Roche, Novartis, Seagen, Agendia, Lilly, MSD, Eisai, Daiichi Sankyo, Hexal, and Pfizer. F.-A.T. received honoraria from Novartis, Tesaro, Genomic Health, Roche, Hexal, and Astra Zeneca. E.-M.G. received honoraria from Lilly Oncology, Pfizer, Astra Zeneca, Leo Pharma, Roche Pharma, MSD, and Novartis. T.E. received honoraria from AstraZeneca, Eli Lilly, Daiichi Sankyo, Gilead, GSK, Novartis, Pfizer, and Roche. S.Y.B., F.-A.T., and A.D.H. received institutional funding from Exact Sciences for conducting the IRMA trial. All other authors report that they do not have any conflict of interest.

References

1. Robert-Koch-Institut. *Krebs in Deutschland für 2017/2018*; Zentrum für Krebsregisterdaten: Berlin, Germany, 2021.
2. Jemal, A.; Center, M.M.; DeSantis, C.; Ward, E.M. Global Patterns of Cancer Incidence and Mortality Rates and Trends. *Cancer Epidemiol. Biomark. Prev.* **2010**, *19*, 1893–1907. [CrossRef] [PubMed]
3. Howlader, N.; Altekruse, S.F.; Li, C.I.; Chen, V.W.; Clarke, C.A.; Ries, L.A.; Cronin, K.A. US Incidence of Breast Cancer Subtypes Defined by Joint Hormone Receptor and HER2 Status. *J. Natl. Cancer Inst.* **2014**, *106*. [CrossRef] [PubMed]
4. Dannehl, D.; Volmer, L.L.; Weiss, M.; Matovina, S.; Grischke, E.-M.; Oberlechner, E.; Seller, A.; Walter, C.B.; Hahn, M.; Engler, T.; et al. Feasibility of Adjuvant Treatment with Abemaciclib—Real-World Data from a Large German Breast Center. *J. Pers. Med.* **2022**, *12*, 382. [CrossRef] [PubMed]
5. Early Breast Cancer Trialists' Collaborative Group (EBCTCG). Effects of chemotherapy and hormonal therapy for early breast cancer on recurrence and 15-year survival: An overview of the randomised trials. *Lancet* **2005**, *365*, 1687–1717.
6. Early Breast Cancer Trialists' Collaborative Group (EBCTCG). Comparisons between different polychemotherapy regimens for early breast cancer: Meta-analyses of long-term outcome among 100,000 women in 123 randomised trials. *Lancet* **2012**, *379*, 432–444. [CrossRef]
7. Martin, M.; Brase, J.C.; Calvo, L.; Krappmann, K.; Ruiz-Borrego, M.; Fisch, K.; Rodriguez-Lescure, A. Clinical validation of the EndoPredict test in node-positive, chemotherapy-treated ER+/HER2− breast cancer patients: Results from the GEICAM 9906 trial. *Breast Cancer Res.* **2014**, *16*, R38. [CrossRef]
8. Cardoso, F.; van't Veer, L.J.; Bogaerts, J.; Slaets, L.; Viale, G.; Delaloge, S.; Piccart, M. 70-Gene Signature as an Aid to Treatment Decisions in Early-Stage Breast Cancer. *N. Engl. J. Med.* **2016**, *375*, 717–729. [CrossRef]
9. Gnant, M.; Filipits, M.; Greil, R.; Stoeger, H.; Rudas, M.; Bago-Horvath, Z.; Mlineritsch, B.; Kwasny, W.; Knauer, M.; Singer, C.; et al. Predicting distant recurrence in receptor-positive breast cancer patients with limited clinicopathological risk: Using the PAM50 Risk of Recurrence score in 1478 postmenopausal patients of the ABCSG-8 trial treated with adjuvant endocrine therapy alone. *Ann. Oncol.* **2014**, *25*, 339–345. [CrossRef]

10. Sparano, J.A.; Gray, R.J.; Makower, D.F.; Pritchard, K.I.; Albain, K.S.; Hayes, D.F.; Sledge, G.W., Jr. Adjuvant Chemotherapy Guided by a 21-Gene Expression Assay in Breast Cancer. *N. Engl. J. Med.* **2018**, *379*, 111–121. [CrossRef]
11. Kalinsky, K.; Barlow, W.E.; Gralow, J.R.; Meric-Bernstam, F.; Albain, K.S.; Hayes, D.F.; Lin, N.U.; Perez, E.A.; Goldstein, L.J.; Chia, S.K.; et al. 21-Gene Assay to Inform Chemotherapy Benefit in Node-Positive Breast Cancer. *N. Engl. J. Med.* **2021**, *385*, 2336–2347. [CrossRef]
12. Paik, S.; Shak, S.; Tang, G.; Kim, C.; Baker, J.; Cronin, M.; Wolmark, N. A multigene assay to predict recurrence of tamoxifen-treated, node-negative breast cancer. *N. Engl. J. Med.* **2004**, *351*, 2817–2826. [CrossRef] [PubMed]
13. Geyer, C.E., Jr.; Tang, G.; Mamounas, E.P.; Rastogi, P.; Paik, S.; Shak, S.; Wolmark, N. 21-Gene assay as predictor of chemotherapy benefit in HER2-negative breast cancer. *NPJ Breast Cancer* **2018**, *4*, 37. [CrossRef] [PubMed]
14. Paik, S.; Tang, G.; Shak, S.; Kim, C.; Baker, J.; Kim, W.; Wolmark, N. Gene expression and benefit of chemotherapy in women with node-negative, estrogen receptor-positive breast cancer. *J. Clin. Oncol.* **2006**, *24*, 3726–3734. [CrossRef] [PubMed]
15. Albain, K.S.; Barlow, W.E.; Shak, S.; Hortobagyi, G.N.; Livingston, R.B.; Yeh, I.T.; Hayes, D.F. Prognostic and predictive value of the 21-gene recurrence score assay in postmenopausal women with node-positive, oestrogen-receptor-positive breast cancer on chemotherapy: A retrospective analysis of a randomised trial. *Lancet Oncol.* **2010**, *11*, 55–65. [CrossRef]
16. Goldhirsch, A.; Winer, E.P.; Coates, A.S.; Gelber, R.D.; Piccart-Gebhart, M.; Thürlimann, B.; Wood, W.C. Personalizing the treatment of women with early breast cancer: Highlights of the St Gallen International Expert Consensus on the Primary Therapy of Early Breast Cancer 2013. *Ann. Oncol.* **2013**, *24*, 2206–2223. [CrossRef]
17. Thill, M.; Anastasiadou, L.; Solbach, C.; Möbus, V.; Baier, P.; Ackermann, S.; Giesecke, D.; Schulmeyer, E.; Gabriel, B.; Mosch, D.; et al. 367 Poster—The REMAR (Rhein-Main-Registry)-Study: Prospective evaluation of oncotype DX® Assay in Addition to Ki-67 for adjuvant treatment decisions in early breast cancer. *Eur. J. Cancer* **2020**, *138*, S92–S93. [CrossRef]
18. Sparano, J.A.; Gray, R.J.; Makower, D.F.; Albain, K.S.; Saphner, T.J.; Badve, S.S.; Sledge, G.W. Clinical Outcomes in Early Breast Cancer With a High 21-Gene Recurrence Score of 26 to 100 Assigned to Adjuvant Chemotherapy Plus Endocrine Therapy: A Secondary Analysis of the TAILORx Randomized Clinical Trial. *JAMA Oncol.* **2020**, *6*, 367–374. [CrossRef]
19. Walter, V.P.; Taran, F.-A.; Wallwiener, M.; Bauer, A.; Grischke, E.-M.; Walter, C.B.; Hahn, M.; Brucker, S.Y.; Hartkopf, A.D. Distribution of the 21-Gene Breast Recurrence Score in Patients with Primary Breast Cancer in Germany. *Geburtshilfe Frauenheilkd.* **2020**, *80*, 619–627. [CrossRef]
20. Bhargava, R.; Clark, B.Z.; Carter, G.J.; Brufsky, A.M.; Dabbs, D.J. The healthcare value of the Magee Decision Algorithm™: Use of Magee Equations™ and mitosis score to safely forgo molecular testing in breast cancer. *Mod. Pathol.* **2020**, *33*, 1563–1570. [CrossRef]
21. Slembrouck, L.; Vanden Bempt, I.; Wildiers, H.; Smeets, A.; Van Rompuy, A.S.; Van Ongeval, C.; Floris, G. Concordance between results of inexpensive statistical models and multigene signatures in patients with ER+/HER2− early breast cancer. *Mod. Pathol.* **2021**, *34*, 1297–1309. [CrossRef]
22. Sparano, J.A.; Crager, M.R.; Tang, G.; Gray, R.J.; Stemmer, S.M.; Shak, S. Development and Validation of a Tool Integrating the 21-Gene Recurrence Score and Clinical-Pathological Features to Individualize Prognosis and Prediction of Chemotherapy Benefit in Early Breast Cancer. *J. Clin. Oncol.* **2021**, *39*, 557–564. [CrossRef] [PubMed]
23. Sparano, J.A.; Gray, R.J.; Ravdin, P.M.; Makower, D.F.; Pritchard, K.I.; Albain, K.S.; Sledge, G.W., Jr. Clinical and Genomic Risk to Guide the Use of Adjuvant Therapy for Breast Cancer. *N. Engl. J. Med.* **2019**, *380*, 2395–2405. [CrossRef] [PubMed]
24. Zhang, S.; Fitzsimmons, K.C.; Hurvitz, S.A. Oncotype DX Recurrence Score in premenopausal women. *Ther. Adv. Med. Oncol.* **2022**, *14*, 17588359221081077. [CrossRef] [PubMed]
25. Haynes, B.P.; Viale, G.; Galimberti, V.; Rotmensz, N.; Gibelli, B.; A'Hern, R.; Dowsett, M. Expression of key oestrogen-regulated genes differs substantially across the menstrual cycle in oestrogen receptor-positive primary breast cancer. *Breast Cancer Res. Treat.* **2013**, *138*, 157–165. [CrossRef] [PubMed]
26. Ditsch, N.; Kolberg-Liedtke, C.; Friedrich, M.; Jackisch, C.; Albert, U.S.; Banys-Paluchowski, M.; Thill, M. AGO Recommendations for the Diagnosis and Treatment of Patients with Early Breast Cancer: Update 2021. *Breast Care* **2021**, *16*, 214–227. [CrossRef]
27. Gradishar, W.J.; Moran, M.S.; Abraham, J.; Aft, R.; Agnese, D.; Allison, K.H.; Kumar, R. NCCN Guidelines® Insights: Breast Cancer, Version 4.2021. *J. Natl. Compr. Cancer Netw.* **2021**, *19*, 484–493. [CrossRef]
28. Mariotto, A.B.; Enewold, L.; Zhao, J.; Zeruto, C.A.; Yabroff, K.R. Medical Care Costs Associated with Cancer Survivorship in the United States. *Cancer Epidemiol. Biomark. Prev.* **2020**, *29*, 1304–1312. [CrossRef]
29. Lux, M.; Minartz, C.; Müller-Huesmann, H.; Sandor, M.-F.; Herrmann, K.; Radeck-Knorre, S.; Neubauer, A. Budget impact of the Oncotype DX® test compared to other gene expression tests in patients with early breast cancer in Germany. *Cancer Treat. Res. Commun.* **2022**, *31*, 100519. [CrossRef]
30. Tesch, M.E.; Speers, C.; Diocee, R.M.; Gondara, L.; Peacock, S.J.; Nichol, A.; Lohrisch, C. AImpact of TAILORx on chemotherapy prescribing and 21-gene recurrence score-guided treatment costs in a population-based cohort of patients with breast cancer. *Cancer* **2022**, *128*, 665–674. [CrossRef]
31. Pawloski, K.R.; Gonen, M.; Wen, H.Y.; Tadros, A.B.; Thompson, D.; Abbate, K.; Morrow, M.; El-Tamer, M. Supervised machine learning model to predict oncotype DX risk category in patients over age 50. *Breast Cancer Res. Treat.* **2022**, *191*, 423–430. [CrossRef]

32. Perou, C.M.; Sørlie, T.; Eisen, M.B.; Van De Rijn, M.; Jeffrey, S.S.; Rees, C.A.; Pollack, J.R.; Ross, D.T.; Johnsen, H.; Akslen, L.A.; et al. Molecular portraits of human breast tumours. *Nature* **2000**, *406*, 747–752. [CrossRef] [PubMed]
33. Nielsen, T.O.; Leung, S.C.Y.; Rimm, D.L.; Dodson, A.; Acs, B.; Badve, S.; Denkert, C.; Ellis, M.J.; Fineberg, S.; Flowers, M.; et al. Assessment of Ki67 in Breast Cancer: Updated Recommendations From the International Ki67 in Breast Cancer Working Group. *JNCI J. Natl. Cancer Inst.* **2021**, *113*, 808–819. [CrossRef] [PubMed]
34. Harbeck, N.; Rastogi, P.; Martin, M.; Tolaney, S.; Shao, Z.; Fasching, P.; Huang, C.; Jaliffe, G.; Tryakin, A.; Goetz, M.; et al. Adjuvant abemaciclib combined with endocrine therapy for high-risk early breast cancer: Updated efficacy and Ki-67 analysis from the monarchE study. *Ann. Oncol.* **2021**, *32*, 1571–1581. [CrossRef] [PubMed]
35. Gluz, O.; Nitz, U.A.; Christgen, M.; Kates, R.E.; Shak, S.; Clemens, M.; Kraemer, S.; Aktas, B.; Kuemmel, S.; Reimer, T.; et al. West German Study Group Phase III PlanB Trial: First Prospective Outcome Data for the 21-Gene Recurrence Score Assay and Concordance of Prognostic Markers by Central and Local Pathology Assessment. *J. Clin. Oncol.* **2016**, *34*, 2341–2349. [CrossRef]

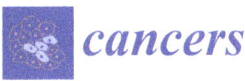

Article

Temporal Heterogeneity of HER2 Expression and Spatial Heterogeneity of ^{18}F-FDG Uptake Predicts Treatment Outcome of Pyrotinib in Patients with HER2-Positive Metastatic Breast Cancer

Chengcheng Gong [1,2,†], Cheng Liu [2,3,4,5,†], Zhonghua Tao [1,2], Jian Zhang [1,2], Leiping Wang [1,2], Jun Cao [1,2], Yannan Zhao [1,2], Yizhao Xie [1,2], Xichun Hu [1,2], Zhongyi Yang [2,3,4,5,*,‡] and Biyun Wang [1,2,*,‡]

1 Department of Breast and Urological Medical Oncology, Fudan University Shanghai Cancer Center, Shanghai 200032, China
2 Department of Oncology, Shanghai Medical College, Fudan University, Shanghai 200032, China
3 Department of Nuclear Medicine, Fudan University Shanghai Cancer Center, Shanghai 200032, China
4 Center for Biomedical Imaging, Fudan University, Shanghai 200032, China
5 Shanghai Engineering Research Center of Molecular Imaging Probes, Shanghai 200032, China
* Correspondence: yangzhongyi21@163.com (Z.Y.); wangbiyun0107@hotmail.com (B.W.); Tel.: +86-21-64175590-86908 (Z.Y.); Fax: +86-21-54520250 (Z.Y.)
† These authors contributed equally to this work.
‡ These authors contributed equally to this work.

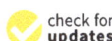

Citation: Gong, C.; Liu, C.; Tao, Z.; Zhang, J.; Wang, L.; Cao, J.; Zhao, Y.; Xie, Y.; Hu, X.; Yang, Z.; et al. Temporal Heterogeneity of HER2 Expression and Spatial Heterogeneity of ^{18}F-FDG Uptake Predicts Treatment Outcome of Pyrotinib in Patients with HER2-Positive Metastatic Breast Cancer. *Cancers* 2022, 14, 3973. https://doi.org/10.3390/cancers14163973

Academic Editor: Naiba Nabieva

Received: 1 July 2022
Accepted: 14 August 2022
Published: 17 August 2022

Publisher's Note: MDPI stays neutral with regard to jurisdictional claims in published maps and institutional affiliations.

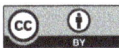

Copyright: © 2022 by the authors. Licensee MDPI, Basel, Switzerland. This article is an open access article distributed under the terms and conditions of the Creative Commons Attribution (CC BY) license (https://creativecommons.org/licenses/by/4.0/).

Simple Summary: Tumor heterogeneity plays an important role in malignant behaviors and treatment responses. This study aimed to evaluate the temporal and spatial heterogeneity in clinical practice and investigate its impact on the treatment outcome of pyrotinib in patients with HER2-positive metastatic breast cancer. Temporal heterogeneity was evaluated by the discordance between primary and metastatic immunohistochemistry results. ^{18}F-FDG uptake heterogeneity on baseline PET/CT scan was assessed to reflect spatial tumor heterogeneity among metastases. Our results showed that heterogeneous HER2 status between primary and metastatic lesions and spatial ^{18}F-FDG uptake heterogeneity were predictive of poorer outcomes of pyrotinib treatment. The best method to evaluate tumor heterogeneity in clinical practice still needs to be identified. Temporal heterogeneity of HER2 expression and spatial heterogeneity of ^{18}F-FDG uptake provided practically applicable methods to assess tumor heterogeneity and potential guidance for treatment decisions.

Abstract: Background: This study aimed to evaluate tumor heterogeneity of metastatic breast cancer (MBC) and investigate its impact on the efficacy of pyrotinib in patients with HER2-positive MBC. Methods: MBC patients who underwent ^{18}F-FDG PET/CT before pyrotinib treatment were included. Temporal and spatial tumor heterogeneity was evaluated by the discordance between primary and metastatic immunohistochemistry (IHC) results and baseline ^{18}F-FDG uptake heterogeneity (intertumoral and intratumoral heterogeneity indexes: HI-inter and HI-intra), respectively. Progression-free survival (PFS) was estimated by the Kaplan–Meier method and compared by a log-rank test. Results: A total of 572 patients were screened and 51 patients were included. In 36 patients with matched IHC results, 25% of them had HER2 status conversion. Patients with homogenous HER2 positivity had the longest PFS, followed by patients with gained HER2 positivity, while patients with HER2 negative conversion could not benefit from pyrotinib (16.8 vs. 13.7 vs. 3.6 months, $p < 0.0001$). In terms of spatial heterogeneity, patients with high HI-intra and HI-inter had significantly worse PFS compared to those with low heterogeneity (10.6 vs. 25.3 months, $p = 0.023$; 11.2 vs. 25.3 months, $p = 0.040$). Conclusions: Temporal heterogeneity of HER2 status and spatial heterogeneity of ^{18}F-FDG uptake could predict the treatment outcome of pyrotinib in patients with HER2-positive MBC, which provide practically applicable methods to assess tumor heterogeneity and guidance for treatment decisions.

Keywords: metastatic breast cancer; heterogeneity; HER2; ^{18}F-fluorodeoxyglucose positron emission tomography/computed tomography; pyrotinib; therapy response

1. Introduction

Breast cancer (BC) remains the most common cancer and the leading cause of cancer-related death in women worldwide. Approximately, 15–20% of BCs are human epidermal growth factor receptor 2 (HER2)-positive, which used to be considered an aggressive phenotype with poor prognosis until the development of anti-HER2 targeted therapy [1–5].

Pyrotinib is an orally available, irreversible pan-Erb receptor tyrosine kinase inhibitor that targets HER1, HER2, and HER4. The phase II study demonstrated that the combination of pyrotinib and capecitabine significantly prolonged the PFS of patients with HER2-positive MBC previously treated with taxanes, anthracyclines, and/or trastuzumab compared with lapatinib and capecitabine (18.1 months vs. 7.0 months, hazard ratio, 0.36; 95% confidence interval [CI], 0.23–0.58; $p < 0.001$) [6]. Based on the impressive improvement in PFS, pyrotinib has been granted accelerated but conditional approval for the treatment of metastatic HER2-positive BC, regardless of prior exposure to trastuzumab, in China in August 2018. PHENIX, a double-blinded, multicenter, randomized phase III study, showed that pyrotinib plus capecitabine significantly prolonged PFS (11.1 months vs. 4.1 months, $p < 0.001$) and had a better overall response rate (ORR) (68.6% vs. 16.0%, $p < 0.001$) than capecitabine monotherapy [7]. PHOBE, another phase III randomized controlled trial of pyrotinib, directly compared pyrotinib and capecitabine with lapatinib and capecitabine in HER2-positive MBC patients who had been previously treated with trastuzumab and taxanes. The median PFS of pyrotinib and capecitabine was 12.5 months, significantly longer than that of 6.8 months in lapatinib ($p < 0.0001$) [8]. Pyrotinib gained full approval in July 2020 based on the results of the PHENIX and PHOBE trials and has been covered by national medical insurance since November 2019.

Due to the fact that trastuzumab emtansine (T-DM1) has not been approved in China for the treatment of MBC until June 2021 and is not covered by national medical insurance till now, pyrotinib has been an important treatment option for HER2-positive MBC. A multicenter, observational, large-scale, real-world study has been conducted to evaluate the efficacy of pyrotinib in China in daily clinical practice [9]. Among 862 MBC patients enrolled in this study, 31.1%, 35.7% and 33.2% received pyrotinib as first-line, second-line and third- or later-line treatment, respectively.

Despite the promising results in clinical trials, not all patients benefited from pyrotinib treatment in real-world clinical practice [10,11]. Therefore, it is important to identify biomarkers to predict response to pyrotinib-based therapy as it may lead to optimization of treatment selection strategy for thousands of patients in China.

Tumor heterogeneity plays an important role in the malignant behaviors and treatment responses of different cancers [12–15]. At an individual level, tumor heterogeneity can manifest as temporal heterogeneity, the molecular evolution of the tumor over time, and as spatial heterogeneity, which describes the uneven distribution of genetically diverse tumor subpopulations across different disease sites or within a single disease site or tumor [16].

Tumor heterogeneity can be detected by conventional immunohistochemistry (IHC), gene expression profiling, or other methods. In breast cancer, the discordance of estrogen receptor (ER), progesterone receptor (PR), and HER2 expression levels between matched primary and metastatic lesions could reflect temporal intratumor heterogeneity. A meta-analysis evaluated receptor discordance rates between primary and metastatic breast cancer in 47 studies with 3384 paired samples. The median discordance rates for ER, PR and HER2 were 14% (0–67%), 21% (0–62%) and 10% (0–44%), respectively [17]. A large-scale real-world study has compared matched IHC results in 1677 MBC patients and reported a change in HR and HER2 expression of 14.2% and 7.8%. In terms of subtypes, more than half of patients (53%) with primary HR+/HER2+ disease showed status change [18]. As a therapeutic target, the evaluation of HER2 is of great importance. Another meta-analysis evaluated the HER2 status in the primary tumor and corresponding distant metastasis in 35 studies. The discordance rate was assessed in 2440 patients for HER2. The studies were subdivided into three groups—studies using FISH only, studies using IHC only, and studies using a combination of IHC and FISH (in case of 2+/equivocal IHC)—to assess receptor status. No significant difference was seen between the total discordance percentages of these groups ($p = 0.25$) [19]. Despite technical reasons that may affect the examination of IHC results, the discordance of ER, PR and HER2 between primary and metastatic disease is considered a truly existing biological phenomenon. Tumor heterogeneity is one of the most important reasons behind this phenomenon. Due to the fact that therapeutic strategy is highly dependent on the IHC evaluation of these markers, the re-biopsy of the metastatic lesion, especially when metastasis is diagnosed for the first time, has been recommended by several international guidelines.

In terms of spatial heterogeneity, however, multiple biopsies of different metastatic sites or multi-region sampling within a single lesion are required for comprehensive assessment, which could not be widely adopted owing to prohibitive risks of biopsy. In this case, functional molecular imaging can serve as an alternative option to characterize tumor spatial heterogeneity noninvasively. ^{18}F- fluorodeoxyglucose (FDG) PET-CT provides the metabolic activity of various lesions, which could reflect regional variation in tumor function in solid tumors. The predictive value of intratumoral heterogeneity of baseline ^{18}F-FDG uptake in various tumors has been proved [20–24]. Common methods to examine this include textural analysis, coefficient of variance (COV), cumulative standardized uptake value (SUV)-volume histogram (CSH), the area under the CSH, and fractal analysis [25–30]. However, these methods are still too complicated to be widely applicable for metastatic disease in clinical practice, particularly if there are multiple metastatic lesions. Our previous study introduced simplified quantitative parameters to represent the inter- and intratumoral heterogeneous characteristics of metastatic disease and proved their value in predicting the response to treatment in patients with triple-negative and hormone receptor (HR)-positive BC [31–34]. In this study, we evaluated ^{18}F-FDG uptake heterogeneity in HER2 positive MBC to reflect spatial tumor metabolic heterogeneity among metastases and explored its predictive value for the treatment outcome of pyrotinib.

This study aimed to evaluate the temporal heterogeneity between primary and metastatic lesions and spatial heterogeneity among metastatic lesions in HER2-positive MBC and to explore their ability to predict patient outcomes under pyrotinib treatment.

2. Materials and Methods

2.1. Patients

A total of 572 patients with MBC treated with pyrotinib in the Fudan University Shanghai Cancer Center (FUSCC) between 1 September 2018 and 24 July 2021 were screened. Patients who underwent whole-body FDG PET/CT within 4 weeks before the initiation of pyrotinib were included in this study. Patients without detailed medical history or who were lost to follow-up were excluded. Data were retrospectively obtained from the patients' medical history.

2.2. IHC Evaluation

The ER, PR and HER2 status was derived from pathological reports. According to the Standard Operating Procedure (SOP) of FUSCC, pathology consultation should be recommended before initiating treatment for patients who were not diagnosed in our center, except for those who were not able to provide archived tumor tissue. Pathology reports were evaluated through an independent review of two committee-certified pathologists with expertise in breast cancer. The discrepancies between the two pathologists were resolved through a review of a third pathologist. Immunohistochemical staining for ER, PR, HER2 was performed with antibodies against ER (SP1, Roche Ventana), PR (IE2, Roche Ventana), HER2 (4B5, Roche Ventana), as previously reported [35]. PathVysion HER2 DNA Probe Kit (Abbott Molecular, Abbott Park, Illinois) was used for HER2 FISH following the manufacturer's instructions [35]. HR positivity was defined according to national guidelines with a cutoff level of 1% [36]. HR status in this article was defined as "positive" or "negative". For further exploration, tumors were stratified into four groups based on the percentage of ER+: ER negative (<1%), low ER (1–10%), intermediate ER (10–50%) and high ER (>50%). "HR expression change" in this article refers to the change between low, intermediate and high expression of HR. HER2 status was interpreted using the updated 2018 ASCO/CAP guideline recommendations for HER2 testing, based on IHC and FISH results [37]. For further exploration, tumors were stratified into four groups based on HER2 IHC results: HER2 negative (0), HER2 low (+, ++ and FISH-), HER2 positive with IHC (+~++, FISH+) and HER2 positive with IHC (+++). "HER2 expression change" in this article refers specifically to the conversion between these groups. The subtype referred to in this study included HR+/HER2+, HR-/HER2+, HR+/HER2- and HR-/HER2- based on the defined thresholds.

2.3. PET/CT Imaging

^{18}F-FDG was produced automatically by cyclotron (Siemens CTI RDS Eclips ST, Siemens, Knoxville, TN, USA) using the Explora FDG4 module in our center. The radiochemical purity was over 95%.

Patients were required to fast for at least 6 h before the ^{18}F-FDG PET/CT scan, and blood glucose levels were to be <200 mg/dL at the time of injection. Sixty minutes following intravenous ^{18}F-FDG administration (mean dose 3.7–7.4 MBq/kg), patients underwent PET/CT from the mid-skull to the mid-thigh (Siemens Biograph 16HR PET/CT or mCT Flow PET/CT scanner, Siemens Medical solutions, USA). Low-dose CT was performed during tidal breathing to correct for attenuation, followed by a PET emission scan that covered the identical transverse field of view.

2.4. Image Interpretation

^{18}F-FDG PET/CT images were reviewed and evaluated independently by two board-certified nuclear medicine physicians using a multimodality computer platform (Syngo, Siemens, Knoxville, TN, USA). In the event of disagreement between the two readers, a consensus was reached on a final reading for the statistical analyses. All hypermetabolic metastatic lesions were picked for analysis, whereas hypermetabolic foci judged to be inflammation or normal physiological activity were not considered.

Semiquantitative analysis of tumor metabolic activity was obtained using SUV normalized to body weight. The maximum SUV (SUVmax) and mean SUV (SUVmean) for each metastatic lesion were recorded by manually placing an individual region of interest (ROI) around each tumor on all consecutive slices that contained the lesion on co-registered and fused transaxial PET/CT images. The SUVmax across all metastatic lesions was then evaluated. Then, the metabolic tumor volume (MTV) was automatically extracted from the software based on an SUV threshold of 40. Total lesion glucose (TLG) was calculated according to the formula: TLG = SUVmean × MTV. A quantitative measure of intratumoral heterogeneity, the intratumoral heterogeneity index (HI-intra), was measured by dividing the SUVmax of each lesion by the SUVmean of that lesion [31,34,38,39]. The mean HI-intra of all lesions was selected to represent the intratumoral heterogeneity for each patient. Intertumoral heterogeneity was evaluated by the COV and intertumoral heterogeneity index (HI-inter), another parameter we proposed. The COV of metastatic lesions was calculated from the SUVmax of every ROI as the ratio of the standard deviation to the mean [40]. The HI-inter was the maximum value of the SUVmax divided by the minimum value of the SUVmax for all metastatic lesions [32]. Considering the partial volume effect and repeatability, only lesions no less than 10 mm in diameter were included in further analysis. Bone lesions with confirmation by CT or magnetic resonance imaging were included.

2.5. Statistical Analyses

Data are presented as medians (ranges) or numbers of patients (percentages). Treatment outcome was assessed as PFS, which was measured from the date of pyrotinib initiation to the first documented disease progression or death. Disease progression was determined by the Response Evaluation Criteria in Solid Tumors version 1.1. Overall survival (OS) was measured from the date of pyrotinib initiation to the date of death or the last follow-up. Kaplan–Meier method was conducted for estimating survivals and log-rank test for comparisons. Mann–Whitney U test was applied for comparison between groups with quantitative variables with non-normal distribution. Analyses of factors potentially associated with temporal and spatial tumor heterogeneity were performed using the Chi-squared test or the Fisher exact test.

Time-dependent survival receiver operating characteristic (ROC) analysis had an advantage in assessing the prognostic value of the biomarkers and determining optimal cutoff values by maximizing both sensitivity and specificity of the event-time outcome [41]. PET/CT parameters cutoff values were determined by survival ROC library in R. Other statistical analyses were conducted by SPSS IBM® version 22 (SPSS Inc., Chicago, IL, USA). All p-values were two-sided, and $p < 0.05$ was considered significant.

3. Results

3.1. Patient Baseline Characteristics and Their Association with PFS

There were 51 MBC patients that met the criteria of undertaking ^{18}F-FDG PET/CT within 4 weeks before the initiation of pyrotinib and were included in the analysis. The demographic and clinical characteristics of the patients are summarized in Table 1.

Table 1. Patients and tumor characteristics.

Characteristics	Patients (n = 51)	
	No.	%
Age (years)		
Median	54	
Range	23–74	
Menopausal status		
Postmenopausal	36	70.6
Premenopausal	15	29.4
HR status [a]		
Positive	20	39.2
Negative	31	60.8
De novo breast cancer		
Yes	6	11.8
No	45	88.2
Histological Grade [b]		
Grade 2	13	25.5
Grade 3	35	68.6
Disease-free interval		
<24 months	31	68.9
>24 months	14	31.1
Number of metastatic sites		
1	16	31.4
2	14	27.5
≥3	21	41.2
Metastatic sites		
Lung	10	19.6
Liver	12	23.5
Bone	23	45.1
Brain	10	19.6

Table 1. Cont.

Characteristics	Patients (n = 51)	
	No.	%
Visceral disease	25	49.0
Treatment line [c]		
1	21	41.2
2	23	45.1
≥3	7	13.7
Previous anti-HER2 treatment		
Trastuzumab	47	92.2
Pertuzumab	13	25.5
Lapatinib	4	7.8
Trastuzumab emtansine	1	2.0

[a] In patients with discordant HR status, the most recent results were presented. [b] Nottingham System, WHO 2019. Three patients did not have results. [c] Treatment line in which pyrotinib was administered. Abbreviations: HR, hormone receptor; No., Number.

The median patient age was 54 years (range 23–74 years). 39.2% of the patients had HR-positive disease. Six patients were diagnosed with de novo stage IV disease. In patients who received radical treatment, 68.9% had disease relapse within two years. Twenty-one patients (41.2%) had ≥3 metastatic sites, and the common sites of metastases were the bone (45.1%), liver (23.5%), brain (19.6%) and lung (19.6%). Around half of the patients (49.0%) had visceral involvement. Most patients received pyrotinib as the first or second treatment (86.3%). Of the patients, 78.4% received pyrotinib and capecitabine and other patients received combinational agents such as vinorelbine. Additionally, 92.2% of the patients had been treated with trastuzumab and 25.5% of the patients had prior pertuzumab exposure.

At the time of analysis, 26 patients had documented disease progression (51%). The median PFS was 13.7 months (95% CI, 9.3–18.2). The data for OS were immature at the time of analysis. In 41 patients with evaluable disease, the objective response rate was 48.8%.

The associations between clinical factors and PFS are shown in Table 2. Patients who received pyrotinib as first or second-line treatment had a significantly longer median PFS than patients who received pyrotinib as third- or later-line treatment (15.7 vs. 10.6 months, $p = 0.017$). Patients with one metastatic site had better outcomes compared with patients with a higher tumor burden (25.3 vs. 11.2 months, $p = 0.015$). HR status did not affect the PFS of pyrotinib treatment (13.7 vs. 13.4 months, $p = 0.930$). Tumors were stratified into four groups based on the percentage of ER+ percentage on the most recent IHC results: ER negative (<1%, $n = 33$), low ER (1–10%, $n = 4$), intermediate ER (10–50%, $n = 5$) and high ER (>50%, $n = 9$). The median PFS for these patients were 13.4 months, 10.2 months, 16.8 months and 15.7 months, respectively ($p = 0.343$). It seems that patients with low ER had the worse outcome. Tumors were stratified into four groups based on HER2 expression on the most recent IHC results: HER2 negative (0, $n = 1$), HER2 low (+, ++ and FISH-, $n = 3$), HER2 positive with IHC (+~++, FISH+) ($n = 12$), HER2 positive with IHC (+++) ($n = 35$). The median PFS for these patients were 3.6 months, 5.8 months, 13.7 months and 16.8 months, respectively ($p < 0.0001$).

Table 2. Analysis of factors associated with PFS.

Factors		No. of Patients	PFS (Months)	95% CI	p-Value
Clinical risk factors					
Age	≥54 years	26	13.4	7.2–19.5	0.456
	<54 years	25	14.4	9.1–19.7	
HR status [a]	Positive	20	13.7	8.9–18.5	0.930
	Negative	31	13.4	8.8–17.9	
Histological Grade	Grade 2	13	10.6	9.7–11.5	0.365
	Grade 3	35	13.7	10.8–16.6	
Disease-free interval	>24 months	14	13.7	1.5–26.0	0.872
	<24 months	31	12.4	9.3–15.6	
Treatment line [b]	First- or second-line	44	15.7	4.1–27.3	0.017 *
	Third- or later-line	7	10.6	10.2–11.1	
Resistance to previous trastuzumab [c]	Yes	26	12.4	3.6–21.2	0.432
	No	25	15.7	9.4–22.06	
No. of metastatic sites	1	16	25.3	NR	0.015 *
	≥2	35	11.2	8.9–13.5	
Visceral disease	Yes	25	11.2	9.6–12.9	0.280
	No	26	16.8	7.4–26.2	
Combinational agent	Capecitabine	40	13.4	7.1–19.6	0.911
	Others	11	14.4	8.7–20.1	
Tumor heterogeneity					
Temporal tumor heterogeneity between primary and metastatic disease					
HR status	heterogeneous	10	11.1	8.6–13.6	0.887
	homogeneous	26	16.8	8.5–25.1	
HR expression	heterogeneous	15	13.7	9.5–18.0	0.541
	homogeneous	21	16.8	8.5–25.1	
HER2 status	heterogeneous	9	5.8	3.0–8.6	0.001 *
	homogeneous	27	16.8	4.5–29.1	
HER2 expression	heterogeneous	12	5.8	3.7–8.0	0.001 *
	homogeneous	24	NR	NR	
Spatial tumor heterogeneity in terms of ^{18}F-FDG uptake					
HI-intra	>1.69	26	10.6	9.5–11.7	0.023 *
	<1.69	25	25.3	5.9–44.8	
HI-inter	>1.15	31	11.2	7.3–15.1	0.040 *
	<1.15	20	25.3	NR	

[a] In patients with discordant HR status, the most recent results were presented. [b] Treatment line in which pyrotinib was administered. [c] Resistance to trastuzumab was defined as relapse during or within 6 months after adjuvant trastuzumab or progression within 3 months of trastuzumab treatment for metastatic disease [8]. Abbreviations: No., Number; PFS, progression-free survival; CI, confidence interval; NR, not reached; HR, hormone receptor; HER2, human epidermal growth factor receptor 2; FDG, fluorodeoxyglucose; HI-intra, intratumoral heterogeneity index; HI-inter, intertumoral heterogeneity index. * $p < 0.05$ is considered significant.

3.2. Temporal Tumor Heterogeneity and Its Association with PFS

Of patients enrolled in this study, 88.2% (45/51) had tumor IHC results confirmed by the Department of Pathology in FUSCC. Among 51 patients enrolled in this study, 46 of them (90.2%) had had re-biopsy before the initiation of pyrotinib and 36 patients (70.6%) had matched primary and metastatic IHC results. Thus, the following evaluation of temporal heterogeneity in terms of IHC was performed in 36 patients with matched IHC results. There were 24 patients' primary sites and metastases IHC results that had both been evaluated in FUSUCC.

The discordance rate for HR and/or HER2 status between primary and metastases was 41.7% (15/36).

The change rate of HER2 status was 25% (9/36), with a positive conversion of 55.6% (5/9) and a negative conversion of 44.4% (Figure 1). Twelve patients (33.3%) showed heterogeneous HER2 expression between primary and metastatic IHC, with a change of gain in 50% and loss in 50%. The change rate for HR status was 27.8% (10/36), with a positive conversion and a negative conversion of 50% each. Fifteen patients (41.7%) showed heterogenous HR expression between primary and metastatic IHC, with a gain of 46.7% and a loss of 53.3%.

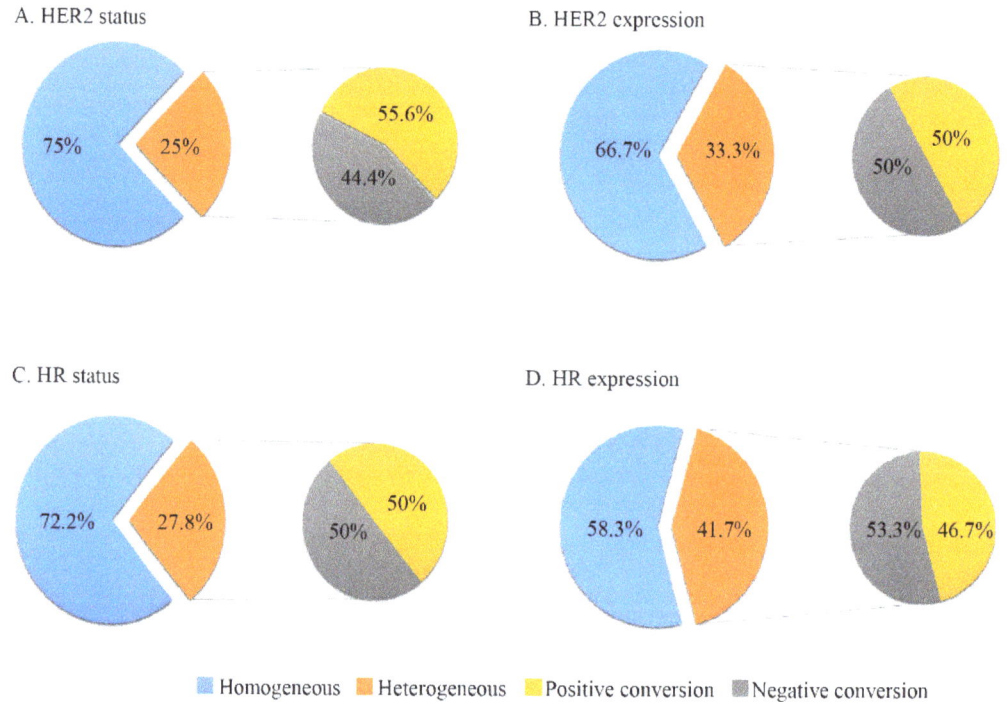

Figure 1. Temporal tumor heterogeneity in terms of IHC discordance between primary and metastatic tumors. (**A**) HER2 status. (**B**) HER2 expression. (**C**) HR status. (**D**) HR expression. Abbreviations: IHC, immunohistochemistry; HR, hormone receptor expression; HER2, human epidermal growth factor receptor 2. HR expression change was defined as conversion between HR negative (<1%), low HR (1–10%), intermediate HR (10–50%) and high HR (>50%). HER2 expression change was defined as conversion between HER2 negative (0), HER2 low (+, ++ and FISH−), HER2 positive with IHC (+~++, FISH+) and HER2 positive with IHC (+++).

In terms of subtype, 41.7% of patients (15/36) showed disordinate subtypes between primary and metastatic lesions. In 21 patients with HR−/HER2+ primary disease, 15 patients (71.4%) showed homogenous IHC results in metastatic sites, while 6 patients changed into HR+/HER2+ (n = 2), HR+/HER2− (n = 2), and HR−/HER2− (n = 2). In 10 patients with HR+/HER2+ breast cancer, 6 patients (60%) remained HR+/HER2+, while 4 patients had HR loss and changed into HR−/HER2+ disease. In addition, 3 of 4 patients with HR+/HER2− primary disease changed into HR+/HER2+ subtype and one patient changed into HR−/HER2+ subtype. One patient with HR−/HER2− breast cancer changed into HR+/HER2+ subtype in metastatic disease.

The association between baseline clinical factors and temporal heterogeneity in terms of HER2 status was evaluated and shown in Table S1. HER2 status discordance was not associated with the treatment line or resistance to previous trastuzumab.

Heterogeneity in HER2 status was significantly associated with shorter PFS of pyrotinib (5.8 vs. 16.8 months, p = 0.001, Figure 2A). Patients with HER2 negative conversion, positive conversion and homogenous status between primary and metastatic disease showed a median PFS of 3.6 months, 13.7 months and 16.8 months (p < 0.0001). Patients with discordant HER2 expression in IHC also showed worse outcomes (5.8 vs. NR, p = 0.001). The PFS for patients with HER2 loss, gain and unchanged were 4.8 months, 13.7 months and not reached, respectively (p < 0.0001).

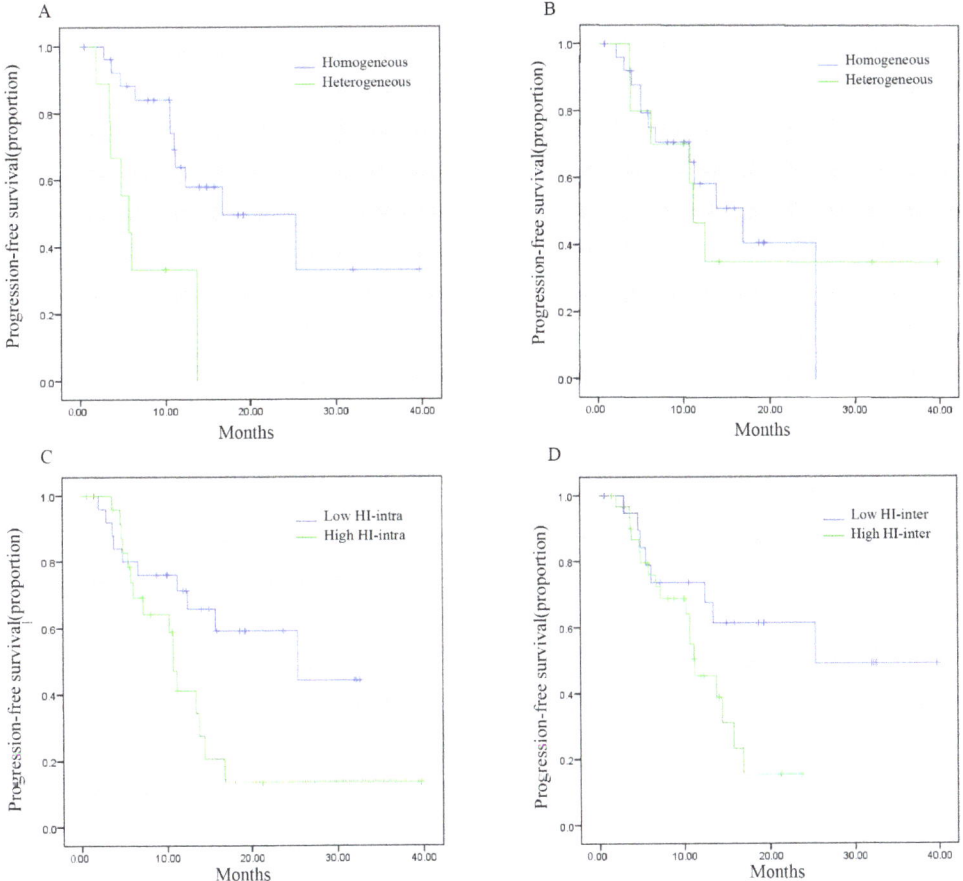

Figure 2. Kaplan–Meier curve of PFS stratified according to the temporal heterogeneity of IHC results (**A,B**) and spatial heterogeneity of ^{18}F-FDG uptake (**C,D**) in patients with HER2-positive metastatic breast cancer. (**A**) HER2 status heterogeneity between primary and metastatic tumors. (**B**) HR status heterogeneity between primary and metastatic tumors. (**C**) Intratumoral heterogeneity of ^{18}F-FDG uptake. (**D**) Intertumoral heterogeneity of ^{18}F-FDG uptake. Abbreviations: PFS, progression-free survival; FDG, fluorodeoxyglucose; IHC, immunohistochemistry; FDG, fluorodeoxyglucose; HER2, human epidermal growth factor receptor 2; HR, hormone receptor; HI-intra, intratumoral heterogeneity index; HI-inter, intertumoral heterogeneity index.

Heterogeneity in HR status did not seem to affect the treatment outcome of pyrotinib-based treatment (11.1 vs. 16.8 months, $p = 0.887$, Figure 2B). Patients with HR negative conversion, positive conversion and homogenous status between primary and metastatic disease showed a median PFS of 11.1 months, 12.4 months and 16.8 months ($p = 0.800$). The discordance of HR expression was not associated with efficacy either ($p = 0.541$). The median PFS for patients with HR loss, gain and unchanged were 13.7 months, 12.4 and 16.8 months, respectively ($p = 0.763$).

Patients with phenotypic heterogeneity between primary and metastatic disease had worse PFS, though not significantly (11.1 vs. 25.3 months, $p = 0.195$). The median PFS for patients with metastatic HR+/HER2+, HR−/HER2+, HR+/HER2− and HR−/HER2− disease was 16.8 months, 11.2 months, 3.6 months and 2.0 months, respectively ($p = 0.0003$).

Seven patients had multiple IHC results of the breast prior and after neoadjuvant therapy. The associations between HR, HER2 conversion and PFS of pyrotinib were consistent if changes during neoadjuvant therapy were also included in temporal tumor heterogeneity analyses.

3.3. Spatial Tumor Heterogeneity and Its Association with PFS

Comprehensive assessment of spatial intratumor heterogeneity required multiple biopsies of different metastatic sites or multi-region sampling within a single lesion, which was difficult to obtain due to practical reasons. Among patients enrolled in this study, only eight patients were able to evaluate spatial tumor heterogeneity in terms of IHC.

Functional molecular imaging offers an alternative option to characterize tumor spatial heterogeneity in a noninvasive way. ^{18}F- FDG PET/CT could demonstrate the metabolic activity of various metastatic lesions at once. A total of 318 metastatic lesions on baseline PET-CT were measured and analyzed. The optimal cutoff values of PET/CT parameters were determined by time-dependent survival ROC analysis.

The association between baseline clinical factors and spatial heterogeneity in terms of FDG uptake was shown in Table S1. HI-intra was not associated with any bassline tumor characteristics. Patients with high HI-inter were more common in those with multiple metastases (≥ 2) and visceral metastasis.

Patients with a high HI-intra (>1.69) had a median PFS of 10.6 months, which was significantly shorter than patients with low HI-intra (PFS: 25.3 months, $p = 0.023$, Figure 2C). Univariate analysis showed that patients with higher intertumoral heterogeneity (measured by classical COV) had worse PFS (11.1 months vs. 25.3 months, $p = 0.026$, Table S2). Simplified measurement of intertumoral heterogeneity- HI -inter could also discriminate patients into two groups (11.2 months and 25.3 months, $p = 0.040$, Figure 2D). Representative examples of patients' images are shown in Figure 3.

Exploratory analysis to investigate the predictive value of other PET parameters was conducted and shown in Table S2. SUVmax uptake and TLG were also significantly associated with PFS. The median PFS of patients with high SUVmax (>7.96) was significantly shorter than that of patients with low SUVmax (11.1 months vs. Not reached, $p = 0.008$). Higher TLG was also associated with significantly shorter PFS (11.2 months vs. Not reached, $p = 0.024$). SUVmean and MTV, on the other hand, were not predictive for PFS.

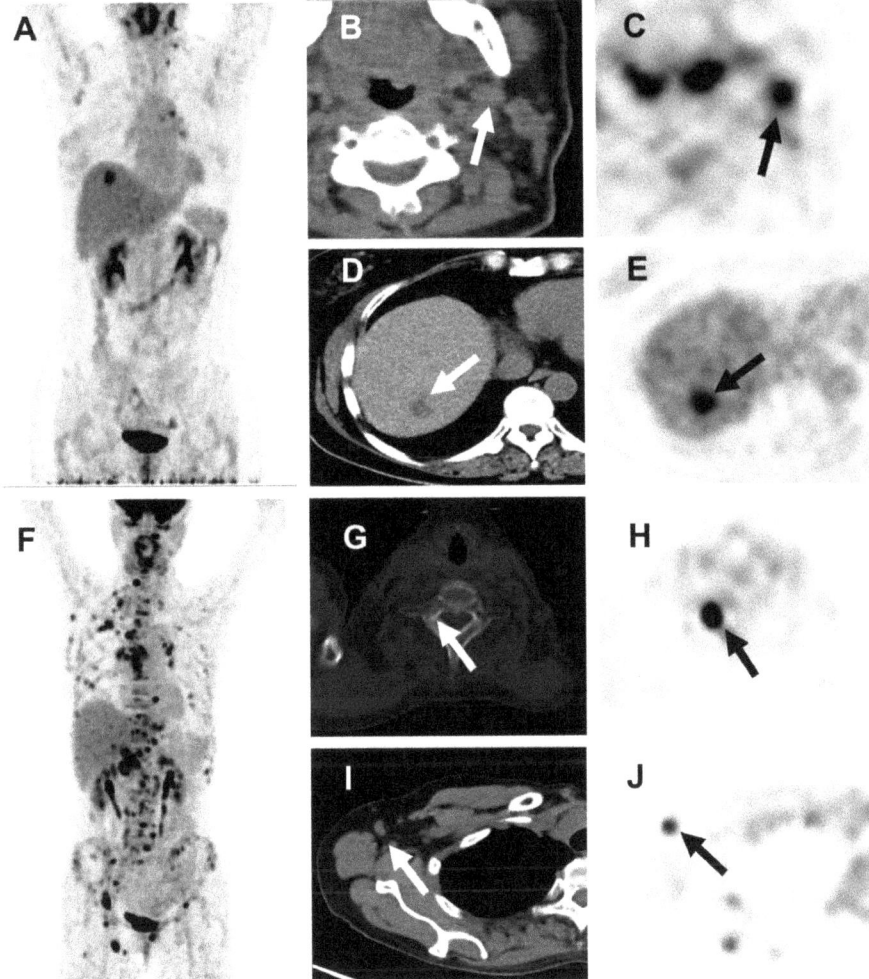

Figure 3. Representative cases of tumoral heterogeneity on ^{18}F-FDG PET/CT and response to pyrotinib. (**A–E**) A 56 year old woman underwent ^{18}F-FDG PET/CT ((**A**), maximum intensity projection [MIP] image). The left cervical lymph node lesion had the highest uptake (**B**), CT image; (**C**), PET image; SUVmax = 7.94, SUVmean = 5.09), whereas the liver lesion had the lowest uptake ((**D**), CT; (**E**), PET, SUVmax = 6.94, SUVmean = 3.84). This patient's median HI-intra was 1.68, and her HI-inter was 1.14. She has received pyrotinib treatment for 39.7 months and has not yet experienced tumor progression. (**F–J**) A 61-year-old woman who underwent ^{18}F-FDG PET/CT ((**F**), MIP) showed multiple bone and lymph nodes metastases, with the highest uptake in the cervical vertebrae ((**G**), CT; (**H**), PET image; SUVmax = 21.72, SUVmean = 13.16) and the lowest uptake in the left axillary lymph node ((**I**), CT; (**J**), PET; SUVmax = 4.73, SUVmean = 3.19). This patient's median HI-intra was 1.70, and her HI-inter was 4.59. She experienced disease progression after 3.6 months of pyrotinib treatment. Abbreviations: FDG, fluorodeoxyglucose; PET/CT, positron emission tomography/computed tomography; SUVmax, maximum standardized uptake value; SUVmean, mean standardized uptake value; HI-intra, intratumoral heterogeneity index; HI-inter, intertumoral heterogeneity index.

3.4. Association between Temporal and Spatial Heterogeneity

The association between temporal and spatial tumor heterogeneity was shown in Table S3. In terms of temporal tumor heterogeneity, patients with heterogeneous HER2 status between primary and metastatic disease showed higher HI-inter value ($z = -2.289$; $p = 0.022$) and similar HI-intra value ($z = -0.785$, $p = 0.432$).

In terms of spatial tumor heterogeneity, 36.4% of patients with high HI-inter showed temporal HER2 discordance compared to 7.1% of patients in the low HI-inter group ($p = 0.062$). In addition, all three patients with synchronous heterogenous IHC results were classified in the high HI-inter group.

Thirteen patients had received circulating tumor DNA (ctDNA) analysis and next generation sequencing (NGS) test before the treatment of pyrotinib and ten of them showed gene abnormalities, including TP53 mutation ($n = 7$), ERBB2 amplification ($n = 6$), PIK3CA mutations ($n = 3$), Myc amplification ($n = 3$) and BRCA2 mutation ($n = 2$). The proportion of abnormal NGS results in patients with high HI-inter and low HI-inter was 90% (9/10) and 33.3% (1/3), respectively ($p = 0.108$).

4. Discussion

Drug resistance has been a heated research topic for decades. Accumulating evidence suggests that tumor heterogeneity resulting from clonal evolution limits the efficacy of BC treatment [42–45]. Therefore, the assessment of tumor clonal heterogeneity could provide important information for the prediction of treatment outcomes. The best method to evaluate tumor heterogeneity in clinical practice still needs to be identified. HR and HER2 expression changes between primary and metastatic lesions may be the most evident demonstration of temporal tumor heterogeneity. Spatial tumor heterogeneity could be hard to evaluate due to the difficulty of multiple biopsies in practice. Functional molecular imaging offers an alternative and noninvasive method for characterizing tumor spatial heterogeneity. FDG uptake among metastatic lesions was under the influence of many factors, such as proliferation, vascularization, cellular hypoxia and necrosis. These factors are also fundamental physiological mechanisms of tumor behaviors and treatment resistance [46]. Thus, FDG uptake heterogeneity could reflect tumor biological heterogeneity to some extent. Our previous work introduced a simplified quantitative index, the HI, to represent the heterogeneous characteristics of metastatic disease and proved the predictive value of the baseline HI in patients with triple-negative breast cancer and HR+/HER2− MBC [32–34]. In this study, we first applied this method to patients with HER2-positive MBC.

HER2-positive BC is a highly heterogeneous disease. Pathologists have noticed cell-to-cell variations in HER2-positive tumors since HER2 was first introduced as a diagnostic marker. Over the years, guidelines of the American Society of Clinical Oncology/College of American Pathologists (ASCO/CAP) are continually making efforts to optimize the thresholds to define HER2 positivity [37]. Multiple studies have reported the intratumoral heterogeneity of HER2 gene amplification. One of the most crucial mechanisms of anti-HER2 treatment therapy resistance was the heterogeneous expression of the therapeutic target within the tumor. The clinical impact of the intratumoral heterogeneity of HER2 copy number levels and regional variation of HER2 gene amplification on the prognosis of patients and the efficacy of anti-HER2 targeted therapy has been studied [47–50]. Neoadjuvant treatment has provided an important platform for exploration. A phase II neoadjuvant trial of T-DM1 and pertuzumab conducted at the Dana-Farber Cancer Institute first defined HER2 heterogeneity as an area with ERBB2 amplification in >5% but <50% of tumor cells, or a HER2-negative area by FISH. Their results showed that none of the 10 patients with HER2 heterogeneity achieved a pathological complete response rate (pCR), whereas 55% of patients not classified as HER2 heterogeneous had a pCR ($p < 0.0001$) [51]. Biomarker analysis from the neoadjuvant KRISTINE study in HER2-positive early breast cancer also showed that pCRs were higher in patients with HER2 IHC (+++) disease than HER2 IHC (++) (60.8% vs. 20.0%). HER2 IHC 2+/3+ fraction, defined as the sum of IHC2+ and IHC3+ staining percentage, was also evaluated. Patients with homogeneous HER2 IHC 2+/3+

fraction (≥80%) had the highest pCR compared to those with focal (<30%) and variable fractions (30–79%) [52]. However, the intratumoral heterogeneity of HER2-positive MBC has not been fully examined.

In this study, we enrolled 51 patients treated with pyrotinib-based therapy with a whole-body PET/CT scan prior to treatment. The treatment lines of patients in this study (1st: 41.2%; 2nd: 45.1%; 3rd or later: 13.7%) were similar to those in the phase III trial of pyrotinib (1st: 43%, 2nd: 42%, 3rd: 16%), but earlier to those reported in real-world study (1st: 31.1%, 2nd: 35.7%, 3rd or later: 33.2%) [8,9]. A possible reason for the high rate of frontlines was selection bias. Only patients who underwent ^{18}F-FDG PET/CT within 4 weeks before the initiation of pyrotinib were included in this study. Whole-body ^{18}F-FDG PET/CT was more likely to be recommended for patients with suspicious metastatic disease, thus the proportion for patients who were first diagnosed was higher. The median PFS was 13.7 months (95% CI, 9.3–18.2) in this study, comparable to that reported in the phase III trial (12.5 months), further proving the efficacy of pyrotinib [9]. Vinorelbine has been an alternative combinational agent for pyrotinib in patients with previous exposure to capecitabine [53].

In this study, tumors were stratified into four groups based on HER2 IHC expression on the most recent IHC results: HER2 negative, HER2 low, HER2 positive with IHC (+~++) and HER2 positive with IHC (+++). The median PFS for these patients were 3.6 months, 5.8 months, 13.7 months and 16.8 months, respectively ($p < 0.0001$). In the MARIANNE study, MBC patients were randomized to first-line trastuzumab plus taxane, T-DM1 plus placebo, or T-DM1 plus pertuzumab. Biomarkers showed that focal HER2 expression (IHC 3+ or IHC 2+) was present in 3.8% of patients and was associated with numerically shorter PFS [54]. We also evaluated the association between ER expression and PFS of pyrotinib. Interestingly, we found that patients with ER low positivity (1–10%) had the shortest PFS, consistent with the previous report of neoadjuvant trastuzumab and chemotherapy [50].

Temporal tumor heterogeneity in this study was evaluated by the IHC conversion between primary and metastatic sites, the most common method used by clinicians in daily practice. In 36 patients with matched primary and metastatic IHC results, the change rate of HER2 status was 25%, with a positive conversion of 55.6% and a negative conversion of 44.4%. Heterogeneity in HER2 status was significantly associated with shorter PFS of pyrotinib (5.8 vs. 16.8 months, $p = 0.001$). Various discordant rates of HER2 status between primary and metastatic breast cancers have been reported [18,19]. Population selection strategy may affect this result since patients with HER2 negative conversion are less likely to be given anti-HER2 treatment in metastatic settings. The association between baseline clinical factors and HER2 status heterogeneity was evaluated (Table S1). HER2 status discordance was not associated with the treatment line or resistance to previous trastuzumab. Another study selected patients who were receiving trastuzumab and reported a HER2 status discordant rate of 37.8%, with 67.9% of patients gaining HER2 amplification and 32.1% losing HER2 expression. Patients with HER2 negative conversion had significantly lower PFS for taxane–trastumab–pertuzumab (PFS 5.5 months), compared to HER2 unchanged patients (PFS 9 months, $p = 0.01$) and patients with HER2 positive conversion (PFS 14 months, $p = 0.01$) [55]. However, patients with positive conversion (PFS =1.0 months) did not seem to benefit from later-line T-DM1 treatment (PFS for HER2 unchanged was 6.0 months, for HER2 negative conversion was 1.5 months). Our study showed that patients with homogenous HER2 positivity throughout the disease had the highest PFS of pyrotinib, followed by positive conversion and negative conversion (16.8 vs. 13.7 vs. 3.6 months, $p < 0.0001$). These studies showed that patients with HER2 gained amplification could benefit from trastuzumab/pertuzumab and pyrotinib treatment but might predict TDM1 resistance. However, both studies were retrospective studies with relatively small sample sizes. Caution should be taken when interpreting these results referring to the treatment outcome of HER2 gained amplifications. Regardless of HER2 status, our study also showed that heterogeneous HER2 expression level between primary and metastatic IHC was also associated with shorter PFS (5.8 vs. Not reached, $p = 0.001$). PFS for patients with HER2

IHC expression loss, gain and unchanged were 4.8 months, 13.7 months and not reached, respectively ($p < 0.0001$).

Spatial tumor heterogeneity was assessed by ^{18}F-FDG uptake on PET/CT scan. Our results showed that baseline spatial heterogeneity could predict the treatment efficacy of pyrotinib in HER2-positive MBC. Patients with a high HI-intra had significantly shorter PFS than patients with a low HI-intra (10.6 months vs. 25.3 months; $p = 0.023$, Figure 1A). In terms of intertumoral heterogeneity, COV is the conventional method for discriminating heterogeneity, but it can be time-consuming to calculate with the presence of multiple metastases. Our results showed that our simplified method of HI-inter can also represent the intertumoral heterogeneity in patients with MBC. Univariate analysis showed that patients with a high HI-inter tended to have worse PFS than those with a low HI-inter (11.2 months and 25.3 months, $p = 0.040$). No significant association was found between HI-intra and baseline tumor characteristics. HI-inter, which reflects the heterogeneity among different metastatic lesions, was higher in patients with multiple metastases (≥ 2) and visceral metastasis (Table S1). Several studies have indicated that SUVmax was higher in visceral metastases but no correlation has been established between visceral metastasis and metabolic heterogeneity [56,57].

Our study demonstrated that tumor heterogeneity had a significant impact on the efficacy of pyrotinib, which was consistent with a previous finding from ctDNA analysis. Translational exploration of the phase I study of pyrotinib performed ctDNA analyses and target-capture deep sequencing in 37 patients with HER2-positive MBC treated with pyrotinib alone or in combination with capecitabine [58]. Patients with three or more mutation clusters (defined as high tumor heterogeneity in this article) had significantly worse PFS, with a median PFS of 30 weeks, compared with 60 weeks for patients with fewer mutation clusters (HR 2.9, 95% CI 1.2–6.4; $p = 0.02$). Moreover, the multivariate analysis further confirmed that high heterogeneity in terms of mutations was a prognosticator of poor PFS [58]. These data suggest that baseline tumor heterogeneity evaluated by ctDNA or ^{18}F-FDG PET/CT could be both used as potential biomarkers of response to pyrotinib in HER2-positive MBC. PET imaging could provide a whole picture of metastatic disease and is a widely accepted diagnostic tool in BC while ctDNA analyses could reflect tumor status more dynamically. There were 13 patients in our study who had received both ctDNA NGS test and PET/CT before the treatment of pyrotinib. 10 of them showed abnormal gene variations. 90% of patients with high HI-inter disease on PET/CT had abnormal NGS results compared with 1/3 of patients in the low HI-inter group. Possible mechanisms for tumor temporal and spatial heterogeneity included differentiation state of cell-of-origin, cell plasticity, genetic evolution of cancer and microenvironment. Gene sequencing analyses offer an important way for a deeper understanding of the nature of tumor heterogeneity.

The SUVmax has been proven to be prognostic in various primary tumors [25,59–62]. Previous studies have shown that the SUVmax has predictive and prognostic value in patients with MBC [57,63,64]. Our study showed that SUVmax and TLG could also serve as potential markers for predicting pyrotinib treatment outcomes in patients with HER2-positive BC.

To the best of our knowledge, our study is the first to evaluate pyrotinib PFS in metastatic breast cancer by temporal HER2 concordance. Our results showed that patients with homogenous HER2 positivity had significantly longer PFS, followed by patients with gained HER2 positivity. Patients with HER2 negative conversion had little benefit from pyrotinib. Clinicians should pay more attention to the changes in a tumor's biological behaviors during a patient's therapeutic journal, which has profound implications for treatment outcomes. ^{18}F-FDG uptake heterogeneity was applied to reflect tumor spatial heterogeneity. In our previous work, we have established novel parameters to represent the intra- and intertumoral heterogeneities among metastatic lesions on PET scans, and they have proven to be effective predictive markers in clinical practice. This study is the first to apply this method in HER2-positive BC. As far as we are concerned, this is also the first research to investigate the predictive value of ^{18}F-FDG heterogeneity in patients with HER2-

positive MBC. Heterogeneity in pretreatment PET/CT could help oncologists gain a better understanding of patients' tumor heterogeneity and identify patients that would benefit from pyrotinib such that they could adapt treatment strategies for individual patients.

There are some limitations to this study. First, this study was an exploratory study based on a small cohort. Furthermore, the temporal heterogeneity in terms of IHC was only performed in patients with matched IHC results, which was 71% of the cohort. Validation is needed for further investigation. In addition, not all primary samples had a central pathology review of IHC results. Differences in the interpretation of IHC might introduce bias. Small changes in HR/HER2 expression were not considered as conversion in order to minimize the effect of technical reasons. In addition, enrollment criteria in this study included whole-body PET/CT scan prior to pyrotinib treatment. There may have been selection bias since PET/CT scans are more likely to be recommended in patients with a more complicated disease. Due to drug availability, only a small percentage of patients had prior pertuzumab or T-DM1 exposure in this population, which was consistent with the case in real-world practice in China. However, results from this study were difficult to be extrapolated directly to MBC patients in other areas. Last, HER2 heterogeneity at the gene level could provide more information. Translational studies investigating the biological mechanisms of inter- and intratumoral heterogeneity in HER2-positive MBC are still needed.

5. Conclusions

This article evaluated tumor heterogeneity in clinically applicable methods and investigated their impact on the efficacy of pyrotinib in MBC patients. Temporal tumor heterogeneity was evaluated by the discordance between primary and metastatic IHC results. Conversion of HER2 status was seen in 25% of these patients. Patients with homogenous HER2 positivity had significantly longer PFS, followed by patients with gained HER2 positivity. HER2 negative conversion, however, was predictive of poor outcome. ^{18}F-FDG uptake heterogeneity was applied to reflect spatial tumor heterogeneity among metastases. Baseline HI-intra and HI-inter could both predict the treatment efficacy of pyrotinib in patients with HER2-positive BC. This study underlines the importance of re-biopsy and adapting treatment with tumor heterogeneity taken into consideration.

Supplementary Materials: The following supporting information can be downloaded at: https://www.mdpi.com/article/10.3390/cancers14163973/s1, Table S1: Associations between clinical factors and tumor heterogeneity; Table S2: Associations between PET parameters and PFS; Table S3: Association between temporal and spatial heterogeneity in terms of IHC results and ^{18}F-FDG uptake.

Author Contributions: Conceptualization, C.G., Z.Y. and B.W.; Formal analysis, C.G. and C.L.; Funding acquisition, Z.Y. and B.W.; Investigation, C.G., C.L. and Z.T.; Methodology, C.G. and C.L.; Resources, C.G., Z.T., J.Z., L.W., J.C., Y.Z., Y.X., X.H., Z.Y. and B.W.; Software, C.G.; Supervision, Z.Y. and B.W.; Validation, Z.Y. and B.W.; Visualization, C.G. and C.L.; Writing—original draft, C.G.; Writing—review and editing, Z.Y. and B.W. All authors have read and agreed to the published version of the manuscript.

Funding: This research was funded by Beijing Medical Award Foundation (grant number: YXJL-2020-0941-0743), the National Natural Science Foundation of China (grant number: 81874114), the Shanghai Sailing Program (grant number: 20YF1408500), and the Shanghai Municipal Health Commission (grant number: No. 202040269).

Institutional Review Board Statement: All procedures performed in studies involving human participants were in accordance with the ethical standards of the institutional research committee and with the 1964 Helsinki declaration and its later amendments or comparable ethical standards. This study was approved by the FUSCC Ethics Committee and Institutional Review Boards for clinical investigation (approval number, 1812195-6; Approval date: 23 January 2019).

Informed Consent Statement: The requirement for written informed consent was waived because of the retrospective nature of the study.

Data Availability Statement: The datasets generated and/or analyzed during the current study are not publicly available due to hospital policy but are available from the corresponding author on reasonable request.

Acknowledgments: The authors would like to thank the doctors, nurses, patients, and their family members for supporting our study.

Conflicts of Interest: The authors declare no conflict of interest.

References

1. Waks, A.G.; Winer, E.P. Breast cancer treatment: A review. *JAMA* **2019**, *321*, 288–300. [CrossRef] [PubMed]
2. Eroglu, Z.; Tagawa, T.; Somlo, G. Human epidermal growth factor receptor family-targeted therapies in the treatment of her2-overexpressing breast cancer. *Oncologist* **2014**, *19*, 135–150. [CrossRef] [PubMed]
3. Slamon, D.J.; Leyland-Jones, B.; Shak, S.; Fuchs, H.; Paton, V.; Bajamonde, A.; Fleming, T.; Eiermann, W.; Wolter, J.; Pegram, M.; et al. Use of chemotherapy plus a monoclonal antibody against her2 for metastatic breast cancer that overexpresses her2. *N. Engl. J. Med.* **2001**, *344*, 783–792. [CrossRef]
4. Swain, S.M.; Baselga, J.; Kim, S.B.; Ro, J.; Semiglazov, V.; Campone, M.; Ciruelos, E.; Ferrero, J.M.; Schneeweiss, A.; Heeson, S.; et al. Pertuzumab, trastuzumab, and docetaxel in her2-positive metastatic breast cancer. *N. Engl. J. Med.* **2015**, *372*, 724–734. [CrossRef]
5. Verma, S.; Miles, D.; Gianni, L.; Krop, I.E.; Welslau, M.; Baselga, J.; Pegram, M.; Oh, D.Y.; Dieras, V.; Guardino, E.; et al. Trastuzumab emtansine for her2-positive advanced breast cancer. *N. Engl. J. Med.* **2012**, *367*, 1783–1791. [CrossRef]
6. Ma, F.; Ouyang, Q.; Li, W.; Jiang, Z.; Tong, Z.; Liu, Y.; Li, H.; Yu, S.; Feng, J.; Wang, S.; et al. Pyrotinib or lapatinib combined with capecitabine in her2-positive metastatic breast cancer with prior taxanes, anthracyclines, and/or trastuzumab: A randomized, phase ii study. *J. Clin. Oncol.* **2019**, *37*, 2610–2619. [CrossRef]
7. Yan, M.; Bian, L.; Hu, X.; Zhang, Q.; Ouyang, Q.; Feng, J.; Yin, Y.; Sun, T.; Tong, Z.; Wang, X.; et al. Pyrotinib plus capecitabine for human epidermal factor receptor 2-positive metastatic breast cancer after trastuzumab and taxanes (phenix): A randomized, double-blind, placebo-controlled phase 3 study. *Transl. Breast Cancer Res.* **2020**, *1*, 13. [CrossRef]
8. Xu, B.; Yan, M.; Ma, F.; Hu, X.; Feng, J.; Ouyang, Q.; Tong, Z.; Li, H.; Zhang, Q.; Sun, T.; et al. Pyrotinib plus capecitabine versus lapatinib plus capecitabine for the treatment of her2-positive metastatic breast cancer (phoebe): A multicentre, open-label, randomised, controlled, phase 3 trial. *Lancet Oncol.* **2021**, *22*, 351–360. [CrossRef]
9. Li, Y.; Tong, Z.; Ouyang, Q.; Wu, X.; Li, L.; Cai, L.; Yu, L.; Han, Z.; Wang, X.; Li, M.; et al. Abstract p2-13-40: Treatment patterns and adverse events of pyrotinib-based therapy in her2-positive breast cancer patients in china: Results from a multicenter, real-world study. *Cancer Res.* **2022**, *82*, P2-13-40.
10. Chen, Q.; Ouyang, D.; Anwar, M.; Xie, N.; Wang, S.; Fan, P.; Qian, L.; Chen, G.; Zhou, E.; Guo, L.; et al. Effectiveness and safety of pyrotinib, and association of biomarker with progression-free survival in patients with her2-positive metastatic breast cancer: A real-world, multicentre analysis. *Front. Oncol.* **2020**, *10*, 811. [CrossRef]
11. Lin, Y.; Lin, M.; Zhang, J.; Wang, B.; Tao, Z.; Du, Y.; Zhang, S.; Cao, J.; Wang, L.; Hu, X. Real-world data of pyrotinib-based therapy in metastatic her2-positive breast cancer: Promising efficacy in lapatinib-treated patients and in brain metastasis. *Cancer Res. Treat.* **2020**, *52*, 1059–1066. [CrossRef]
12. Shipitsin, M.; Campbell, L.L.; Argani, P.; Weremowicz, S.; Bloushtain-Qimron, N.; Yao, J.; Nikolskaya, T.; Serebryiskaya, T.; Beroukhim, R.; Hu, M.; et al. Molecular definition of breast tumor heterogeneity. *Cancer Cell* **2007**, *11*, 259–273. [CrossRef] [PubMed]
13. Junttila, M.R.; de Sauvage, F.J. Influence of tumour micro-environment heterogeneity on therapeutic response. *Nature* **2013**, *501*, 346–354. [CrossRef] [PubMed]
14. Rottenberg, S.; Vollebergh, M.A.; de Hoon, B.; de Ronde, J.; Schouten, P.C.; Kersbergen, A.; Zander, S.A.; Pajic, M.; Jaspers, J.E.; Jonkers, M.; et al. Impact of intertumoral heterogeneity on predicting chemotherapy response of brca1-deficient mammary tumors. *Cancer Res.* **2012**, *72*, 2350–2361. [CrossRef]
15. Vasan, N.; Baselga, J.; Hyman, D.M. A view on drug resistance in cancer. *Nature* **2019**, *575*, 299–309. [CrossRef]
16. Zardavas, D.; Irrthum, A.; Swanton, C.; Piccart, M. Clinical management of breast cancer heterogeneity. *Nat. Rev. Clin. Oncol.* **2015**, *12*, 381–394. [CrossRef] [PubMed]
17. Yeung, C.; Hilton, J.; Clemons, M.; Mazzarello, S.; Hutton, B.; Haggar, F.; Addison, C.L.; Kuchuk, I.; Zhu, X.; Gelmon, K.; et al. Estrogen, progesterone, and her2/neu receptor discordance between primary and metastatic breast tumours-a review. *Cancer Metastasis Rev.* **2016**, *35*, 427–437. [CrossRef]
18. Grinda, T.; Joyon, N.; Lusque, A.; Lefevre, S.; Arnould, L.; Penault-Llorca, F.; Macgrogan, G.; Treilleux, I.; Vincent-Salomon, A.; Haudebourg, J.; et al. Phenotypic discordance between primary and metastatic breast cancer in the large-scale real-life multicenter french esme cohort. *NPJ Breast Cancer* **2021**, *7*, 41. [CrossRef]
19. Schrijver, W.; Suijkerbuijk, K.P.M.; van Gils, C.H.; van der Wall, E.; Moelans, C.B.; van Diest, P.J. Receptor conversion in distant breast cancer metastases: A systematic review and meta-analysis. *J. Natl. Cancer Inst.* **2018**, *110*, 568–580. [CrossRef]

20. Tixier, F.; Le Rest, C.C.; Hatt, M.; Albarghach, N.; Pradier, O.; Metges, J.P.; Corcos, L.; Visvikis, D. Intratumor heterogeneity characterized by textural features on baseline 18f-fdg pet images predicts response to concomitant radiochemotherapy in esophageal cancer. *J. Nucl. Med.* **2011**, *52*, 369–378. [CrossRef]
21. Kang, S.R.; Song, H.C.; Byun, B.H.; Oh, J.R.; Kim, H.S.; Hong, S.P.; Kwon, S.Y.; Chong, A.; Kim, J.; Cho, S.G.; et al. Intratumoral metabolic heterogeneity for prediction of disease progression after concurrent chemoradiotherapy in patients with inoperable stage iii non-small-cell lung cancer. *Nucl. Med. Mol. Imaging* **2014**, *48*, 16–25. [CrossRef] [PubMed]
22. Kidd, E.A.; Grigsby, P.W. Intratumoral metabolic heterogeneity of cervical cancer. *Clin. Cancer Res.* **2008**, *14*, 5236–5241. [CrossRef] [PubMed]
23. Ha, S.; Park, S.; Bang, J.I.; Kim, E.K.; Lee, H.Y. Metabolic radiomics for pretreatment 18f-fdg pet/ct to characterize locally advanced breast cancer: Histopathologic characteristics, response to neoadjuvant chemotherapy, and prognosis. *Sci. Rep.* **2017**, *7*, 1556. [CrossRef] [PubMed]
24. Son, S.H.; Kim, D.H.; Hong, C.M.; Kim, C.Y.; Jeong, S.Y.; Lee, S.W.; Lee, J.; Ahn, B.C. Prognostic implication of intratumoral metabolic heterogeneity in invasive ductal carcinoma of the breast. *BMC Cancer* **2014**, *14*, 585. [CrossRef]
25. Cook, G.J.; Yip, C.; Siddique, M.; Goh, V.; Chicklore, S.; Roy, A.; Marsden, P.; Ahmad, S.; Landau, D. Are pretreatment 18f-fdg pet tumor textural features in non-small cell lung cancer associated with response and survival after chemoradiotherapy? *J. Nucl. Med.* **2013**, *54*, 19–26. [CrossRef]
26. Vaidya, M.; Creach, K.M.; Frye, J.; Dehdashti, F.; Bradley, J.D.; El Naqa, I. Combined pet/ct image characteristics for radiotherapy tumor response in lung cancer. *Radiother. Oncol.* **2012**, *102*, 239–245. [CrossRef]
27. Watabe, T.; Tatsumi, M.; Watabe, H.; Isohashi, K.; Kato, H.; Yanagawa, M.; Shimosegawa, E.; Hatazawa, J. Intratumoral heterogeneity of f-18 fdg uptake differentiates between gastrointestinal stromal tumors and abdominal malignant lymphomas on pet/ct. *Ann. Nucl. Med.* **2012**, *26*, 222–227. [CrossRef]
28. El Naqa, I.; Grigsby, P.; Apte, A.; Kidd, E.; Donnelly, E.; Khullar, D.; Chaudhari, S.; Yang, D.; Schmitt, M.; Laforest, R.; et al. Exploring feature-based approaches in pet images for predicting cancer treatment outcomes. *Pattern Recognit.* **2009**, *42*, 1162–1171. [CrossRef]
29. Van Velden, F.H.; Cheebsumon, P.; Yaqub, M.; Smit, E.F.; Hoekstra, O.S.; Lammertsma, A.A.; Boellaard, R. Evaluation of a cumulative suv-volume histogram method for parameterizing heterogeneous intratumoural fdg uptake in non-small cell lung cancer pet studies. *Eur. J. Nucl. Med. Mol. Imaging* **2011**, *38*, 1636–1647. [CrossRef]
30. Miwa, K.; Inubushi, M.; Wagatsuma, K.; Nagao, M.; Murata, T.; Koyama, M.; Koizumi, M.; Sasaki, M. Fdg uptake heterogeneity evaluated by fractal analysis improves the differential diagnosis of pulmonary nodules. *Eur. J. Radiol.* **2014**, *83*, 715–719. [CrossRef]
31. Yang, Z.; Sun, Y.; Xu, X.; Zhang, Y.; Zhang, J.; Xue, J.; Wang, M.; Yuan, H.; Hu, S.; Shi, W.; et al. The assessment of estrogen receptor status and its intratumoral heterogeneity in patients with breast cancer by using 18f-fluoroestradiol pet/ct. *Clin. Nucl. Med.* **2017**, *42*, 421–427. [CrossRef] [PubMed]
32. Gong, C.; Ma, G.; Hu, X.; Zhang, Y.; Wang, Z.; Zhang, J.; Zhao, Y.; Li, Y.; Xie, Y.; Yang, Z.; et al. Pretreatment (18)f-fdg uptake heterogeneity predicts treatment outcome of first-line chemotherapy in patients with metastatic triple-negative breast cancer. *Oncologist* **2018**, *23*, 1144–1152. [CrossRef] [PubMed]
33. Xie, Y.; Gu, B.; Hu, X.; Zhang, Y.; Zhang, J.; Wang, Z.; Zhao, Y.; Gong, C.; Li, Y.; Yang, Z.; et al. Heterogeneity of targeted lung lesion predicts platinum-based first-line therapy outcomes and overall survival for metastatic triple-negative breast cancer patients with lung metastasis: A "pet biopsy" method. *Cancer Manag. Res.* **2019**, *11*, 6019–6027. [CrossRef] [PubMed]
34. Zhao, Y.; Liu, C.; Zhang, Y.; Gong, C.; Li, Y.; Xie, Y.; Wu, B.; Yang, Z.; Wang, B. Prognostic value of tumor heterogeneity on 18f-fdg pet/ct in hr+her2- metastatic breast cancer patients receiving 500 mg fulvestrant: A retrospective study. *Sci. Rep.* **2018**, *8*, 14458. [CrossRef]
35. Shaoxian, T.; Baohua, Y.; Xiaoli, X.; Yufan, C.; Xiaoyu, T.; Hongfen, L.; Rui, B.; Xiangjie, S.; Ruohong, S.; Wentao, Y. Characterisation of gata3 expression in invasive breast cancer: Differences in histological subtypes and immunohistochemically defined molecular subtypes. *J. Clin. Pathol.* **2017**, *70*, 926–934. [CrossRef]
36. Hammond, M.E.; Hayes, D.F.; Dowsett, M.; Allred, D.C.; Hagerty, K.L.; Badve, S.; Fitzgibbons, P.L.; Francis, G.; Goldstein, N.S.; Hayes, M.; et al. American society of clinical oncology/college of american pathologists guideline recommendations for immunohistochemical testing of estrogen and progesterone receptors in breast cancer. *J. Clin. Oncol.* **2010**, *28*, 2784–2795. [CrossRef]
37. Wolff, A.C.; Hammond, M.E.H.; Allison, K.H.; Harvey, B.E.; Mangu, P.B.; Bartlett, J.M.S.; Bilous, M.; Ellis, I.O.; Fitzgibbons, P.; Hanna, W.; et al. Human epidermal growth factor receptor 2 testing in breast cancer: American society of clinical oncology/college of american pathologists clinical practice guideline focused update. *J. Clin. Oncol.* **2018**, *36*, 2105–2122. [CrossRef]
38. Salamon, J.; Derlin, T.; Bannas, P.; Busch, J.D.; Herrmann, J.; Bockhorn, M.; Hagel, C.; Friedrich, R.E.; Adam, G.; Mautner, V.F. Evaluation of intratumoural heterogeneity on (1)(8)f-fdg pet/ct for characterization of peripheral nerve sheath tumours in neurofibromatosis type 1. *Eur. J. Nucl. Med. Mol. Imaging* **2013**, *40*, 685–692. [CrossRef]
39. Tahari, A.K.; Alluri, K.C.; Quon, H.; Koch, W.; Wahl, R.L.; Subramaniam, R.M. Fdg pet/ct imaging of oropharyngeal squamous cell carcinoma: Characteristics of human papillomavirus-positive and -negative tumors. *Clin. Nucl. Med.* **2014**, *39*, 225–231. [CrossRef]

40. Bundschuh, R.A.; Dinges, J.; Neumann, L.; Seyfried, M.; Zsoter, N.; Papp, L.; Rosenberg, R.; Becker, K.; Astner, S.T.; Henninger, M.; et al. Textural parameters of tumor heterogeneity in (1)(8)f-fdg pet/ct for therapy response assessment and prognosis in patients with locally advanced rectal cancer. *J. Nucl. Med.* **2014**, *55*, 891–897. [CrossRef]
41. Adams, H.; Tzankov, A.; Lugli, A.; Zlobec, I. New time-dependent approach to analyse the prognostic significance of immunohistochemical biomarkers in colon cancer and diffuse large b-cell lymphoma. *J. Clin. Pathol.* **2009**, *62*, 986–997. [CrossRef]
42. Aparicio, S.; Caldas, C. The implications of clonal genome evolution for cancer medicine. *N. Engl. J. Med.* **2013**, *368*, 842–851. [CrossRef]
43. Gerlinger, M.; Rowan, A.J.; Horswell, S.; Math, M.; Larkin, J.; Endesfelder, D.; Gronroos, E.; Martinez, P.; Matthews, N.; Stewart, A.; et al. Intratumor heterogeneity and branched evolution revealed by multiregion sequencing. *N. Engl. J. Med.* **2012**, *366*, 883–892. [CrossRef]
44. Arnedos, M.; Vicier, C.; Loi, S.; Lefebvre, C.; Michiels, S.; Bonnefoi, H.; Andre, F. Precision medicine for metastatic breast cancer–limitations and solutions. *Nat. Rev. Clin. Oncol.* **2015**, *12*, 693–704. [CrossRef]
45. Beca, F.; Polyak, K. Intratumor heterogeneity in breast cancer. *Adv. Exp Med. Biol.* **2016**, *882*, 169–189.
46. Asselin, M.C.; O'Connor, J.P.; Boellaard, R.; Thacker, N.A.; Jackson, A. Quantifying heterogeneity in human tumours using mri and pet. *Eur. J. Cancer* **2012**, *48*, 447–455. [CrossRef]
47. Liu, Z.H.; Wang, K.; Lin, D.Y.; Xu, J.; Chen, J.; Long, X.Y.; Ge, Y.; Luo, X.L.; Zhang, K.P.; Liu, Y.H.; et al. Impact of the updated 2018 asco/cap guidelines on her2 fish testing in invasive breast cancer: A retrospective study of her2 fish results of 2233 cases. *Breast Cancer Res. Treat.* **2019**, *175*, 51–57. [CrossRef]
48. Bartlett, A.I.; Starczynski, J.; Robson, T.; Maclellan, A.; Campbell, F.M.; van de Velde, C.J.; Hasenburg, A.; Markopoulos, C.; Seynaeve, C.; Rea, D.; et al. Heterogeneous her2 gene amplification: Impact on patient outcome and a clinically relevant definition. *Am. J. Clin. Pathol.* **2011**, *136*, 266–274. [CrossRef]
49. Seol, H.; Lee, H.J.; Choi, Y.; Lee, H.E.; Kim, Y.J.; Kim, J.H.; Kang, E.; Kim, S.W.; Park, S.Y. Intratumoral heterogeneity of her2 gene amplification in breast cancer: Its clinicopathological significance. *Mod. Pathol.* **2012**, *25*, 938–948. [CrossRef]
50. Rye, I.H.; Trinh, A.; Saetersdal, A.B.; Nebdal, D.; Lingjaerde, O.C.; Almendro, V.; Polyak, K.; Borresen-Dale, A.L.; Helland, A.; Markowetz, F.; et al. Intratumor heterogeneity defines treatment-resistant her2+ breast tumors. *Mol. Oncol.* **2018**, *12*, 1838–1855. [CrossRef]
51. Filho, O.M.; Viale, G.; Stein, S.; Trippa, L.; Yardley, D.A.; Mayer, I.A.; Abramson, V.G.; Arteaga, C.L.; Spring, L.M.; Waks, A.G.; et al. Impact of her2 heterogeneity on treatment response of early-stage her2-positive breast cancer: Phase ii neoadjuvant clinical trial of t-dm1 combined with pertuzumab. *Cancer Discov.* **2021**, *11*, 2474–2487. [CrossRef]
52. De Haas, S.L.; Hurvitz, S.A.; Martin, M.; Kiermaier, A.; Lewis Phillips, G.; Xu, J.; Helms, H.J.; Slamon, D.; Press, M.F. Abstract nr P6-07-09: Biomarker analysis from the neoadjuvant kristine study in her2-positive early breast cancer (ebc). *Cancer Res.* **2017**, *77*, P6-07. [CrossRef]
53. Li, Y.; Qiu, Y.; Li, H.; Luo, T.; Li, W.; Wang, H.; Shao, B.; Wang, B.; Ge, R. Pyrotinib combined with vinorelbine in her2-positive metastatic breast cancer: A multicenter retrospective study. *Front. Oncol.* **2021**, *11*, 664429. [CrossRef]
54. Perez, E.A.; de Haas, S.L.; Eiermann, W.; Barrios, C.H.; Toi, M.; Im, Y.H.; Conte, P.F.; Martin, M.; Pienkowski, T.; Pivot, X.B.; et al. Relationship between tumor biomarkers and efficacy in marianne, a phase iii study of trastuzumab emtansine +/- pertuzumab versus trastuzumab plus taxane in her2-positive advanced breast cancer. *BMC Cancer* **2019**, *19*, 517.
55. Van Raemdonck, E.; Floris, G.; Berteloot, P.; Laenen, A.; Vergote, I.; Wildiers, H.; Punie, K.; Neven, P. Efficacy of anti-her2 therapy in metastatic breast cancer by discordance of her2 expression between primary and metastatic breast cancer. *Breast Cancer Res. Treat.* **2021**, *185*, 183–194. [CrossRef]
56. Bural, G.; Torigian, D.A.; Houseni, M.; Basu, S.; Srinivas, S.; Alavi, A. Tumor metabolism measured by partial volume corrected standardized uptake value varies considerably in primary and metastatic sites in patients with lung cancer. A new observation. *Hell. J. Nucl. Med.* **2009**, *12*, 218–222.
57. Zhang, J.; Hu, X.-C.; Jia, Z.; Ragaz, J.; Zhang, Y.-J.; Zhou, M.; Zhang, Y.-P.; Li, G.; Wang, B.-Y.; Wang, Z.-H. The maximum standardized uptake value of [sup 18] f-fdg pet scan to determine prognosis of hormone-receptor positive metastatic breast cancer. *BMC Cancer* **2013**, *13*. [CrossRef]
58. Ma, F.; Guan, Y.; Yi, Z.; Chang, L.; Li, Q.; Chen, S.; Zhu, W.; Guan, X.; Li, C.; Qian, H.; et al. Assessing tumor heterogeneity using ctdna to predict and monitor therapeutic response in metastatic breast cancer. *Int. J. Cancer* **2020**, *146*, 1359–1368. [CrossRef]
59. Cacicedo, J.; Fernandez, I.; Del Hoyo, O.; Navarro, A.; Gomez-Iturriaga, A.; Pijoan, J.I.; Martinez-Indart, L.; Escudero, J.; Gomez-Suarez, J.; de Zarate, R.O.; et al. Prognostic value of maximum standardized uptake value measured by pretreatment 18f-fdg pet/ct in locally advanced head and neck squamous cell carcinoma. *Clin. Transl. Oncol.* **2017**, *19*, 1337–1349. [CrossRef]
60. Lee, S.W.; Nam, S.Y.; Im, K.C.; Kim, J.S.; Choi, E.K.; Ahn, S.D.; Park, S.H.; Kim, S.Y.; Lee, B.J.; Kim, J.H. Prediction of prognosis using standardized uptake value of 2-[(18)f] fluoro-2-deoxy-d-glucose positron emission tomography for nasopharyngeal carcinomas. *Radiother. Oncol.* **2008**, *87*, 211–216. [CrossRef]
61. Zhang, S.; Li, S.; Pei, Y.; Huang, M.; Lu, F.; Zheng, Q.; Li, N.; Yang, Y. Impact of maximum standardized uptake value of non-small cell lung cancer on detecting lymph node involvement in potential stereotactic body radiotherapy candidates. *J. Thorac. Dis.* **2017**, *9*, 1023–1031. [CrossRef]
62. Aogi, K.; Kadoya, T.; Sugawara, Y.; Kiyoto, S.; Shigematsu, H.; Masumoto, N.; Okada, M. Utility of (18)f fdg-pet/ct for predicting prognosis of luminal-type breast cancer. *Breast Cancer Res. Treat.* **2015**, *150*, 209–217. [CrossRef]

63. Cokmert, S.; Tanriverdi, O.; Karapolat, I.; Demir, L.; Bayoglu, V.; Can, A.; Akyol, M.; Yilmaz, Y.; Oktay Tarhan, M. The maximum standardized uptake value of metastatic site in 18 f-fdg pet/ct predicts molecular subtypes and survival in metastatic breast cancer: An izmir oncology group study. *J. BUON* **2016**, *21*, 1410–1418.
64. Ohara, M.; Shigematsu, H.; Tsutani, Y.; Emi, A.; Masumoto, N.; Ozaki, S.; Kadoya, T.; Okada, M. Role of fdg-pet/ct in evaluating surgical outcomes of operable breast cancer–usefulness for malignant grade of triple-negative breast cancer. *Breast* **2013**, *22*, 958–963. [CrossRef]

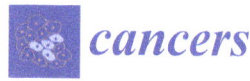

Article

Chemotherapy Shows a Better Efficacy Than Endocrine Therapy in Metastatic Breast Cancer Patients with a Heterogeneous Estrogen Receptor Expression Assessed by ^{18}F-FES PET

Yizhao Xie [1,2,†], Xinyue Du [2,3,4,5,†], Yannan Zhao [1,2], Chengcheng Gong [1,2], Shihui Hu [1,2], Shuhui You [1,2], Shaoli Song [2,3,4,5], Xichun Hu [1,2], Zhongyi Yang [2,3,4,5,*,‡] and Biyun Wang [1,2,*,‡]

1. Department of Breast Cancer and Urological Medical Oncology, Fudan University Shanghai Cancer Center, Shanghai 200032, China; vermouth1993@126.com (Y.X.); 14211230018@fudan.edu.cn (Y.Z.); gcckino@163.com (C.G.); 20211230025@fudan.edu.cn (S.H.); 21211230028@m.fudan.edu.cn (S.Y.); huxichun2017@163.com (X.H.)
2. Department of Oncology, Shanghai Medical College, Fudan University, Shanghai 200032, China; xinyuedu2020@163.com (X.D.); 16211230029@fudan.edu.cn (S.S.)
3. Department of Nuclear Medicine, Fudan University Shanghai Cancer Center, Shanghai 200032, China
4. Center for Biomedical Imaging, Fudan University, Shanghai 200032, China
5. Shanghai Engineering Research Center of Molecular Imaging Probes, Shanghai 200032, China
* Correspondence: yangzhongyi21@163.com (Z.Y.); wangbiyun0107@hotmail.com (B.W.); Tel.: +86-21-64175590-86908 (B.W.); Fax: +86-21-54520250 (B.W.)
† These authors contributed equally to this work.
‡ These authors contributed equally to this work.

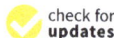

Citation: Xie, Y.; Du, X.; Zhao, Y.; Gong, C.; Hu, S.; You, S.; Song, S.; Hu, X.; Yang, Z.; Wang, B. Chemotherapy Shows a Better Efficacy Than Endocrine Therapy in Metastatic Breast Cancer Patients with a Heterogeneous Estrogen Receptor Expression Assessed by ^{18}F-FES PET. *Cancers* **2022**, *14*, 3531. https://doi.org/10.3390/cancers14143531

Academic Editor: Naiba Nabieva

Received: 31 May 2022
Accepted: 14 July 2022
Published: 20 July 2022

Publisher's Note: MDPI stays neutral with regard to jurisdictional claims in published maps and institutional affiliations.

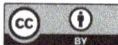

Copyright: © 2022 by the authors. Licensee MDPI, Basel, Switzerland. This article is an open access article distributed under the terms and conditions of the Creative Commons Attribution (CC BY) license (https://creativecommons.org/licenses/by/4.0/).

Simple Summary: About 10–20% of breast cancer patients have a heterogeneous estrogen receptor expression. The diagnosis and treatment strategy remains controversial in these patients, especially regarding the metastatic pattern. The aim of our study was to investigate the occurrence and properties of estrogen receptor heterogeneity and to evaluate the following treatment efficacy among a certain group of metastatic breast cancer patients. We found the novel ^{18}F-FES PET/CT method could identify patients with estrogen receptor heterogeneity, and chemotherapy showed a better efficacy compared with endocrine therapy in these patients. Our findings could give valuable suggestions to physicians and researchers in clinical practice.

Abstract: Background: The heterogeneity of estrogen receptor (ER) expression has long been a challenge for the diagnosis and treatment strategy of metastatic breast cancer (MBC). A novel convenient method of ER detection using ^{18}F-fluoroestradiol positron emission tomography/computed tomography (^{18}F-FES PET/CT) offers a chance to screen and analyze MBC patients with ER uncertainty. Methods: MBC patients who received ^{18}F-FES PET/CT were screened and patients with both FES positive (FES+) and negative (FES-) lesions were enrolled in this study. Progression-free survival (PFS) was estimated using the Kaplan–Meier method and was compared using the log-rank test. Results: A total of 635 patients were screened and 75 of 635 (11.8%) patients showed ER uncertainty; 51 patients received further treatment and were enrolled in this study. Among them, 20 (39.2%) patients received chemotherapy (CT), 21 (41.2%) patients received endocrine-based therapy (ET), and 10 (19.6%) patients received combined therapy (CT + ET). CT showed a better progression-free survival (PFS) compared with ET (mPFS 7.1 vs. 4.6 months, HR 0.44, 95% CI 0.20–0.93, p = 0.03). CT + ET did not improve PFS compared with either CT or ET alone (mPFS 4.4 months, p > 0.2). All three treatment options were well tolerated. Conclusions: ^{18}F-FES PET/CT could identify patients with ER heterogeneity. Patients with bone metastasis are more likely to have ER heterogeneity. Patients with ER heterogeneity showed better sensitivity to CT rather than ET. Combined therapy of CT + ET did not improve the treatment outcome.

Keywords: breast cancer; ER heterogeneity; ^{18}F-FES PET/CT; diagnosis; treatment pattern

1. Introduction

Breast cancer is the most common malignancy accounting for 30% of female cancers and is the second leading cause of cancer death in women [1]. Estrogen receptor positive (ER+) breast cancer constitutes more than 70% of all breast cancers [2]. Normally, ER+ breast cancer patients have lower rates of recurrent disease and a better prognosis compared with other molecular subtypes [3]. However, more and more research points out that the heterogeneity of ER could affect the treatment response and overall prognosis [4–6]. Furthermore, whether traditional endocrine therapy (ET) is still applicable in tumors with ER uncertainty remains controversial.

Novel methods of detection for ER heterogeneity are warranted because multiple pathological punctures are often infeasible, especially for metastatic patients. ^{18}F-fluoroestradiol (^{18}F-FES) positron emission tomography/computed tomography (PET/CT) is a non-invasive, molecular imaging technique to observe and quantify ER status in vivo [7]. ^{18}F-FES is now widely used in the diagnosis and treatment prediction of breast cancer patients [8,9]. Moreover, studies have demonstrated that ^{18}F-FES uptake correlates well with ICH scoring for ER [10,11]. It has been reported that a conspicuous number of patients present with discordant ER expression between primary tumor and metastasis, and ^{18}F-FES PET/CT is used to reveal the existence and prognostic effects of ER heterogeneity [7,12–14].

Previous studies indicate that patients with low positive ER (ER expression 1–10%) have unique molecular features and thus are more sensitive to chemotherapy (CT) rather than endocrine therapy (ET) [15]. We considered whether a similar situation happens in patients with ER heterogeneity.

Few studies focus on ER heterogeneity among MBC patients because of the difficulties in ER detection among multiple lesions. Therefore, the purpose of our study is to investigate the occurrence and properties of ER heterogeneity using ^{18}F-FES PET/CT and to evaluate the following treatment efficacy among a certain group of MBC patients.

2. Methods

2.1. Patients

We screened all MBC patients who received ^{18}F-FES PET/CT in Fudan University Shanghai Cancer Center from 2017–2021. Patients who had both FES positive (FES+) and negative (FES−) lesions were enrolled in this study. Patients who did not receive further treatments or who had incomplete medical records were excluded.

MBC was defined as unresectable, recurrent, or metastatic breast cancer. Medical and PET/CT data were collected retrospectively from the electronic medical database system.

Fudan University Shanghai Cancer Center Ethics Committee and Institutional Review Boards approved this clinical study. All of the techniques and methods were conducted in accordance with the Declaration of Helsinki and the relevant guidelines. This research is registered under clinicaltrials.gov (NCT05392985).

2.2. ^{18}F FES PET/CT Imaging

All of the chemicals were obtained from commercial sources and were used without further purification. The MMSE precursor and the authentic ^{18}F-FES was purchased from Jiangsu Huayi Chemical Co, Ltd. (Suzhou, Jiangsu, China). ^{18}F-FES was prepared according to the published methods [16]. To prevent ^{18}F-FES false-negative results, ER antagonists were discontinued for a minimum of 5 weeks before the study. The use of aromatase inhibitors was allowed [17]. All of the patients received an injection of approximately 222 MBq (6 mCi) of ^{18}F-FES over 2 min. Scanning consisted of a whole-body PET/CT examination (2–3 min per table position) initiated 1 h after the administration of the tracer on a Siemens biograph ^{16}HR PET/CT scanner. The transaxial intrinsic spatial resolution was 4.1 mm (full width at half maximum) in the center of the field of view. The PET/CT data acquisition protocol was as follows: CT scanning was first acquired from the proximal thighs to the head using a low-dose technique (120 kV, 80–250 mA, pitch 3.6, rotation time 0.5 ms). Immediately after the CT scan, a PET emission scan that covered the identical transverse field-of-view was obtained. We used a Gaussian-filter iterative reconstruction method to reconstruct the PET images. The coregistered images were displayed on a workstation.

2.3. Image Interpretation

A multimodality computer platform (Syngo, Siemens, Knoxville, TN, USA) was utilized for image review and manipulation. Two experienced board-certified nuclear medicine physicians evaluated the images independently and reached a consensus in cases of discrepancy. Lesions in ^{18}F-FES PET/CTs were identified using paired ^{18}F-FDG PET/CT images. Semiquantitative analysis of the tumor metabolic activity was obtained using SUV normalized to body weight. The maximum SUV (SUVmax) for each metastatic lesion was recorded by manually placing an individual ROI around each tumor on all consecutive slices that contained the lesion on coregistered and fused transaxial PET/CT images. We used a cut-off value of SUVmax $\geq$ 1.82 or SUVmean $\geq$ 1.21 to dichotomize the results as either ER positive and negative [18,19]. Patients with both ER positive and negative lesions were defined as having ER heterogeneity.

2.4. Outcome Measurements

The primary outcome measurement was PFS of different treatment groups (ET, CT, and ET + CT); secondary measurements were the incidence and characteristics of ER heterogeneity as well as treatment safety. PFS was defined as the time from the first dose of treatment to disease progression or death from any cause. The National Cancer Institute Common Terminology Criteria for Adverse Events (CTCAE) version 4.03 was used to evaluate safety. Response Evaluation Criteria in Solid Tumors (RECIST) version 1.1 was used for the tumor response: complete response (CR), partial response (PR), stable disease (SD), and progressive disease (PD).

2.5. Statistical Analysis

The quantitative data were presented as medians (range) or number of patients, and the categorical data were shown as counts (percentage). Descriptive statistics were used in the clinicopathologic characteristics and the Chi square test was used to compare between groups. Descriptive statistics were also used to depict the secondary outcomes. The survival analyses were evaluated with Kaplan–Meier method, and the hazard ratios (HRs) and corresponding 95% confidence intervals (CIs) were estimated using the Cox proportional hazard model. Prognostic factors were investigated using the Cox regression model with a 95% confident interval in both the univariate and multivariate models. A p value less than 0.05 was considered statistically significant. All statistical analyses were managed using SPSS (IBM) version 23.0 or R language (R i386 4.0.2).

3. Results

3.1. FES Results and Treatment Options

A total of 635 MBC patients who received ^{18}F-FES PET/CT were screened, and 560 patients had confirmed ER positive or negative expression, while 75 of 635 (11.8%) patients showed ER heterogeneity. Among the 75 patients with a heterogeneous ER expression, 51 patients received further treatment, met our inclusion criteria, and were enrolled in our study. With regards to the treatment alternatives, 20 (39.2%) patients received chemotherapy (CT), 21 (41.2%) patients received endocrine-based therapy (ET), and 10 (19.6%) patients received combined therapy (CT + ET) (Figure 1).

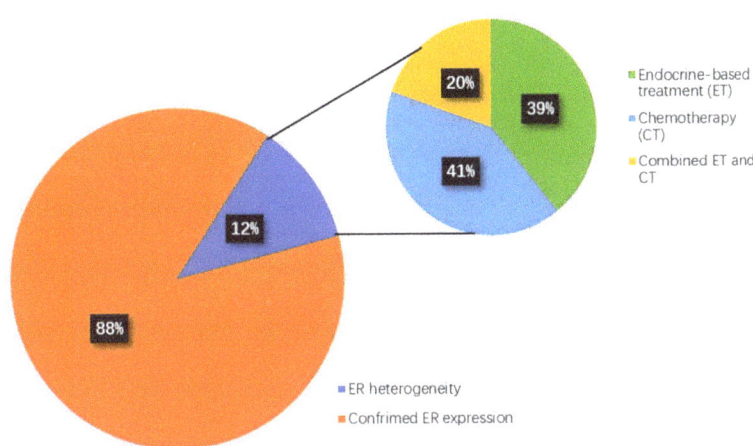

Figure 1. Incidence and treatment pattern of patients with ER heterogeneity.

3.2. Patient Characteristics

The baseline patient characteristics between the three treatment groups are summarized in Table 1. The median ages of the ET and CT groups were 55, and the ET + CT group was 48. A majority of patients had surgery before, while 14%, 10%, and 20% of patients were de novo stage IV patients in the ET, CT, and ET + CT groups, respectively. Most of the patients were in good status. Visceral metastasis occupied about half of patients, while the majority of patients had bone metastasis (over 80%). The median treatment lines were the first and second lines for three groups. Overall, no significant differences were observed in the baseline characteristics between the three groups.

Table 1. Baseline characteristics of the patients.

Characteristics	Endocrine-Based Therapy (ET) N = 21 n (%)	Chemotherapy (CT) N = 20 n (%)	ET + CT N = 10 n (%)	p Values
Median age	55	55	48	0.39
(range)	(29–73)	(39–70)	(32–68)	
Age > 48	16	15	7	0.93
Median disease-free interval	3	3	2	0.76
(range)	(0–13)	(0–12)	(0–15)	
De novo stage IV	3 (14)	2 (10)	2 (20)	
ECOG score				0.84
0–1	19 (90)	19 (95)	9 (90)	
≥2	2 (10)	1 (5)	1 (10)	
Number of metastatic sites				0.78
1	10 (48)	11 (55)	6 (60)	
2	8 (38)	7 (35)	4 (40)	
≥3	3 (14)	2 (10)	0 (0)	
Metastatic sites				
Visceral	11 (52)	10 (50)	4 (40)	0.81
Liver	3 (14)	3 (15)	1 (10)	0.92
Lung	10 (48)	6 (30)	2 (20)	0.26
Bone	18 (85)	16 (80)	10 (100)	0.32
Median treatment lines	1	1	2	0.12
(range)	(1–4)	(1–6)	(1–5)	

3.3. Treatment Efficacy

The most frequently applied (>20%) CT regimens were the combined treatment of two chemotherapy regimens (55%) and capecitabine (30%); ET regimens were aromatase inhibitor/fulvestrant (42.8%) and CDK4/6 inhibitors plus aromatase inhibitor/fulvestrant (28.6%); and the ET + CT regimens were capecitabine plus aromatase inhibitor/fulvestrant (90%).

At the median 18-month follow-up, 38 of the 51 patients experienced progressive disease. The median PFS of the CT group was 7.1 months (95% CI 3.8–10.5), the ET group was 4.6 months (95% CI 1.8–7.4), and the ET + CT group was 4.4 months (95% CI 0.5–8.3). CT showed better mPFS compared with ET (HR 0.44, 95% CI 0.20–0.93, p = 0.03, Figure 2A). CT + ET did not improve the PFS compared with either CT (HR 1.32, 95% CI 0.81–2.17, p = 0.26) or ET alone (HR 0.66, 95% CI 0.24–1.81, p = 0.42) (Figure 2B,C). The multivariate analysis showed CT treatment as an independent prognostic factor, even after balancing the DFI, age, visceral metastasis, number of metastatic sites, and prior MBC treatment lines (adjusted HR 0.46, 95% CI 0.22–0.98, p = 0.043). The analysis examples of the CT and ET group are shown in Figures 3 and 4.

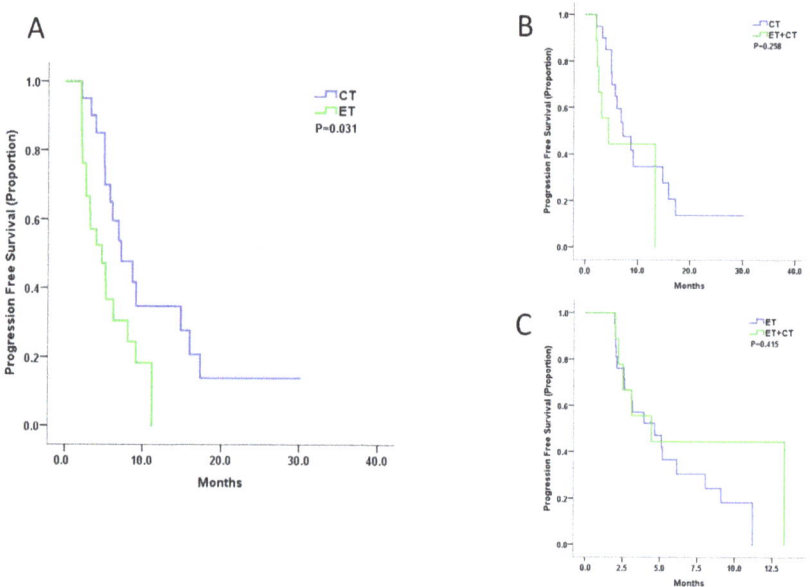

Figure 2. Kaplan–Meier curves for progression-free survival by treatment arm: (**A**). ET versus CT; (**B**) CT versus ET + CT; (**C**) ET versus ET + CT.

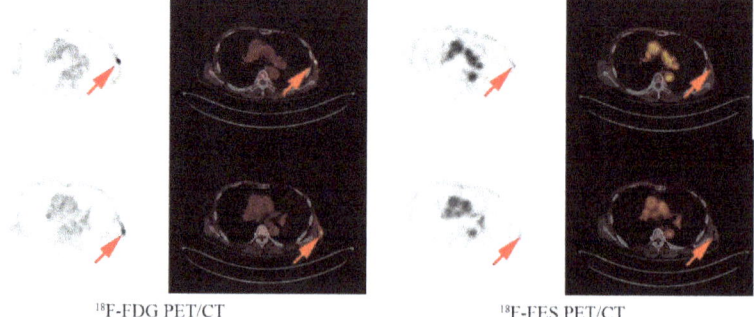

Figure 3. Analysis examples: A 73 year old female had an FES positive lesion in the chest wall and a FES negative lesion in the axillary lymph nodes and received fulvestrant treatment with a PFS of 4 months.

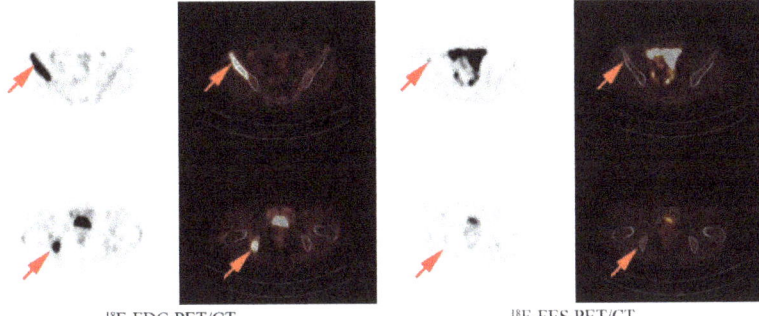

Figure 4. Analysis examples: A 53 year old female had both FES positive and negative lesions in the bone and received capecitabine treatment with a PFS of 15 months.

3.4. Safety

We collected and analyzed the grade 3/4 adverse events of different treatment groups (Table 2). Only one diarrhea and leukopenia case were seen in the ET group, while more hematologic toxicity and peripheral neurotoxicity were observed in the CT group. Palmar-plantar erythrodysesthesia syndrome was seen in both the CT and ET + CT groups. Overall, the three groups all showed an acceptable safety profile without a significant statistical difference ($p = 0.14$).

Table 2. Adverse events (grade 3/4).

Adverse Events (Grade 3/4)	ET N = 21 n (%)	CT N = 20 n (%)	ET + CT N = 10 N (%)
Diarrhea	1 (4.8)	0	1 (10)
Leukopenia	1 (4.8)	4 (20)	0
Anemia	0	1 (5)	0
Thrombocytopenia	0	1 (5)	
Palmar-plantar erythrodysesthesia syndrome	0	1 (5)	1 (10)
Peripheral neurotoxicity	0	2 (10)	0
All	2 (9.5)	7 (35)	2 (20)

4. Discussion

This study uncovered the real-world prevalence of MBC patients with ER heterogeneity using the ^{18}F FES PET/CT method and evaluated the strategy, efficacy, and safety of the following treatments. As far as we know, this is the first investigation in ER heterogeneity using ^{18}F-FES PET/CT method.

In terms of the incidence of ER heterogeneity, among all 635 MBC patients who received an FES scan, 11.8% patients had ER heterogeneity, which was lower than a previous study showing a 32.4% change in ER status in recurrent tumors compared with the primary tumors [20]. It is reasonable that for traditional study, only one metastatic site could be evaluated using the IHC method, thus increasing the false positive and false negative results. Interestingly, the incidence is similar to patients with a ER low expression reported before (6–11%), which might suggest a similar biological feature between ER heterogeneity and a low ER expression [15].

We found a majority of patients with ER heterogeneity had bone metastasis (86%). Previous preclinical study demonstrated that the osteogenic niche could reversibly reduce ER expression and activities in bone micrometastases, thus leading to endocrine resistance [21]. Our data, to some extent, proved this phenomenon in a clinical setting, which should further remind physicians to double check the ER status of MBC patients with bone metastasis in the case of ER heterogeneity in clinical practice.

With regards to treatment alternatives, about 40% patients received ET or CT, and the remaining 20% patients chose ET combined with CT. The current data fully indicated the clinical dilemma in patients with ER heterogeneity. Endocrine therapy remains to be the first choice for the first line treatment of luminal type MBC patients, both in guidelines and clinical practice [22,23]. However, among patients with a low ER expression, endocrine therapy seems to be less effective [15]. Traditionally, we tend not to use combined treatment of ET and CT because of the antagonism of chemotherapy-induced cytotoxicity by antiestrogens [24]. However, more and more research hint to the synergistic effect of ET plus CT, making it a relatively reasonable choice [25].

The current study revealed the superiority of CT over ET with regards to PFS. As for ER positive MBC patients, real-world data from Holland indicate that initial ET had an overwhelming advantage compared with CT in both PFS and OS settings [26]. Another propensity score analysis revealed that ET was not inferior to CT in first line treatment of ER positive MBC patients [27]. Our results showed the opposite results, which further demonstrated that patients with ER heterogeneity had a completely different biological behavior and treatment response from ER positive patients. On the other hand, besides the fact that ET is not suitable for ER/PR negative patients, researchers also found that patients with a ER low expression had worse treatment outcomes for ET and overall survival compared with a ER high expression [15]. This phenomenon, to some extent, suggests that patients with ER heterogeneity might be similar to those with a low ER expression or negative ER expression.

In our study, the combined treatment of ET and CT did not improve the treatment efficacy compared with either ET or CT alone. Although ET plus CT is not a common treatment option clinically, some studies have explored its feasibility. First, the SWOG-8814 trial revealed that the sequential use of cyclophosphamide, doxorubicin, fluorouracil (CAF), and tamoxifen (CAF-T) was better than concurrent CAF and tamoxifen (CAFT), although not reaching statistical significance [28]. However, the exploratory analysis of the TEXT/SOFT study showed that the concurrent use of triptorelin with chemotherapy was not associated with a significant difference in breast cancer-free interval compared with sequential triptorelin post-chemotherapy [29]. In an advanced setting, a phase II trial used fulvestrant with metronomic capecitabine on luminal-type MBC patients and found a mPFS of 15 months, which gave confidence on this treatment pattern [25]. Our study suggested little benefit gained from ET in patients with ER heterogeneity.

As expected, more 3/4 adverse events were observed in the CT group, although this did not reach statistical difference, partly because of the sample limits. Capecitabine plus aromatase inhibitors/fulvestrant were well tolerated in the ET + CT group. All adverse events were reversed after symptomatic treatment. Notably, patients needed to suspend or reduce the treatment dose after the diagnosis of grade 3 peripheral neurotoxicity, which were mostly caused by capecitabine according to previous study [30].

In conclusion, this study revealed the incidence and treatment pattern of patients with ER heterogeneity using the ^{18}F-FES PET/CT method. Patients with bone metastasis are more likely to have ER heterogeneity. Patients with ER heterogeneity showed better sensitivity to CT rather than ET. The combined therapy of CT + ET did not improve the treatment outcome. Capecitabine-based treatments were well tolerated.

As this study is exploratory, more randomized controlled trials (RCT) are warranted to give more evidence regarding treatment among ER heterogenous patients. In this era of precision medicine, more and more novel methods in multidisciplinary cooperation will bring about the best benefit to patients.

5. Conclusions

This study revealed the incidence and treatment pattern of patients with ER heterogeneity using the ^{18}F-FES PET/CT method. Patients with bone metastasis are more likely to have ER heterogeneity. Patients with ER heterogeneity showed better sensitivity to CT rather than ET. The combined therapy of CT + ET did not improve the treatment outcome. Capecitabine-based treatments were well tolerated. Our findings not only provided a novel way of detecting ER heterogeneity, but also suggested a better efficacy of CT compared with ET among patients with ER heterogeneity, which could help physicians to make decisions.

Author Contributions: Y.X. collected all of the data, performed statistical analysis, and finished the manuscript. X.D., Z.Y. and S.S. analyzed and confirmed the PET figures. C.G., Y.Z., S.H. and S.Y. participated in the data collection. X.H., B.W. and Z.Y. designed, carried out the study and revised the manuscript. All authors have read and agreed to the published version of the manuscript.

Funding: This work was supported by grants from National Natural Science Foundation of China (82102722).

Institutional Review Board Statement: The study was conducted in accordance with the Declaration of Helsinki. Ethical review and approval were waived from Institutional Review Board of Fudan University Cancer Hospital (SCCIRB) because it's a retrospective study (waived by SCCIRB, 1812195-6).

Informed Consent Statement: Patient consent was waived as it's a retrospective study.

Data Availability Statement: The datasets generated and/or analyzed during the current study are not publicly available due to hospital policy, but are available from the corresponding author upon reasonable request.

Acknowledgments: The authors would like to thank the patients, nurses, and clinicians for their participation in this study.

Conflicts of Interest: The authors declare no conflict of interest.

References

1. Siegel, R.L.; Miller, K.D.; Fuchs, H.E.; Jemal, A. Cancer Statistics, 2021. *CA Cancer J. Clin.* **2021**, *71*, 7–33. [CrossRef] [PubMed]
2. Khongthong, P.; Roseweir, A.K.; Edwards, J. The NF-KB pathway and endocrine therapy resistance in breast cancer. *Endocr.-Relat. Cancer* **2019**, *26*, R369–R380. [CrossRef] [PubMed]
3. Waks, A.G.; Winer, E.P. Breast Cancer Treatment: A Review. *JAMA* **2019**, *321*, 288–300. [CrossRef] [PubMed]
4. Zattarin, E.; Leporati, R.; Ligorio, F.; Lobefaro, R.; Vingiani, A.; Pruneri, G.; Vernieri, C. Hormone Receptor Loss in Breast Cancer: Molecular Mechanisms, Clinical Settings, and Therapeutic Implications. *Cells* **2020**, *9*, 2644. [CrossRef]
5. Lindström, L.S.; Yau, C.; Czene, K.; Thompson, C.K.; Hoadley, K.; Veer, L.J.V.; Balassanian, R.; Bishop, J.W.; Carpenter, P.M.; Chen, Y.-Y.; et al. Intratumor Heterogeneity of the Estrogen Receptor and the Long-term Risk of Fatal Breast Cancer. *JNCI J. Natl. Cancer Inst.* **2018**, *110*, 726–733. [CrossRef] [PubMed]
6. Yeo, S.K.; Guan, J. Breast Cancer: Multiple Subtypes within a Tumor? *Trends Cancer* **2017**, *3*, 753–760. [CrossRef]
7. Boers, J.; Loudini, N.; Brunsch, C.L.; Koza, S.A.; de Vries, E.F.; Glaudemans, A.W.; Hospers, G.A.; Schröder, C.P. Value of (18)F-FES PET in Solving Clinical Dilemmas in Breast Cancer Patients: A Retrospective Study. *J. Nucl. Med.* **2021**, *62*, 1214–1220. [CrossRef]
8. Brien, S.R.O.; Edmonds, C.E.; Katz, D.; Mankoff, D.A.; Pantel, A.R. 18F-Fluoroestradiol (FES) PET/CT: Review of current practice and future directions. *Clin. Transl. Imaging* **2022**, *10*, 1–11.
9. Kurland, B.F.; Wiggins, J.R.; Coche, A.; Fontan, C.; Bouvet, Y.; Webner, P.; Divgi, C.; Linden, H.M. Whole-Body Characterization of Estrogen Receptor Status in Metastatic Breast Cancer with 16α-18F-Fluoro-17β-Estradiol Positron Emission Tomography: Meta-Analysis and Recommendations for Integration into Clinical Applications. *Oncologist* **2020**, *25*, 835–844. [CrossRef]
10. Gemignani, M.L.; Patil, S.; Seshan, V.E.; Sampson, M.; Humm, J.L.; Lewis, J.S.; Brogi, E.; Larson, S.M.; Morrow, M.; Pandit-Taskar, N. Feasibility and predictability of perioperative PET and estrogen receptor ligand in patients with invasive breast cancer. *J. Nucl. Med.* **2013**, *54*, 1697–1702. [CrossRef]
11. Yang, Z.; Sun, Y.; Xu, X.; Zhang, Y.; Zhang, J.; Xue, J.; Wang, M.; Yuan, H.; Hu, S.; Shi, W.; et al. The Assessment of Estrogen Receptor Status and Its Intratumoral Heterogeneity in Patients with Breast Cancer by Using 18F-Fluoroestradiol PET/CT. *Clin. Nucl. Med.* **2017**, *42*, 421–427. [CrossRef] [PubMed]
12. Bottoni, G.; Piccardo, A.; Fiz, F.; Siri, G.; Matteucci, F.; Rocca, A.; Rocca, O.; Monti, M.; Brain, E.; Alberini, J.L.; et al. Heterogeneity of bone metastases as an important prognostic factor in patients affected by oestrogen receptor-positive breast cancer. The role of combined [18F]Fluoroestradiol PET/CT and [18F]Fluorodeoxyglucose PET/CT. *Eur. J. Radiol.* **2021**, *141*, 109821. [CrossRef] [PubMed]
13. Currin, E.; Peterson, L.M.; Schubert, E.K.; Link, J.M.; Krohn, K.A.; Livingston, R.B.; Mankoff, D.A.; Linden, H.M. Temporal Heterogeneity of Estrogen Receptor Expression in Bone-Dominant Breast Cancer: 18F-Fluoroestradiol PET Imaging Shows Return of ER Expression. *J. Natl. Compr. Canc. Netw.* **2016**, *14*, 144–147. [CrossRef] [PubMed]

14. Hao, W.; Li, Y.; Du, B.; Li, X. Heterogeneity of estrogen receptor based on 18F-FES PET imaging in breast cancer patients. *Clin. Transl. Imaging* **2021**, *9*, 599–607. [CrossRef]
15. Yu, K.D.; Cai, Y.; Wu, S.; Shui, R.; Shao, Z. Estrogen receptor-low breast cancer: Biology chaos and treatment paradox. *Cancer Commun.* **2021**, *41*, 968–980. [CrossRef]
16. Mori, T.; Kasamatsu, S.; Mosdzianowski, C.; Welch, M.J.; Yonekura, Y.; Fujibayashi, Y. Automatic synthesis of 16 alpha-[(18)F]fluoro-17beta-estradiol using a cassette-type [(18)F]fluorodeoxyglucose synthesizer. *Nucl. Med. Biol.* **2006**, *33*, 281–286. [CrossRef]
17. Linden, H.M.; Kurland, B.F.; Peterson, L.M.; Schubert, E.K.; Gralow, J.R.; Specht, J.M.; Ellis, G.K.; Lawton, T.J.; Livingston, R.B.; Petra, P.H.; et al. Fluoroestradiol positron emission tomography reveals differences in pharmacodynamics of aromatase inhibitors, tamoxifen, and fulvestrant in patients with metastatic breast cancer. *Clin. Cancer Res.* **2011**, *17*, 4799–4805. [CrossRef]
18. Sun, Y.; Yang, Z.; Zhang, Y.; Xue, J.; Wang, M.-W.; Shi, W.; Zhu, B.; Hu, S.; Yao, Z.; Pan, H.; et al. The preliminary study of 16α-[18F]fluoroestradiol PET/CT in assisting the individualized treatment decisions of breast cancer patients. *PLoS ONE* **2015**, *10*, e0116341. [CrossRef]
19. Yang, Z.; Sun, Y.; Zhang, Y.; Xue, J.; Wang, M.; Shi, W.; Zhu, B.; Hu, S.; Yao, Z.; Pan, H.; et al. Can fluorine-18 fluoroestradiol positron emission tomography-computed tomography demonstrate the heterogeneity of breast cancer in vivo? *Clin. Breast Cancer* **2013**, *13*, 359–363. [CrossRef]
20. Lindström, L.S.; Karlsson, E.; Wilking, U.M.; Johansson, U.; Hartman, J.; Lidbrink, E.K.; Hatschek, T.; Skoog, L.; Bergh, J. Clinically Used Breast Cancer Markers Such As Estrogen Receptor, Progesterone Receptor, and Human Epidermal Growth Factor Receptor 2 Are Unstable Throughout Tumor Progression. *J. Clin. Oncol.* **2012**, *30*, 2601–2608. [CrossRef]
21. Bado, I.L.; Zhang, W.; Hu, J.; Xu, Z.; Wang, H.; Sarkar, P.; Li, L.; Wan, Y.-W.; Liu, J.; Wu, W.; et al. The bone microenvironment increases phenotypic plasticity of ER(+) breast cancer cells. *Dev. Cell* **2021**, *56*, 1100–1117.e9. [CrossRef] [PubMed]
22. Gradishar, W.J.; Moran, M.S.; Abraham, J.; Aft, R.; Agnese, D.; Allison, K.H.; Anderson, B.; Burstein, H.J.; Chew, H.; Dang, C.; et al. Breast Cancer, Version 3.2022, NCCN Clinical Practice Guidelines in Oncology. *J. Natl. Compr. Canc. Netw.* **2022**, *20*, 691–722. [CrossRef]
23. Zanotti, G.; Hunger, M.; Perkins, J.J.; Horblyuk, R.; Martin, M. Treatment patterns and real world clinical outcomes in ER+/HER2- post-menopausal metastatic breast cancer patients in the United States. *BMC Cancer* **2017**, *17*, 393. [CrossRef]
24. Osborne, C.K.; Kitten, L.; Arteaga, C.L. Antagonism of chemotherapy-induced cytotoxicity for human breast cancer cells by antiestrogens. *J. Clin. Oncol.* **1989**, *7*, 710–717. [CrossRef] [PubMed]
25. Schwartzberg, L.S.; Wang, G.; Somer, B.G.; Blakely, L.J.; Wheeler, B.M.; Walker, M.S.; Stepanski, E.J.; Houts, A.C. Phase II trial of fulvestrant with metronomic capecitabine for postmenopausal women with hormone receptor-positive, HER2-negative metastatic breast cancer. *Clin. Breast. Cancer* **2014**, *14*, 13–19. [CrossRef] [PubMed]
26. Lobbezoo, D.J.A.; van Kampen, R.; Voogd, A.; Dercksen, M.; Berkmortel, F.V.D.; Smilde, T.; van de Wouw, A.; Peters, F.; van Riel, J.; Peters, N.; et al. In real life, one-quarter of patients with hormone receptor-positive metastatic breast cancer receive chemotherapy as initial palliative therapy: A study of the Southeast Netherlands Breast Cancer Consortium. *Ann. Oncol.* **2016**, *27*, 256–262. [CrossRef]
27. Bonotto, M.; Gerratana, L.; Di Maio, M.; DE Angelis, C.; Cinausero, M.; Moroso, S.; Milano, M.; Stanzione, B.; Gargiulo, P.; Iacono, D.; et al. Chemotherapy versus endocrine therapy as first-line treatment in patients with luminal-like HER2-negative metastatic breast cancer: A propensity score analysis. *Breast* **2017**, *31*, 114–120. [CrossRef]
28. Albain, K.S.; Barlow, W.E.; Ravdin, P.M.; Farrar, W.B.; Burton, G.V.; Ketchel, S.J.; Cobau, C.D.; Levine, E.G.; Ingle, J.N.; Pritchard, K.I.; et al. Adjuvant chemotherapy and timing of tamoxifen in postmenopausal patients with endocrine-responsive, node-positive breast cancer: A phase 3, open-label, randomised controlled trial. *Lancet* **2009**, *374*, 2055–2063. [CrossRef]
29. Regan, M.M.; Walley, B.; Francis, P.A.; Fleming, G.F.; Gomez, H.; Colleoni, M.; Tondini, C.; Pinotti, G.; Salim, M.; Spazzapan, S.; et al. Concurrent and sequential initiation of ovarian function suppression with chemotherapy in premenopausal women with endocrine-responsive early breast cancer: An exploratory analysis of TEXT and SOFT. *Ann. Oncol.* **2017**, *28*, 2225–2232. [CrossRef]
30. Martin, M.; Campone, M.; Bondarenko, I.; Sakaeva, D.; Krishnamurthy, S.; Roman, L.; Lebedeva, L.; Vedovato, J.C.; Aapro, M. Randomised phase III trial of vinflunine plus capecitabine versus capecitabine alone in patients with advanced breast cancer previously treated with an anthracycline and resistant to taxane. *Ann. Oncol.* **2018**, *29*, 1195–1202. [CrossRef]

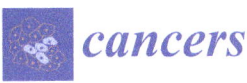

Article

High PANX1 Expression Leads to Neutrophil Recruitment and the Formation of a High Adenosine Immunosuppressive Tumor Microenvironment in Basal-like Breast Cancer

Wuzhen Chen [1,2,3,†], Baizhou Li [4,†], Fang Jia [1,2,3], Jiaxin Li [1,2,3], Huanhuan Huang [1,2,3], Chao Ni [1,2,3,*] and Wenjie Xia [5,*]

1. Department of Breast Surgery (Surgical Oncology), Second Affiliated Hospital, Zhejiang University School of Medicine, Hangzhou 310009, China; chenwuzhen@zju.edu.cn (W.C.); jiaf@zju.edu.cn (F.J.); 22018203@zju.edu.cn (J.L.); huanghuanhuanth@163.com (H.H.)
2. Key Laboratory of Tumor Microenvironment and Immune Therapy of Zhejiang Province, Hangzhou 310009, China
3. Cancer Institute, Zhejiang University, Hangzhou 310009, China
4. Department of Pathology, Second Affiliated Hospital, Zhejiang University School of Medicine, Hangzhou 310009, China; alexlibz@gmail.com
5. General Surgery, Cancer Center, Department of Breast Surgery, Zhejiang Provincial People's Hospital (Affiliated People's Hospital, Hangzhou Medical College), Hangzhou 310014, China
* Correspondence: nicaho428@zju.edu.cn (C.N.); xiawenjie1031@zju.edu.cn (W.X.)
† These authors contributed equally to this work.

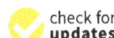

Citation: Chen, W.; Li, B.; Jia, F.; Li, J.; Huang, H.; Ni, C.; Xia, W. High PANX1 Expression Leads to Neutrophil Recruitment and the Formation of a High Adenosine Immunosuppressive Tumor Microenvironment in Basal-like Breast Cancer. *Cancers* 2022, 14, 3369. https://doi.org/10.3390/cancers14143369

Academic Editor: Naiba Nabieva

Received: 11 June 2022
Accepted: 5 July 2022
Published: 11 July 2022

Publisher's Note: MDPI stays neutral with regard to jurisdictional claims in published maps and institutional affiliations.

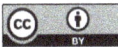

Copyright: © 2022 by the authors. Licensee MDPI, Basel, Switzerland. This article is an open access article distributed under the terms and conditions of the Creative Commons Attribution (CC BY) license (https://creativecommons.org/licenses/by/4.0/).

Simple Summary: A high adenosine level is an important characteristic of the tumor microenvironment (TME) in breast cancer. Pannexin 1 (PANX1) can release intracellular ATP to the extracellular space and elevate extracellular ATP (exATP) levels under physiological conditions. PANX1 has been found to be a poor prognostic factor in breast cancer, however, the role of PANX1 in breast cancer remains unknown. In this study, we performed RNA sequencing, bioinformatics analysis, surgical specimen histological validation, and exATP/extracellular adenosine (exADO) assays to reveal the role of PANX1 in regulating the immune microenvironment of basal-like breast cancer. The results revealed that PANX1 acted as a poor prognostic factor for breast cancer and had high expression in basal-like breast cancer. PANX1 expression was positively correlated with exATP and exADO levels in basal-like breast cancer TME. PANX1 expression was also positively correlated with tumor-associated neutrophil (TAN) infiltration in breast cancer TME, and TANs highly expressed CD39/CD73, which synergistically build a high exADO immunosuppressive TME and promote tumor progression. This study suggests that high PANX1 expression is associated with high TAN infiltration and adenosine production to induce local immunosuppression in basal-like breast cancer TME.

Abstract: Background: A high adenosine level is an important characteristic of the tumor microenvironment (TME) in breast cancer. Pannexin 1 (PANX1) can release intracellular ATP to the extracellular space and elevate extracellular ATP (exATP) levels under physiological conditions. **Methods:** We performed public database bioinformatics analysis, surgical specimen histological validation, RNA sequencing, and exATP/extracellular adenosine (exADO) assays to reveal the role of PANX1 in regulating the immune microenvironment of basal-like breast cancer. **Results:** Our results revealed that PANX1 acted as a poor prognostic factor for breast cancer and had high expression in basal-like breast cancer. PANX1 expression was positively correlated with exATP and exADO levels in basal-like breast cancer TME. PANX1 expression was also positively correlated with tumor-associated neutrophil (TAN) infiltration in breast cancer TME and TANs highly expressed ENTPD1 (CD39)/NT5E (CD73). **Conclusions:** This study suggests that high PANX1 expression is associated with high TAN infiltration and adenosine production to induce local immunosuppression in basal-like breast cancer TME.

Keywords: pannexin 1 (PANX1); neutrophils; adenosine; tumor microenvironment (TME); breast cancer

1. Introduction

Breast cancer is the most common malignant tumor in women. Basal-like breast cancer, as an important breast subtype, is a heterogeneous group of tumors defined by negative immunohistochemical staining for estrogen receptor (ER) and progesterone receptor (PR) and a lack of overexpression of human epidermal growth factor receptor 2 (HER2) with different levels of expression in basal cell keratins and myoepithelial markers [1,2]. Basal-like breast cancer is prone to recurrence and metastasis and has a poor prognosis due to the lack of specific treatments [3,4]. According to the PAM50 algorithm, 71% of triple negative breast cancer (TNBC) was found to be basal-like breast cancer [2]. Basal-like breast cancer is a clinically exclusive diagnosis that needs to be more precisely characterized at the molecular level. Compared with other subtypes, the immune status of the tumor microenvironment (TME) has a significant impact on the treatment and prognosis in basal-like breast cancer [5,6]. Therefore, it is of clinical importance to investigate the key regulatory genes related to the immune TME of basal-like breast cancer.

Pannexin 1 (PANX1), a member of the gap junction protein family, mediates the release of intracellular ATP to the extracellular microenvironment in its full-length form [7]. Extracellular ATP (exATP) and its metabolite extracellular adenosine (exADO) are important factors that regulate local immune TME [8]. Under physiological conditions, exATP released by PANX1 promotes innate and adaptive immune responses by attracting immune cells [9]. In the TME, this process is disrupted, and exATP is rapidly metabolized by nucleotidases ENTPD1 (CD39) and NT5E (CD73) to generate exADO [10]. In the TME, exADO is a key factor that contributes to local immunosuppression [11]. Recently, PANX1 expression was found to be important in suppressing airway inflammation in the asthma mouse model, and the knockdown of PANX1 resulted in increased airway inflammation [12]. In breast cancer, PANX1 was overexpressed and promoted the transformation of tumor cells to the epithelial-to-mesenchymal transition (EMT) phenotype; breast cancer patients with high PANX1 expression had a poor clinical prognosis [13]. However, the way in which PANX1 affects tumor-infiltrating immune cells (TIICs) and the immune TME by regulating exATP levels has not been reported.

This study revealed that basal-like breast cancer tissues had high PANX1 expression, which was positively correlated with tumor-associated neutrophils (TANs) and the accumulation of exADO, forming an immunosuppressive TME.

2. Materials and Methods

2.1. Data Acquisition

The TCGA-BRCA RNA-Seq gene expression matrix data with clinical information were downloaded from the TCGA data portal (https://portal.gdc.cancer.gov/) (accessed on 5 April 2021) and normalized using R package TCGAbiolinks [14–16]. METABRIC [17] microarray (Illumina HT-12 v3) normalized gene expression data were downloaded from the cBioPortal website (https://www.cbioportal.org) (accessed on 7 April 2021) [18]. The GSE103091 dataset (normalized gene expression data, GPL570, Affymetrix Human Genome U133 Plus 2.0 Array) [19,20] was downloaded from the GEO database (https://www.ncbi.nlm.nih.gov/geo/query/acc.cgi?acc=GSE103091) (accessed on 12 April 2021) using R package GEOquery for further CIBERSORT analysis. The METABRIC and TCGA-BRCA samples were classified into molecular subtypes using the PAM50 algorithm [21] using R package genefu [22].

2.2. Clinical Specimen Collection

Formalin-fixed paraffin-embedded (FFPE) sections from 12 TNBC patients who underwent surgery at the Second Affiliated Hospital of Zhejiang University School of Medicine (SAHZU) were collected from March 2020 to December 2020. Fresh surgical tumor specimens from 21 patients with TNBC and 12 patients with Luminal A cancer who underwent surgery at SAHZU were collected from March 2020 to April 2022 (with paired peripheral blood samples in 6 patients). Clinicopathological and survival information was also collected after receipt of informed consent and approval from the ethics committee. Clinical baseline characteristics of the included patients and corresponding experimental procedures for the surgical specimens have been summarized in Table 1, and detailed patient information was included in Supplementary Table S1. The percentage of stromal tumor-infiltrating lymphocytes (TILs) in breast cancer was evaluated under recommendations of the International TILs Working Group [23].

Table 1. Clinical baseline characteristics of the included patients and corresponding experimental procedures for the specimens.

No.	Age	ER	PR	HER2	Ki-67	Subtype	WHO Grade	Stage	Stromal TILs%	Bulk RNA-Seq	PAM50	Barcode	IHC	IF	TAN RNA-seq	Paired PBN RNA-seq	ATP/ADO Assay
PT01	50	Neg	Neg	Neg	20%	TNBC	3	IIA	5.0%		NA						Yes
PT02	37	Neg	Neg	Neg	70%	TNBC	3	IIA	30.0%		NA						Yes
PT03	41	Neg	Neg	Neg	40%	TNBC	3	IIIC	7.0%		NA						Yes
PT04	48	Neg	Neg	1+	50%	TNBC	3	IIB	30.0%	Yes	Basal-like	TNBC08					Yes
PT05	62	Neg	Neg	Neg	40%	TNBC	3	IIA	65.0%	Yes	Basal-like	TNBC02	Yes	Yes	Yes	Yes	
PT06	61	Neg	Neg	1+	30%	TNBC	3	IIA	10.0%	Yes	Basal-like	TNBC07		Yes	Yes	Yes	
PT07	44	Neg	Neg	Neg	70%	TNBC	3	IIA	20.0%		NA						Yes
PT08	47	Neg	Neg	Neg	70%	TNBC	3	IIA	7.0%		NA						Yes
PT09	54	Neg	Neg	1+	15%	TNBC	2	IIA	3.0%	Yes	Basal-like	TNBC06	Yes				
PT10	48	Neg	Neg	Neg	15%	TNBC	3	I	60.0%	Yes	Basal-like	TNBC05			Yes	Yes	
PT11	59	Neg	Neg	Neg	30%	TNBC	2	I	10.0%	Yes	Basal-like	TNBC09			Yes	Yes	
PT12	53	Neg	Neg	1+	40%	TNBC	3	IIA	40.0%	Yes	Basal-like	TNBC03	Yes				
PT13	61	Pos	Pos	1+	8%	Luminal A	2	IIA	5.0%		NA						Yes
PT14	59	Pos	Pos	1+	5%	Luminal A	2	IIA	5.0%		NA						Yes
PT15	87	Pos	Pos	1+	5%	Luminal A	2	IIA	5.0%		NA						Yes
PT16	61	Pos	Pos	1+	10%	Luminal A	3	IIA	5.0%	Yes	Luminal-A	LUM03					
PT17	47	Pos	Pos	1+	10%	Luminal A	3	IIB	4.0%		NA						Yes
PT18	51	Pos	Pos	1+	15%	Luminal A	2	IIA	10.0%	Yes	Luminal-A	LUM01					
PT19	66	Pos	Pos	1+	5%	Luminal A	2	I	5.0%		NA						Yes
PT20	61	Pos	Pos	Neg	5%	Luminal A	2	IIA	7.0%		NA						Yes
PT21	73	Pos	Pos	1+	15%	Luminal A	3	IIA	5.0%	Yes	Luminal-A	LUM02					
PT22	61	Pos	Pos	Neg	5%	Luminal A	2	IIA	2.0%		NA						Yes
PT23	76	Pos	Pos	Neg	10%	Luminal A	3	IIA	2.0%		NA						Yes
PT24	52	Pos	Pos	Neg	10%	Luminal A	2	IIA	5.0%		NA						Yes
PT25	55	Neg	Neg	Neg	40%	TNBC	2	IIA	55.0%	Yes	Basal-like	TNBC04	Yes		Yes	Yes	Yes
PT26	35	Neg	Neg	1+	10%	TNBC	2	IIB	20.0%	Yes	Basal-like	TNBC10	Yes	Yes			Yes
PT27	52	Neg	Neg	Neg	15%	TNBC	2	IIA	12.0%	Yes	Basal-like	TNBC01	Yes		Yes	Yes	Yes
PT28	45	Neg	Neg	Neg	70%	TNBC	3	IIB	25.0%	Yes	Basal-like	TNBC11					
PT29	51	Neg	Neg	Neg	65%	TNBC	3	I	15.0%	Yes	Basal-like	TNBC12					
PT30	28	Neg	Neg	Neg	40%	TNBC	3	IIA	50.0%	Yes	Basal-like	TNBC13					
PT31	60	Neg	Neg	Neg	75%	TNBC	3	IIB	30.0%	Yes	Basal-like	TNBC14					
PT32	71	Neg	Neg	Neg	45%	TNBC	3	IIB	10.0%	Yes	Basal-like	TNBC15					
PT33	43	Neg	Neg	Neg	50%	TNBC	2	IIA	7.0%	Yes	Basal-like	TNBC16					

ER: estrogen receptor; PR: progesterone receptor; HER2: human epidermal growth factor receptor 2; IHC: immunohistochemistry; IF: immunofluorescence; TAN: tumor-associated neutrophil; PBN: peripheral blood neutrophil.

2.3. Cell Lines and Culture Conditions

The MDA-MB-231, HCC-1937, and MCF-7 human breast cancer cell lines were all obtained from the American Type Culture Collection (ATCC, Manassas, VA, USA). MDA-MB-231 and MCF-7 cells were cultured in DMEM with 10% fetal bovine serum, while HCC-1937 cells were cultured in RPMI 1640 medium with 10% fetal bovine serum. All cell lines were grown with 5% CO_2 at 37 °C.

2.4. RNA Sequencing

Total RNA was isolated using Trizol (Invitrogen, Carlsbad, CA, USA) and RNeasy mini kit (Qiagen, Valencia, CA, USA) according to the manufacturer's protocol. For clinical samples, single-end libraries were subsequently constructed using the standard protocol provided by BGI (BGI, Shenzhen, China) and were then sequenced on the BGISEQ-500 platform. Clinical sample RNA sequencing was performed in 19 fresh surgical samples (TNBC: 16; Luminal A: 3) and tumor-associated neutrophils with paired peripheral blood neutrophils sorted from 6 TNBC patients (Table 1). For cell lines, RNASeq library was prepared using Illumina TruSeq RNA sample preparation kit (Illumina, San Diego, CA, USA) and RNA sequencing was performed by Illumina HiSeq 2500 platform in MDA-MB-231 and HCC-1937 cells (WT/shPANX1/shCTRL).

2.5. Bulk Transcription Data Analysis

The relative proportions of tumor-infiltrating immune cells were inferred using TIMER (TCGA-BRCA data and own data) [24,25] (V1: https://cistrome.shinyapps.io/timer; V2: http://timer.comp-genomics.org/) (accessed on 21 March 2021) and CIBERSORT LM22 (TCGA-BRCA data) (accessed on 9 April 2021) [26] (22 immune cell reference profiles: https://cibersort.stanford.edu/). For CIBERSORT processed data relating to neutrophil infiltration, we screened for and removed all outliers (2 standard deviations above or below the mean) for further linear regression analysis. For RNA-seq data of fresh surgical specimens, the fractions of tumor-infiltrating immune cells were inferred using TIMER V2 and quanTIseq [27] (http://timer.comp-genomics.org/) (accessed on 3 May 2021). GEPIA2 [28] was used to detect the top 250 genes related to PANX1 (https://gepia2.cancer-pku.cn/) (accessed on 2 May 2021). A list of human immune-related genes was derived through the Immunology Database and Analysis Portal (ImmPort) [29] (https://www.immport.org/) (accessed on 2 May 2021). The Lehmann's TNBC typing had been adopted to evaluate the PANX1 expression in different TNBC subtypes by using the webtool TNBCtype [30,31] (https://cbc.app.vumc.org/tnbc/) (accessed on 12 April 2022). The enriched gene ontology (GO) immune-related pathways were identified via the ClueGO v2.5.8 plugin in Cytoscape 3.8.2 software [32,33]. Using TCGA-BRCA and METABRIC data with clinical information, the overall survival (OS) status in different PAM50 subtypes of breast cancer under PANX1 high/low expression (median as the cut-off) was analyzed by R package Survminer and Survival. All packages used in this study were run in R environment 4.0.5.

2.6. Single Cell Transcription Data Analysis

The TNBC single-cell dataset [34] was downloaded from the Broad Institute Single Cell Portal (https://singlecell.broadinstitute.org/single_cell/study/SCP1106/) (accessed on 7 September 2021). The dataset was analyzed using the Seurat R package. Nonlinear dimensional reduction (tSNE) was used to visualize clustering results. Epithelial cell clusters with highly variable CNVs were determined to be malignant by the inferCNV R package. The SingleR R package was used for cell type annotation, and the default annotated file (Wu_EMBO_metadata.csv) was used as a reference. The single-cell dataset was divided into PANX1 high and low expression groups according to the PANX1 expression of each tumor sample in the count matrix. We calculate the average PANX1 expression for each tumor sample and choose the median value as the cut-off (PANX1 low expression tumor group: CID4513, CID4515, and CID44971 (included cell number = 9623); PANX1 high expression tumor group: CID44041 and CID44991 (included cell number = 4252)).

2.7. Immunofluorescence Staining

Gene colocalization was validated by monoclonal antibody-based immunofluorescence. FFPE sections were subjected to antigen retrieval by heating the slides in citrate buffer for 2 min, after which they were incubated with primary antibodies (anti-human PANX1 (#AB139715, 1:500, Abcam, Cambridge, MA, USA) and anti-human MPO (#AF3667,

1:300, R&D Systems, Minneapolis, MN, USA) antibodies) at 4°C overnight. Then, the slides were incubated with fluorescein-labeled secondary antibodies (Cy3-conjugated donkey anti-rabbit IgG (#AP182C, 1:200, Merck, Darmstadt, Germany), Alexa Fluor 488-conjugated donkey anti-goat IgG (#A11055, 1:100, ThermoFisher, Waltham, MA, USA)) at room temperature, stained with DAPI, and photographed under a laser confocal microscope (OLYMPUS IX83-FV3000-OSR).

2.8. Immunohistochemical Staining

Gene expression was validated by monoclonal antibody-based immunohistochemistry. Immunohistochemical staining of FFPE slides, which were deparaffinized and rehydrated before the antigen retrieval step, was performed using the Envision method. Endogenous peroxidase was blocked by incubating the slides with 3% H_2O_2. FFPE slides were heated in citrate buffer for 2 min, incubated with primary antibodies (rabbit anti-human PANX1(#AB139715, 1:500, Abcam, Cambridge, MA, USA)/mouse anti-human ENTPD1 (clone A1, 1:300, Biolegend, San Diego, CA, USA)/anti-human NT5E antibodies (clone AD2, 1:300, Biolegend, San Diego, CA, USA)) at 4 °C overnight, and then incubated with the secondary antibody (HRP-conjugated goat anti-mouse IgG, #AB205719, 1:2000, Abcam; HRP-conjugated goat anti-rabbit IgG, AB205718, 1:5000, Abcam, Cambridge, MA, USA) for 30 min at room temperature. 3,3′-Diaminobenzidine (DAB) chromogen (Zhongshan Jinqiao Biotech, Beijing, China) was used for visualization. The intensity and frequency were used as evaluation indexes based on PANX1 staining. The expression intensity was divided into 4 subgroups: negative (0), weakly positive (1), positive (2), and strong positive (3). The expression frequency was divided into 5 subgroups: 0–10% (1), 11–30% (2), 31–50% (3), 51–75% (4), and 76–100% (5). PANX1 comprehensive score = intensity*frequency. The TNBC specimens included in immunofluorescence and immunohistochemical staining were subjected to transcriptomic analysis and confirmed to be basal-like subtype using the PAM50 algorithm (Table 1). The samples with the upper 50% of PANX1 comprehensive scores were defined as the PANX-high group (n = 3), while the samples with the lower 50% of PANX1 comprehensive scores were defined as the PANX-low group (n = 3). We quantitatively assessed the ENTPD1 and NT5E protein expression levels by ImageJ FIJI software [35] using the method developed by Alexandra Crowe and Wei Yue [36].

2.9. Neutrophil Isolation

Fresh surgical specimens were cut into small pieces and digested in medium containing 1 mg/mL collagenase IV (#V900893, Sigma-Aldrich, Saint Louis, MO, USA) at 37 °C in a constant temperature shaker for 2 h. The cell suspension was filtered through 40 μm nylon mesh (BD FALCON, #352340) for subsequent detection or culture. The separation of neutrophils from surgical specimens and peripheral blood was performed with a human neutrophil isolation kit according to the manufacturer's protocol (Miltenyi Biotec, Auburn, CA, USA). For the neutrophils RNA-seq data, key immune-related gene expression was analyzed, and the heatmap was generated by the ComplexHeatmap R package.

2.10. ShRNA Knockdown of PANX1

MDA-MB-231 and HCC-1937 cells were transfected using the PANX1 human shRNA plasmid kit (OriGene, Rockville, MD, USA) (sequence: 5′-CGCAATGCTACTCCTGACAAA CCTTGGCATGTCAAGAGCATGCCAAGGTTTGTCAGGAGTAGCATTGTT-3′). The PANX1/ENTPD1/NT5E expression was evaluated by RNA sequencing using Illumina HiSeq 2500 platform in MDA-MB-231 and HCC-1937 cells (WT/shPANX1/shCTRL). Single-cell colonies of PANX shRNA-expressing cells were selected with puromycin and examined for PANX1 knockdown. Stable knockdown samples showed a 70–90% reduction in PANX1 expression. Cells were maintained under puromycin selection pressure and were periodically examined for effective PANX1 knockdown using western blot.

2.11. Extracellular ATP/ADO Assay

In 24-well plates, 2×10^4 cells (MDA-MB-231/MDA-MB-231 shPANX1/MDA-MB-231 shControl/HCC-1937/HCC-1937 shPANX1/HCC-1937 shControl/MCF-7) per well were allowed to adhere overnight after which they were removed by centrifugation at 4 °C for 10 min (MCF-7 as a representative of luminal breast cancer cell lines). For probenecid (PRB) treatment group, the MDA-MB-231/HCC-1937 cells were pretreated for 10 min with 1 mM PRB (#P8761, Sigma-Aldrich, Saint Louis, MO, USA). The supernatant was then collected for ATP/ADO detection assays. Fresh surgical TNBC tissues and normal breast tissue specimens were cut into small pieces and digested in medium containing 1 mg/mL collagenase IV (#V900893, Sigma-Aldrich, Saint Louis, MO, USA) at 37 °C at a constant temperature. The cell suspension was then filtered through 40 μm nylon mesh (#352340, BD FALCON) for subsequent ATP/ADO detection assays. ATP/ADO levels were measured using the ATP/ADO Assay Kit (fluorometric) (Abcam, Cambridge, MA, USA) according to the manufacturer's protocol.

2.12. Statistical Analyses

Statistical significance was determined using unpaired two-tailed Student's *t*-tests or analysis of variance (ANOVA) followed by Tukey's test. Pearson's correlation and Spearman's rank correlation statistics were used to determine the correlation for linear regression. A log-rank test was performed to assess PANX1 as a survival biomarker. For all in vitro assays, data are representative of at least three independent experiments, which each included three technical replicates unless otherwise stated. Differences in PANX1 expression in different subtypes were assessed using one-way ANOVA (Tukey's test). Paired differences in ATP/ADO levels and ENTPD1/NT5E expression between different groups were assessed using two-tailed *t*-tests. Statistical analyses were performed using GraphPad Prism software (version 9.0) and R software (version 4.0.5, R Core Team, http://www.R-project.org/) (accessed on 5 April 2021). The results are given as mean ± S.D. and *p* values < 0.05 were considered significant (unless otherwise stated). The details of the statistical analysis are provided in the results section and figure legends.

3. Results

3.1. PANX1 Was Highly Expressed in Basal-like Breast Cancer

Compared with normal tissues, we found that PANX1 was highly expressed in breast cancer (BRCA), colon adenocarcinoma (COAD), esophageal carcinoma (ESCA), head and neck squamous cell carcinoma (HNSC), kidney chromophobe (KICH), lung adenocarcinoma (LUAD), lung squamous cell carcinoma (LUSC), and stomach adenocarcinoma (STAD) based on the web tool TIMER (TCGA-BRCA data) ($p < 0.001$ was significant) (Figure 1A). Using TCGA-BRCA (n = 1083) and METABRIC (n = 1699) data, high PANX1 expression suggested poor prognosis for basal-like breast cancer in terms of overall survival (OS) ($p < 0.05$), while not for Luminal A, Luminal B, HER2-enriched, or normal-like subtype (PAM50 algorithm) (Figures 1B and S1A). To further investigate the role of PANX1 expression in breast cancer, we analyzed TCGA-BRCA and METABRIC transcriptome data and confirmed that PANX1 was highly expressed in the basal-like subtype (TCGA-BRCA (n = 1083) and METABRIC (n = 1699) data, PAM50 algorithm) (Figure 1C,D). We also explored PANX1 expression in different TNBC subtypes (Lehmann's TNBC typing; TCGA-BRCA-TNBC (n = 157) and METABRIC-TNBC (n = 158) data) and found there was no significant difference of PANX1 expression among different TNBC subtypes ($p > 0.05$) (Supplementary Figure S1B). Using TCGA-BRCA data, we further explored the relationship between PANX1 expression and tumor stage and found no significant differences in PANX1 expression across stages in all breast cancer samples or basal subtype ($p > 0.05$) (Supplementary Figure S1C). The above results suggested that, as a poor prognostic factor in breast cancer, PANX1 was highly expressed in basal-like breast cancer.

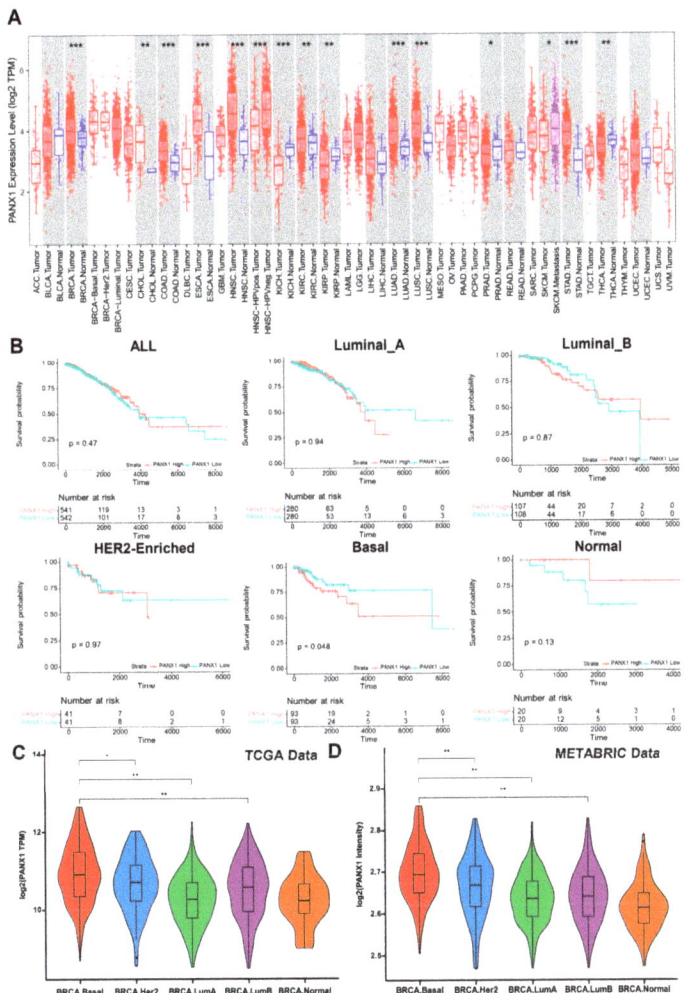

Figure 1. (**A**) PANX1 was highly expressed in breast cancer (BRCA), colon adenocarcinoma (COAD), esophageal carcinoma (ESCA), head and neck squamous cell carcinoma (HNSC), kidney chromophobe (KICH), lung adenocarcinoma (LUAD), lung squamous cell carcinoma (LUSC), and stomach adenocarcinoma (STAD) compared with normal tissues ($p < 0.001$ as significant; Student's t test) (TCGA-BRCA data; red bar: tumor tissue; blue bar: normal tissue); (**B**) correlation between PANX1 expression and overall survival (OS) in breast cancer under PAM50 molecular intrinsic subtypes (All (n = 1083), Luminal A (n = 560), Luminal B (n = 215), HER2-enriched (n = 82), Basal (n = 186), and Normal (n = 40)); (**C**,**D**) PANX1 expression under different PAM50 breast cancer molecular intrinsic subtype (TCGA-BRCA (n = 1083) and METABRIC (n = 1699) data, PAM50 algorithm; Turkey's test) (* $p < 0.05$; ** $p < 0.01$; *** $p < 0.001$).

3.2. PANX1 Expression Positive Correlated with ENTPD1/NT5E Expression in the TME

PANX1 is acknowledged as a dominant regulator of exATP release, while exATP and its metabolite exADO are believed to induce an immune-suppressive TME [10]. An analysis of TCGA-BRCA and METABRIC basal-like subtype transcriptome data revealed that the group with high expression of PANX1 (top 50%) had higher ENTPD1 and NT5E expression levels than the group with low expression (bottom 50%) ($p < 0.001$, TCGA-BRCA (n = 186) and METABRIC (n = 199)) (Figure 2A). Further linear analysis suggested a positive correlation between PANX1 expression and ENTPD1 (R^2 = 0.47 (TCGA) and 0.14 (METABRIC); $p < 0.001$) and NT5E (R^2 = 0.39 (TCGA) and 0.08 (METABRIC); $p < 0.001$) expression in TCGA-BRCA and METABRIC basal-like subtype transcriptome data (Figure 2B). The RNA-seq data of surgical breast cancer specimens (basal-like PANX1 high: n = 6; basal-like PANX1 low: n = 6; Luminal subtype: n = 3) suggested a higher expression of ENTPD1 and NT5E in the basal-like PANX1-high group compared to basal-like PANX1-low and Luminal group ($p < 0.05$) (Figure 2C). According to immunohistochemistry of basal-like surgical specimens, the expressions of ENTPD1 and NT5E were higher in the PANX1 high group (n = 3) than in the PANX1 low group (n = 3) (Table 2, Figures 2D and S2A,B). The above results indicated that PANX1 expression was positive correlated with ENTPD1 and NT5E expression in the basal-like breast cancer TME.

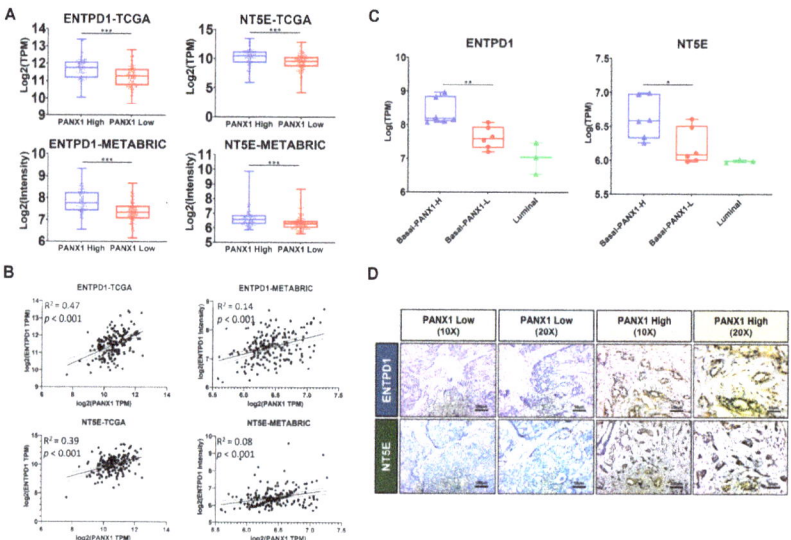

Figure 2. (A) ENTPD1 and NT5E expression in basal-like breast cancer under high and low level of PANX1 expression ($p < 0.01$) (TCGA-BRCA (n = 186) and METABRIC (n = 199) basal-like subtype data; Student's t test); (B) ENTPD1 and NT5E expression was positively correlated with PANX1 expression in basal-like breast cancer ($p < 0.001$) (TCGA-BRCA and METABRIC basal-like subtype data; Pearson's correlation); (C) ENTPD1 and NT5E expression in breast cancer specimens (Basal-like PANX1 high subgroup: n = 6; basal-like PANX1 low subgroup: n = 6; Luminal subtype: n = 3) ($p < 0.05$; Turkey's test); (D) ENTPD1 and NT5E expression in basal-like breast cancer surgical specimens with different PANX1 expression levels by immunohistochemistry at 10× and 20× magnifications (* $p < 0.05$; ** $p < 0.01$; *** $p < 0.001$).

Table 2. Clinical characteristics of the included samples for immunohistochemistry.

No.	Age	Subtypes	Ki-67	WHO Grade	Stage	Stromal TILs%	Bulk RNA-Seq	PAM50	Barcode	IHC	IHC-PANX1
PT05	62	TNBC	40%	3	IIA	65.0%	Yes	Basal-like	TNBC02	Yes	High
PT25	55	TNBC	40%	2	IIA	55.0%	Yes	Basal-like	TNBC04	Yes	High
PT27	52	TNBC	15%	2	IIA	12.0%	Yes	Basal-like	TNBC01	Yes	High
PT09	54	TNBC	15%	2	IIA	3.0%	Yes	Basal-like	TNBC06	Yes	Low
PT12	53	TNBC	40%	3	IIA	40.0%	Yes	Basal-like	TNBC03	Yes	Low
PT26	35	TNBC	10%	2	IIB	20.0%	Yes	Basal-like	TNBC10	Yes	Low

TILs: tumor infiltrating lymphocytes; IHC: immunohistochemistry.

3.3. PANX1 Expression Was Positively Correlated with TAN Infiltration in Basal-like Breast Cancer

Using CIBERSORT LM22, we analyzed the effect of PANX1 expression on basal-like breast cancer immune microenvironment in TCGA-BRCA (n = 186) data and GSE103091 (n = 238) dataset. We found that the abundances of infiltrating neutrophils ($p < 0.05$), resting memory CD4$^+$ T cells ($p < 0.05$), follicular helper T cells ($p < 0.05$), monocytes ($p < 0.05$), CD8$^+$ T cells ($p < 0.05$), and activated natural killer (NK) cells ($p < 0.05$) were significantly different between PANX1 high expression (top 50%) and low expression (bottom 50%) tumors (Figure 3A). Coexpressed PANX1-related genes were obtained using GEPIA2; the immune-related GO analysis suggested that PANX1 and its coexpressed genes were related to granulocyte migration, neutrophil activation, etc. ($p < 0.01$) (Figure 3B). Furthermore, the relationship between PANX1 expression and TIICs was assessed using TIMER in the TCGA-BRCA basal-like subtype data, and a positive correlation was indicated between PANX1 and the infiltration level of TANs and CD4$^+$ T cells ($p < 0.05$) (Figure 3C). Using TCGA-BRCA data and the CIBERSORT algorithm, we verified the positive correlation between PANX1 expression and TANs infiltration in the basal-like subtype (n = 25, outliers have been filtered; $R^2 = 0.32$; $p = 0.003$; Pearson's correlation) (Figure 3D).

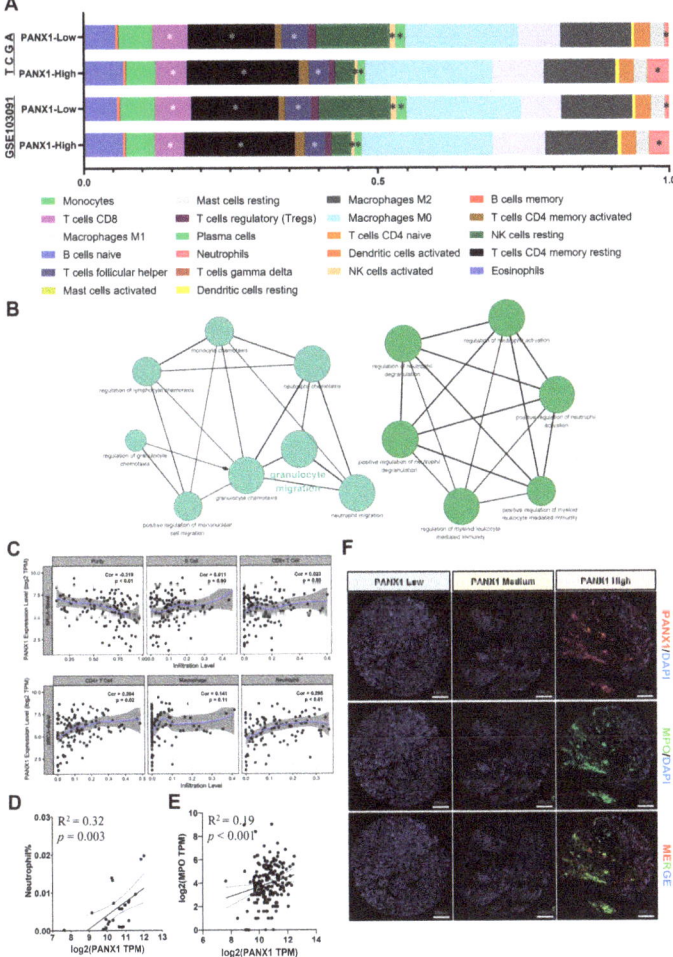

Figure 3. (**A**) CIBERSORT evaluated tumor-infiltrating immune cell (TIIC) differences under high

(top 50%)/low (bottom 50%) PANX1 expression in basal-like subtype breast cancer (The key difference immune cells are shown by star (* $p < 0.05$); TCGA-BRCA basal-like subtype (n = 186) and GSE103091(n = 238) data); (**B**) GO analysis of PANX1 and its coexpression immune-related genes; (**C**) TIMER analysis of PANX1 expression and TIIC correlation (TCGA-BRCA data; n = 1083; Spearman's rank correlation); (**D**) neutrophil abundance was positively correlated with PANX1 expression in METABRIC basal-like subtype data ($R^2 = 0.32$; $p = 0.003$; Pearson's correlation) (CIBERSORT algorithms; n = 25, outliers have been filtered); (**E**) MPO (neutrophil marker) expression was positively correlated with PANX1 expression in TCGA-BRCA basal-like subtype data (n = 186; $R^2 = 0.19$; $p < 0.001$; Pearson's correlation); (**F**) immunofluorescence detection of PANX1/MPO coexpression in basal-like breast cancer paraffin-embedded pathological specimens (DAPI, 4′,6-diamidino-phenylindole; MPO, myeloperoxidase).

In addition, the PANX1 expression was positively correlated with myeloperoxidase (MPO) expression in the TCGA-BRCA basal-like subtype ($R^2 = 0.19$; $p < 0.001$) (Figure 3E). Moreover, the coexpression of PANX1 and MPO in basal-like breast cancer paraffin-embedded surgical specimens was also observed using immunofluorescence (Figure 3F). PANX1 and MPO expression was positive correlated, indicating that high PANX1 expression might promote TAN infiltration in basal-like breast cancer TME. However, the way in which PANX1 establishes an immunosuppressive microenvironment with TANs should be further explored.

3.4. Immunosuppressive TANs Demonstrated More Infiltration in Basal-like Breast Cancer with High PANX1 Expression

quanTIseq and TIMER deconvolution methods were reported to have high deconvolution performance for RNA-seq data from different tumor types and could be suitable tools for the further exploration of tumor-infiltrating neutrophils [37]. RNA-seq data from fresh surgical specimens were converted into infiltrating immune cell information by quanTIseq and TIMER. The results revealed that basal-like breast cancer with high PANX1 expression (n = 6) had more infiltrating TANs than basal-like breast cancer with low PANX1 expression (n = 6) and Luminal subtype (n = 3) ($p < 0.05$ for TIMER and quanTIseq method) (Figure 4A–C). In addition, the relationship between ENTPD1/NT5E expression and the infiltration level of TANs in basal-like subtype was evaluated. In TCGA-BRCA data, ENTPD1/NT5E expression was positively correlated with the infiltration level of TANs in basal-like subtype ($p < 0.05$) (Figure 4D: CIBERSORT method; Figure 4E: TIMER method). Neutrophils were purified from fresh basal-like breast cancer surgical specimens (n = 6) and paired peripheral blood samples (n = 6). Transcriptome analysis revealed TANs had higher expressions of nucleotidases ENTPD1 and NT5E ($p < 0.05$) and higher expressions of immunosuppressive cell recruitment-related cytokines CCL2 and CCL17 ($p < 0.05$) compared with peripheral blood neutrophils (Figure 4F). The above results suggested that PANX1 expression was positively associated with the TANs infiltration in TME, and TANs could convert exATP to exADO by highly expressing ENTPD1 and NT5E.

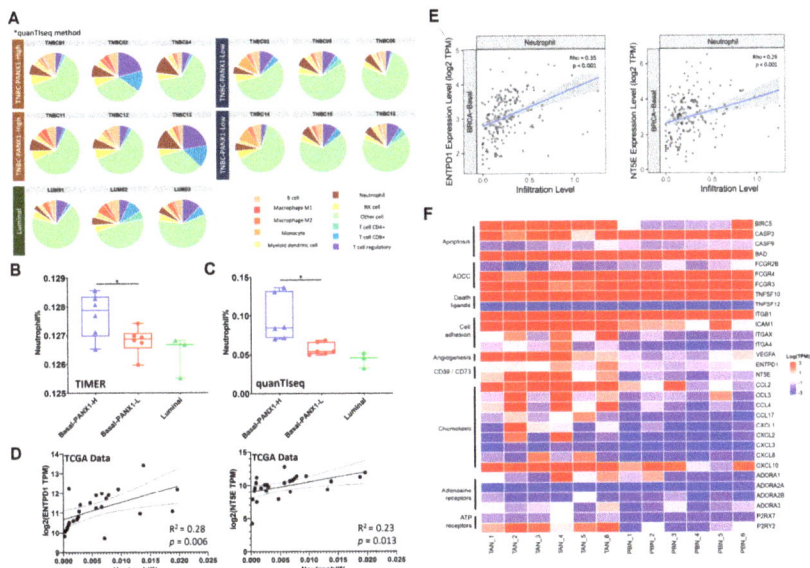

Figure 4. (**A**) The proportion of infiltrating TANs in Luminal (n = 3) and basal-like subtype (High PANX1 expression: n = 6; low PANX1 expression: n = 6) surgical specimens; (**B,C**) basal-like breast cancer with high PANX1 expression had more infiltrating TANs than basal-like breast cancer with low PANX1 expression and the Luminal subtype ($p < 0.05$ for TIMER; $p = 0.11$ for quanTIseq; Student's t test); (**D**) the correlation between ENTPD1/NT5E expression and TAN infiltration in basal-like breast cancer (n = 25; $p < 0.05$; R^2 = 0.28 (ENTPD1) and 0.23 (NT5E); Pearson's correlation; TCGA-BRCA data; CIBERSORT-LM22 algorithms; outliers have been filtered); (**E**) TIMER analysis suggested a positive correlation between ENTPD1/NT5E expression and TAN infiltration in the basal-like subtype (n = 186; $p < 0.01$; Rho = 0.35 (ENTPD1) and 0.26 (NT5E); Spearman's rank correlation; TCGA-BRCA data); (**F**) heatmap of the transcriptome analysis of TANs (n = 6) and PBNs (n = 6) in basal-like breast cancer (TANs, tumor-associated neutrophils; PBNs, peripheral blood neutrophils) (* $p < 0.05$).

3.5. High PANX1 Expression Induced a High exADO Immunosuppressive TME in Basal-like Breast Cancer

To clarify whether high PANX1 expression in basal-like breast cancer could establish an immunosuppressive TME with local high exADO levels, we measured exATP and exADO levels in the supernatant of cultured breast cancer cell lines and found that exATP and exADO levels in MDA-MB-231 and HCC-1937 (basal-like subtype cell lines) cell culture media were significantly higher than those in MCF-7 (Luminal subtype cell line) cell culture media (n = 19 for each group; $p < 0.05$) (Figure 5A). Knocking down PANX1 and probenecid treatment in MDA-MB-231 and HCC-1937 cell lines led to a downregulation of exATP and exADO levels in the cell culture media (n = 19 for each group; $p < 0.05$) (Figure 5A). Moreover, exATP and exADO levels in digested tissue supernatant of basal-like breast cancer surgical samples were significantly higher than those in Luminal A breast cancer surgical samples (n = 9 for each group; $p < 0.05$) (Figure 5B). In MDA-MB-231 and HCC-1937 cell lines (WT/shPANX1/shCTRL), we explored the relationship between PANX1 expression and ENTPD1/NT5E expression and found no significant correlation between PANX1 expression and ENTPD1/NT5E expression at the cell line level ($p > 0.05$; Turkey's test; Supplementary Figure S2C,D). The above results suggest that the correlation between PANX1 expression and ENTPD1/NT5E expression at the tissue level may be due to the recruitment of immune cells with high expression of ENTPD1/NT5E in TME. The correlation between PANX1 expression and TIIC infiltration in TCGA-BRCA basal-like subtype was analyzed by TIMER. The results indicated that PANX1 expression was positively correlated with the infiltration level of neutrophils, regulatory T cells (Tregs), M2-like macrophages, and myeloid-derived suppressor cells (MDSCs) ($p < 0.05$) and was negatively correlated with the infiltration level of CD8$^+$ T cells and NK cells ($p < 0.05$) (Figure 5C) in basal-like breast cancer. For HER2-enriched and Luminal B subtypes, PANX1 expression was also positively correlated with the infiltration level of neutrophils ($p < 0.05$), but it was negatively correlated with the infiltration level of CD8$^+$ T cells and NK cells only in HER2 enriched subtype ($p < 0.05$) (Figure 5C). The single-cell transcriptome data revealed that TNBC tumor samples with high PANX1 expression had lower infiltration of B cells, CD4$^+$ T cells, CD8$^+$ T cells, myeloid cells, NK cells, and NK T cells and higher infiltration of cancer-associated fibroblasts (CAFs), plasma cells, and Tregs (Supplementary Figure S2E,F). The above results suggested that PANX1 might be a key gene responsible for exADO accumulation and establishment of an immunosuppressive TME in basal-like breast cancer.

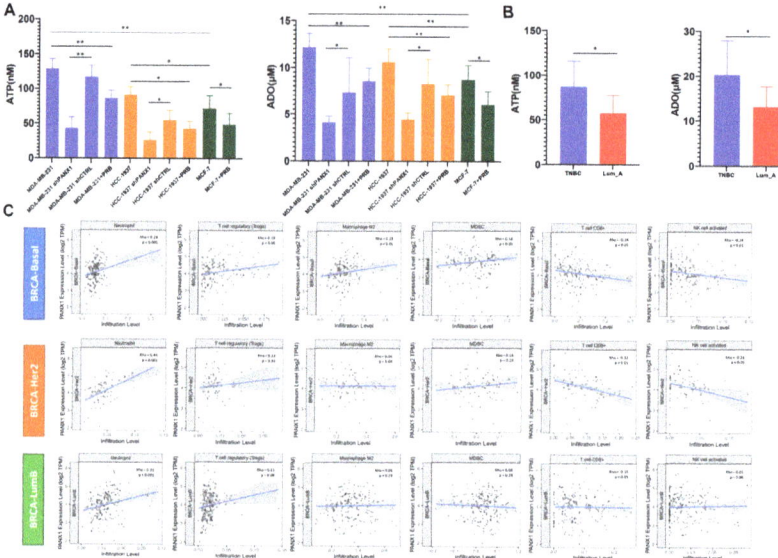

Figure 5. (**A**) Levels of exATP and exADO in MDA-MB-231, HCC-1937 and MCF-7 cell culture media; PANX1 knock down and probenecid (PRB) treatment reduced the levels of exATP and exADO in the supernatant of MDA-MB-231 and HCC-1937 cells (n = 19 for each group; $p < 0.05$; Student's t test); (**B**) levels of exATP and exADO in the supernatant of digested tissue from triple-negative and Luminal A breast cancer surgical specimens ($p < 0.05$; n = 9 for each group; Student's t test); (**C**) the correlation between PANX1 expression and infiltration levels of neutrophils, Tregs, M2-like macrophages, MDSC cells, CD8$^+$ T cells, and NK cells in the tumor microenvironment for Luminal B, HER2 enriched and basal-like breast cancer by TIMER (TCGA-BRCA data; Spearman's rank correlation). (* $p < 0.05$; ** $p < 0.01$).

4. Discussion

Malignant tumors are known as "never healing wounds", and chronic inflammation is one of the key features of malignancy. Chronic inflammatory processes are involved in tumorigenesis and tumor progression. Purine nucleosides (ATP and ADO) exert a strong immunomodulatory ability in TME, and exATP/exADO can regulate local immune responses by activating immune cell purinergic P2 receptors. This study suggested that PANX1 was highly expressed in basal-like breast cancer and might be a poor prognostic factor. High PANX1 expression was associated with high TANs infiltration. PANX1 might play an important role in promoting TAN infiltration by increasing exATP levels. TANs could highly express ENTPD1/NT5E, which synergistically contributes to an immunosuppressive environment with high exADO levels in basal-like breast cancer.

In this study, we investigated the effect of PANX1 in basal-like breast cancer primary lesions. We found that PANX1 was highly expressed in basal-like breast cancer and could increase the exATP level in the TME and that high PANX1 expression was associated with poor prognosis in basal-like breast cancer. PANX1 knock down and probenecid (PRB) treatment reduced the levels of exATP and exADO. Although the relationship between PANX1 and exATP/exADO has been reported [38,39], the immunomodulatory role of PANX1 in the tumor microenvironment still requires further investigation. It was reported that PANX1 had certain effect on the prognosis and metastasis of various tumor, such as pro-carcinogenic effects in pancreatic adenocarcinoma [40], breast cancer [13,41], hepatocellular carcinoma [42], testicular carcinoma [43], melanoma [44], and anticarcinogenic effects in rhabdomyosarcoma [45]. Stewart et al. found that PANX1 expression was required for breast development during lactation and that high PANX1 expression was associated with worse clinical outcomes in breast cancer [13]. However, previous studies were mainly focused on the effects of PANX1 on breast cancer tumor cells [13,41], and the role of PANX1 in the formation of the immunosuppressive microenvironment has not been fully explored. Our study first proposed that the high expression of PANX1 might be one of the reasons for high infiltration of immune cells but local immunosuppression in basal breast cancer, indicating PANX1 might play an important role in constructing pro-tumor TME.

In addition, the key target cells of PANX1 in breast cancer TME need to be further explored. We found that the TANs infiltration was significantly higher in PANX1 high expression basal-like breast cancer and that the genes coexpressed with PANX1 were related to granulocyte migration and neutrophil activation. In the early stage of tumor development, as the first immune cells to enter the tumor microenvironment, neutrophils mediate subsequent immune responses and regulatory processes [46,47]. The exATP secreted by PANX1 was considered to be an important damage-associated molecular pattern (DAMP) signal [48]. Neutrophils, as the target cells of PANX1, could respond to elevated ATP concentrations [9]. exATP could exacerbate the local immune response by mediating NLRP3 inflammasome activation and IL-1β secretion via the P2Y7 receptor (P2×7R) on neutrophils [49]. Moreover, exATP could also delay neutrophil apoptosis via the P2Y11 receptor (P2Y11R) [50].

This study demonstrated that TANs expressing high levels of ENTPD1/NT5E could promote the hydrolysis of exATP to exADO to aggravate the immunosuppressive TME. This result was consistent with the results of studies in lipopolysaccharide (LPS)-induced inflammatory states [51,52]. Chen et al. demonstrated that neutrophils were chemotactic to exATP and hydrolyzed exATP to exADO by NT5E to promote cell migration [52,53]. In addition, exADO inhibits neutrophil adhesion and the release of TNF-α and chemokines from LPS-stimulated neutrophils [54]. Neutrophil-expressed adenosine A2A receptor (A2AR) could inhibit the neutrophil recruitment cascade [55]. Previous studies also revealed that the purinergic receptor P2Y6 receptor (P2Y6R) [56], adenosine A2B receptor (A2BR) [57], and adenosine A3 receptor (A3R) [58] on neutrophils were involved in the regulation of neutrophil extracellular traps (NETs) in inflammatory states. Whether exATP/exADO can regulate NETs or the N1/N2-like subtype transition of TANs through purinergic receptors and further affect the development and metastasis of breast cancer requires further investigation. In addition, our study results also suggested some CCLs, such as CCL3 and CCL4 as well as vascular endothelial growth factor (VEGF) and baculoviral IAP repeat containing 5 (BIRC5), were highly expressed in TANs transcriptome analysis. CCLs were reported to have played an important role of breast tumor cell–neutrophil interactions in regulating pro-tumor characteristics in neutrophils [59,60]. VEGF was known as a primary stimulant of angiogenesis, and it was a macrophage chemotactic cytokine [61]. It was reported that VEGF level was correlated with MPO [62]. Moreover, BIRC5 was reported to play an important role in carcinogenesis by influencing cell division and proliferation and inhibiting apoptosis [63].

Our study demonstrated that ENTPD1 and NT5E expressions were higher in the PANX1 high expression basal-like breast cancer and PANX1 upregulated exADO levels in the TME. At the tissue level, there was a positive correlation between the expression of PANX1 and the expression of ENTPD1 and NT5E. At the cell line level, the expression of ENTPD1 and NT5E was not affected by the expression of PANX1. This suggests that a high expression of PANX1 may lead to high expression of ENTPD1 and NT5E at the tissue level by recruiting high expression of ENTPD1 and NT5E immune cells. PANX1 was an important immunomodulator in the TME. When combining the results of single-cell transcriptome data analysis with TCGA-BRCA data analysis in basal-like breast cancer, we found that PANX1 expression was negatively correlated with the infiltration levels of CD8$^+$ T cells and NK cells, and it was positively correlated with the infiltration levels of Tregs. Higher PANX1 expression caused an increase in exATP, which was further catabolized by ENTPD1 and then converted to adenosine by NT5E [64]. Thus, the prognostic value of PANX1 was not independent of NT5E/ENTPD1. Previous studies mainly focused on the role of the nucleotidases ENTPD1 and NT5E in exADO production [65,66]. As the upstream source of exATP, PANX1 could be a potential and effective therapeutic target. Previous studies also showed that PANX1 promoted the activation of NLRP3 (NOD-, LRR- and pyrin domain-containing protein 3) inflammasome and increased the level of interleukin 1β (IL-1β) in the local microenvironment [67]. In-depth investigations of PANX1 may help elucidate tumor-inflammation interactions.

There are also some limitations in our study. First, we selected representative PAM50 basal-like subtype for analysis rather than TNBC. As a group with strong heterogeneity, TNBC can be further divided into more subtypes. As the subtype with the highest proportion in TNBC, studying the TME characteristics of basal-like subtype could help deepen our understanding of TNBC. Second, although our study results indicated that high PANX1 expression was closely related to high ENTPD1/NT5E expression in the basal-like breast cancer TME, we could not draw definitive conclusions on cause-effect correlations, as the sample size for verifying the bioinformatics analysis was relatively small and we did not perform in vivo experiments. However, a correlation could spawn hypotheses, which then can be tested in future studies. The cause–effect correlations need to be confirmed by further experimental validation in vivo and in vitro in the future. Third, we mainly focused on the effect of PANX1 expression levels on breast cancer TME in this study. However, as a channel protein, the structure and activity of PANX1 are crucial for its function. The effects of different structures and different activation levels of PANX1 on the state of the breast cancer TME deserve further investigation.

5. Conclusions

In summary, the expression of PANX1 was positively correlated with TANs infiltration through exATP secretion in basal-like breast cancer. The high expression of ENTPD1/NT5E in TANs could synergistically establish an immunosuppressive TME with high exADO levels. In this study, the relationship between high exATP/exADO levels and TANs was investigated to elucidate the properties of PANX1 and its ability to reshape the metabolic-immunosuppressive TME and provide new targets and strategies for breast cancer treatment.

Supplementary Materials: The following supporting information can be downloaded at: https://www.mdpi.com/article/10.3390/cancers14143369/s1, Figures S1, S2; Table S1: Detailed patient information included in the study.

Author Contributions: Conceptualization, W.C. and C.N.; data curation, B.L., F.J. and W.X.; formal analysis, B.L., F.J. and W.X.; funding acquisition, W.C. and W.X.; investigation, J.L.; project administration, H.H.; validation, C.N.; writing—original draft, W.C. and W.X.; writing—review and editing, C.N. and W.X. All authors have read and agreed to the published version of the manuscript.

Funding: This work was supported by the Zhejiang Medical and Health Science and Technology Plan Project (No: 2019RC040), the Natural Science Foundation of Zhejiang Province (No: LQ20H160064 and LR19H160001), the Fundamental Research Funds for the Central Universities (No:

2021FZ203-02-08), the Public Welfare Technology Application Research Project of Zhejiang Province (No: LGF21H160030) and the Natural Science Foundation of China (No: 82073151).

Institutional Review Board Statement: The study was conducted in accordance with the Declaration of Helsinki, and ethical approval for this study was received from the Ethical Committee of Second Affiliated Hospital, Zhejiang University School of Medicine (No. SHENYAN 2020-337, approved March 2020) (scanned original file has been uploaded Zenodo: https://doi.org/10.5281/zenodo.6806339). Written informed consent was obtained from all clinical sample donors according to the guidelines approved by the Ethical Committee of the Second Affiliated Hospital, Zhejiang University School of Medicine, and all methods were carried out in accordance with relevant guidelines and regulations.

Informed Consent Statement: Informed consent was obtained from all subjects involved in the study.

Data Availability Statement: The data from previously reported studies and datasets, which support this research, have been cited in the manuscript. All raw data and results generated during and/or analyzed during the current study have been publicly deposited in the Zenodo repository and can be accessed at https://doi.org/10.5281/zenodo.6806339.

Acknowledgments: The authors thank Jian Huang, Zhigang Chen, Pu Chen, Ke Wang, and Zhigang Zhang for their helpful advice.

Conflicts of Interest: The authors declare no conflict of interest.

References

1. Alluri, P.; Newman, L.A. Basal-like and triple-negative breast cancers: Searching for positives among many negatives. *Surg. Oncol. Clin. N. Am.* **2014**, *23*, 567–577. [CrossRef] [PubMed]
2. Bertucci, F.; Finetti, P.; Cervera, N.; Esterni, B.; Hermitte, F.; Viens, P.; Birnbaum, D. How basal are triple-negative breast cancers? *Int. J. Cancer* **2008**, *123*, 236–240. [CrossRef] [PubMed]
3. Abramson, V.G.; Lehmann, B.D.; Ballinger, T.J.; Pietenpol, J.A. Subtyping of triple-negative breast cancer: Implications for therapy. *Cancer* **2015**, *121*, 8–16. [CrossRef] [PubMed]
4. Badve, S.; Dabbs, D.J.; Schnitt, S.J.; Baehner, F.L.; Decker, T.; Eusebi, V.; Fox, S.B.; Ichihara, S.; Jacquemier, J.; Lakhani, S.R.; et al. Basal-like and triple-negative breast cancers: A critical review with an emphasis on the implications for pathologists and oncologists. *Mod. Pathol.* **2011**, *24*, 157–167. [CrossRef]
5. Gao, G.; Wang, Z.; Qu, X.; Zhang, Z. Prognostic value of tumor-infiltrating lymphocytes in patients with triple-negative breast cancer: A systematic review and meta-analysis. *BMC Cancer* **2020**, *20*, 179. [CrossRef]
6. Bayraktar, S.; Batoo, S.; Okuno, S.; Glück, S. Immunotherapy in breast cancer. *J. Carcinog.* **2019**, *18*, 2. [CrossRef]
7. Lohman, A.W.; Leskov, I.L.; Butcher, J.T.; Johnstone, S.R.; Stokes, T.A.; Begandt, D.; DeLalio, L.J.; Best, A.K.; Penuela, S.; Leitinger, N.; et al. Pannexin 1 channels regulate leukocyte emigration through the venous endothelium during acute inflammation. *Nat. Commun.* **2015**, *6*, 7965. [CrossRef]
8. Jacob, F.; Perez Novo, C.; Bachert, C.; Van Crombruggen, K. Purinergic signaling in inflammatory cells: P2 receptor expression, functional effects, and modulation of inflammatory responses. *Purinergic Signal* **2013**, *9*, 285–306. [CrossRef]
9. Yang, D.; He, Y.; Muñoz-Planillo, R.; Liu, Q.; Núñez, G. Caspase-11 Requires the Pannexin-1 Channel and the Purinergic P2X7 Pore to Mediate Pyroptosis and Endotoxic Shock. *Immunity* **2015**, *43*, 923–932. [CrossRef]
10. Vijayan, D.; Young, A.; Teng, M.W.L.; Smyth, M.J. Targeting immunosuppressive adenosine in cancer. *Nat. Rev. Cancer* **2017**, *17*, 709–724. [CrossRef]
11. Feng, L.L.; Cai, Y.Q.; Zhu, M.C.; Xing, L.J.; Wang, X. The yin and yang functions of extracellular ATP and adenosine in tumor immunity. *Cancer Cell Int.* **2020**, *20*, 110. [CrossRef] [PubMed]
12. Medina, C.B.; Chiu, Y.H.; Stremska, M.E.; Lucas, C.D.; Poon, I.; Tung, K.S.; Elliott, M.R.; Desai, B.; Lorenz, U.M.; Bayliss, D.A.; et al. Pannexin 1 channels facilitate communication between T cells to restrict the severity of airway inflammation. *Immunity* **2021**, *54*, 1715–1727.e7. [CrossRef]
13. Jalaleddine, N.; El-Hajjar, L.; Dakik, H.; Shaito, A.; Saliba, J.; Safi, R.; Zibara, K.; El-Sabban, M. Pannexin1 Is Associated with Enhanced Epithelial-To-Mesenchymal Transition in Human Patient Breast Cancer Tissues and in Breast Cancer Cell Lines. *Cancers* **2019**, *11*, 1967. [CrossRef] [PubMed]
14. Colaprico, A.; Silva, T.C.; Olsen, C.; Garofano, L.; Cava, C.; Garolini, D.; Sabedot, T.S.; Malta, T.M.; Pagnotta, S.M.; Castiglioni, I.; et al. TCGAbiolinks: An R/Bioconductor package for integrative analysis of TCGA data. *Nucleic. Acids. Res.* **2016**, *44*, e71. [CrossRef]
15. Mounir, M.; Lucchetta, M.; Silva, T.C.; Olsen, C.; Bontempi, G.; Chen, X.; Noushmehr, H.; Colaprico, A.; Papaleo, E. New functionalities in the TCGAbiolinks package for the study and integration of cancer data from GDC and GTEx. *PLoS Comput. Biol.* **2019**, *15*, e1006701. [CrossRef] [PubMed]

16. Silva, T.C.; Colaprico, A.; Olsen, C.; D'Angelo, F.; Bontempi, G.; Ceccarelli, M.; Noushmehr, H. TCGA Workflow: Analyze cancer genomics and epigenomics data using Bioconductor packages. *F1000Research* **2016**, *5*, 1542. [CrossRef]
17. Curtis, C.; Shah, S.P.; Chin, S.F.; Turashvili, G.; Rueda, O.M.; Dunning, M.J.; Speed, D.; Lynch, A.G.; Samarajiwa, S.; Yuan, Y.; et al. The genomic and transcriptomic architecture of 2,000 breast tumours reveals novel subgroups. *Nature* **2012**, *486*, 346–352. [CrossRef]
18. Wu, Z.; Liu, W.; Jin, X.; Ji, H.; Wang, H.; Glusman, G.; Robinson, M.; Liu, L.; Ruan, J.; Gao, S. NormExpression: An R Package to Normalize Gene Expression Data Using Evaluated Methods. *Front. Genet.* **2019**, *10*, 400. [CrossRef]
19. Jézéquel, P.; Loussouarn, D.; Guérin-Charbonnel, C.; Campion, L.; Vanier, A.; Gouraud, W.; Lasla, H.; Guette, C.; Valo, I.; Verrièle, V.; et al. Gene-expression molecular subtyping of triple-negative breast cancer tumours: Importance of immune response. *Breast Cancer Res.* **2015**, *17*, 43. [CrossRef]
20. Jézéquel, P.; Kerdraon, O.; Hondermarck, H.; Guérin-Charbonnel, C.; Lasla, H.; Gouraud, W.; Canon, J.L.; Gombos, A.; Dalenc, F.; Delaloge, S.; et al. Identification of three subtypes of triple-negative breast cancer with potential therapeutic implications. *Breast Cancer Res.* **2019**, *21*, 65. [CrossRef]
21. Jørgensen, C.L.T.; Larsson, A.M.; Forsare, C.; Aaltonen, K.; Jansson, S.; Bradshaw, R.; Bendahl, P.O.; Rydén, L. PAM50 Intrinsic Subtype Profiles in Primary and Metastatic Breast Cancer Show a Significant Shift toward More Aggressive Subtypes with Prognostic Implications. *Cancers* **2021**, *13*, 1592. [CrossRef] [PubMed]
22. Gendoo, D.M.; Ratanasirigulchai, N.; Schröder, M.S.; Paré, L.; Parker, J.S.; Prat, A.; Haibe-Kains, B. Genefu: An R/Bioconductor package for computation of gene expression-based signatures in breast cancer. *Bioinformatics* **2016**, *32*, 1097–1099. [CrossRef]
23. Salgado, R.; Denkert, C.; Demaria, S.; Sirtaine, N.; Klauschen, F.; Pruneri, G.; Wienert, S.; Van den Eynden, G.; Baehner, F.L.; Penault-Llorca, F.; et al. The evaluation of tumor-infiltrating lymphocytes (TILs) in breast cancer: Recommendations by an International TILs Working Group 2014. *Ann. Oncol.* **2015**, *26*, 259–271. [CrossRef] [PubMed]
24. Li, T.; Fu, J.; Zeng, Z.; Cohen, D.; Li, J.; Chen, Q.; Li, B.; Liu, X.S. TIMER2.0 for analysis of tumor-infiltrating immune cells. *Nucleic Acids Res.* **2020**, *48*, W509–W514. [CrossRef]
25. Li, T.; Fan, J.; Wang, B.; Traugh, N.; Chen, Q.; Liu, J.S.; Li, B.; Liu, X.S. TIMER: A Web Server for Comprehensive Analysis of Tumor-Infiltrating Immune Cells. *Cancer Res.* **2017**, *77*, e108–e110. [CrossRef] [PubMed]
26. Newman, A.M.; Liu, C.L.; Green, M.R.; Gentles, A.J.; Feng, W.; Xu, Y.; Hoang, C.D.; Diehn, M.; Alizadeh, A.A. Robust enumeration of cell subsets from tissue expression profiles. *Nat. Methods* **2015**, *12*, 453–457. [CrossRef]
27. Finotello, F.; Mayer, C.; Plattner, C.; Laschober, G.; Rieder, D.; Hackl, H.; Krogsdam, A.; Loncova, Z.; Posch, W.; Wilflingseder, D.; et al. Molecular and pharmacological modulators of the tumor immune contexture revealed by deconvolution of RNA-seq data. *Genome Med.* **2019**, *11*, 34. [CrossRef]
28. Tang, Z.; Kang, B.; Li, C.; Chen, T.; Zhang, Z. GEPIA2: An enhanced web server for large-scale expression profiling and interactive analysis. *Nucleic Acids Res.* **2019**, *47*, W556–W560. [CrossRef]
29. Bhattacharya, S.; Dunn, P.; Thomas, C.G.; Smith, B.; Schaefer, H.; Chen, J.; Hu, Z.; Zalocusky, K.A.; Shankar, R.D.; Shen-Orr, S.S.; et al. ImmPort, toward repurposing of open access immunological assay data for translational and clinical research. *Sci. Data* **2018**, *5*, 180015. [CrossRef]
30. Chen, X.; Li, J.; Gray, W.H.; Lehmann, B.D.; Bauer, J.A.; Shyr, Y.; Pietenpol, J.A. TNBCtype: A Subtyping Tool for Triple-Negative Breast Cancer. *Cancer Inform.* **2012**, *11*, 147–156. [CrossRef]
31. Lehmann, B.D.; Bauer, J.A.; Chen, X.; Sanders, M.E.; Chakravarthy, A.B.; Shyr, Y.; Pietenpol, J.A. Identification of human triple-negative breast cancer subtypes and preclinical models for selection of targeted therapies. *J. Clin. Investig.* **2011**, *121*, 2750–2767. [CrossRef] [PubMed]
32. Bindea, G.; Mlecnik, B.; Hackl, H.; Charoentong, P.; Tosolini, M.; Kirilovsky, A.; Fridman, W.H.; Pagès, F.; Trajanoski, Z.; Galon, J. ClueGO: A Cytoscape plug-in to decipher functionally grouped gene ontology and pathway annotation networks. *Bioinformatics* **2009**, *25*, 1091–1093. [CrossRef] [PubMed]
33. Shannon, P.; Markiel, A.; Ozier, O.; Baliga, N.S.; Wang, J.T.; Ramage, D.; Amin, N.; Schwikowski, B.; Ideker, T. Cytoscape: A software environment for integrated models of biomolecular interaction networks. *Genome Res.* **2003**, *13*, 2498–2504. [CrossRef] [PubMed]
34. Wu, S.Z.; Roden, D.L.; Wang, C.; Holliday, H.; Harvey, K.; Cazet, A.S.; Murphy, K.J.; Pereira, B.; Al-Eryani, G.; Bartonicek, N.; et al. Stromal cell diversity associated with immune evasion in human triple-negative breast cancer. *EMBO J.* **2020**, *39*, e104063. [CrossRef]
35. Schindelin, J.; Arganda-Carreras, I.; Frise, E.; Kaynig, V.; Longair, M.; Pietzsch, T.; Preibisch, S.; Rueden, C.; Saalfeld, S.; Schmid, B.; et al. Fiji: An open-source platform for biological-image analysis. *Nat. Methods* **2012**, *9*, 676–682. [CrossRef]
36. Crowe, A.R.; Yue, W. Semi-quantitative Determination of Protein Expression using Immunohistochemistry Staining and Analysis: An Integrated Protocol. *Bio-Protocol* **2019**, *9*, e3465. [CrossRef]
37. Finotello, F.; Trajanoski, Z. Quantifying tumor-infiltrating immune cells from transcriptomics data. *Cancer Immunol. Immunother.* **2018**, *67*, 1031–1040. [CrossRef]
38. Velasquez, S.; Eugenin, E.A. Role of Pannexin-1 hemichannels and purinergic receptors in the pathogenesis of human diseases. *Front. Physiol.* **2014**, *5*, 96. [CrossRef]
39. Dahl, G. ATP release through pannexon channels. *Philos. Trans. R. Soc. Lond. B Biol. Sci.* **2015**, *370*, 20140191. [CrossRef]

40. Bao, L.; Sun, K.; Zhang, X. PANX1 is a potential prognostic biomarker associated with immune infiltration in pancreatic adenocarcinoma: A pan-cancer analysis. *Channels* **2021**, *15*, 680–696. [CrossRef]
41. Furlow, P.W.; Zhang, S.; Soong, T.D.; Halberg, N.; Goodarzi, H.; Mangrum, C.; Wu, Y.G.; Elemento, O.; Tavazoie, S.F. Mechanosensitive pannexin-1 channels mediate microvascular metastatic cell survival. *Nat. Cell Biol.* **2015**, *17*, 943–952. [CrossRef] [PubMed]
42. Shi, G.; Liu, C.; Yang, Y.; Song, L.; Liu, X.; Wang, C.; Peng, Z.; Li, H.; Zhong, L. Panx1 promotes invasion-metastasis cascade in hepatocellular carcinoma. *J. Cancer* **2019**, *10*, 5681–5688. [CrossRef] [PubMed]
43. Liu, H.; Yuan, M.; Yao, Y.; Wu, D.; Dong, S.; Tong, X. In vitro effect of Pannexin 1 channel on the invasion and migration of I-10 testicular cancer cells via ERK1/2 signaling pathway. *Biomed. Pharmacother* **2019**, *117*, 109090. [CrossRef]
44. Penuela, S.; Gyenis, L.; Ablack, A.; Churko, J.M.; Berger, A.C.; Litchfield, D.W.; Lewis, J.D.; Laird, D.W. Loss of pannexin 1 attenuates melanoma progression by reversion to a melanocytic phenotype. *J. Biol. Chem.* **2012**, *287*, 29184–29193. [CrossRef]
45. Xiang, X.; Langlois, S.; St-Pierre, M.E.; Blinder, A.; Charron, P.; Graber, T.E.; Fowler, S.L.; Baird, S.D.; Bennett, S.A.L.; Alain, T.; et al. Identification of pannexin 1-regulated genes, interactome, and pathways in rhabdomyosarcoma and its tumor inhibitory interaction with AHNAK. *Oncogene* **2021**, *40*, 1868–1883. [CrossRef] [PubMed]
46. Eruslanov, E.B. Phenotype and function of tumor-associated neutrophils and their subsets in early-stage human lung cancer. *Cancer Immunol. Immunother.* **2017**, *66*, 997–1006. [CrossRef] [PubMed]
47. Shaul, M.E.; Fridlender, Z.G. Cancer-related circulating and tumor-associated neutrophils—subtypes, sources and function. *FEBS J.* **2018**, *285*, 4316–4342. [CrossRef] [PubMed]
48. Di Virgilio, F.; Sarti, A.C.; Coutinho-Silva, R. Purinergic signaling, DAMPs, and inflammation. *Am. J. Physiol. Cell Physiol.* **2020**, *318*, C832–C835. [CrossRef]
49. Karmakar, M.; Katsnelson, M.A.; Dubyak, G.R.; Pearlman, E. Neutrophil P2X7 receptors mediate NLRP3 inflammasome-dependent IL-1β secretion in response to ATP. *Nat. Commun.* **2016**, *7*, 10555. [CrossRef]
50. Vaughan, K.R.; Stokes, L.; Prince, L.R.; Marriott, H.M.; Meis, S.; Kassack, M.U.; Bingle, C.D.; Sabroe, I.; Surprenant, A.; Whyte, M.K. Inhibition of neutrophil apoptosis by ATP is mediated by the P2Y11 receptor. *J. Immunol.* **2007**, *179*, 8544–8553. [CrossRef]
51. Antonioli, L.; Pacher, P.; Vizi, E.S.; Haskó, G. CD39 and CD73 in immunity and inflammation. *Trends. Mol. Med.* **2013**, *19*, 355–367. [CrossRef]
52. Wang, X.; Chen, D. Purinergic Regulation of Neutrophil Function. *Front. Immunol.* **2018**, *9*, 399. [CrossRef] [PubMed]
53. Chen, Y.; Corriden, R.; Inoue, Y.; Yip, L.; Hashiguchi, N.; Zinkernagel, A.; Nizet, V.; Insel, P.A.; Junger, W.G. ATP release guides neutrophil chemotaxis via P2Y2 and A3 receptors. *Science* **2006**, *314*, 1792–1795. [CrossRef] [PubMed]
54. Barletta, K.E.; Ley, K.; Mehrad, B. Regulation of neutrophil function by adenosine. *Arter. Thromb. Vasc. Biol.* **2012**, *32*, 856–864. [CrossRef] [PubMed]
55. Yago, T.; Tsukamoto, H.; Liu, Z.; Wang, Y.; Thompson, L.F.; McEver, R.P. Multi-Inhibitory Effects of A2A Adenosine Receptor Signaling on Neutrophil Adhesion Under Flow. *J. Immunol.* **2015**, *195*, 3880–3889. [CrossRef] [PubMed]
56. Sil, P.; Hayes, C.P.; Reaves, B.J.; Breen, P.; Quinn, S.; Sokolove, J.; Rada, B. P2Y6 Receptor Antagonist MRS2578 Inhibits Neutrophil Activation and Aggregated Neutrophil Extracellular Trap Formation Induced by Gout-Associated Monosodium Urate Crystals. *J. Immunol.* **2017**, *198*, 428–442. [CrossRef] [PubMed]
57. Barletta, K.E.; Cagnina, R.E.; Burdick, M.D.; Linden, J.; Mehrad, B. Adenosine A(2B) receptor deficiency promotes host defenses against gram-negative bacterial pneumonia. *Am. J. Respir. Crit. Care Med.* **2012**, *186*, 1044–1050. [CrossRef]
58. Corriden, R.; Self, T.; Akong-Moore, K.; Nizet, V.; Kellam, B.; Briddon, S.J.; Hill, S.J. Adenosine-A3 receptors in neutrophil microdomains promote the formation of bacteria-tethering cytonemes. *EMBO Rep.* **2013**, *14*, 726–732. [CrossRef]
59. Wu, L.; Saxena, S.; Goel, P.; Prajapati, D.R.; Wang, C.; Singh, R.K. Breast Cancer Cell-Neutrophil Interactions Enhance Neutrophil Survival and Pro-Tumorigenic Activities. *Cancers* **2020**, *12*, 2884. [CrossRef]
60. Abrahamsson, A.; Rzepecka, A.; Dabrosin, C. Equal Pro-inflammatory Profiles of CCLs, CXCLs, and Matrix Metalloproteinases in the Extracellular Microenvironment In Vivo in Human Dense Breast Tissue and Breast Cancer. *Front. Immunol.* **2017**, *8*, 1994. [CrossRef]
61. Queen, M.M.; Ryan, R.E.; Holzer, R.G.; Keller-Peck, C.R.; Jorcyk, C.L. Breast cancer cells stimulate neutrophils to produce oncostatin M: Potential implications for tumor progression. *Cancer Res.* **2005**, *65*, 8896–8904. [CrossRef] [PubMed]
62. Coelho, B.A.; Belo, A.V.; Andrade, S.P.; Amorim, W.C.; Uemura, G.; da Silva Filho, A.L. N-acetylglucosaminidase, myeloperoxidase and vascular endothelial growth factor serum levels in breast cancer patients. *Biomed. Pharmacother.* **2014**, *68*, 185–189. [CrossRef] [PubMed]
63. Dai, J.B.; Zhu, B.; Lin, W.J.; Gao, H.Y.; Dai, H.; Zheng, L.; Shi, W.H.; Chen, W.X. Identification of prognostic significance of BIRC5 in breast cancer using integrative bioinformatics analysis. *Biosci. Rep.* **2020**, *40*, BSR20193678. [CrossRef] [PubMed]
64. Poudel, N.; Okusa, M.D. Pannexins in Acute Kidney Injury. *Nephron Exp. Nephrol.* **2019**, *143*, 158–161. [CrossRef]
65. Buisseret, L.; Pommey, S.; Allard, B.; Garaud, S.; Bergeron, M.; Cousineau, I.; Ameye, L.; Bareche, Y.; Paesmans, M.; Crown, J.P.A.; et al. Clinical significance of CD73 in triple-negative breast cancer: Multiplex analysis of a phase III clinical trial. *Ann. Oncol.* **2018**, *29*, 1056–1062. [CrossRef]
66. Allard, B.; Allard, D.; Buisseret, L.; Stagg, J. The adenosine pathway in immuno-oncology. *Nat. Rev. Clin. Oncol.* **2020**, *17*, 611–629. [CrossRef] [PubMed]
67. Laird, D.W.; Penuela, S. Pannexin biology and emerging linkages to cancer. *Trends Cancer* **2021**, *7*, 1119–1131. [CrossRef]

MDPI
St. Alban-Anlage 66
4052 Basel
Switzerland
www.mdpi.com

Cancers Editorial Office
E-mail: cancers@mdpi.com
www.mdpi.com/journal/cancers

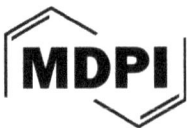

Disclaimer/Publisher's Note: The statements, opinions and data contained in all publications are solely those of the individual author(s) and contributor(s) and not of MDPI and/or the editor(s). MDPI and/or the editor(s) disclaim responsibility for any injury to people or property resulting from any ideas, methods, instructions or products referred to in the content.

www.ingramcontent.com/pod-product-compliance
Lightning Source LLC
LaVergne TN
LVHW070140100526
838202LV00015B/1854